HEALTH MANAGEMENT – DIFFERENT APPROACHES AND SOLUTIONS

Edited by **Krzysztof Śmigórski**

Health Management – Different Approaches and Solutions
Edited by Krzysztof Śmigórski

Published by InTech

Janeza Trdine 9, 51000 Rijeka, Croatia

Publishing Process Manager Iva Simcic

Technical Editor Teodora Smiljanic

Cover Designer InTech Design Team

Additional hard copies can be obtained from orders@intechopen.com

Health Management – Different Approaches and Solutions, Edited by Krzysztof Śmigórski
p. cm.
ISBN 978-953-307-296-8

For EU product safety concerns:
IN TECH d.o.o., Prolaz Marije Krucifikse Kozulić 3, 51000 Rijeka, Croatia,
info@intechopen.com or visit our website at intechopen.com.

Meet the editor

Dr. Krzysztof Śmigórski, PhD, is a psychologist; he graduated on Catholic University of Lublin (MSc and PhD). He worked as a clinical psychologist at the Medical University of Wroclaw Research Institute for Dementia-Related Diseases. At present he is employed at an international company specialized in conducting psychological assessments for clinical trials purposes. His scientific interests are: cognitve neuropsychology (semantic priming paradigm), neuropsychological rehabilitation in dementia, and the theory of psychological measurement.

Contents

Preface

Advances in modern medicine have enabled the ability to significantly prolong the average lifespan expectancy. The development of this knowledge ensures unprecedented possibilities in terms of explaining the causes of diseases and effective treatment. However, increased capabilities create new issues. Both, researchers and clinicians, as well as managers of healthcare units face new challenges: increasing validity and reliability of clinical trials, effectively distributing medical products, managing hospitals and clinics flexibly, and managing treatment processes efficiently.

In the past decades, the development of a new, fascinating discipline of science has been observed. This discipline is called "health management". For the purposes of this book, the report by the Canadian Minister of National Health and Welfare, Marc LaLonde, has been taken as a point of reference. The report proclaimed in 1974 is considered to be "the first modern government document in the western world to acknowledge that our emphasis upon a biomedical health care system is wrong, and that we need to look beyond the traditional health care (sick care) system if we wish to improve the health of the public". It has offered new prospects for the issues of health care. It emphasizes the responsibility of an individual in developing behaviors conducive to keeping her/him in good health.

LaLonde assumes that there are four main factors of health: human biology, the environment, the lifestyle, and health care services. He contended that health cannot be secured only by development of medical sciences, but by making wise and rational decisions by individuals and the whole society too. His legacy includes a recommendation according to which health care interventions should focus on groups at risk of a disease development and point health inequalities out. LaLonde's work widened significantly as the range of actions related to health care services by incorporating categories had not been associated with it before. At present, thanks to LaLonde, health management strategies are highly differentiated with respect to its recipients and dimensions of constituting areas of their activities.

Many great authors have contributed to this book. Their work is divided in the three following sections:

1. **Wellness and Lifestyle** – In this section, readers will find chapters describing interventions that are designed to support the generally healthy before they exhibit symptoms of chronic or catastrophic disease.

2. **Disease Management** – Programs requiring the identification of population sub-groups that are already exhibiting some elements of chronic disease are put here. The interventions described in this section are less individualized and should tend to address the characteristics of the larger population with risk factors.

3. **General Issues** – Readers interested in methodology of clinical trials and general findings that widen our understanding of human health determinants should pay special attention to this section.

This book is a direct legacy of Marc LaLonde's report. The aim of it is to present issues relating to health management in a way that would be satisfying to academicians and practitioners. The book is designed to be a forum for the experts in the thematic area to exchange viewpoints, and to present health management's state-of-art as a scientific and professional domain. I hope it will provide readers with new valuable information and they will enjoy reading it.

Dr. Krzysztof Śmigórski
Medical University of Wroclaw
Research Institute for Dementia-Related Diseases
Poland

Part 1

Wellness and Lifestyle

1

A Future for Integrated Diagnostic Helping

Mathieu Thevenin and Anthony Kolar
CEA, LIST, Embedded Computing Laboratory
France

1. Introduction

Medical systems used for exploration or diagnostic helping impose high applicative constraints such as real time image acquisition and displaying. This is especially the case when they are used in surgical room where a high reactivity is required from operators. Large computing capacity is required in order to obtain valuable results. Integrators mainly prefer the use of general purpose architectures such as workstations (Gomes, 2011). They have to cope with manufacturing cost and setup simplicity. As general purpose devices need a large amount of space, the main part of the processing is deported from the handled diagnostic tools to an external unit. For example, this is the case of endoscopic device. Today, dedicated rooms are usually used for this purpose in many hospitals. Their associated external computers that are used for diagnostic system are cumbersome and are also energy consumers. These issues are too problematic to use efficiently these systems in a limited space. Indeed, they restrain the movements of the medical staff and complexify the deployment on the ground for military or humanitarian operations. Therefore it seems logical to integrate the maximum computing capacities diagnostic into helping devices themselves to make them completely handleable.

A large part of computing requirement of these systems is devoted to image processing. They can be quite simple like images reconstruction and enhancement, features detector or 3D reconstruction. Today, a large part of these processing is mainly embedded inside handled consumer's devices such as digital cameras or advanced driving assistance systems (ADAS). By the analysis of both medical and consumer's applications systems, it is possible to notice that they rely on similar algorithmic approaches. Also, most of integration constraints are similar if someone wants to miniaturize these consumer devices. This mainly concerns the chips silicon areas, their power consumption and their computing capacities. For example, a digital video sensor and image processor integrated to a cell phone cannot reach more than a half watt of power consumption for a silicon area of less than a dozen square millimeters. This is also the case for one of the most integrated medical diagnostic device which is the endocapscule. It form factor (Harada, 2008) limits components size while its autonomy is driven by energies efficiency. The whole device may not exceed a Watt of power consumption. About a half Watt is devoted to the part dedicated to computation for diagnostic, especially based on image processing. However, this part depends on the device features, such as communication systems and mechanical elements that may be used for mobility or biopsy.

Integrators also demands versatility in order to design unique products that can be used for different targets. For example, endoscopic exploration of larynx or intestinal and lung exploration do not uses the same devices, but these applications are all based on similar image processing with minor variations. Moreover, these systems should be updatable to follow the science developments.

These requirements are also valid for large market devices such as cell phones and cameras. For example, general purposes or specific embedded processors are widely used like ARM microprocessors and Texas Instrument Digital Signal Processors (DSP) which are integrated into transportation, photonics, communications or entertainment (Texas Instrument, 2006). These markets drive both academic and industrial researches. The background knowledge is present inside laboratories; however its transfer to medical applications is not yet completely industrially ready.

This chapter provides clues to transfer consumers computing architecture approaches to the benefit of medical applications. The goal is to obtain fully integrated devices from diagnostic helping to autonomous lab on chip while taking into account medical domain specific constraints.

This expertise is structured as follows: the first part analyzes vision based medical applications in order to extract essentials processing blocks and to show the similarities between consumer's and medical vision based applications. The second part is devoted to the determination of elementary operators which are mostly needed in both domains. Computing capacities that are required by these operators and applications are compared to the state-of-the-art architectures in order to define an efficient algorithm-architecture adequation. Finally this part demonstrates that it's possible to use highly constrained computing architectures designed for consumers handled devices in application to medical domain. This is based on the example of a high definition (HD) video processing architecture designed to be integrated into smart phone or highly embedded components.

This expertise paves the way for the industrialisation of intergraded autonomous diagnostic helping devices, by showing the feasibility of such systems. Their future use would also free the medical staff from many logistical constraints due the deployment of today's cumbersome systems.

2. Video processing in diagnosis helping system

Since many years, the research about diagnosis helping devices is very active. This is true in both academic and industrial world. This can be explained by the fact that the possibilities of data analysis systems are becoming more and more complex and can extract a large amount of information. The helping in diagnosis can provide a solution to decrease the response time of the practitioner in urgent case or to help him in the preparation of the patient operation. This section firstly presents endocapsules as an example of one of the most constrained integrated diagnostic devices. It also representative of some of the major research domains in biomedical technology: image and signal processing, robotics and in-vivo communication. Next, the needs for diagnosis helping for such devices are presented, followed by an introduction about low level image processing in both consumers and medical components. Finally similarities between these two applications are developed and clues are given to appreciate required capacity for these embedded algorithms.

2.1 Researches in diagnostic helping devices

Researches in diagnostic helping devices cover a large number of domains, however one can focus on three items that emphasize the conception of an autonomous device. This is illustrated by Lab-On-Chips projects (Harada, 2008) that are able to do an auto diagnostic.

1. The video processing:
In the case of endocapsule (Karargyris, 2010), the main goal of video processing is to analyse a video sequence in order to find different features like bleeding, polyps, tumours, etc. Theses kinds of diagnosis helping are usually done in two steps. First a camera equipped device grab images to diagnostic, these images are then transmitted through a wireless connection to a workstation that analyzes them during an off-line processing. Figure 2.1 depicts the PillCam by GivenImaging, and the Endocam by Olympus can also be cited;

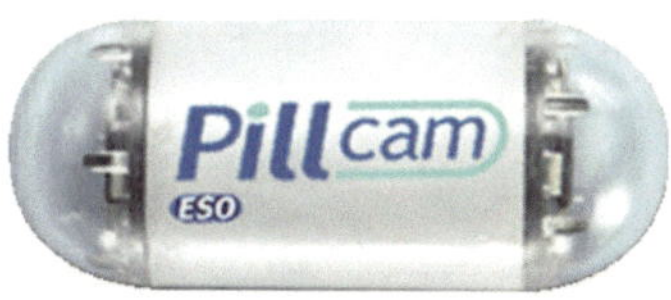

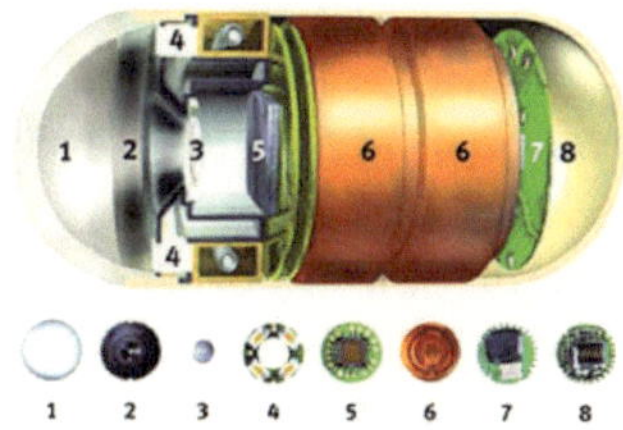

Fig. 2.1. PillCam by GivenImaging

2. The mechanical systems for autonomous devices:
Some researches focus on the integration of mechanicals devices to endocapsules in order to give them the ability to surgery using micro-instrumentation such as biopsy. An example of such an endocapsule is "Miro" (Kim and al., 2007) under Korea's Frontier 21 project as shown on Figure 2.2. The "Scuola Superiore Sant'Anna" (Quirini, 2007) also tries to integrate small mechanic legs to a video-capsule in order to give the practitioner the ability to move freely in the intestinal system.

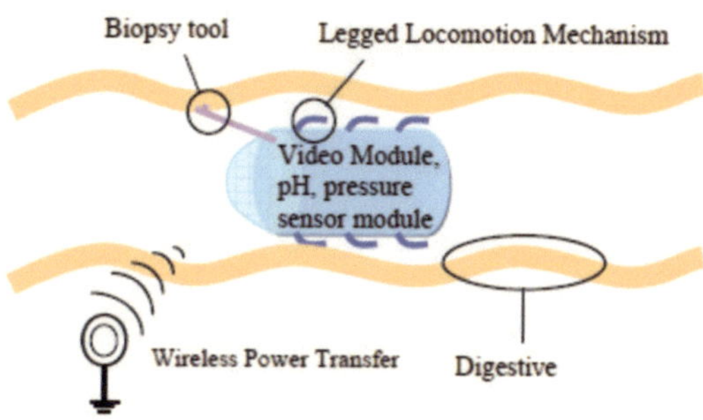

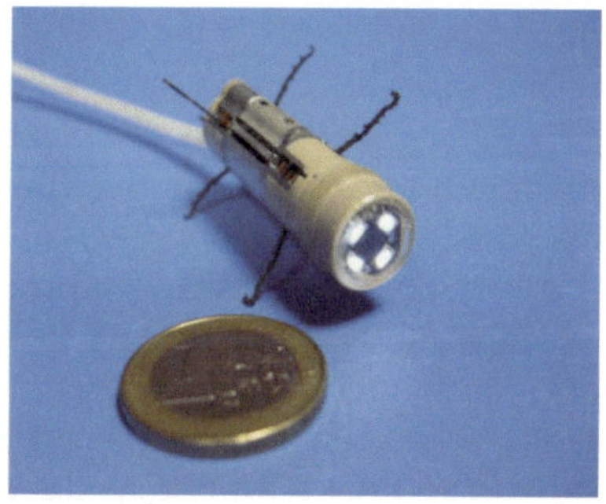

Fig. 2.2. Principe of the endocapsule "Miro" and prototypes of a mobile endo-capsule

3. The communication and transfer protocol:
Communication protocol in human body is defined by the norm IEEE 820.15. Its frequency is 403 MHz. This is defined by the norm for in-vivo electronic devices. Antennas for this band are small while low emitting power is required due to limited loss of the signal in the environment. Moreover this frequency should not infers with usual communications devices. Energy efficiency is a critical point for the energetic life of an integrated and autonomous system. For this reason, many researchers work in order to find an optimal way to communicate between the device and the external world. There are three aspects of this research: the first one focuses on the silicon device technologies and materials. The second one focuses on the architecture trying to define the most efficient hardware architecture for

embedded computing integration. Finally, the third one focuses on communication protocol, as well at hardware level - antennas, computing, power consumption - at system level - soft radio, compression, computing complexity reduction.
The most important part of required computing capacity is devoted to video processing. It is crucial for a diagnostic helping device such an endocapsule. The practitioners have to visualize the body exploration which requires large computing capacity to ensure a confortable real-time high resolution video. Video processing is also essential for the control of mechanical parts of endocapsules that enable movement or biopsy. For example its purpose is to extract features from the image for positioning. Consequently, the video processing block usually requires large silicon area on the component. For this reason this chapter will focus in the video processing part.

2.2 Diagnostic helping devices: The needs

One of the domains that requires an efficient and accurate exploration is the endoscopy. The length of the digestive system causes many limitations. However they are drastically reduced from a decade thanks to the conception of the endoscopic video capsule.
Video endocapsules are shown to be useful in many cases:

- Unexplained digestive bleeding:

They represent about 5% of the digestive bleeding. general's methods offer very poor result. Profitability of radiological examination is only between 5 and 10% because no direct visualization of the mucous membrane is possible. Using enteroscopy, the profitability diagnosis for the lesions of hail is between 15 and 30% which is far from 100%. Using an endocapsule the profitability diagnosis are higher than that of the thorough enteroscopy, up to 70% (Maieron et al, 2004) (Fireman et al, 2004) (Selby et al, 2004).

- Crohn syndrom and hemorrhagic recto-colitis:

Chohn symdrom concerns about 2.5 billion patient in the world. This number increases each year. In this case, literature also shows that the endocapsule is a good choice for first intention exploration of clinical suspicion when traditional methods such as fibroscopy coloscopy and biopsies are negative (Bernardini, 2008).

- Polyps and hail tumors:

On 1042 examinations carried out, it was diagnosed 6-8% of tumors of hail (malignant 50%) (Lewis, Miami 2004). Endocapsule is especially efficient in the detection of small tumors (< 1 cm) which are difficult to see by general exploration such as simple radiological examination. There is also an interest like examination of tracking in the event of clinical suspicion (carcinoïde, lymphoma) due to the non-invasive nature of the technique and its simplicity of implementation for the patient.
By the literature, state of art, contact with practitioners and the study of diagnosis methods, diagnostic helping devices can benefit from following applications.

- Vision and real time 3D reconstruction of the scene is used to determine precisely the size of the lesions. This is used to find the optimal solution to treat the patient. At this time, the size of an anomaly is determined by the experience of the practitioner.
- Real time and autonomous detection of tumors, polyps, lesions and bleeding. Sometime, an anomaly can be very difficult to detect due to its localisation or its little size. The goal is to have the higher profitability diagnoses possible. This kind of processing is also very useful to determinate the region of interest - the region where an abnormally is seen - in the image. An autonomous detection should allow a better management of the power consumption by sending to the external world the image of the anomaly only.

- Spectrography is a possible solution to define the nature of a tumor when the biopsy not easily feasible. Spectrography is based on the spectral response of the organic fabric to a laser operating at a specific wavelength (Péry, 2008).

2.3 Algorithms used for general image processing in consumer's devices and diagnostic helping

The importance of the consumer devices market pushes the academic and industrial labs to innovate. This is required by the integration of brand new features in order to create new products, while maintaining the production cost as low as possible. Most of these new features require high computing capacities while silicon area must be kept under control and power consumption need to be sustained as low as possible. First, silicon area has a direct impact on production cost; moreover, too large components may be incompatible with a product form factor. Power consumption has a direct impact on battery life, which is crucial for handled products.

For example, on 2010, cell phones' image sensor represented about 80% of the overall sensor market for about 5 000 millions Dollar . These sensors are systematically associated with a digital Image and Signal Processor (ISP) to reconstruct and enhance the images from raw format. Cell phone integrators need video module, which include a video sensor and ISP at a price of about one dollar. Lenses and sensor costs are reduced as most as possible by reduction of the matrix and pixel size (today 2µm pixel are the state of the art). In addition to traditional color image reconstruction from raw data, this pixel size reduction implies an image quality degradation that must be corrected using digital ISP. An example of traditional image correction and reconstruction pipeline is presented in Figure 2.3. However to keep production costs low, their silicon area must be maintained under a few square millimetres using today's technologies. This forbids the use of traditional image processing approaches such as the use of a frame memory which may require more than times of silicon area budget.

Additional computing resources are used for high level application such as face recognition or augmented reality. Digital cameras and security cameras represent another part of the market of embedded image processing. Depending on their usage, they can embed low level to complex high level algorithms, from simple image enhancement to face recognition or motion detection and tracking.

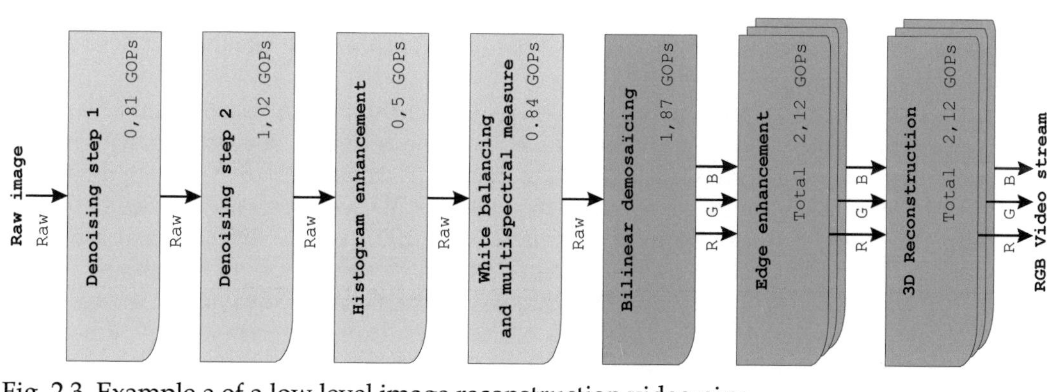

Fig. 2.3. Example a of a low level image reconstruction video pipe.

Todays handled video games and digital cameras are able to handle 3D as well for image grabbing and displaying. Designers now consider this feature must be integrated into devices. This feature requires specific algorithms to process images, especially when they are grabbed by a stereoscopic pair.
Basic image enhancement algorithms are used as well for image grabbing as for image displaying. Depending on the nature of the targeted application, high level algorithms may be used in addition. For example, interest point detection is widely used for face detection or augmented reality. Stereoscopy may be also used for this last purpose.

2.4 Algorithms used for diagnosis helping

By the analysis of the applications needed to enhance the diagnosis, it is possible to define a selection of video-processing algorithms. If we let on the side the most common processing used for image reconstruction and enhancement, which is the first step of all image acquisition, one can extract the following algorithms:

- Shape detector:

In order to define a region of interest in the image, this kind of detector is very common. In a simplifying way, we can summarize this algorithm by the analysis of the reflectance or depth discontinuity in an image; actually, the intensity discontinuity allows the edge definition. The principle of edge detection is based on the study of the derivative of the intensity function in the image: local extrema of the gradient and passages by zero of the Laplacian. This can normally be achieved by convolution like approaches;

- Colour analysis:

This technique allows to fetch the information about the incident spectrum wave. This is similar to spectroscopy. The base of this method is to record a certain color profile and to compare it to a matching table, which contains the known color profile. This enables to find the needed information for example the nature of a tumor - considering that each tumor has a specific color response.

- Labelling:

The goal is to give an identification code to each region of interest in the image in order to process them separately; the labelling is one of the most important processing with the form recognition. If we simplify to the maximum, this method is based on the scanning of the image, each time that a region of interest is found, which was defined by a previous processing like form recognition, a label can be attributed. There are many different technique of labelling, depending of the complexity of the image. Graba (Graba, 2006) proposes a solution to integrate labelling in a small 3D vision sensor. Lacassagne (Lacassagne, 2009) proposes an extremely fast method to process the labelling.

- 3D reconstruction:

The depth reconstruction is usually based on three different solutions: the so called active one, based pattern projection read by a camera. The second one is passive stereoscopy, with two or more cameras allowing a triangulation from the images (Darouich, 2010). N. Ventroux and R. Schimit (Ventroux, 2009) defines a solution to achieve a 3D reconstruction device based on stereoscopic method for autonomous cars. Kolar (Kolar, 2007) (Kolar, 2009) defines a way to integrate the 3D reconstruction into an integrated vision sensor for an endoscopic video capsule. Ruben Machucho-Cadena and Eduardo Bayro-Corrochano (Machucho-Cadena, 2010) present a solution to create a 3D model of a brain tumor from endoscopic and ultra-sound images. The processing will depend on the complexity of the scene and the required precision. The third solution is based on the time of fly of an energetic wave (Oggier, 2004).

- Form recognition and classification:

The form recognition allows finding a certain object from the raw data in order to classify it and to take a decision; this can be to stop your camera-equipped car when an obstacle is detected (Ponsa and al., 2005). This method is based on two different steps: firstly, the system needs to learn what kind of object it has to detect. This is usually done by a method called AdaBoost. A database that contains the objects to recognize is used to define classifier coefficients in order to obtain the good set of output. Finally, a classifier is able to determinate what kind of object is present on the raw data and to classify it.

The analysis of diagnostic helping algorithms shows that simple algorithms such as pattern recognition or stereo reconstruction are required. These approaches require a computing capacity of hundred billion of operations (GOPs) in order to be executed. Moreover, some of them also may require a frame memory to be correctly executed. Figure 2.4 shows an approximation of computing capacity required expressed in GOPs of the previously presented algorithms.

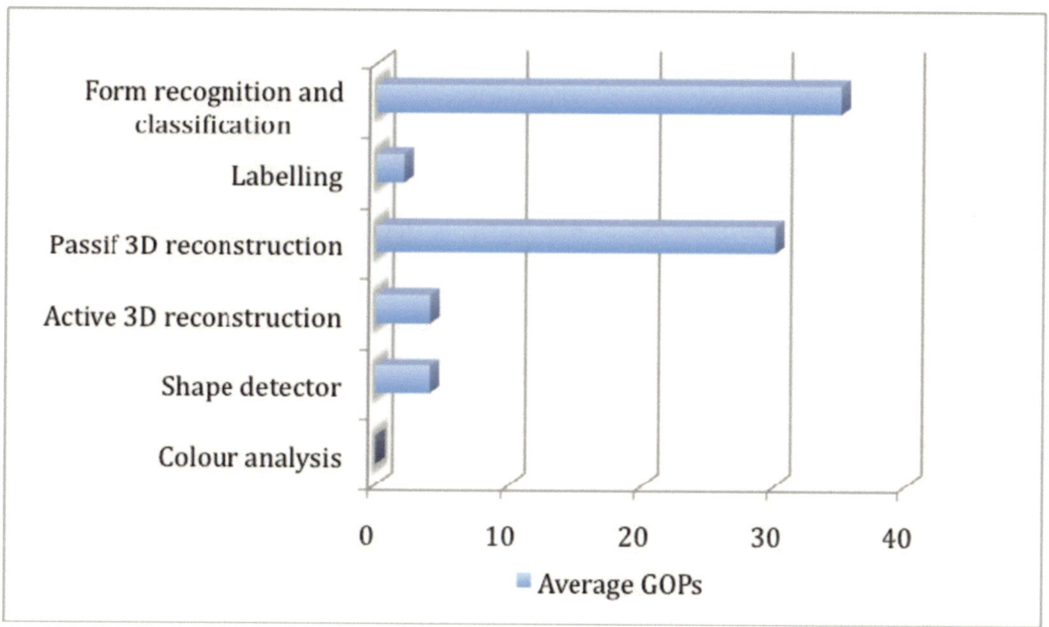

Fig. 2.4. GOPs consumption of diagnosis helping algorithms

But one of the most interesting thing that we can see after the analysis of the algorithms used for the diagnosis helping, is that we can find the same algorithms in consumers devices likes smartphone, camera, game station, etc. Innovations concern architecture design as well as algorithmic definition. Researches also involve co-design and high level synthesis in order to match embedded systems constrains. The expertise of image processing community and embedded devices is widely used for consumers devices researches.

3. Application to endoscopic imaging

A co-design approach is required in order to meet the computing resources requirement of handled diagnostic devices. These approaches are widely used in the community of consumer's devices. First, the whole application set is studied in order to define computing intensive blocks from image processing applications. The first section presents them and their operators that can be ported to hardware resources for both medical and consumer's application. The second section presents a brief state of the art of hardware components known to be efficient for embedded computing intensive image processing from both industrial and academic works. Finally, third section presents a feasibility study of an autonomous endoscopic capsule which has not only the ability to grab and outcast videos like today's one, but also to process them in order to emphasize specific medical abnormality.

3.1 Required operations for image processing

Study of the applications done in previous part of this chapter gives a set of atomic operators. The first processing level needed for every sensed picture consists in a low level image reconstruction and enhancement as previously presented in Figure 2.3. It is realized by algorithms that are pipelined downstream of the image sensor.

In order to capture a correct image, exposure metering and system for auto-focusing must take place. The second step is devoted to the elimination of the electronic noise, which degrades the signal. A contrast enhancement step permits a better usage the sensor dynamic range. Because many types of illuminant sources induce color variation, white balancing makes image colors look natural. The demosaicing step interpolates a complete color image from raw data produced by a color-filtered sensor such as Bayer filter. Finally, various image enhancement processes, such as distortion correction or adaptive edge and contrast enhancement can be applied. The last step (not discussed in this paper) is devoted to the compression and the storage of the image, or to detect points of interest such as corners facilitating object recognition.

- Image capture

Fine exposure-metering methods are required to ensure a correct use of the sensor dynamic range. Similar methods can be employed to ensure that the subject is correctly focused and suitably sharp.

- Exposure control

This step consists in defining exposure parameters which are exposure time, optical aperture, linear ISO sensor sensitivity, and scene luminance.

In smart phones, but also in non Single Lens Reflex (SLR) cameras and camcorders, exposure control can be achieved by direct analysis of the stream of pictures from the sensor as done by Shimizu et al. (Shimizu, 1992).

- Auto-focusing

Auto-focusing consists in measuring image sharpness in a region of interest while displacing certain optical elements. The most common methods are either gradient-based or Laplacian-based such as (Lee, 1980). The region of interest is conventionally considered to be the centre of the image.

- Noise reduction

The use of multiple mega-pixel sensors is encouraged by the current market trends for mobile devices. This tendency has also led to reduction in pixel size, thereby limiting both SNR and overall image quality as explained in Chen et al. (Chen, 2000). Some of the correctible noise is especially due to the CMOS technologies used in image sensors.

    - Pixel noise is directly correlated with photo site area, since photodiode voltage following exposure must be comparable to voltage value after reset (if the latter is more than zero, reset is incomplete). The resulting noise, which can be significant, takes the form of a residual current generated when a pixel is read quickly. Pixel noise is also caused by thermal excitation and leakage. Spatial and temporal disparities caused by such noise are observable and can be statistically characterized.

- Amplification and quantization noise is directly due to ADC sampling. In CMOS sensors, an amplifier and an ADC are present for each column. As in any other electronic device, the signal generated by them includes thermal noise to which quantization noise must also be added.

It is possible to reduce the impact of amplification and quantization noise on images in various ways. The first is to cancel Fixed Pattern Noise (FPN) by deleting characterized noise pixel-per-pixel or column-per-column. The second is to replace any absurd pixel values, which are also those most visible to the human eye. This can be done using Gaussian-kernel convolution or adaptive filtering, for example with bilateral filters (Tomasi, 1998).

- Contrast enhancement

This step allows an optimum use of the full dynamic range of the image. Histogram equalization can be applied to the whole image. The existing literature also describes various embeddable, local adaptive methods. These methods, like High Dynamic Range Imaging (HDRi), are used to extract high and low light values that are not visible on standard displays. Numerous signals are recorded by the sensors in dark and bright areas of the image. Without tone mapping, these signals are not visible on a standard monitor due to saturation effect. Adaptive methods ensure local contrast enhancement using local gamma, local histogram or Retinex-like approaches.

- White balancing and multispectral analysis

Sensor pixels are covered by a color filter such as the well known Bayer one that they "grab" signals corresponding to each primary color. This allows measurement of the absolute luminance values for each color component. These values depend on the scene illuminant color, which induces a global image color—yellow-orange for tungsten and blue-violet for fluorescent light sources. This step aims to determine illuminant color and obtain realistic image colors. The best known method is the grey world assumption, which is used in numerous applications and may vary to other methods like the grey-edge one as proposed by van de Weijer and Gevers (Weijer, 2007).

Multispectral analysis consists in lighting the scene using different wavelength. Nature of the object may be determined by analysis of its response to these different lights. For example a some kind of tumour would be revealed by a 1200 to 1400 nm wavelength.

- Color plan interpolation

The crucial demosaicing step computes each RGB or YUV plan from a single raw image "grabbed" by the sensor, like any camera. There is literature available on a large number of research projects relating to this step, such as. While simple bilinear interpolation calls for computing pixel values by averaging the neighbourhood, other methods use channel-to channel correlations or edge-of-neighbourhood to adapt the demosaicing method to neighbourhood content.

- Image enhancement

Enhancement is necessary to ensure a high quality image. A good contrast balance and sharp edges are two essential parameters for visual perception of an image. Therefore, they can be corrected at the same time. Although correct exposure allows efficient use of the sensor dynamic range, histogram-based processing, like normalization and equalization, are also used to enhance dynamic range. Such processing usually takes place after noise reduction. Edge enhancement can then be performed with a high-pass filter. For this purpose, convolution-based filters like the Sobel filter, unsharp mask or Canny Deriche can be used, as can local adaptive filters, which serve to sharpen images. Image enhancement is traditionally executed in spatial domain, but new approaches tends to execute process in wavelet domains (Courroux, 2010).

- Pattern Recognition

Any device that need to detect specific feature in an image such as face recognition and smile detection like most digital cameras must detect interest points or shape (red eye, face, smile). Traditional methods can be used, however, new approaches based on dynamic neural network are under study (Bichler, 2011).

- Tracking

Many consumer devices are able to detect and to track moving objects such as faces. This is the case for video-conferences devices or digital cameras that uses this feature to enhance auto-focusing. Methods that allow object tracking can be based on feature detection. For example the Harris (Harris, 1998) corner detector. This algorithm is based on three convolutions that process horizontally and vertically edge filtering. The detection of the corner is allowed by the overlapping of the previous results. A final step consists in a cleaning filter to keep only the righteous interest points.

Global exposure control	< 1 MOPs
Autofocus (spot)	< 1 MOPs
FPN removal	0.210 GOPs
White balancing and multispectral detection	20 MOPs
Convolution 3×3	2.5 GOPs
Demosaicing	1.2 to 3 GOPs
Image enhancement	3 GOPs
Active 3D reconstruction	1.5 GOPs
Labelling	2 GOPs + frame memory
Object recognition (tumor, polyp etc)	4 to 30 GOPs + frame memory
TOTAL	~40 GOPs

Table 2.1. Example of the required computing capacity for low level image processing.

Previous approaches have presented image and signal processing algorithmic. They can be ported onto programmable or configurable components on the shelves, Application Specific Processors (ASIPs) may be designed for the execution of the algorithms, or they can be hardwired. The choice of the hardware implementation depends on the constraints to meet for the targeted design. Table 2.1 shows an example of different computing resources that are required to process some of most common low level image processing. It shows the variety of approaches and the variety of required resources.

3.2 A brief survey of embedded computing architectures

Consumers devices such as smart phone, cameras and handled devices drive a large market. This is especially the case for embedded real-time video processing that is the subject of both academic and industrial researches. These researches are driven by the market constraints. First the silicon area infers the component cost, next the power consumption determines if this component can cope with battery powered devices. Finally, flexibility is a feature that is more and more required by integrators. This allows them to use the same component in different generation of devices by simply reconfiguring the hardware or by an update of the firmware or the software of the devices' components. As the choice of an hardware implementation for signal processing can be complex depending on the silicon area constraints, power consumption and computing capacity requirement of the applications. This section presents some of the architectures that may enable image enhancement on smart phone, considering their complexity in terms of gates count or silicon area, their power consumption and their ability to run different kind of processing. Many classifications of these signal processing architectures can be done. For didactic purposes, this section split them into three parts. Dedicated architectures are firstly presented, followed by reconfigurable architectures and by programmable architecture.

A. Dedicated architectures

Are considered as dedicated architecture, components that are made of specialized wired operators grouped together in order to realize more complex hardwired functionalities. These architectures are low silicon footprints and are usually low-power, thus enabling them to be used inside embedded systems such as cell phones. Indeed, their fully wired design is optimized for the applications integration constraints. Today, they are often used by integrators for low level pixel processing such as contrast and color correction, demosacing (Garcia-Lammond, 2008) or denoising (P.Y. Chen, 2008). Designers group these Intellectual Properties (IPs) to forms complete signal processing architecture such as a video pipe image enhancement. For example (Zhou 2003) architecture is able to process Video Gate Array (640×480 pixels (VGA) video stream at 30 frames per second (fps), while Hitachi (Nakano 1998) proposes a component that is able to process Super eXtended Gate Array (SXGA) pictures. However, these more complex systems require an external memory acting as a frame buffer to work properly. Videantis proposes two processors (Videantis inc., 2007) (Videantis inc., 2008) that are able to process High Definition (HD) video stream conforming to standards HD 720p and HD 1080p. The most powerful of them requires large silicon area and power consumption which is not compatible with their integration into low-cost components. As dedicated operators cannot be autonomous, they need to be used in association with embedded processors (e.g. ARMs or MIPSs) and an external memory or finite state machines. This is a common solution for low-power mobile devices like cell phones or compact cameras. Despite the high computational efficiency of these solutions, they lack flexibility due to their hardwired implementation that allows to the customers to configure only a set of limited predefined parameters, these solutions are widely used thanks to a short time to market.

B. Reconfigurable architectures

Reconfigurable architectures may be seen as evolutions of dedicated operators, especially when they are used in complex System-on-Chips (SoCs). SoCs need of flexibility and operator reuse for different applications pushes the architect to define methods for this purpose. For example, the Coarse Grained Reconfigurable Image Processor (CRISP) architecture (Chen, 2008a) can handle HD 1080p video streams. It was specifically designed in order to run image processing and enhancement application downstream the image sensor with more flexibility than dedicated IPs. However supported processes are limited by hardwired modules that compose the design. It also was designed to limit its silicon area usage and power consumption in order to be embeddable into smart phones. Its implementation requires approximately 170 kGates and 74 kb of memory. This correspond to a 400 kGates and 5 mm2 when implemented in 180 nm technology - an extrapolation gives about 1 mm2 of silicon area in Taiwan SeMi Conductor (TSMC) 65 nm. Its given power consumption is 218 mW at 115 MHz while it can run a complete image processing on HD 1080p video streams at 55 fps. Unfortunately, its flexibility is limited by its hard-wired embedded processes. Moreover, to run algorithms properly, it must be associated with memory resources. DART (David, 2002), MORA, MorphoSys or ADRES approaches can be cited, however, more flexible reconfigurable architectures are, and more fine grained their reconfigurability is. The reconfigurability elements of such architecture, especially interconnects, implies an important silicon area overcost, thus can be larger than the computing elements themselves making their integration into low-cost devices difficult.

C. Programmable architectures

Programmable architectures can be seen as specifically designed fine grained reconfigurable architectures. In order to maintain a low silicon area and high computing performance over power consumption, architects have to specialize their design for an application predefined set. Spiral Gateway, for example, proposes RICA, a configurable System on Chip (SoC), which is based on algorithm analysis (Khawam, 2008) and is thus programmable within the scope of the initial application set. Tensilica provides another product that is extended instruction set processors (Tensilica). SiliconHive markets a processor template that is customized by application code analysis. Its type and number of operators - from 4 to 128 - can be customized at the time of chip design. For the automotive market, NEC has devised the ImapCar processor (Kyo, 2005) containing 128 SIMD - Single Instruction Multiple Data means that every processor executes the same instruction on different data, for example each processor do the same job on each pixel of an image - parallel arithmetic and logic units with a power consumption of more than one Watt. Xetal also proposes a programmable, massively-parallel processor integrating 320 computing units (Abbo, 2008). SIMPil (Gentile, 2005) architecture calls for parallelized 4096 processors, each of which is intended to compute a single pixel block. Stream Processors Inc., a commercial spinoff of Stanford's Imagine project (Stream, 2007) and Massashusset Institute of Technology (MIT), proposes STORM, a family of parallel chips that can handle video streams. These components are not directly embeddable in cell phones due to their high power consumption and large area. An acceptable silicon "budget" is about 1 to 2 mm2 in a typical 65 nm technology with a power consumption of less than half a watt. These constraints is lacking for programmable architectures in this competitive market niche.

However, the common feature in all these programmable components is the use of different forms of parallelism such Single Instruction Multiple Data (SIMD) and Very Long Instruction Word (VLIW), making them efficient for computing regular data patterns. This is especially the case for stream processors. This brief study of the state of the art architecture shows that many of the most efficient flexible machines are based on multiple programmable processors running in SIMD mode. Moreover, VLIW processors are often used allowing the ILP of programs to be exploited. In this fact, the proposed architecture includes these features (programmability, SIMD and VLIW). However, data access remains an important bottleneck that limits computing bandwidth. In order to get a high computing capacity, the proposed architecture is designed to separate data access and computing, in this way, we can achieve the computation directly on incoming video stream without needing an external frame buffer.

3.3 Proposed vision architecture for integrated diagnostic helping devices

The proposed architecture is based on the eISP (Thevenin, 2010) processor that is designed for smart phone embedded video and is derived to give enough computing capacity to support diagnostic helping image processing algorithms that could be required in an endocapsule. Our study established an approximation of the required computing capacity of about 50 GOPs for an average power consumption of less than a half Watt, and a maximum silicon area of 15 mm² dedicated to computations.

As shown previously, algorithms can easily be divided in elementary stages and pipelined. One of the most efficient architecture models consists in splitting a whole multiprocessor architecture into elementary computing tiles as shown in Figure 3.1. Each of them acts as an autonomous SIMD computer that can execute a process. Figure 3.2 depict a *P* processors computing tile. Each computing tiles is connected using a bus, allowing the execution of different kind of processes. For example, video processing are chained as shown in the first section can be mapped onto each computing tile.

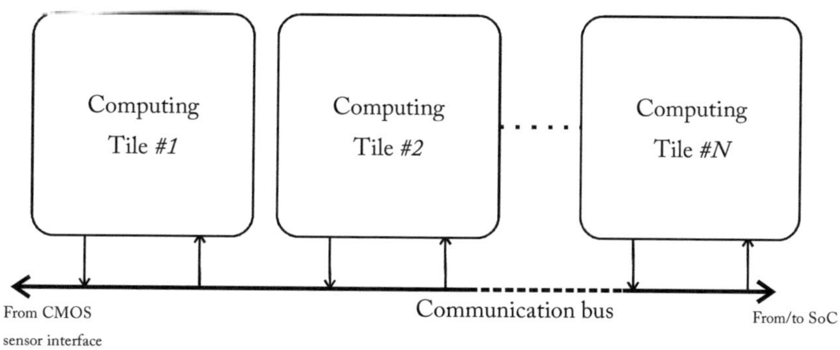

Fig. 3.1. eISP, a computile tile architecture.

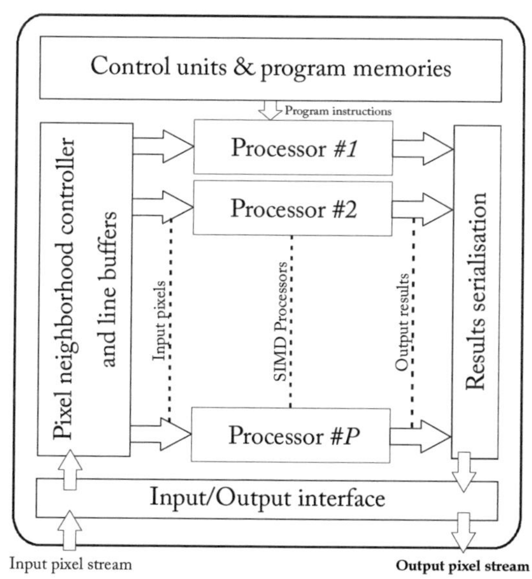

Fig. 3.2. A *P* processors computing tile.

Different instances of computing tiles are characterized in terms of computing capacity, power consumption, silicon area in function of their number of processor and memory resources. An example characterization of the architecture is shown on Figure 3.3. This work gives a normalized performance measure expressed in MOPs/mW and GOPs/mm². Standard instance of the eISP architecture gives a computing capacity of about 25GOPs/mm² for 100mW. Reaching a computing capacity of 100 GOPs that would be required for image processing in diagnostic helping device would require 4mm² of silicon area and 400mW of power consumption.
Each computing tile can be generated with a set of parameters that are given by the designer. For example the data-path width, usually 8 to 32 bits and its operators, memory maps, that is distributed in each processor or that is shared with all processor of a same computing tile.
Sizing the whole architecture depends on the total required computing capacity, but also on the computing capacity that the designer need for each task that will be ported on each computing tile. Designer may uses results of the characterization, as the example shown on Figure 3.3 to size its architecture. He can generate computing tiles and connect them to the communication bus. Final synthesizes and simulations are required to check the designed architecture. Finally, the eISP can be integrated into a complete System on Chip or to a Lab on Chip that include control and communication components.

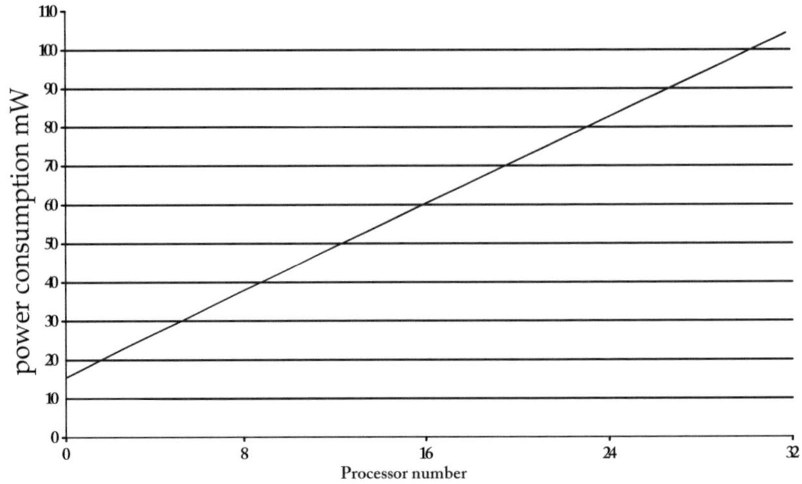

Fig. 3.3. Characterization of the power consumption of a single computing tile eISP architecture versus number of processors.

A complete characterization of the eISP architecture in TSMC 65nm was done allowing an accurate design space exploration. We can add up to two frame buffer for HD 720p require that would require 4 mm² for each frame. Thus, allow high level processing such as video compression and labelling that requires up to several dozen GOPs and a frame memory depending on the selected implementation.

4. Conclusion

This chapter has presented the algorithms that could be used for digital image processing in handled diagnostic devices, and more precisely in the case of endoscopy. As research in consumer devices imaging is intense, a comparisons of the algorithms that are used in that domain is done in this chapter. This work shows similarities between the approaches. These similarities can be exploited in order to transfer the hardware processors initially designed for consumers market - such as cell phone or gaming - to integrated medical domain. The case of the endoscopic video capsule is used due to its highly constrained integrability, as well in terms of silicon area or power consumption and computational capacity. A state of the art of the architectures that could match these constraints is described. It shows that the existent architectures do not to perfectly cope with computational requirement, silicon area or power consumption. A computing architecture derived from the eISP, an image signal processor designed for low level image enhancement is proposed. With less than 5 mm^2 and 0.5 Watt of power consumption, this can integrate the required computing and memory resources for handled diagnostic device in limited constraints inherent to this domain. Due to its programmability, it can be used not only as image enhancement architecture, but also as a high-level diagnostic helping processor by executing processes like form recognition, 3D-reconstruction, shape detector etc.

The use of such signal processing architecture in conjunction with complete robotized diagnostic helping platforms as (Valdastri, 2009) may allows the conception of an autonomous lab-on-chip that would be able to execute simple tasks like free move and biopsy.

5. References

A.A. Abbo, R.P. Kleihorst, V. Choudhary, L. Sevat, P.Wielage, S.Mouy, B. Vermeulen and M. Heijligers. (2008) Xetal-II: A 107 GOPS, 600 mW Massively Parallel Processor for Video Scene Analysis. Solid-State Circuits, *IEEE Journal of, vol. 43, no. 1*, pp 192–201, Jan. 2008.

F. Bernardini, M. Cerbo, T. Jefferson, A. Lo Scalzo, M. Ratti, (2008). Age.na.s HTA Report - Wireless Capsule Endoscopy in the diagnosis of small bowel disease, Rome, September 2008.

O. Bichler, D. Querlioz, S.J. Thorpe, J.P Bourgoin, C. Gamrat. (2011) A wavelet-based demosaicking algorithm for embedded applications; *International Joint Conference on Neural Networks (IJCNN - 2011)*, San José, Etats-unis, 31/07/2011 - 05/08/2011.

T. Chen, Peter Catrysse, Abbas E Gamal and Brian W. (2008) How small should pixel size be ? In *Proceedings of SPIE, April 2000, vol 7, no. 9*, pp 451–459, 2000.

J.C. Chen and Shao-Yi Chien (2008). CRISP: Coarse-Grained Reconfigurable Image Stream Processor for Digital Still Cameras and Camcorders. *IEEE Trans. Circuits Syst. Video Technol.*, vol. 18, no. 9, pp 1223–1236, Sept 2008.

P.Y. Chen, Chih-Yuan Lien and Yi-Ming Lin. (2008) A real-time image denoising chip. In Circuits and Systems, *ISCAS 2008. IEEE International Symposium on*, pp 3390–3393, May 2008.

S. Courroux, S. Guyetant, S. Chevobbe S., M. Paindavoine. (2010), Reconfigurable Computing: Architectures, Tools and Applications, *International Conference on*

Design and Architectures for Signal and Image Processing (DASIP – 2010), Edimbourg ; Royaume-uni, 2010.

M. Darouich, S. Guyetant and D. Lavenier. (2010) A Reconfigurable Disparity Engine for Stereovision in Advanced Driver Assistance Systems *Lecture Notes in Computer Science*, , Volume 5992, 2010.

R. David, D. Chillet, S. Pillement, O. Sentieys. (2002) DART: a dynamically reconfigurable architecture dealing with future mobile telecommunications constraints, *Proceedings International Parallel and Distributed Processing Symposium, IPDPS 2002*, pp. 156, 2002.

Fireman and al (2004), *Eur J GEH* 2004

J. Garcia-Lamont, M. Aleman-Arce and J. Waissman-Vilanova. (2008) A Digital Real Time Image Demosaicking Implementation for High Definition Video Cameras. *In Electronics, Robotics and Automotive Mechanics Conference, 2008. CERMA '08*, pp 565–569, 30 2008-Oct.

A. Gentile, S. Vitabile, L. Verdoscia and F. Sorbello. (2005) Image processing chain for digital still cameras based on the SIMPil architecture. *Parallel Processing, 2005. ICPP 2005 Workshops. International Conference Workshops on*, pp 215–222, June 2005.

P. Gomes, (2011) Surgical robotics: Reviewing the past, analysing the present, imagining the future, *Robot. Comput.-Integr. Manuf.*, vol. 27, no. 2, pp. 261-266, Apr. 2011.

T. Graba (2009), Etude d'une architecture de traitement pour un capteur intégré de vision 3D, *Phdthesis, Université Pierre and Marie Curie*, 2009.

K. Harada, E. Susilo, N. Ng Pak, A. Menciassi, and P. Dario, (2008) Design of a Bending Module for Assembling Reconfigurable Endoluminal Surgical System Pisa, *ISG conference*, Tuscany, Italy - June 4-6, 2008.

Harris and Stephans, (1988) A Combined Corner and Edge Detector. *In Alvey Vision Conference*, pp 147–152, 1988.

M. Hartmann, V. Pantazis, T. Vander Aa, M. Berekovic, C. Hochberger and B. de Sutter, (2007) Still Image Processing on Coarse-Grained Reconfigurable Array Architectures. *In Embedded Systems for Real-Time Multimedia, 2007. ESTIMedia 2007. IEEE/ACM/IFIP Workshop on*, pp 67–72, Oct. 2007.

R. Machucho-Cadena and E. Bayro-Corrochano, (2010) 3D Reconstruction of Brain Tumors from Endoscopic and Ultrasound Images, *Pattern Recognition Recent Advances, InTech,* Adam Herout (Ed.), ISBN: 978-953-7619-90-9, , 2010.

A. Menciassi, C. Stefanini, G. Orlandi, M. Quirini, P. Dario, (2006) Towards active capsular endoscopy: preliminary results on a legged platform, *28th Annual International Conference of the IEEE Engineering in Medicine and Biology Society, EMBS '06*, Page(s): 2215 - 2218, 2006.

M. Katona, A. Pižurica, N. Teslic, V. Kovacevic and W. Philips. (2006) A real-time wavelet-domain video denoising implementation in FPGA. *EURASIP J. Embedded Syst., vol. 2006, no. 1*, pages 6–6, 2006.

A. Karargyris, N. Bourbakis, (2010) Wireless Capsule Endoscopy and Endoscopic Imaging: A Survey on Various Methodologies Presented, *IEEE Engineering in Medicine and Biology Magazine, Vol. 29 Issue:1* ,pages 72 - 83 , Jan.-Feb. 2010

S. Khawam, I. Nousias, M. Milward, Ying Yi, M. Muir and T. Arslan. (2008) The Reconfigurable Instruction Cell Array. Very Large Scale Integration (VLSI) Systems, IEEE Transactions on, vol. 16, no. 1, pages 75–85, Jan. 2008.

T. S. Kim, S. Y. Song, H. Jung, J. Kim and E.-S. Yoon (2007), Micro Capsule Endoscope for Gastro Intestinal Trac, *IEEE EMBS*, 2007, pp 2823-2826.

A. Kolar, O. Romain , T. Graba, T. Ea and B. Granado, (2008) The Integrated Active Stereoscopic Vision Theory, *Integration and Application Stereo Vision, InTech*, ISBN 978-953-7619-22-0, November 2008

A. Kolar, A. Pinna, O. Romain, S. Viateur, T. Ea, E. Belhaire, T. Graba and B. Granado (2009), A multi shutter time sensor for multi-spectral imaging in a 3D Reconstruction integrated sensor, *IEEE Sensor Journal*, vol 9, pp 478-484, 2009

S. Kyo, S. Okazaki and T. Arai, (2005) An integrated memory array processor architecture for embedded image recognition systems. *Computer Architecture, 2005. ISCA '05. Proceedings. 32nd International Symposium on*, pp 134–145, June 2005.

J.S. Lee. (1980) Digital image enhancement and noise filtering by use of local statistics. *IEEE Transactions on Pattern Analysis and Machine Intelligence., vol. PAMI-2*, pp 165–168, March 1980.

L. Lacassagne, B. Zavidovique, (2009) Light Speed Labeling for RISC architectures, *16th IEEE International Conference on Image Processing (ICIP)*, 2009 , Page(s): 3245 - 3248

Ming-Hau Lee, Hartej Singh, Guangming Lu, Nader Bagherzadeh, Fadi J. Kurdahi, Fadi and J. Kurdahi. (2000) Design and Implementation of the MorphoSys Reconfigurable Computing Processor. *In Journal of VLSI and Signal Processing-Systems for Signal, Image and Video Technology*. Kluwer Academic Publishers, 2000.

Maieron and al, (2004) *Endoscopy* 2004

N. Nakano, R. Nishimura, H. Sai, A. Nishizawa and H. Komatsu, (1998) Digital still camera system for megapixel CCD. *Consumer Electronics, IEEE Transactions on, vol. 44, no. 3*, pages 581–586, Aug 1998.

T. Oggier, M. Lehmann, R. Kaufmann, M. Schweizer, M. Richter, P. Metzler, G. Lang, Lustenberger, F. & Blanc, N., (2004) An all-solid-state optical range camera for 3D real-time imaging with sub-centimeter depth resolution (SwissRanger),*SPIE, Optical Design and Engineering*, pp534-545, 2004.

E. Péry, (2008) Spectroscopie bimodale en diffusion élastique and autofluorescence résolue spatialement: instrumentation, modélisation des interactions lumiére-tissus and application à la caractérisation de tissus biologiques ex vivo and in vivo pour la détection de cancers, *Phdthesis, Institut National Polytechnique de Lorraine*, 2008.

D. Ponsa, A. L´opez, F. Lumbreras, J. Serrat, T. Graf, (2005) 3D Vehicle Sensor based on Monocular Vision, *IEEE Conference on Intelligent Transportation Systems*, 2005.

M. Quirini, S. Scapellato, P. Valdastri, A. Menciassi and P. Dario, (2007), An Approach to Capsular Endoscopywith Active Motion *IEEE EMBS*, 2007, pp 2827-2830.

Selby and al, Gastrointest Endosc 2004.

Tensilica Co. (2007) 388VDO Video *DSP Product Brief.*, Tensilica Co., 2007.

S. Shimizu, T. Kondo, T. Kohashi, M. Tsurata, T. Komuro, (1992), A new algorithm for exposure based on fuzzy logic for video cameras , *IEEE Transactions on Consumer Electronics Volume: 38 , Issue: 3*, 1992 , Page(s): 617 - 623.

Stream Processors, Inc. (2007) Storm-1 Stream Processors, SP16HP-G220 *Product Brief. Stream Processors, Inc.*, Apr. 2007.

M. Thevenin, M. Paindavoine, L. Letellier, R. Schmit, and B. Heyrman, (2010) The eISP a low-power and tiny silicon footprint programmable video architecture, *Journal of Real-Time Image Processing*, pp. 1–14, Jun. 2010.

Texas Instruments (2006) Texas Instrument TMS320DSC21 : A High-Performance, Programmable, Single Chip Digital Signal Processing Solution to Digital Still Cameras.

C. Tomasi and R. Manduchi, (1998) Bilateral Filtering for Gray and Color Images, Proceedings of the *1998 IEEE International Conference on Computer Vision*, Bombay, India, 1998.

P. Valdastri, R. J. Webster III, C. Quaglia, M. Quirini, A. Menciassi, and P. Dario (2009) A New Mechanism for Meso-Scale Legged Locomotion in Compliant Tubular Environments. *IEEE Transactions on Robotics*, 2009.

Videantis Inc. (2007) v-MP2000SD, Dual-Core Multi-Standard Video Codec IP Solution. *Technical Report, Videantis Inc.*, 2007.

Videantis Inc. (2008) v-MP4180HDX, Full HD 1080p Video Codec Integrated Solution. *Technical Report, Videantis Inc.*, 2008.

J. van de Weijer, A. Gijsenij and Th. Gevers. (2007) Edge-based color constancy. *IEEE Transactions on Image Processing*, 2007.

Rongzheng Zhou, Xuefeng Chen, Feng Liu, Jie He, Tiankang Liao, Yanfeng Su, Jinghua Ye, Yajie Qin, Xiaofeng Yi and Zhiliang Hong. (2003) System-on-chip for mega-pixel digital camera processor with auto control functions. *In ASIC, 2003. Proceedings. 5th International Conference on, volume 2*, pp 894–897 Vol.2, Oct. 2003.

Rongzheng Zhou, Xuefeng Chen, Feng Liu, Jie He, Tiankang Liao, Yanfeng Su, Jinghua Ye, Yajie Qin, Xiaofeng Yi and Zhiliang Hong. (2003) System-on-chip for mega-pixel digital camera processor with auto control functions. *In ASIC, 2003. Proceedings. 5th International Conference on, volume 2*, pp 894–897 Vol.2, Oct. 2003.

N. Ventroux, R. Schmit, F. Pasquet, P.-E. Viel, S. Guyetant. (2009) Stereovision-based 3D detection for automotive safety driving assistance, *12th International IEEE Conference on Intelligent Transportation Systems, 2009. ITSC '09*, pp 1, 4-7 Oct. 2009.

2

A Mobile-Phone-Based Health Management System

Yu-Chi Wu et al.*
National United University,
Taiwan

1. Introduction

"Prevention is better than cure." The system proposed in this chapter aims to achieve this.
According to the bulletin report of Taiwan Ministry of Interior, the elder population in Taiwan at the end of 2008 was 2.4 million, about 10.4% of the total Taiwan population. This percentage has already exceeded the standard for aging society set by the World Health Organization (WHO). Furthermore, it is estimated that in 2025 the elder population in Taiwan will reach more than 20% of the total population; therefore, the "long-distance home health care service" has become one of the key emerging businesses in Taiwan. It was estimated that the market revenue of home health care for these elders reached 300 million dollars in 2010.

In recent years, several studies integrating communication and sensor technologies for home health monitoring system have been discussed (Chang, 2004; Chen, 2008; Lee, 2006a, 2006b, 2007a, 2007b; J.L. Lin, 2005; T.H. Lin, 2004, Shu, 2005; Wu, 2004; Ye, 2006; Yu et al., 2005), such as monitoring long-term health data to find out the abnormal signs and monitoring the medical record regularly for chronic patients to cut down their treatment frequency, to save doctor's treatment time, and to reduce medical expenses. Based on the sensor and communication technologies used, these systems can be categorized into two systems: immobile and mobile long-distance health monitoring systems. Our previous works all focused on mobile long-distance physiological signal measuring based on either a single-chip-microprocessor or a smart phone. The physiological sensor used was a RFID ring-type pulse/temperature sensor. The measured data can be transmitted via different communication protocols, such as Bluetooth, ZigBee, HSDPA, GPRS, and TCP/IP. In order to meet the requirement for mobile health monitoring system (MHMS), the system design needs to adopt light modular sensors for data collection and wireless communication technology for mobility. The popular smart phones used in people's daily life are the best devices for MHMS.

In this chapter, a different mobile e-health-management system based on mobile physiological signal monitoring is presented to practice the idea of "Prevention is better than cure." This system integrates a wearable ring-type pulse monitoring sensor and a portable biosignal

* Chao-Shu Chang[1], Yoshihito Sawaguchi[2], Wen-Ching Yu[1], Men-Jen Chen[3], Jing-Yuan Lin[1], Shih-Min Liu[1], Chin-Chuan Han[1], Wen-Liang Huang[1] and Chin-Yu Su[1]
1 *National United University, Taiwan,*
2 *Kisarazu National College of Technology, Japan,*
3 *National Kaohsiung University of Applied Science, Taiwan.*

recorder with a smart phone. The ring-type pulse monitoring sensor can measure pulse and temperature, while the biosignal recorder can record electroencephalogram (EEG), electrocardiogram (ECG), and body 3-axis acceleration during daily lives. The smart phone provides mobile "exercise-333" health management mechanisms. The user can monitor his/her own pulse and temperature from the smart phone where the "exercise-333" health management mechanism can help him/her to develop a healthy life style: taking exercise 3 or more times a week, at least 30 minutes per time, raising heart rate to 130 per minute. With the popularity and mobility of smart phones, this system effectively provides the needs for mobile health management.

2. System architecture, hardware, and software

2.1 System architecture

The proposed monitoring system architecture is shown as Fig. 1 where the ring-type sensor measures pulse/temperature and transmits the physiological data to the reader using wireless RF, the biosignal recorder collects EEG/ECG/body-acceleration data and sends data to the

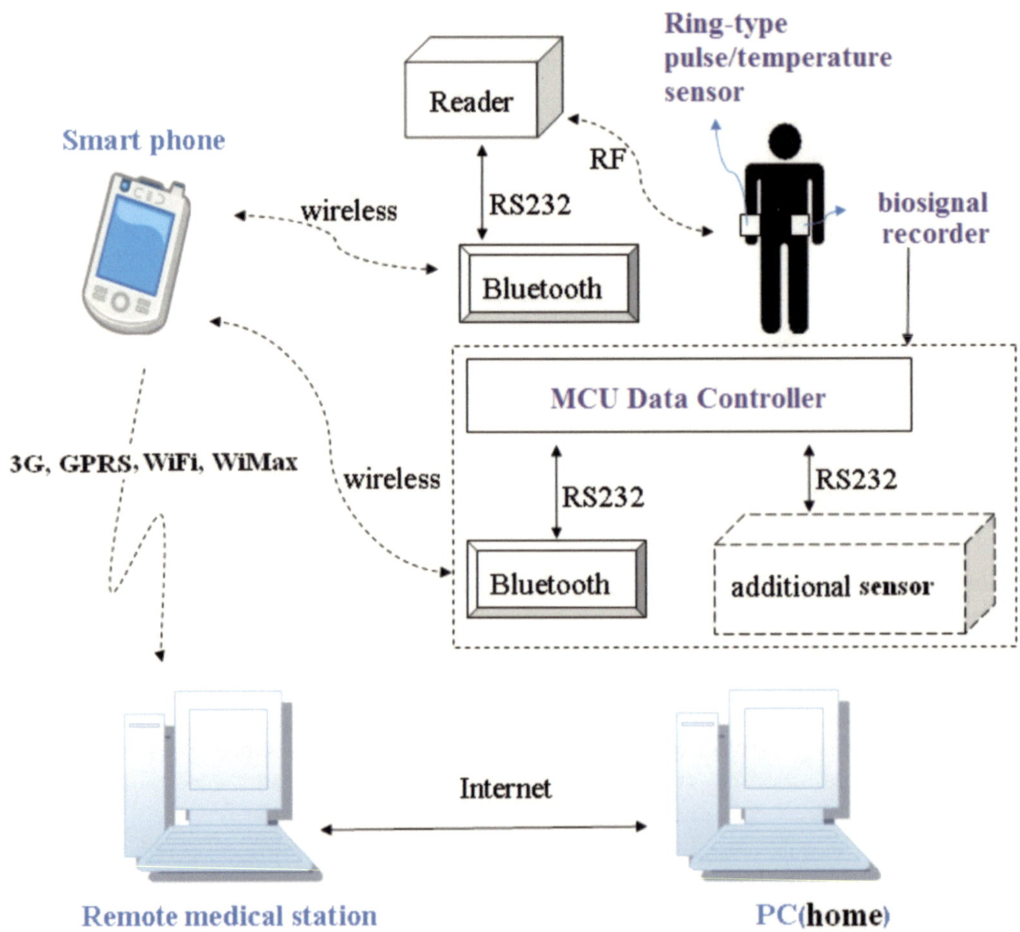

Fig. 1. MHMS Architecture

MCU data controller, the Bluetooth adaptors connected to the reader and the MCU data controller pass the data to the smart phone, and the smart phone records/displays the physiological data and also transmits data to the remote medical station using GPRS, HSDPA (3.5G), WiFi, or WiMax. The GPS built in the smart phone can provide the position information of the monitored person so that the medical personnel can be dispatched to the right location more promptly in an emergency situation. The proposed system architecture is capable of integrating additional physiological sensors via the MCU data controller. Therefore, it can be used as an e-coach to keep the user having healthy life style. It also can be applied to the baby-caring by detecting baby's pulse and/or ECG to identify whether the baby is being suffocated by pillow or blanket.

2.2 Hardware

The hardware used in MHMS includes RFID pulse/temperature sensor tag (Ring) and RFID reader, Bluetooth RS232 adaptor, biosignal recorder, and smart phone.

2.2.1 RFID pulse/temperature sensor

Although there is a ring-type pulse monitoring sensor in the market, shown as Fig. 2, the measured data are displayed in the LCD and cannot be transmitted out of the ring. In this paper, a RFID wearable ring-type sensor designed by Sinopulsar Technology Inc., Taiwan was adopted, instead. Fig. 3 shows this RFID ring (tag). This ring sensor is non-invasive, portable, and mobile. It can measure pulse and temperature signals which are processed by a built-in microcontroller. It uses optical sensors to detect heart rate and has anti data collision mechanism. Physiological data are then transmitted by RF wireless transmission with FSK modulation using UHF ISM band (up to 50 meters) to a RFID reader shown as Fig. 4. Fig. 5 illustrates the integration of Bluetooth adaptor, RFID ring (tag), and RFID reader.

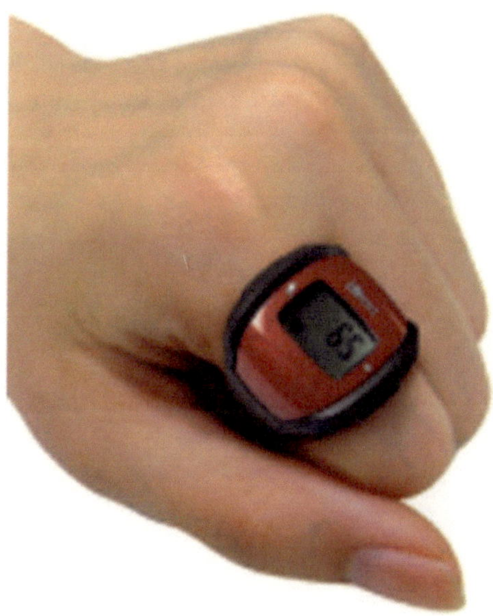

Fig. 2. A commercial ring-type pulse sensor

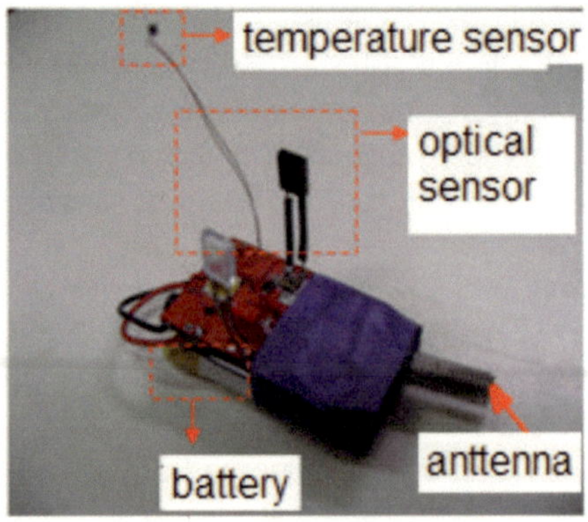

Fig. 3. RFID ring (tag)

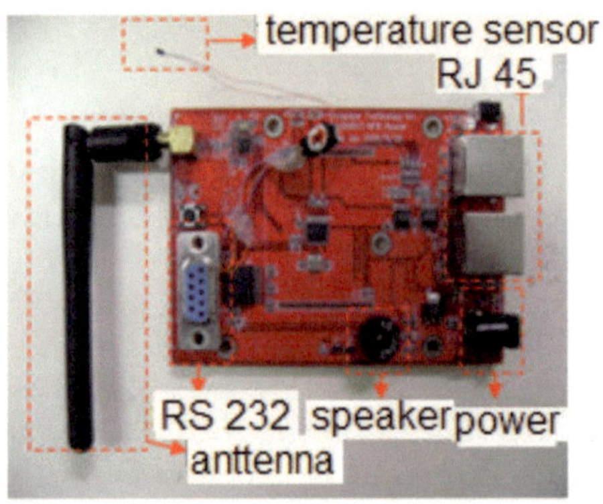

Fig. 4. RFID reader

2.2.2 Bluetooth RS232 adaptor

The data communication between RFID reader and the smart phone is through Bluetooth. HL-MD08A (Bluetooth RS232 Adaptor manufactured by Hotlife Technology) is used in the presented system. It supports a wide range of Baud rates from 1.2K to 921.6K bps. Fig. 5 shows the picture of HL-MD08A, and Fig. 6 shows the picture of the RFID ring (tag) and the connection of HL-MD08A to the RFID reader.

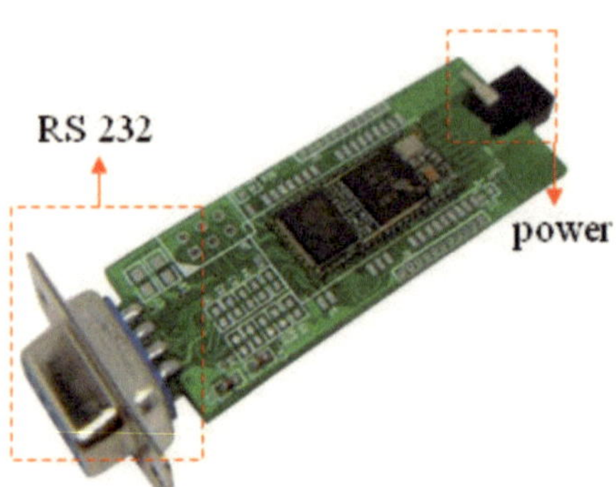

Fig. 5. Bluetooth RS232 Adaptor

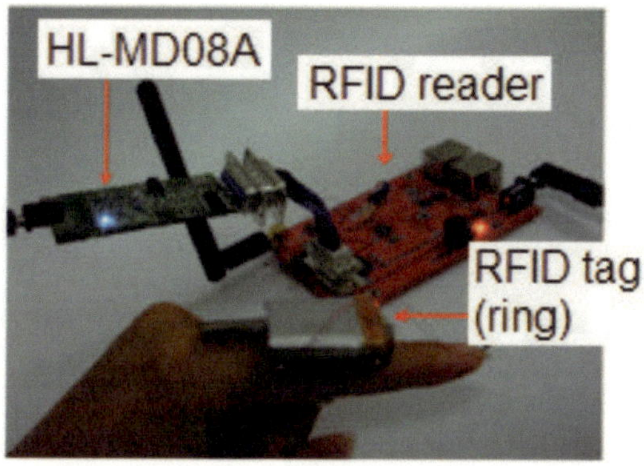

Fig. 6. Bluetooth adaptor, RFID ring (tag) & RFID reader

2.2.3 Biosignal recorder

The biosignal recorder, developed in this system for assessment of sleep depth and physical activities during daily lives, can measure electroencephalogram (EEG), electrocardiogram (ECG) and body acceleration signals. The size of this developed device (45mm × 25mm × 65mm, 62.5g) is more appropriate for ambulatory recoding than that of the well-known devices such as LifeGuard (Mundt et al., 2005) (129mm × 100mm × 20mm, 166g), AMON (Anliker et al., 2004) (286g) and Smart Vest (Pandian et al., 2008) (460g). Fig. 7 shows photographs of the developed device. The device consists of an analog part, a digital part and a power supply, as in Fig. 8.

The analog part has five electrodes. Two of them are placed on the forehead and ear lobe for EEG acquisition. Another two electrodes are patched on upper-right and lower-left breast for ECG acquisition. The last electrode is put on back neck for right-leg-driving. The acquired signals are amplified by instrumentation amplifiers (Analog Devices AD627) and operational amplifiers (Texas Instruments TLV2254). The amplification factors are 60dB for EEG and 46dB for ECG. These amplification circuits also have bandpass characteristics with the passband from 0.5Hz to 100Hz. Then the conditioned signals are sent to the digital part.

The digital part consists of a mixed-signal microcontroller, an accelerometer and a memory card. The mixed-signal microcontroller (Texas Instruments MSP430F4270) converts the conditioned signals (EEG and ECG) to digital signals with 16-bit resolution at the sampling rate of 256Hz. This microcontroller also collects three-axis acceleration values from the accelerometer (Freescale MMA7456L). This accelerometer provides 10-bit digital values whose range and sampling frequency are ± 8g and 8Hz, respectively. The microcontroller records these digital data into the memory card. The memory card can store digital data up to 2GBytes, large enough for 2-week recordings. The power supply provides regulated voltage to other parts. The power source is one-cell lithiumion polymer battery (3.7V, 900mAh) and connected to a voltage regulator (Texas Instruments TPS73130) through a diode-OR circuit. This diode-OR circuit enables us to hotswap batteries. The principal parts of the developed device is enclosed in an ABS plastic case (Takachi SW-65S) whose size is 45mm × 25mm × 65mm. The overall weight of the device is 62.5g. Since the current consumption is 29mA in the steady state, the device can record EEG, ECG and three-axis accelerogram for up to 31 hours with the fully-charged battery. Furthermore, the measurement duration can be prolonged up to 2-weeks when two or more batteries are used, swapped and charged alternately once a day.

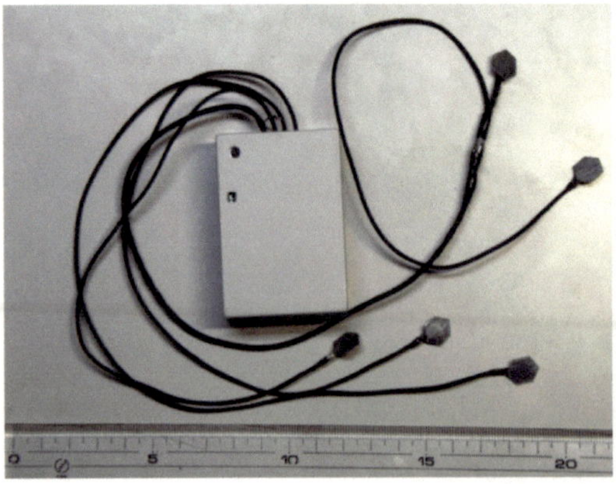

(a)

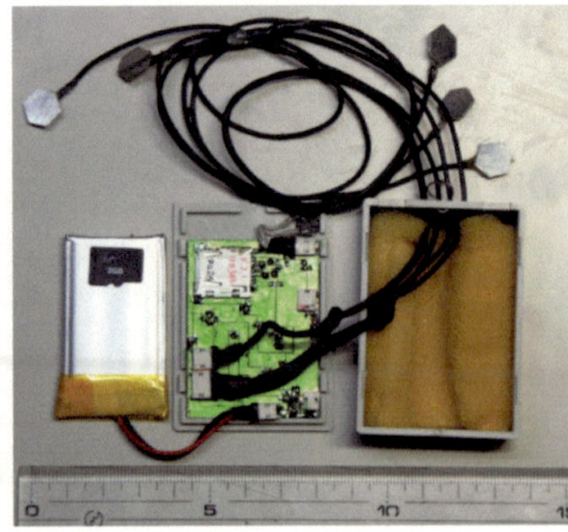

(b)

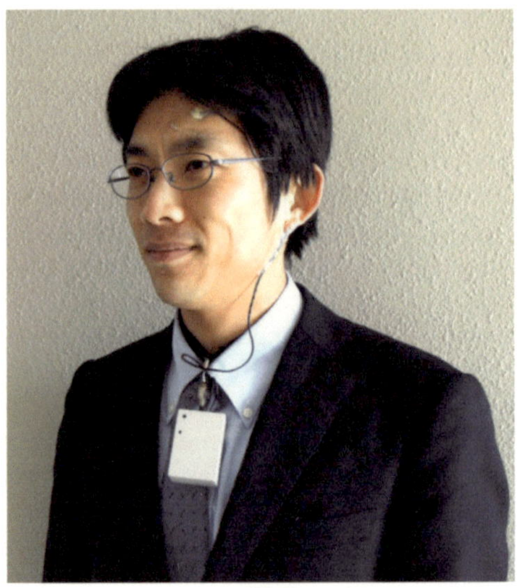

(c)

Fig. 7. Biosignal recorder (a) recorder with case closed, (b) recorder with case opened, (c) portable recorder with wires attached to user's body

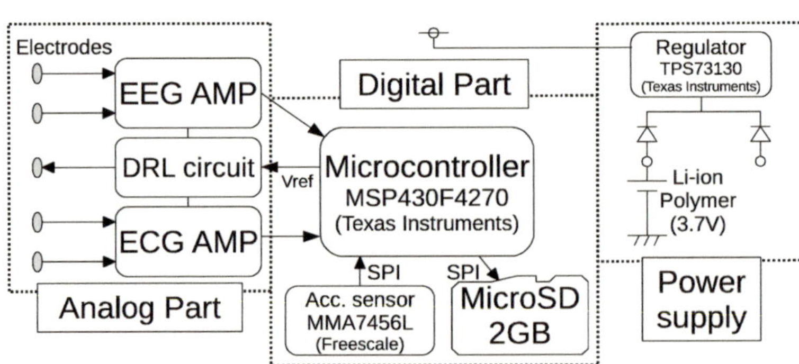

Fig. 8. Block diagram of developed biosignal recorder

2.2.4 MCU data controller

The data controller consists of a MCU (Philips P89C51RD2HBP microcontroller), a multiplexer (Hitachi HD74LS153P, Dual 4-line to one-line Data Selectors), a demultiplexer (SN74LS156N, Dual one-line to 4-line Data Decoder), and a RS232-TTL voltage conversion IC (Intersil HIN232CP). Fig. 9 shows the developed data controller circuit on a breadboard. The function of this data controller is like a data switch to bridge the biosignal recorder and additional sensor to the Bluetooth adaptor. It alternately transmits the data from these two different sensors to the smart phone via Bluetooth.

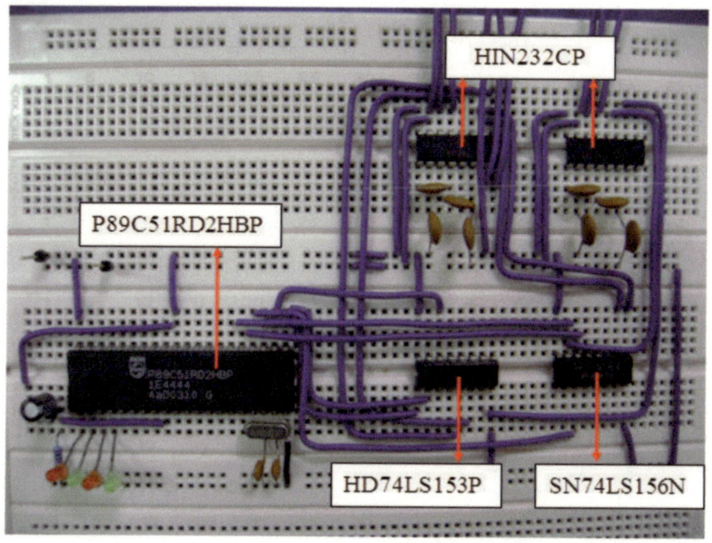

Fig. 9. MCU Data Controller

2.2.5 Smart phone

Any smart phone which operating system is Windows Mobile 6.1 is suitable for the presented system. The smart phone used in this system is ASUS P552W with built-in GPS. It supports HSDPA 3.6Mbps/EDGE/GPRS/GSM 900/1800/1900. Fig. 10 shows the picture of this smart phone.

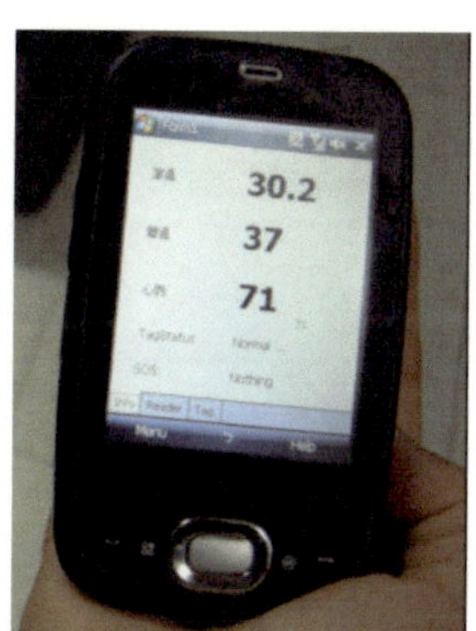

Fig. 10. ASUS P552W smart phone

2.3 Software

The GUI programs developed on the smart phone and on the remote medical station were coded in Visual C#. Microsoft .Net compact framework 3.5 was installed on the smart phone for running the client APs, and Windows Mobile 6 SDK, smart phone emulator, and Cellular Emulator were installed on the PC for developing the client APs.

Several GUIs were developed to communicate with the RFID reader/tag and then were packaged into a DLL file for ARM-based embedded systems (smart phones). The reason of using DLL file is for the security reason so that the physical data format can be hidden in the DLL file. Table 1 shows the commands developed for the APs. The shaded area in Fig. 11 illustrates the flow chart of the AP on the smart phone. After the hardware devices are set up properly, the user is ready to run the developed AP by starting the setup procedures: 1. Open Bluetooth ComPort, 2. Execute ReaderReset command to initialize the RFID reader, 3. Execute ReaderQuery command to search for available RFID Reader, 4. Execute AllReset command, 5. Execute SearchTag command to search for available ring tag. Then, the user can start receiving data from the ring tag to the smart phone by executing the Access command. The GPS data can also be received to the smart phone by executing the "Open" command. These collected data on the smart phone can be transmitted to the remote server through 3.5G Internet communication by performing the following procedures: 1. Check connection manager, 2. Check available network , 3. Establish Internet connection, and 4. Send out data using Socket class.

Command (for Reader)	Descriptor
ReaderReset	Reset RFID Reader
ReaderQuery	Search for all available RFID Readers
Command (for Tag)	**Descriptor**
SearchTag	Search for all available ring Tags 。
Access	Read back data from ring Tag
StopAccess	Stop reading back data from ring Tag
Command (for Reader and Tag)	**Descriptor**
AllReset	Reset both RFID Reader and ring Tag
Command (for GPS)	**Descriptor**
Open	Open GPS receiver
Command (for SMS)	**Descriptor**
SendSMS	Send SMS text message

Table 1. Commands for APs

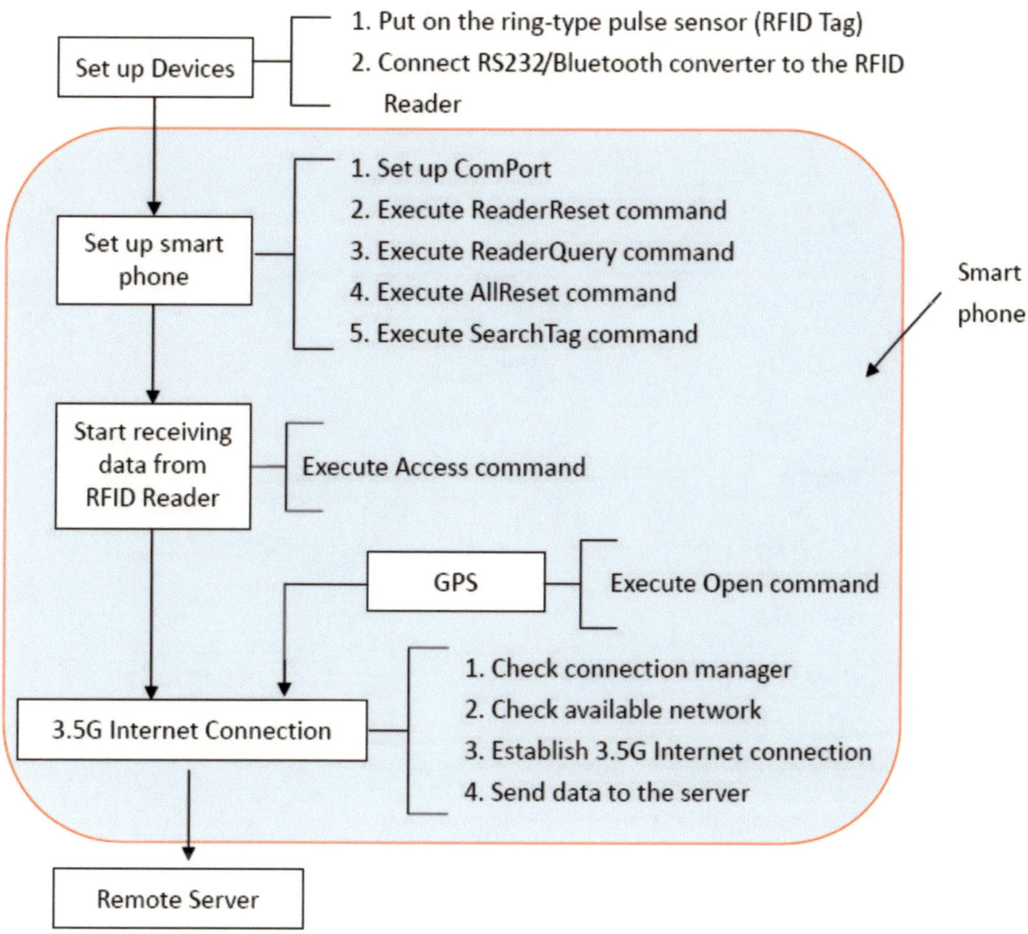

Fig. 11. Flowchart of MHMS under normal situation

Fig. 12 shows the interactions among the smart phone, RFID reader, and ring Tag for those commands used on smart phone. For instance, the SearchTag command instructs the RFID reader (action 1) to search for available ring Tag (action 2), and the available ring Tag responds Tag ID back to the reader (action 3) and the reader sends the received Tag ID to the smart phone(action 4). Fig. 13 depicts the flow chart of sending SMS text message to the emergency contact's phone under emergency situation when the SOS button on the Tag is pressed.

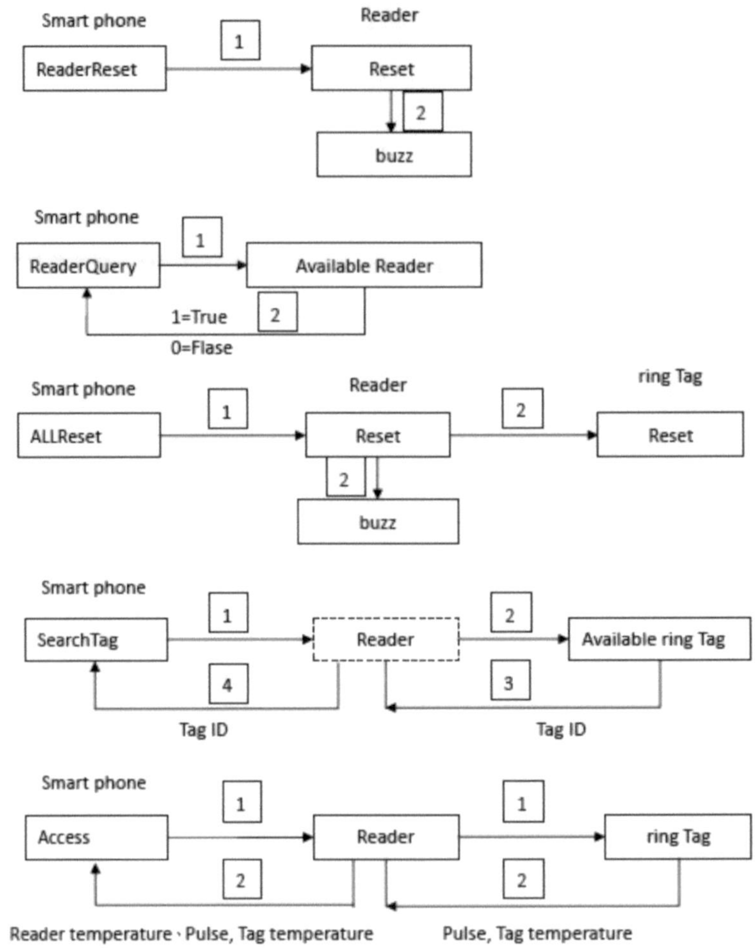

Fig. 12. Interactions among smart phone, Reader, and Tag

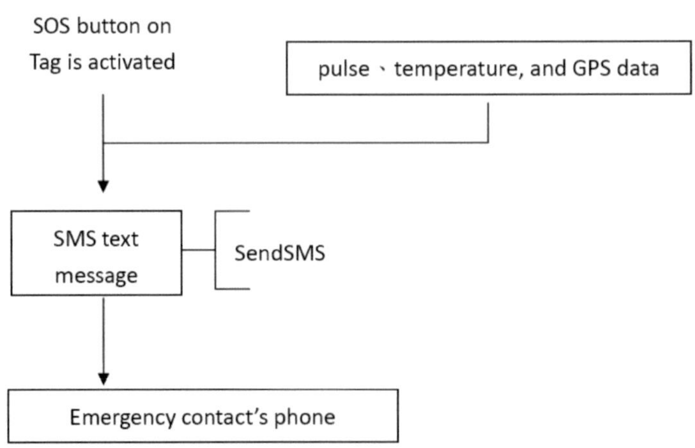

Fig. 13. Flow chart of sending SMS text message under emergency situation

3. Physiological data presentation

The hardware is implemented as Fig. 6. The Bluetooth adaptor is connected to the RFID reader and the ring Tag is worn on the user's finger. The setup steps for communication between the smart phone and the RFID reader/Tag can be executed either on the smart phone emulator (on PC) or on the smart phone using the Cellular Emulator. Fig. 14 illustrates these steps on the smart phone emulator.

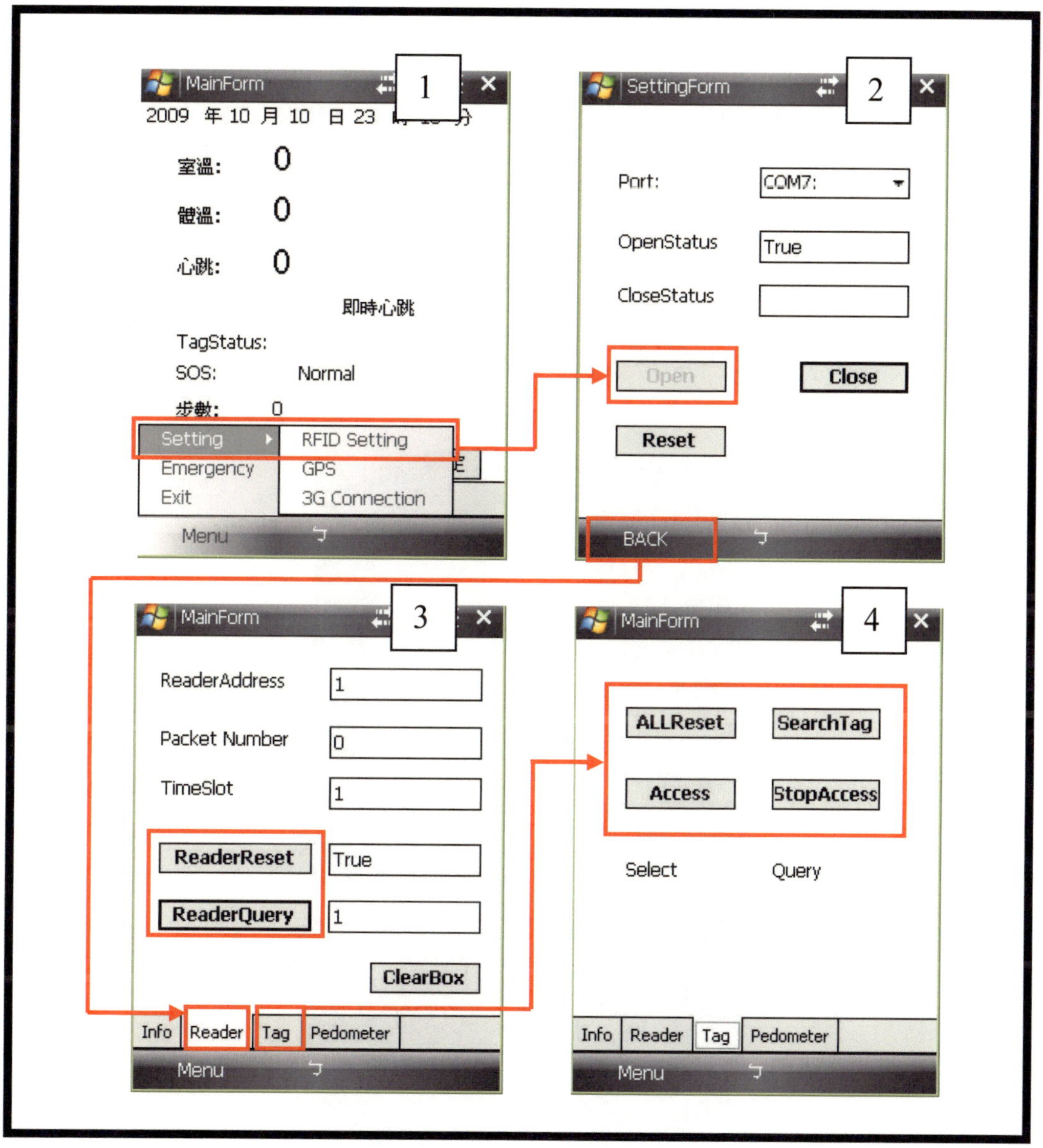

Fig. 14. Setup steps for communication between the smart phone and RFID reader/tag

Step 1. On the main page, click the "Menu," go to "Setting," and then choose "RFID setting." RS232 COM port setup page will pop up.

Step 2. Choose the correct COM port and click "OPEN." Then, click "BACK" to return to the main page.

Step 3. Click "Reader" and "Reader setup" page will pop up. Click "ReaderReset" to reset the RFID reader, and the RFID reader beeps and "True" is shown on the message box. Then click "ReaderQuery" to search for the Reader's address. The message box of ReaderQuery shows the address number.

Step 4. Click Tag and the "Tag setup" page will pop up. First click "ALLReset" and turn on the power of the ring Tag. Then click "SearchTag" to search for the ring Tag around the RFID reader. Once the ring Tag is detected, the Tag ID number will be shown on the page and finally click "Access" to go to the physiological data monitoring GUI.

Fig. 15 depicts the physiological data monitoring GUI on the smart phone emulator. The same GUI on the smart phone is shown in Fig. 10. On this page, two temperature values measured by RFID reader and Tag and pulse data are shown. The SOS message box indicates the status of the SOS button on the ring Tag. If this button is pressed, the smart phone will dial the pre-set emergency phone number(s) to send out SMS with the GPS position information to other people for help. Fig. 16 shows the GUI for setting up pre-set emergency phone number(s). Fig. 17 shows the GPS information.

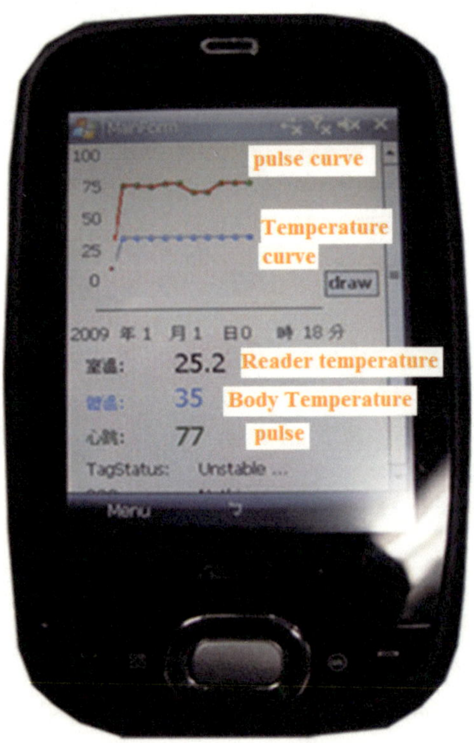

Fig. 15. Physiological data monitoring GUI

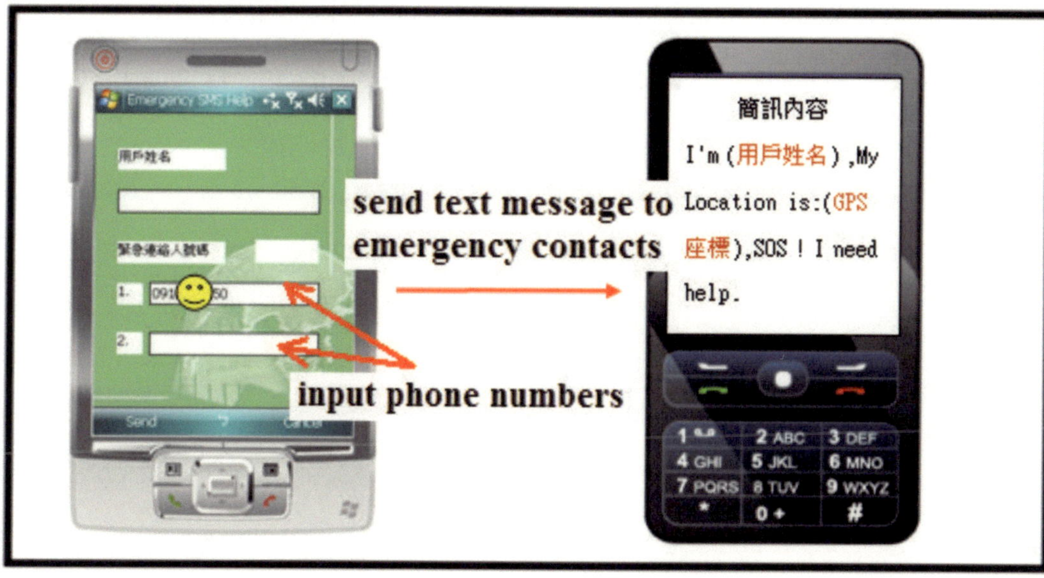

Fig. 16. GUI for emergency numbers

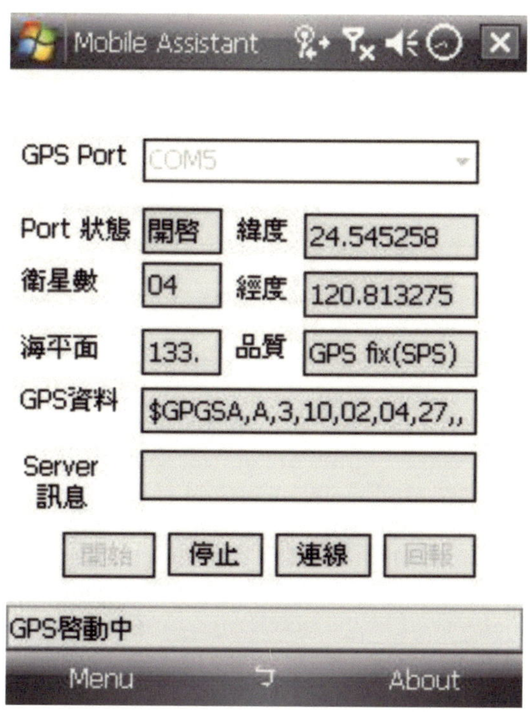

Fig. 17. GPS information

Fig. 18 presents the 3G communication of smart phone and the webpage of remote medical station. The 3G connection setup page of the smart phone is shown on the left side and the webpage of the server is on the right side where temperature values, pulse, and Google map are displayed. Based on the GPS position information sent from the smart phone, the Google map helps the medical staff to locate promptly the monitored user who needs further assistance.

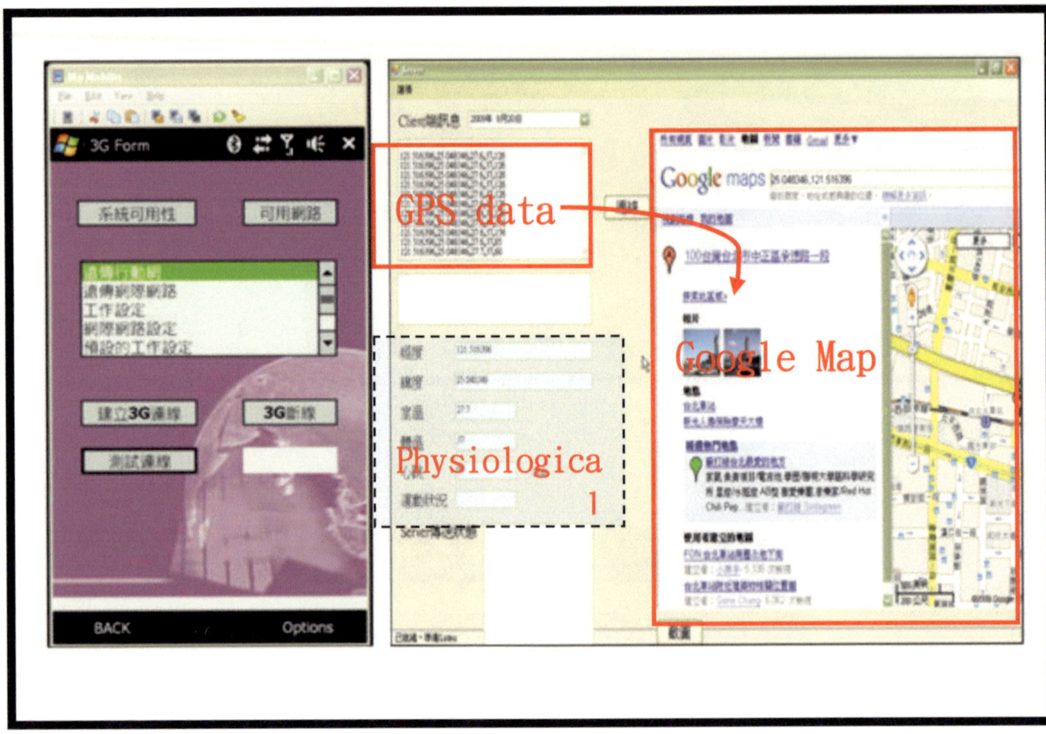

Fig. 18. 3G communication setup and the webpage of remote medical station

For evaluation of the developed biosignal recorder, a 4-day measurement was performed. Figures 19–21 show typical waveforms of EEG, ECG and accelerogram during the 4-day measurement. Fig. 19 represents waveforms during deep sleep. In the EEG waveform, sleep spindles appeared frequently. The heart rate was very slow (42 bpm) as seen in ECG waveform. The accelerogram did not change during this period. Fig. 20 was acquired during shallow sleep. The ECG and accelerogram are almost same to these in Fig. 19. On the other hand, sleep spindles are not seen in EEG waveform. In Fig. 21, waveforms during deskwork are shown. The heart rate (50 bpm) was faster than that during sleep. The accelerogram denotes that subject's body is upstand. In EEG waveform, large artifacts generated by eye blinks appear. Fig. 22 shows waveforms during walk movements. Up and down movements of the walking cycle are observed in the accelerogram. The heart rate was moderately fast (about 90 bpm) due to the walking movements. In Fig. 23, waveforms during meal are indicated. The EEG waveform was disturbed by chewing movements. This phenomenon was not desirable for true EEG recording, however, this characteristic waveform is useful for activity estimation The characteristics of these waveforms suggest some indices for estimation of sleep depth and physical activities. In Fig. 24, four indices listed below are shown for the waveforms during the 4-day measurement:

1. Median value of heart rate derived from 3-minute ECG waveform,
2. Standard deviation for 3-minute absolute values of accelerogram,
3. EEG power ratio of gamma band (30~128 Hz) to delta band (below 4 Hz) derived from 128-second EEG waveform,
4. EEG power ratio of alpha band (8~13 Hz) to beta band (13~30 Hz) derived from 128-second EEG waveform.

These indices are calculated for every 3-minute periods, and time courses of them are shown. Note that the index value for a particular 3-minute period disappears if more than 5% of the raw waveform exceeds the A/D conversion range during the period, for example in the EEG ratios at the first day's night (from about 20 to midnight).

From examination of Fig. 24 and subject's handwritten note, the availability of these indices for activity and sleep depth estimation can be pointed out. Both the median of heart rate and the standard deviation of accelerogram are low during sleep. Therefore these indices are useful for estimation of sleep/wake state. More complicated algorithm may enable us to estimate physical activities from these biosignals. The EEG power ratio of gamma band to delta band shows sharp peaks. The peak times coincide with mealtimes of subject's record. This EEG ratio surges when chewing EMG appears and is useful for estimation of mealtime. The EEG power ratio of alpha band to beta band changes periodically during sleep periods. This phenomenon suggests that this index may reflect changes in sleep depth. However, further investigation is required for more rigorous conclusions.

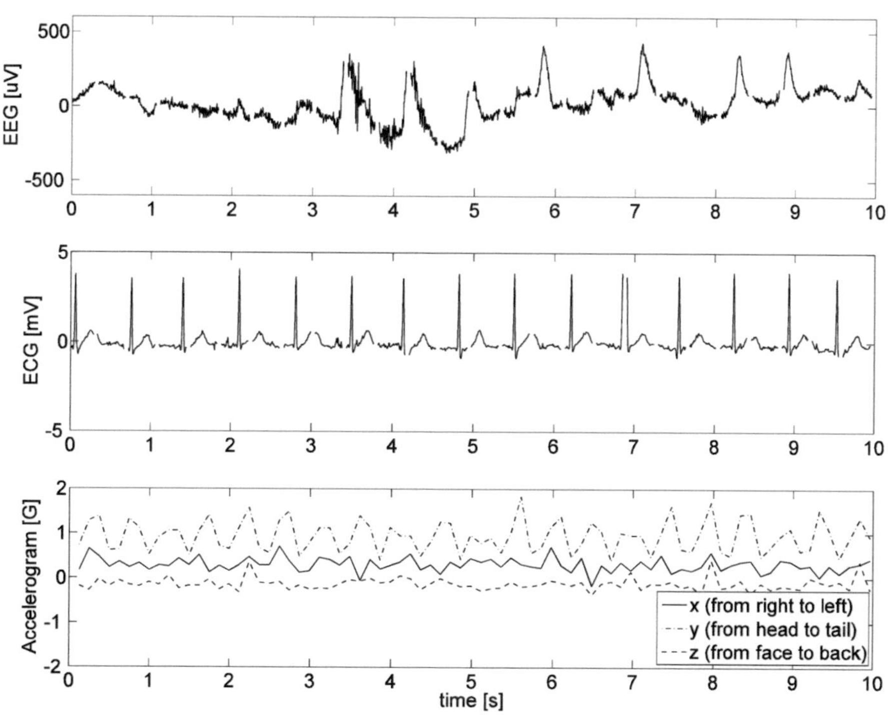

Fig. 19. Waveforms during deep sleep

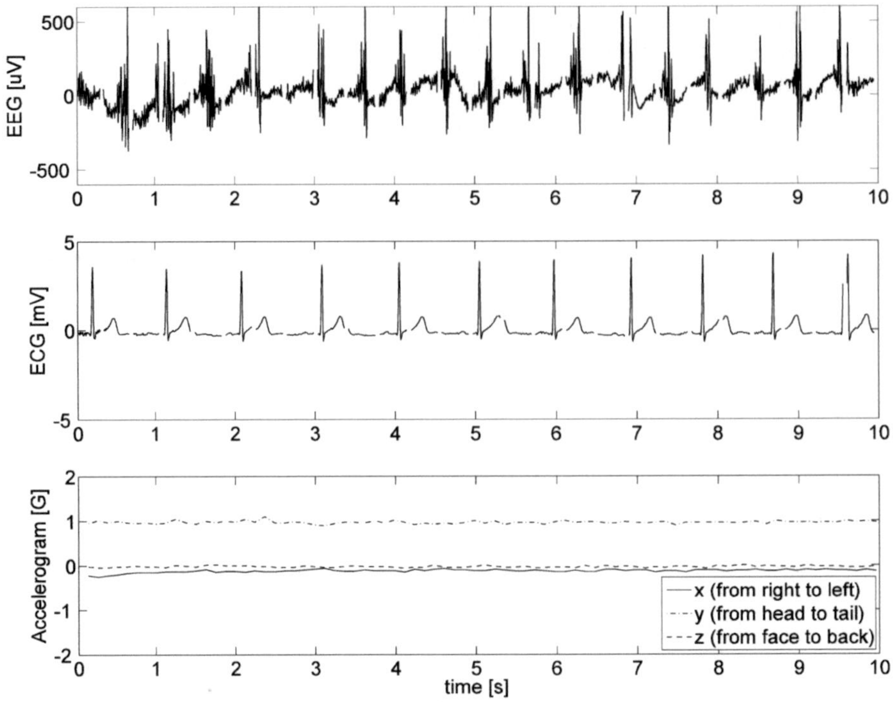

Fig. 20. Waveforms during shallow sleep

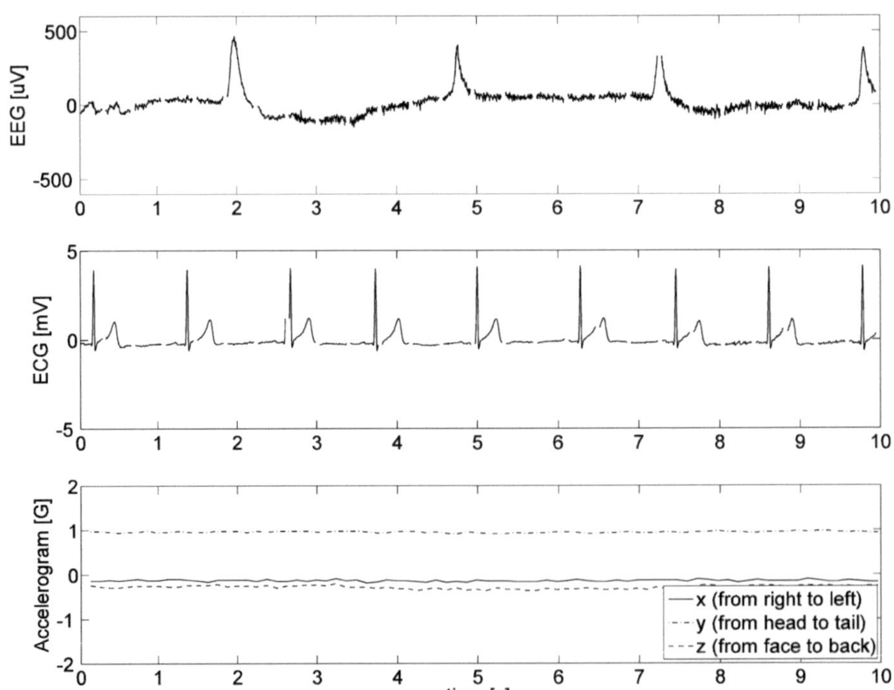

Fig. 21. Waveforms during deskwork

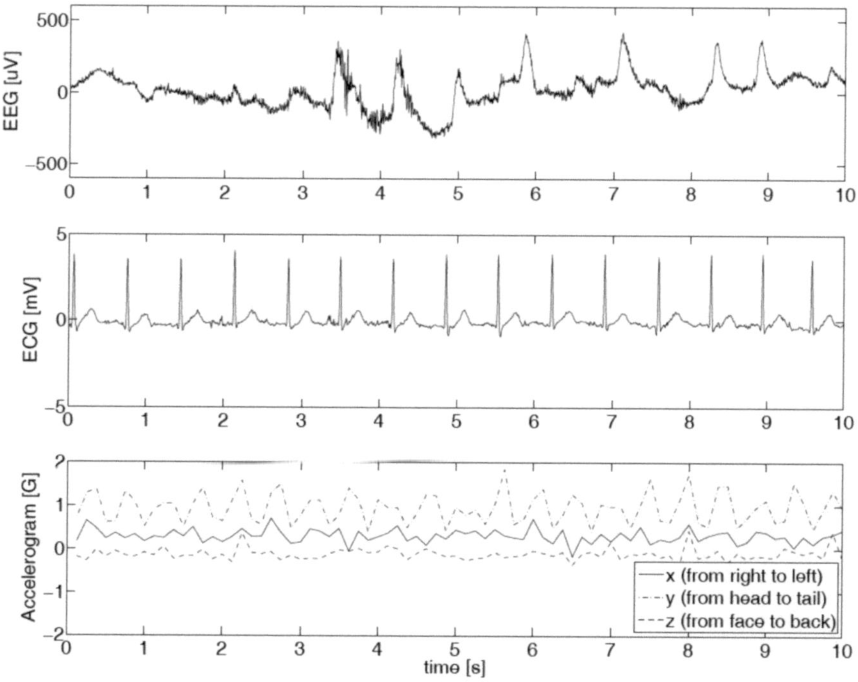

Fig. 22. Waveforms during walk

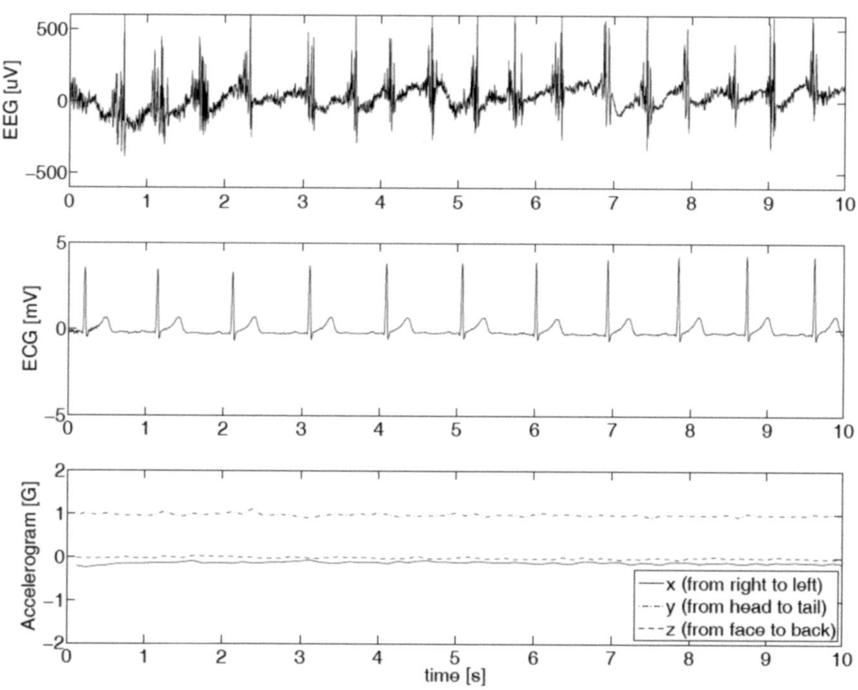

Fig. 23. Waveforms during meal

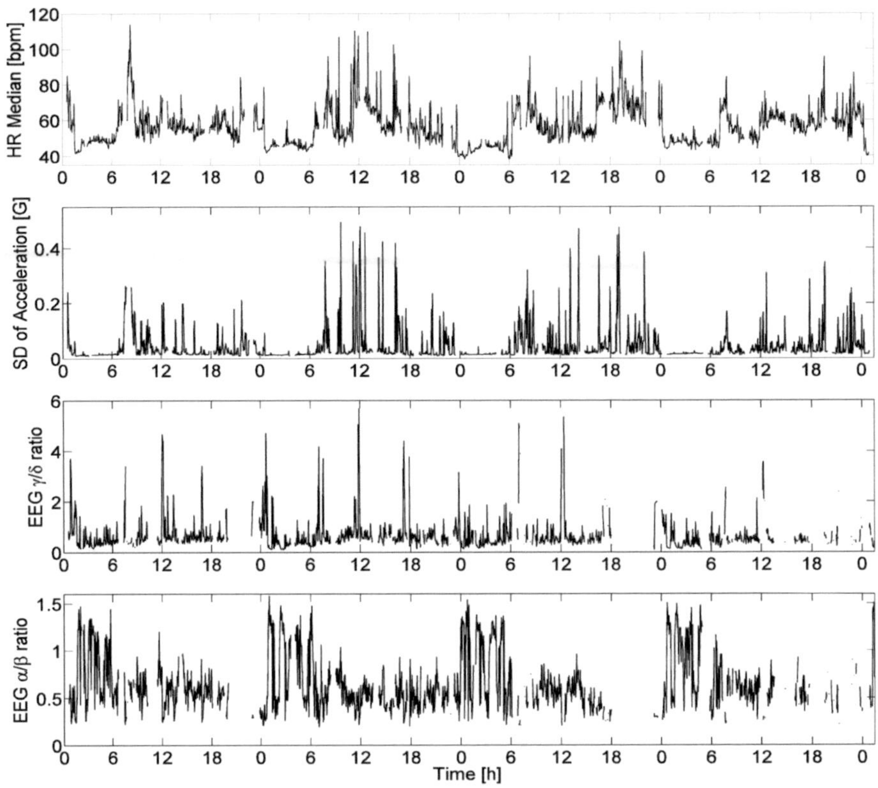

Fig. 24. Indices for activity estimation

4. "Exercise 333" health management mechanism

Compared to the traditional medical care that people receive medical treatment after they feel ill, an effective health management program can provide prevention of illness in a more aggressive manner—prevention is better than cure. Especially for people working in present modern high-tech society under lots of pressures and lacking exercise, such a preventive health management becomes essential. According to the report conducted by a hospital in Taiwan (Cheng-Ching Hospital Medical Center, 2010), exercise-333 can effectively prevent cardiovascular diseases. The concept of "exercise-333" is quite simple; i.e., taking exercise 3 or more times a week, at least 30 minutes per time, raising heart rate to 130 per minute. The health management mechanism presented here, based on "exercise 333", can help to remind the user to develop such a healthy life style.

Fig. 25 depicts the exercise-333 health management GUIs on the smart phone. In the first GUI, the user can set up 3 weekdays as checking points and at each checking point it will show the progress status to remind the user. In the second GUI, at the end of each day it will show the user whether his/her heart rate has ever been over 130 for more than 30 minutes. And at the end of each week, this GUI also shows the condition whether the user has accomplished exercise-333. With these two smart-phone GUIs, the user can constantly receive reminders and check his/her exercise status.

Based on the fact that in Taiwan every 100 people have 108 cellular phone numbers (Y.S. Lin, 2008), the high popularity of smart phone makes the presented health management system effective and convenient to help people on developing a healthy life style.

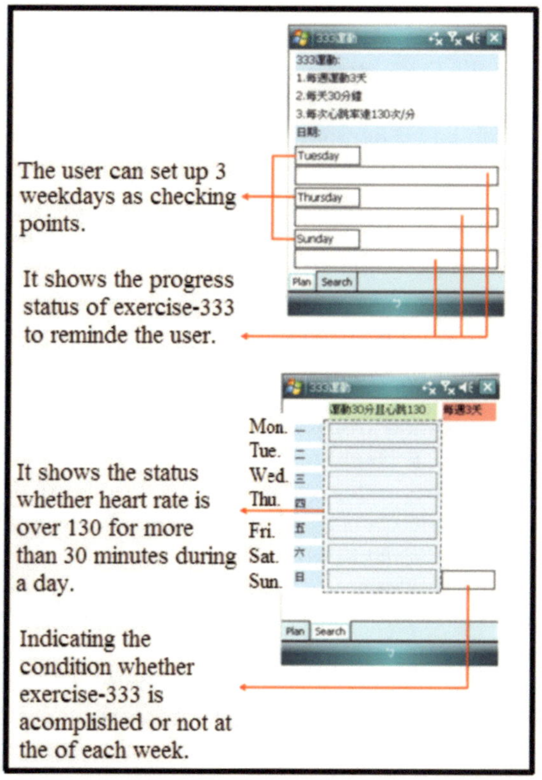

Fig. 25. Exercise-333 health management GUIs

5. Conclusions

In this chapter, a mobile e-health-management system has been presented. This system integrates a wearable ring-type pulse monitoring sensor and a portable biosignal recorder with a smart phone. The ring-type pulse monitoring sensor can measure pulse and temperature, while the biosignal recorder can record electroencephalogram (EEG), electrocardiogram (ECG), and body 3-axis acceleration during daily lives. Based on these EEG, ECG, and acceleration data, several indices can be evaluated to estimate the user's physical activities. With the help of the mobile "exercise-333" health management mechanism developed on the smart phone, the user can monitor his/her own physiological data to practice the idea of "Prevention is better than cure," developing a healthier life style. The presented system, with the popularity and mobility of smart phones, effectively provides the needs for mobile health management.

6. Acknowledgement

The authors would like to express their gratitude to Sinopulsar Technology Inc., Taiwan for free use of their RFID ring pulse sensor in this work. Financial support from the National Science Council, Taiwan are acknowledged as well.

7. References

Anliker, U, et al. (2004). AMON: A wearable multiparameter medical monitoring and alert system, *IEEE Trans. Inf. Technol. Biomed.*, Vol. 8, pp. 415-427

Chang, K.S. (2004). *Embedded Electrocardiogram Measurement System Design and Its Application to Personal Remote Health Care*, Master thesis, National Cheng Kung University, Taiwan (in Chinese)

Chen, C.M., et al. (2008). Web-based Remote Human Pulse Monitoring System with Intelligent Data Analysis for Home Healthcare, *IEEE International Conference on Cybernetics and Intelligent Systems*

Cheng-Ching Hospital Medical Care Center, (2010). Exercise-333 and Vegie-579 Can Prevent Cardiovascular Diseases, Available from: http://www.uho.com.tw/hotnews.asp?aid=5628 (in Chinese)

Lee, R.G., et el. (2006a). A Mobile-care System Integrated with Bluetooth Blood Pressure and Pulse Monitor, and Cellular phone. *IEICE Transactions on Information and Systems*, Vol. E89-D, No. 5, pp. 1702-1711

Lee, R.G., et el. (2006b). Design and Implementation of a Mobile-care System over Wireless Sensor Network for Home Healthcare Applications, *Proceedings of Annual International Conference of the IEEE Engineering in Medicine and Biology*, pp. 6004-6007

Lee, R.G., et el. (2007a). A Mobile Care System with Alert Mechanism, *IEEE Transactions on Information Technology in Biomedicine*, Vol 11, No 5, pp. 507-517

Lee, R.G., et el. (2007b). A Mobile-care System over Wireless Sensor Network for Home Healthcare Applications, *Biomedical Engineering-Applications, Basis and Communications*, Vol. 19, No. 2, pp. 85-90

Lin, J.L. (2005). *Development of Wireless Sensor Network for Home Health Care*, Master thesis, National Chiao Tung University, Taiwan (in Chinese)

Lin, T.H. (2004). *A Mechanism Integrating Electrocardiogram Compression and Error Protection and Its Application to the Bluetooth Transmission in the Home Care System*, Mater thesis, Chung Yuan Christian University, Taiwan (in Chinese)

Lin, Y.S. (2008). High Ownership Rate of Mobile Phones Brings New Media Era. Electronic Commerce Times, Available from: www.ectimes.org.tw/ shownews.aspx?id=080622225140 (2008)

Mundt, C.W., et al. (2005). A multiparameter wearable physiological monitoring system for space and terrestrial applications, *IEEE Trans. Inf. Technol. Biomed.*, Vol. 9, pp. 382-391

Pandian, P.S., et al. (2008). Smart vest: Wearable multiparameter remote physiological monitoring system, Med. Eng. Phys., vol. 30, pp. 466-477

Shu, Y.L. (2005). Development of Intelligent Maintenance System for Establishing the Quality of the Elder's Life, Engineering, *Science and Technology Communication*, Vol. 84 (in Chinese)

Wu, J.L. (2004). *Implementation of a Portable Wireless Physiological Signal Measurement System*, Master thesis, Southern Taiwan University, Taiwan (in Chinese)

Ye, C.F. (2006). *A PDA-based Home Care System*, Master thesis, National Chiao Tung University, Taiwan (in Chinese)

Yu, S.A., Lu, S.S., Lin, C.W., & Wang, Y.H. (2005). Personal Electronic Nurse, *Scientific Development*, Vol. 393, (Sept. 2005) (in Chinese)

3

Health Care with Wellness Wear

Hee-Cheol Kim[1], Yao Meng[1] and Gi-Soo Chung[2]
[1]*Inje University,*
[2]*Korea Institute of Technology,*
South Korea

1. Introduction

As the new medical practice paradigm of ubiquitous health care has gradually evolved, "smart" clothes with noninvasive sensors that obtain biosignals, such as ECG, respiration, SpO_2, and blood pressure data, have great potential (Axisa et al., 2005; Lauter, 2003). We call such clothes "*wellness wear*." A wellness wear system is an integration of biosensors that attach to clothes, digital yarns that transmit biosignals and other data, integrated circuits and microprocessors that process those signals, wired and wireless communication, and software applications that process and analyze vital signs obtained from the biosensors.

The need for wellness wear systems is clear. Wellness wear enables the continuous monitoring of health conditions at any time and place because the clothing is worn continuously. Thus, the use of wellness wear can promote easier home care. Both patients and nonpatients experience efficient and comfortable health care and disease prevention (Saranummi, 2002). This is particularly important because as the aging population increases, the interest in quality of life grows quickly. Undoubtedly, the physical boundaries and distances that restrict doctors' treatments can be reduced. Generally, wearable systems provide real-time feedback about one's long-term health condition, and can even provide alarms in potentially health-threatening situations (Pantelopoulos and Bourbakis, 2010). From an economic point of view, the increasing cost of medicine will be also reduced by the usage of wellness wear because some portion of expensive traditional health-care practices will be replaced.

Despite the need, however, there is not yet a stable market for wellness wear. Additionally, it has not achieved its goal of providing either low-cost or ubiquitous health-care services. One critical reason for this is that biosensors attached to clothes cause motion artifacts; thus, the quality of biosignals may be unreliable. This means that they have not yet been validated clinically. Many sensors can also cause skin irritation or allergies. Further, wellness wear is not of sufficient quality in terms of fashion, usability, and acceptability in consumer culture. There are probably more reasons that wellness wear has not been successful nor actively commercialized; the major reason is likely that wellness wear is still in its infancy. We believe that the currently immature technical, clinical, and cultural aspects of wellness wear will gradually improve, eventually increasing its use.

In this chapter, we shed some light on health care with smart clothes. First, we briefly review previously introduced smart health clothes. Second, as an example, we present a wellness wear system that we are developing that assists with weight loss by using software called the Calorie Tracker, which works together with wellness wear.

2. Wellness wear and related medical services

This section presents a survey of the state of research and development of smart clothes for health care. The general architecture and basic design considerations of smart clothes are introduced briefly. Research prototypes and commercial products of the main smart clothes that have been developed so far are then reviewed.

2.1 An overview

Figure 1 shows the general architecture of smart clothes for health care (Park and Jayaraman, 2010). The miniature *sensors* that are integrated into the textile measure biosignals from the wearer and the environment to provide physiological and contextual information. The *signal processing system*, which serves as the system's central node and usually takes the form of a hand-held device or carry-on electronics, provides temporary data storage and may also preliminarily process sensory data to acquire appropriate parameters, including vital signs. The *communication system* transmits the raw data and extracted parameters to a remote station for long-term storage and further analysis. The *decision support system* installed in the station obtains and interprets the data to assist in the diagnosis and treatment by health-care professionals.

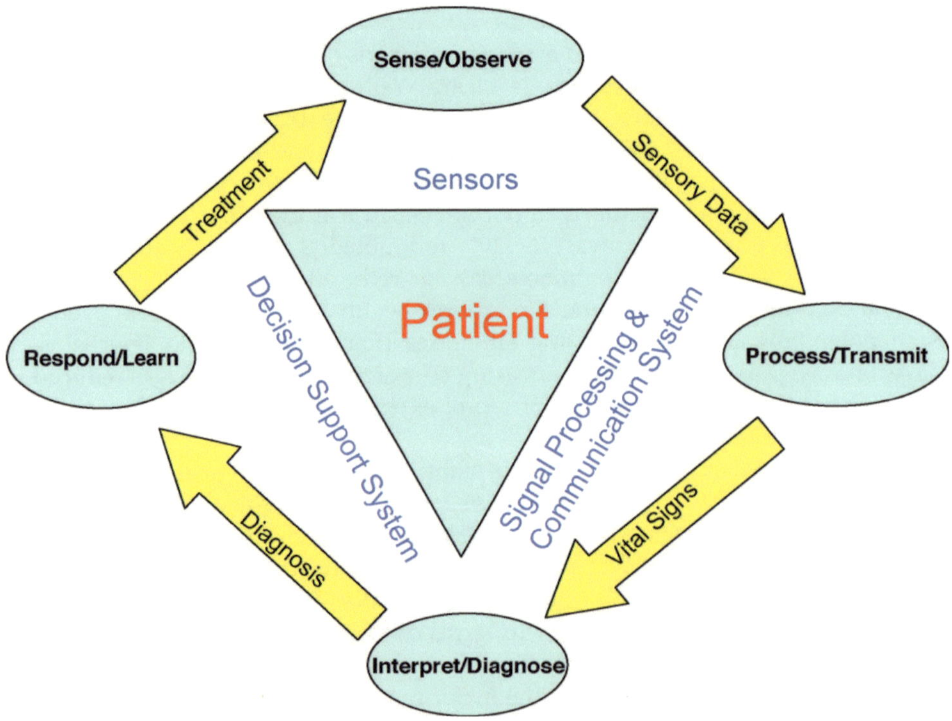

Fig. 1. Architecture of smart clothes (from Park and Jayaraman, 2010, p. 87)

This smart clothes framework shows that the design and implementation of such a system is a challenging task. Many constraining and sometimes conflicting requirements must be considered in enabling smart clothes to become an efficient and applicable health-care solution in real-life situations. More specifically, smart clothes should:

1. satisfy the need of wearability (low weight and small size to enable a comfortable experience);
2. provide an easy-to-use interface to minimize the cognitive effort of the user;
3. incorporate noninvasive biomedical sensors, which allow for biosignal measurements on humans without radiation or infection concerns, to comprehensively estimate and evaluate the wearer's health status;
4. enable real-time processing to facilitate use and track the timing of emergencies, which could be lifesaving;
5. possess a certain level of intelligence to aid health-care professionals in identifying and addressing health problems
6. acquire biosignals with high accuracy and low distortion and present results with a high degree of reliability to gain the trust of professionals;
7. deploy appropriate security and privacy solutions that mainly focus on data transmission and storage to protect the status information and personal medical data of the user;
8. provide reliable communication channels for transmission of biosignals from the sensors to the system's central node and then from the smart clothes to a remote medical station (or to a physician's hand-held device);
9. enable low power consumption to support extended operation times and system miniaturization
10. enable scalability and reconfigurability to improve system applicability and user acceptance, such as adding or removing sensors; and
11. undergo testing in clinical situations to demonstrate validity and practicability, the outcome of which can help to convince stakeholders.

2.2 Research and development of smart health clothes

As one of the most important applications of wearable technology, smart clothes for health care started in early 2000 (Lymberis and Olsson, 2003). Since then, this promising area has attracted much attention from both the research and business communities. In the following two subsections, we review the main achievements from both research and commercial aspects.

2.2.1 Research prototypes

The VTAMN (Vêtement de Télé Assistance Médicale Nomade—Undergarment for Nomad Medical Tele-assistance) project was supported, in part, by the French government and aims to measure physiological information on the wearer as well as environmental and activity parameters in daily life situations (Fig. 2). Six-lead ECG signals (from 4 textile electrodes), breathing frequency (from 2 coil pneumographs), and ambient and mid-temperature (from 2 I_2C temperature sensors) are transmitted automatically or on demand to the remote station using a GSM placed onto the belt. This enables remote detection and tracing of cardiac arrhythmias. The system also incorporates a fall detection module (a 2-axis accelerometer and a microcontroller embedded on an electronic board) to enable an alarm to launch by a cell phone and subsequent rescue to occur with the help of GPS localization. Evaluation has shown simple and comfortable wearing, significant ECG readings, correct breathing frequency and temperature, and functional activity sensing during normal activities. However, some shortcomings also exist, including bulky batteries and electronics and a QRS issue (Noury et al., 2004).

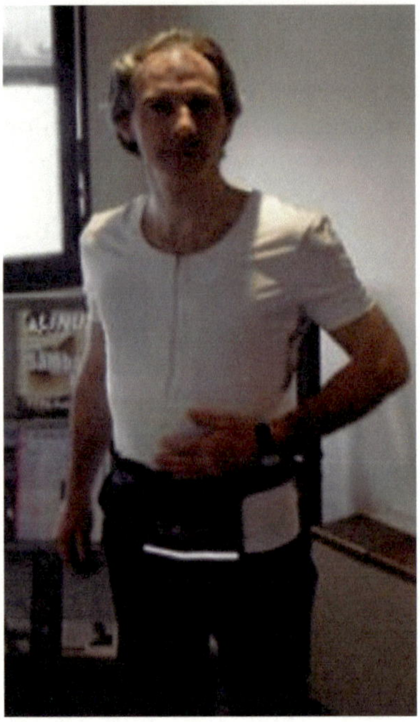

Fig. 2. VTAMN garment with the belt

The HealthWear (Remote Health Monitoring with Wearable non-Invasive Mobile System) project is supported by the European Commission and is based on the WEALTHY prototype with improved thermal and wearing comfort of the textile. The HealthWear system aims to deliver a service that provides uninterrupted and ubiquitous monitoring of the health condition of patients undergoing rehabilitation, patients out of the hospital with chronic diseases or after an acute event, high-risk people, such as the elderly, and others. The measurement capabilities of the system include ECG signals and deduced parameters such as heart rate (HR) and QRS duration (from 6 textile electrodes), oxygen saturation (SpO_2, by oximetry), respiration (by impedance pneumography), activity (from a 3-axis accelerometer integrated into the portable unit), and temperature (from 4 I_2C skin temperature sensors).

Figure 3 shows the HealthWear portable unit and garment. The portable unit is responsible for deciphering and transmitting (to the remote station through GPRS) the sensory data, which are collected from the sensors integrated into the garment (Paradiso et al., 2008).

The MagIC (Maglietta Interattiva Computerizzata) system was developed by researchers in Milan, Italy, and aims to unobtrusively monitor cardiorespiratory and motion signals during spontaneous behavior in clinical practice and daily life. The system consists of a washable sensorized vest and portable electronic board (Fig. 4). Two electrodes made by conductive fibers are woven at the thoracic level of the vest to obtain an ECG lead. A textile transducer is also included in the vest to measure respiratory activity. The obtained ECG and respiratory signals are transmitted by conductive fiber connections to the vest's portable electronic board, which is responsible for motion detection through a 2-axis accelerometer and wireless data transmission to the remote station. Tests performed on patients in bed and during physical exercise showed good signal quality (except in the case of maximal physical activity), correct identification of arrhythmic events, and correct estimation of the average HR (Di Rienzo et al., 2005).

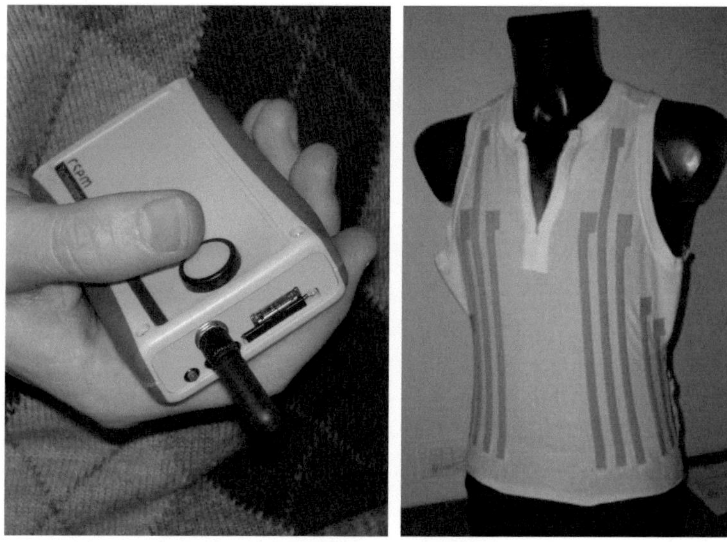

Fig. 3. Portable unit (left) and garment (right) of HealthWear

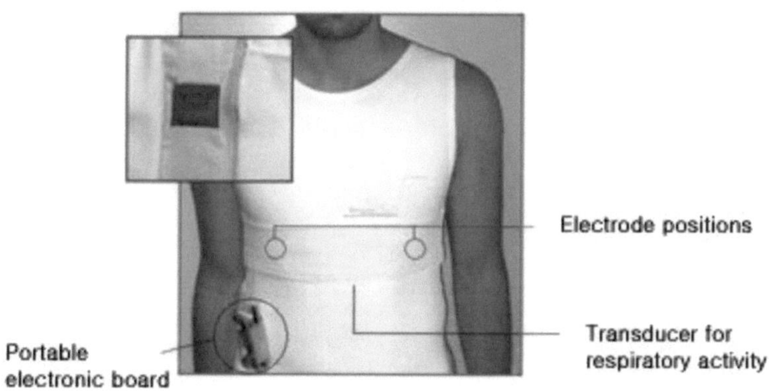

Fig. 4. The MagIC system

The MyHeart project (Fig. 5) is supported by the European Commission and involves 33 partners from 10 countries, including industrial partners such as Philips, Nokia, Vodafone, and Medtronic. It aims to systematically fight cardiovascular diseases by promotion of a preventive lifestyle, early diagnosis of acute events, and interaction with various stakeholders (e.g., local feedback to the wearer and remote feedback to professionals) (Habetha, 2006). An on-body sensor network is applied using integrated or embedded sensors and conductive wires knitted like normal textile yarns to reduce the size of sensor nodes and avoid the presence of both a local battery and an additional wireless module. On-body signal processing is performed to estimate HR from textile-ECG and continuously classify ambulatory activity (resting, lying, walking, running, and going up/down stairs) based on a 1-axis accelerometer within the on-body electronics. Bluetooth wireless communication is also established between the on-body electronics and a cell phone, which is then used to forward the processed signals to a remote monitoring station (Luprano et al., 2006).

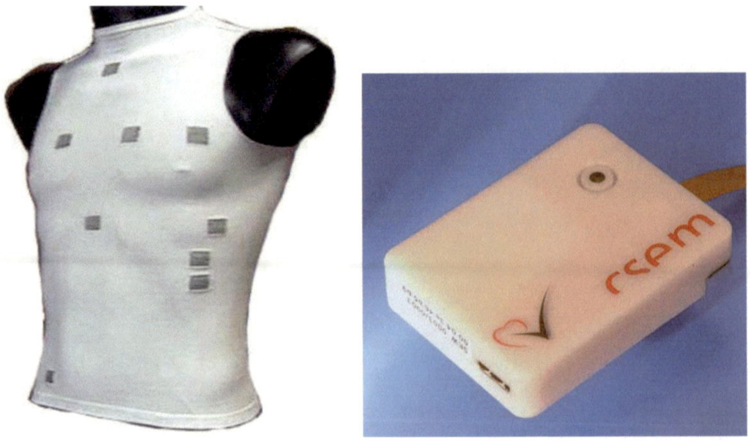

Fig. 5. Inner layer of MyHeart shirt (left) and first prototype of the on-body electronics (right)

SmartVest, a wearable physiological monitoring system, consists of a vest, data acquisition and processing hardware, and a remote monitoring station. The sensors (Fig. 6), integrated into the vest, can sense vital parameters, such as ECG signals, photoplethysmography (PPG) readings, HR, blood pressure, body temperature, and galvanic skin response (GSR). Good ECG quality (no baseline wander or motion artifact) is obtained without the use of gel. Blood pressure is measured by a non-invasive, cuffless method. Data fusion provides a more comprehensive picture of the wearer's health state (Pandian et al., 2008).

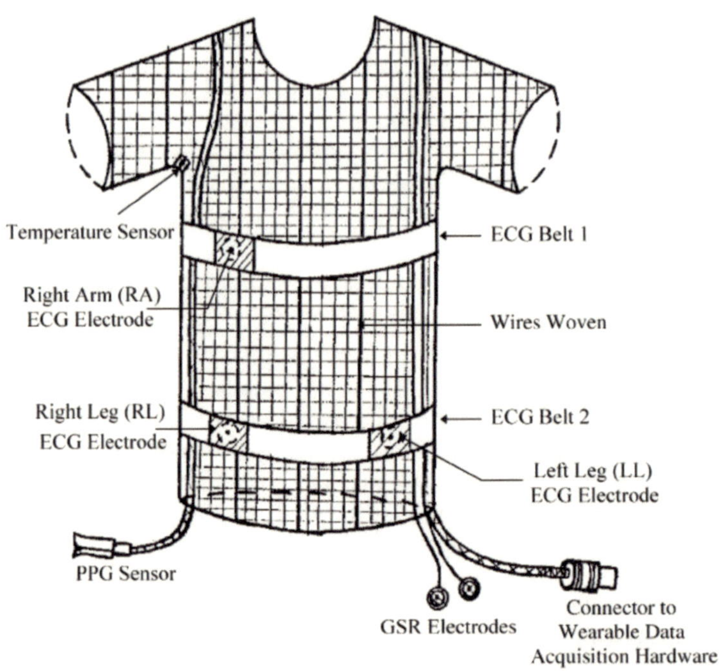

Fig. 6. Sensors integrated at specific locations in the vest

The BIOTEX (Biosensing Textile for Health Management) project is partly funded by the European Commission and aims to develop biochemical-sensing techniques that can be integrated into textiles for medical applications, including the monitoring of diabetes, sports activity, and obesity. The capabilities of BIOTEX include monitoring of pH, conductivity, sweat rate, electrolyte concentrations in sweat, SpO_2, and protein levels in blood and plasma (Luprano et al., 2007). The results of BIOTEX will be also used in the PROETEX project, the applications of which target at-risk professionals.

2.2.2 Commercial products

The LifeShirt, released by Vivometrics, is the first commercially available piece of smart clothing. It consists of a washable lightweight vest, a data recorder, and PC-based software. Its capabilities include continuous monitoring of the ECG, respiration, activity, and posture (Fig. 7) (Grossman, 2004). It has been used in various studies, and its potential applicability in future studies has been acknowledged. Additionally, its performance, such as HR detection, has been demonstrated to be accurate (Heilman and Porges, 2007). Foster-Miller's Watchdog physiological monitoring tool is a comfortable, garment-based system for monitoring HR, respiration rate, posture, activity, skin temperature, and GPS location. The Smart Shirt, manufactured by Sensatex, contains sensors that monitor vital signs, such as ECG, HR, respiration, and blood pressure (Pantelopoulos and Bourbakis, 2010).

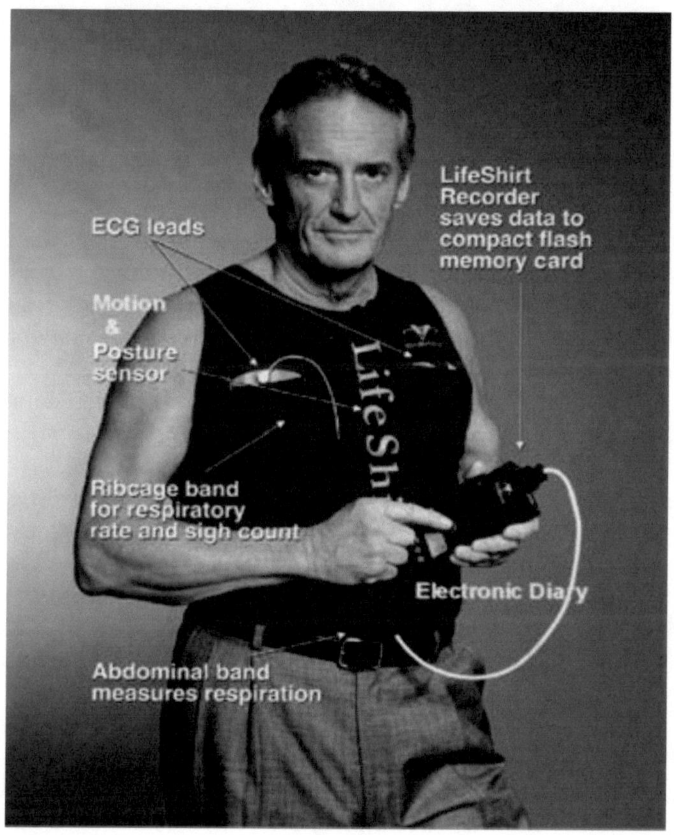

Fig. 7. The LifeShirt system

The Zephyr BioHarness technology is well-known because it was used in connection with the rescue operation of 33 trapped miners in northern Chile's San Jose mine (Zephyr Technology, 2010). It has also been adopted by NASA for use by astronauts in training. The BioHarness, a chest strap with sensors and wireless technology, monitors and transmits the wearer's vital signs, such as ECG data, HR, breathing rate, skin temperature, posture, activity, acclerometry, blood pressure, and pulse oximetry. Vital signs are transmitted with ISM or Bluetooth for remote monitoring anywhere in the world. The software platform OmniSense is used to display the BioHarness data.

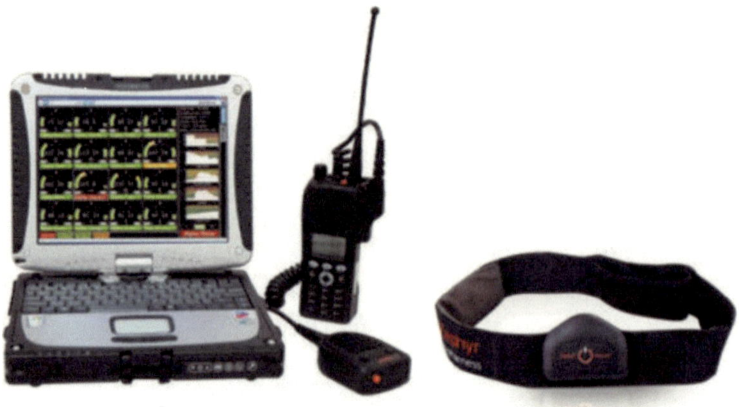

Fig. 8. The Zephyr BioHarness technology

3. A wellness wear system

A wellness wear system is an integrated system consisting of wellness wear, biosensors, hardware, and software. One of its advantages is easy aquisition of vital signs at any time and anywhere, which provide important basic data for monitoring health status. In this respect, advanced sensor technology is recommended to ensure the accuracy of the signals. The development of digital or conductive yarns also plays a crucial role in the formation of a body area network (BAN) within the clothes. These special yarns enable wired transmission of the data over the clothes. Further, hardware is used for digital signal processing (DSP), wired and wireless communication, and integration of multiple biosensors. However, another important technology is software.
In particular, the success of wellness wear systems depends highly on the quality of the medical information extracted from that data by the software and the medical content that is provided. In this section, we present a nanofiber technique-based wellness wear system that we are developing as an example of wellness wear. This system has a particular emphasis on software applications, including a fundamental service framework as an infrastructure and an application called Calorie Tracker, which runs on Android-based smartphones and enables weight loss and exercise management (Kim et al., 2011).

3.1 An overview

Here, we introduce a wellness wear system that we are currently developing. A primitive but fundamental scenario that we assume is that the user wears smart clothes with noninvasive and comfortable biosensors that typically measure ECG, respiration, body temperature, and the like. While the subject is sitting, sleeping, walking, running, exercising, or performing any other activity, biosignals are recorded and transmitted to the terminal and/or the server. Smart phones can be both terminals that transmit the data and devices that enable the application software to run. The software system analyzes the signals and other general data such as age and gender, and provides the user with a relevant medical recommendation. Figure 9 illustrates the scenario described.

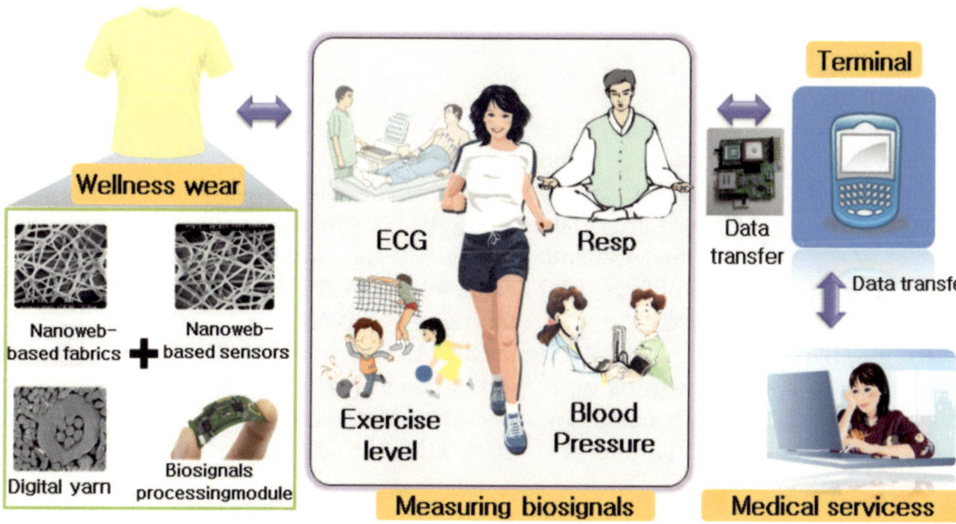

Fig. 9. Use scenario of a wellness wear system

Using calorie tracking as an example, here, we describe four of the important elements required for the development of the wellness wear system that we are implementing: biosensors, digital yarns, a software framework, and communication and medical services.

3.2 Biosensors

When we develop biosensors that are attachable to wellness wear, two crucial factors are accuracy of the obtained signals and user comfort. However, a tradeoff is typically required between them. Generally, the more accurate wearable biosensors are, the less comfortable they are, and *vice versa*. Thus, a future goal concerns how to overcome this. Comfort is a particularly important element. Because biosensors are adhered to smart clothes and touch the skin, they should be small, comfortable, and noninvasive. This is one of the reasons for the requirement for nanofiber. In fact, nanofiber is comfortable even when sensors are attached to smart clothes. For example, the physiological sensor belt (PSB), which detects the breath and pulse (Kim et al., 2009), is poromeric and protected from electromagnetic waves. It is much more comfortable than ordinary hospital devices that sense vital signs.

Several typical vital signs can be detected by biosensors attached to wellness wear. As we saw in the previous section, the ECG is one biosignal that most smart medical clothes aim to detect. It is ideal to detect life-threatening diseases early and to monitor patients and manage health through wireless communications (Taylor and Sharif, 2006). HR variability (HRV) extracted from ECG is also an important biosignal that helps in diagnosing heart-related illnesses and can check the efficiency of exercise and even stress. Respiration monitoring is also required to monitor walking and detect sleep apnea. Recently, fabric-based respiration sensors for wellness wear have been developed, and the quality of the signal has improved (Catrysse et al., 2004). Accelerometers have become popular to evaluate the amount of exercise. The number of steps taken can be identified by accelerometers. Together with GPS, one can determine the distance walked or run. For the elderly, accelerometers can support fall detection. They are also used to monitor chronic obstructive pulmonary disease patients (Mathie et al., 2004). Additionally, researchers are making efforts to develop wellness wear-based biosensors to obtain skin temperature, SpO_2, and blood pressure.

3.3 Digital yarns

To produce wellness wear, several technologies are needed, such as sewing, knitting, and embroidering technologies. More importantly, however, digital yarns that require highly advanced technologies play an important role in the transmission of biosignal data. In fact, conductive or digital yarns that transmit data within the clothes form a BAN. Dr. Gi-Soo Chung at the Korea Institute of Industrial Technology (KITECH) developed a digital yarn in which the major material is a copper alloy (Chung et al., 2006; Chung, 2007). His digital yarn is divided into two parts: a core and an outer part. As seen in Figure 10, its core consists of 7 microwires and a special resin. Its outer part is covered with dyed normal yarn. Electric resistance of the digital yarn is fairly low, at 7.5 Ω/m, compared with previously developed conductive yarns (Bekaert, 2011; Linz et al., 2005; TEXTILE, 2005).

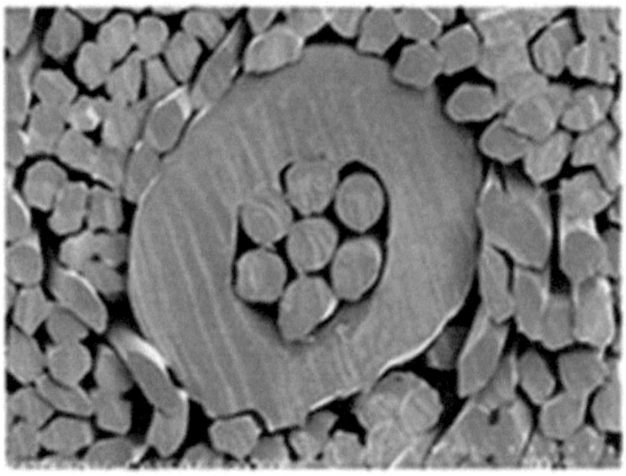

Fig. 10. A digital yarn

A digital garment is made with both ordinary yarns and digital bands for data transmission. Here, a digital band is a set of 10 to 30 digital yarns that are used as a communication line. The transmission speed of the yarn is very high (approximately 80 Mbps). This indicates that it could transmit an 800-MB movie file within approximately 1.5 min (Chung and Kim, 2011).

3.4 Software: Framework and software solution

Software aspects consist of a framework and a software solution. The framework is a foundation on which software applications are built, and the software solution concerns everything related to the software that is implemented on the framework.

3.4.1 Framework

Applications to provide medical service content are more complex and larger to build than many realize. This is because issues such as standardization, interoperability, reusability, reduction of maintenance cost, and readability must be addressed, which requires a sustainable and flexible infrastructure before application development. For this purpose, we have developed a framework that underlies all wellness wear application systems (Kim et al., 2009).

The primary idea is that vital signs from the wellness clothes are transformed into a metamodel-based abstract tree on which health-care services are defined through Object Constraint Language (OCL) (OMG-OCL, 2009) with the help of medical specialists and engineers. This idea implies that each service must be clearly defined and that integrated management is much easier when a repository of biosignal data is constructed. It also helps to make additions, deletions, and updates of services convenient. In particular, because the framework expresses the biosignal data as an HL7 (HL7, 2009) metamodel. based on MetaObject Facility (MOF), the M3 level, defined by the Object Management Group (OMG), standardization of the data and interoperability and integration between the biosignal data. is achieved.

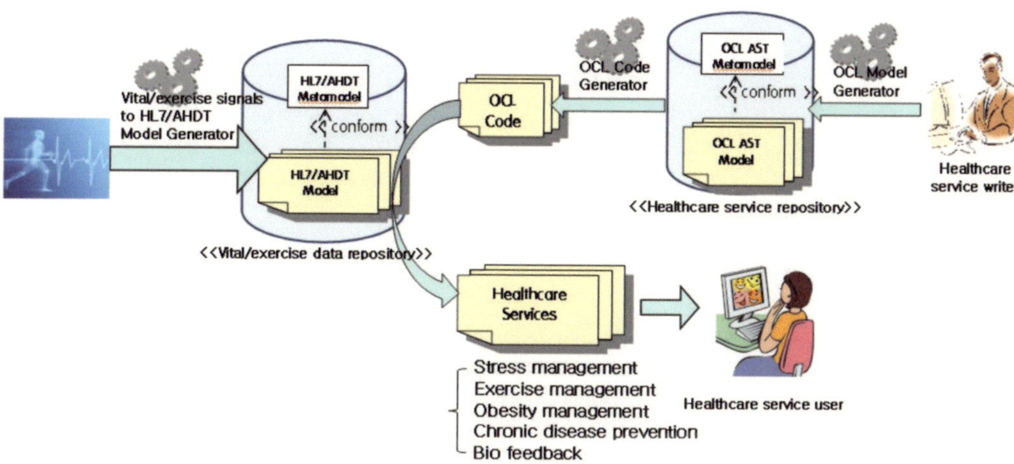

Fig. 11. Framework for a software solution in the wellness wear system

3.4.2 Software solution

Once the biosignal data obtained from sensors are accurate and stable, what is then important is how to support proper health management services, such as stress management, food control, an exercise plan, and general health management. When these services are perceived as useful by different stakeholders, the whole system, including other technologies such as the digital garments, DSP, and biosensors, will eventually succeed. In this respect, software and related medical services are primary elements for the success of the wellness wear system.

We consider that the software solution has four critical areas. First, algorithms and data mining techniques to process and analyze the given biosignals are required. Noise detection and filtering must be very basic techniques, and analysis of the biosignals, including both single and multiple biosignals, is important. In particular, multiple-signal analysis is a relatively new and important research field that involves understanding stress and the amount of exercise by analyzing the relationship between ECG and respiration. Second, development of health-care service content by medical specialists is key. Their roles are to plan and organize health-care service content using their expertise and cooperating with engineers. They will also develop health indices in the context of wellness wear systems, such as a wellness index and HR variation index. Third, both wired and wireless communication are required for the wellness wear system. For example, Bluetooth or ZigBee is used for short-distance wireless communication of vital signs. Another important task is to accept the international standard ISO/IEEE 11073 communication model and add its related communication protocols for processing vital signs information in different medical devices. A standardized protocol is not urgently needed in the near future; however, many experts anticipate that communication between personal health devices (PHDs) will be standardized eventually. It is also meaningful to follow a communication standard. Finally, an application service system provides health-care services. It is the central system that integrates various modules, including the biosignal analysis module, service components, and communication. Next, we present a software program called Calorie Tracker, which works together with the wellness wear system.

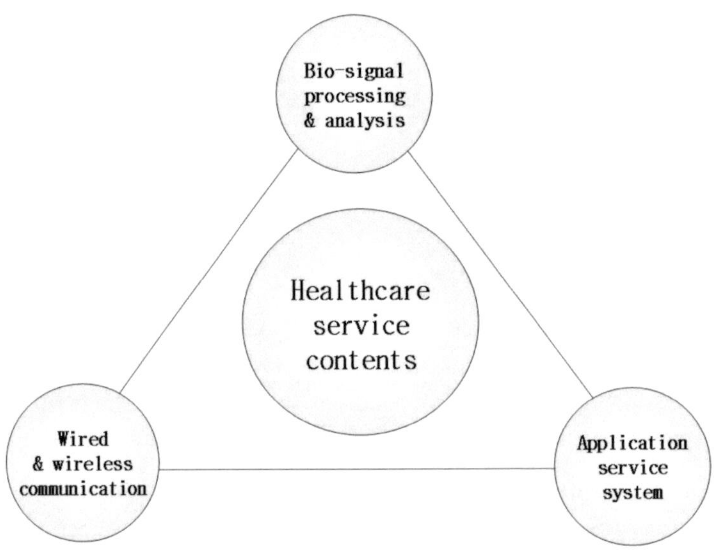

Fig. 12. Software solution in the wellness wear system

3.5 Calorie tracker: A medical service example

There must be a large number of potential medical services supported by a wellness wear system. We have developed a software application involving a calorie tracker (Kim et al., 2011) and herein describe how wellness wear is used with the software for health care.

3.5.1 Why calorie tracker?

The calorie tracker, which runs on an Android-based smartphone, analyzes HRV extracted from the ECG data obtained by wellness wear and provides a weight-loss program. The calorie tracker is useful in managing obesity. As we know, obesity reduction is a top priority in most developed countries. Obesity not only affects one's physical appearance, but also leads to a number of weight-related diseases, such as insulin resistance syndrome, cardiovascular disease, and type 2 diabetes. It is also leads to various chronic diseases. Generally, obesity is treated with food control and exercise. The calorie tracker was designed to evaluate the amount of exercise, show the number of calories burned during the exercise, and recommend simple exercise plans.

The choice of Android as an operating system was made primarily because of its multitasking performance, which is important for real-time continuous transmission of ECG data. If multitasking is not supported, ECG data transmission will suddenly cease when another application begins running or when the user initiates or receives a telephone call. The smartphone is both a device that handles client programs and a terminal that exchanges data with a server. The ECG data acquired from the wellness wear are transferred to the smartphone using Bluetooth, and the system on the smartphone transmits the data to the server using the XML form that conforms to the HL7 standard.

3.5.2 Usage scenario

The calorie tracker is best understood in terms of its four phases of use. First, it acquires ECG data from the wellness wear. More specifically, ECG data are obtained while the user is performing an activity such as running, walking, or sitting for a certain period of time; for example, 5 min. Figure 13 shows an ECG signal obtained from wellness wear. The user also provides the calorie tracker with other general data, such as the user's weight, height, age, gender, and more. Additionally, the user must provide information regarding whether he/she is at rest or active, is taking medications, or is diabetic.

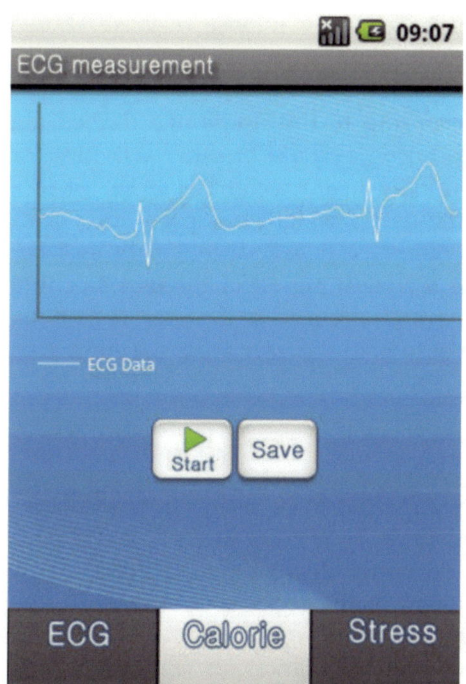

Fig. 13. Screenshot of the user interface of the calorie tracker

Second, the system measures HRV from the ECG data. ECGs consist of waves of P-Q-R-S-T, with R peaks being the highest of the five. Figure 14 illustrates an ideal ECG signal, showing adjacent R peaks and the R-R interval. Here, the HRV indicates the variablity of intervals between R waves, which are called R-R intervals. Thus, HRV is a time series of intervals between successive R peaks in the ECG. HRV has relevance for physical, emotional, and mental functions. The variability in HR is an adaptive quality in a healthy body. Generally, HRV is useful for evaluating functions of the autonomous nervous system, whereas ECG is better for the diagnosis of various heart-related diseases. Well-known HRV indices include the normalized beat-to-beat interval (NN), the standard deviation of those intervals (SDNN), and the percentage of the interbeat intervals differing from neighboring intervals by 50 ms or more.

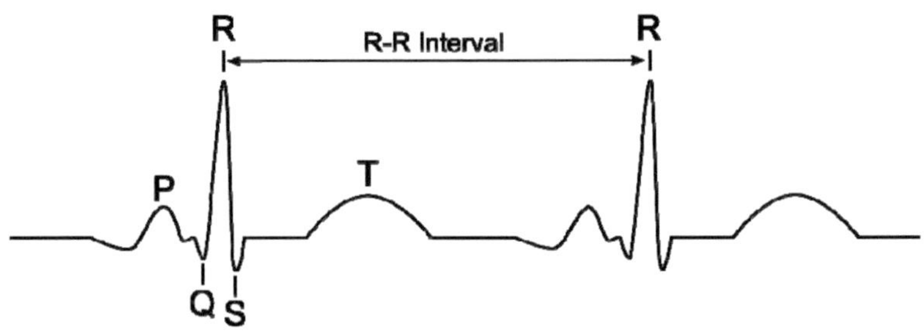

Fig. 14. R peaks and R-R intervals on an ECG

Third, the system calculates the number of calories burned (energy expenditure) and the body mass index using the HRV and other general data. Energy expenditure is crucial to the determination of how much and how intense exercise should be for each person. To determine calorie consumption, the maximal oxygen consumption per min (%VO_2max) is obtained using HRV measurements, including the average resting HRV (HRV_R) and the maximal HRV (HRV_M), according to the user's age (Lubell and Marks, 1986). Next, the number of calories burned during exercise or other activities for a given period of time is calculated from %VO_2max and the user's weight.

Finally, the system offers the user a weight-loss program. For example, it may state, "You need light exercise for two hours a day to reduce weight by 1 kg in a month." Based on the HRV data recorded during a certain period of the user's activity (e.g., 5 min), the system determines the intensity of exercise related to the user. It then makes a recommendation for an appropriate exercise level to help the user reduce weight according to his or her weight loss goals (Fig. 15).

4. Conclusions

Wellness wear systems are expected to be used for health care in the near future. In this chapter, we described wellness wear systems in general and introduced in detail a wellness wear system that we are currently developing. In doing so, we have demonstrated the potential for health care using wellness wear. Additionally, we presented a weight loss program called Calorie Tracker, which works together with wellness wear, as an example of a medical service. Although a stable market for wellness wear has not yet developed, we believe that a healthy life with wellness wear will eventually be realized as certain technological problems are resolved.

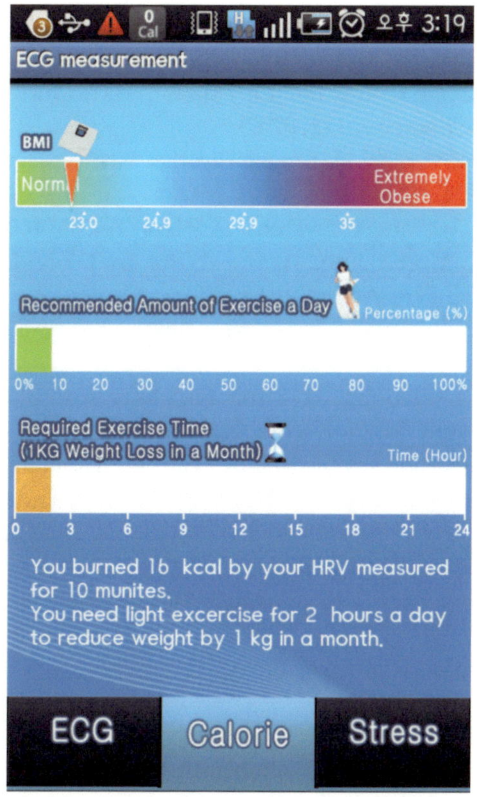

Fig. 15. The calorie tracker's evaluation and recommendation

5. Acknowledgment

This work is funded by the Korean Ministry of Knowledge Economy (#10033321 and #10033443).

6. References

Axisa, F., Schmitt, P. M., Gehin, C., Delhomme, G., McAdams, E. and Dittmar, A. (2005). Flexible Technologies and Smart Clothing for Citizen Medicine, Home Healthcare, and Disease Prevention, *IEEE Transactions on Information Technology in Biomedicine*, vol. 9, no. 3, September, 2005, pp. 325-336.

Bekaert (a firm in Belgium), (2011). April, 2011. http://www.swicofil.com/bekintex.

Catrysse M., Puers R., Hertleer C., Van Langenhove L., van Egmond H., and Matthys D. (2004). Towards the integration of textile sensors in a wireless monitoring suit. *Sensors and Actuators. A: Physical.* 114(2-3), pp. 302-311.

Chung, G. S., An, J. S., Lee, D. H. and Hwang, C. S. (2006). A Study on the Digital Yarn for the High Speed Data Communication, *The 2nd International Conference on Clothing and Textiles*, 2006, pp. 207~210.

Chung, G. S. (2007). Wearable Computer for Protective Clothing, *8th European Seminar on Personal Protective Equipment*, 2007.03

Chung, G. S. and Kim, H. C. (2011). Smart Clothes Are Neew Interactive Devices. *HCI International 2011*, To appear.

Di Rienzo, M. et al. (2005). MagIC System: A New Textile-based Wearable Device for Biological Signal Monitoring. Applicability in Daily Life and Clinical Setting, *Proceedings of IEEE 27th Annual International Conference on Engineering in Medicine and Biology Society*, pp. 7167-7169, ISBN 0-7803-8741-4, Shanghai, China, September, 2005.

Grossman, P. (2004). The LifeShirt: A Multi-Function Ambulatory System Monitoring Health, Disease, and Medical Intervention in the Real World, *Studies in Health Technology and Informatics*, Vol. 108, pp. 133-141, ISBN 978-1-58603-449-8.

Habetha, J. (2006). The MyHeart Project - Fighting Cardiovascular Diseases by Prevention and Early Diagnosis, *Proceedings of IEEE 28th Annual International Conference on Engineering in Medicine and Biology Society*, Vol. Supplement, pp. 6746-6749, ISBN 1-4244-0032-5, New York, USA, August 30-September 3, 2006.

Heilman, K.J. & Porges, S.W. (2007). Accuracy of the Lifeshirt® (Vivometrics) in the Detection of Cardiac Rhythms, *Biological Psychology*, Vol. 75, No. 3,(April 2007), pp. 300-305.

HL7, Inc. (2009). What is HL7?, http://www.hl7.org/about/hl7about.htm

Kim, H. -C., Chung, G. -S., and Kim. T. -W. (2009). A Framework for Health Management Services in Nanofiber Technique-based Wellness Wear Systems, *IEEE Healthcom 2009*. Decmber 16-18, Sydney, Australia, 2009, pp. 70-73.

Kim, H., Kim, T., M. Joo, S. Yi, C. Yoo, K. Lee, J. Kim, and G. Chung (2011). Design of a Calorie Tracker Utilizing Heart Rate Variability Obtained by a Nanofiber Technique-based Wellness Wear System, *Applied Mathematics and Information Science*. Special Issue, Vol. 5, No. 2, pp. 70-73. To appear.

Kim, K. J., Chang, Y. M., Yoon, S. and Kim, H. J. (2009). A Novel Piezoelectric PVDF Film-based Physiological Sensing Belt for a Complementary Respiration and Heartbeat Monitoring System, *Integrated Ferroelectrics, 107*, pp. 53-68.

Lauter, L. (2003). Personal Health Care in Philips: Status and Ambition, *Proceedings of 25th Annual International Conference on IEEE-EMBS*, Cancun, Mexico, September. 17-21, 2003, pp. 3748.

Linz, T., Kallmayer, C., Aschenbrenner, R. and Reichl, H. (2005). Embroidering Electrical Interconnects with Conductive Yarn for the Integration of Flexible Electronic Modules into Fabric, *IEEE International Symposium on Wearable Computing*, October 19-21, 2005, Osaka, Japan.

Lubell, M. and Marks, S. (1986) Health Fitness Monitor. U.S. Patent 4,566,461, Jan 28, 1986.

Luprano, J. et al. (2006). Combination of Body Sensor Networks and On-Body Signal Processing Algorithms: the practical case of MyHeart project, *International Workshop on Wearable and Implantable Body Sensor Networks*, pp. 76-79, ISBN 0-7695-2547-4, Cambridge, Massachusetts, USA, April 3-5, 2006.

Luprano, J. et al. (2007). New Generation of Smart Sensors for Biochemical and Bioelectrical Applications, *Proceedings of 2007 pHealth Conference*, Chalkidiki, Greece, June, 2007.

Lymberis, A. & Olsson S. (2003). Intelligent Biomedical Clothing for Personal Health and Disease Mangement : State of the Art and Future Vision, *Telemediciane Journal and e-Health*, Vol. 9, No. 4, (December 2003), pp. 379-386, ISSN 1530-5627.

Mathie M. J., Coster A. C., Lovell N. H., and Celler B. G. (2004). Accelerometry: providing an integrated, practical method for long-term, ambulatory monitoring of human movement. *Physiol. Meas.* 25(2), pp. 1-20.

McCann, J., Hurford, R. And Martin, A. (2005). A Design Process for the Development of Innovative Smart Clothing that Addresses End-User Needs from Technical, Functional, Aesthetic and Cultureal View points. *Proceedings of the IEEE International Symposium on Wearable Computers (ISWC'05).*

Noury, N. et al. (2004). A Smart Cloth for Ambulatory Telemonitoring of Physiological Parameters and Activity: the VTAMN Project, *Proceedings of 6th International Workshop on Enterprise Networking and Computing in Healthcare Industry*, pp. 155-160, ISBN 0-7803-8453-9, Odawara, Japan, June 28-29, 2004.

OMG-OCL, (2009). "Object Constraint Language Specification, Version 2.0", http://www.omg.org/technology/documents/formal/ocl.htm

Pandian, P.S. et al. (2008). Smart Vest: Wearable Multi-parameter Remote Physiological Monitoring System, *Medical engineering & Physics*, Vol. 30, No. 4, (May 2008), pp. 466-477, ISSN 1350-4533.

Pantelopoulos, A. & Bourbakis, N.G. (2010). A Survey on Wearable Sensor-Based Systems for Health Monitoring and Prognosis, *IEEE Trans. on Systems, Man, and Cybernetics, Part C: Applications and Reviews*, Vol. 40, No. 1, (January 2010), pp. 1-12, ISSN 1094-6977.

Paradiso, R. et al. (2008). Remote Health Monitoring with Wearable Non-Invasive Mobile System: the HealthWear Project, *Proceedings of IEEE 30th Annual International Conference on Engineering in Medicine and Biology Society*, pp. 1699-1702, ISBN 1557-170X, Vancouver, British Columbia, Canada, August 20-24, 2008.

Park, S. & Jayaraman S. (2010). Smart Textile-based Wearable Biomedical Systems: A Transition Plan for Research to Reality, *IEEE Transactions on Information Technology in Biomedicine*, Vol. 14, No. 1, (January 2010), pp. 86-92, ISSN 1089-7771.

Saranummi, N. (2002). Information Technology in Biomedicine, *IEEE Trans. Biomed. Eng.*, vol. 49, no. 12, pp. 1385–1386.

Taylor S. A. and Sharif H. (2006). Wearable Patient Monitoring Application (ECG) using Wireless Sensor Networks. *Proc IEEE Eng Med Biol Soc.* pp. 5977-5980.

"TEXTILE WIRE version 03.01-e", (2005). ELEKTRO-FEINDRHAT-AG, Switzerland.

Zephyr-Technology (2010). Case Study: Zephyr Provides Physiological Monitoring of Chilean Miners During San Jose Mine Rescue Operation. http://www.zephyr-technology.com/wp-content/uploads/2010/10/Case-Study-Chilean-Miner-Rescue-Operation.pdf

4

Smart Health Management Technology

Hiroshi Nakajima
Omron Corporation
Japan

1. Introduction

The notion of health management technology (HMT) is simple but powerful because it employs the ideas of cyclical evolution and synergetic integration of devices and services based on causality and human machine collaboration (Nakajima, 2008a). It can be applied for the different entities of human beings, artifacts, and nature environment as following discussions.

An essential and simple observation and understanding of our world reveals that it can be considered as comprising humans, artifacts, and nature environments shown in Fig.1. Even though the values of the entities are given by humans, they have obviously different directions. Examples of such values are comfort and safety for humans, efficiency and effectiveness for artifacts, and environmental enhancement for nature. The problem is that these values come into conflict with each other. Examples of conflicts in a factory are as follows. Productivity related to efficiency and effectiveness is the most important value in manufacturing lines. However, the focus only on productivity will increase the emission of carbon dioxide and other contaminants that will negatively influence to the sustainability of nature environment, and the safety and comfort of human operators in the manufacturing line. Thus, the conflicts of values among the respective entities cause serious problems in important areas such as the environment, agriculture and food, security and safety, and human health these days. In this sense, harmonization among them should be realized with keeping good health condition of each entity for realizing a desired next society. Although this vision might look grandiloquent, health management of each entity is considered as important activity as steady steps toward the bright future.

Because of recent development of information and communication technology (ICT), sensory networks have been pervading various fields such as home security, healthcare, condition-based maintenance for manufacturing equipment, and environment monitoring. They require the suitable integration of both sensing devices and valuable services.

HMT is designed for providing basic four kinds of functions by centering causality. The functions are measurement, recognition, estimation, and evolution. The functions provide the solution of cyclical evolvement based on causality which abstractly illustrates conditions of target systems and is used as problem solving knowledge, which is composed of feature attributes extracted from sensory data and intermediate characteristics. In this sense, causality could evolve and be updated according to sophistication of sensing and control mechanisms. Because the nature of causality is transparent to humans, the structure can be easily improved through human-machine collaboration. This feature of the technology is quite important because the integration of human knowledge and sensory data will bring a powerful and sophisticated solution for complex problems. HMT has been applied to various types of applications such as human healthcare, machine health monitoring in manufacturing process, and energy management systems. Some case studies of human health care are introduced in the article.

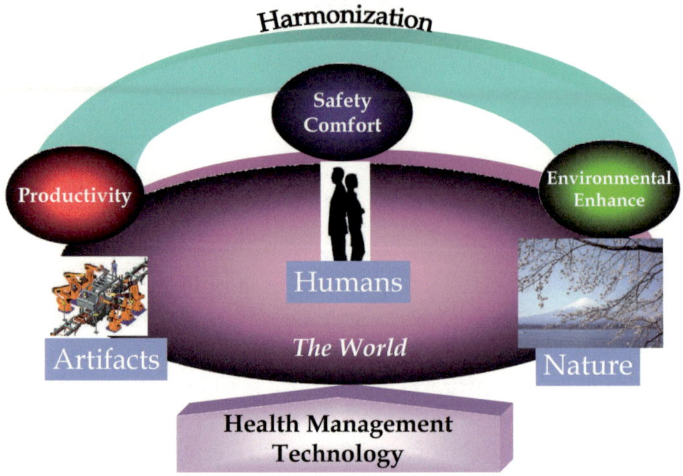

Fig. 1. The world consists of humans, artifacts, and nature environment

The rest of this chapter is organized as follows; Section 2 proposes Health Management Technology; Section 3 and 4 introduce the applications of visceral fat estimation and heart rate estimation respectively; Section 5 concludes this chapter.

2. Health management technology

In this section, the notion of the health management technology (HMT) is introduced to discuss its basic mechanisms and the four functions defined in the technology framework. It employs causality as an essential solution component in the technology. Fig.2 shows the structure of the target systems and HMT.

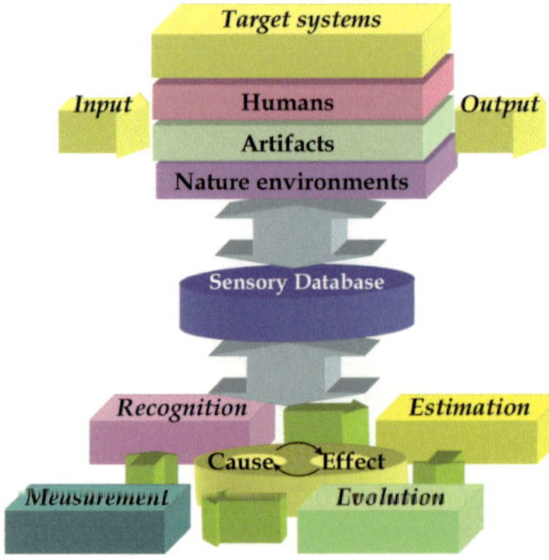

Fig. 2. Structure of the target systems and health management technology centering sensory database and causality

2.1 Overviews

Fig.3 shows an overview of HMT based on causality. The objective of the technology is to estimate the health condition of humans, artifacts, and nature to improve their health. Because the target system continuously changes and their health management systems must adapt to these changes, the cause-effect structure must evolve cyclically and continuously according to sophistication of both the target system and its management side. In HMT, four functions are defined for cyclically evolving the model as shown in Fig.3.

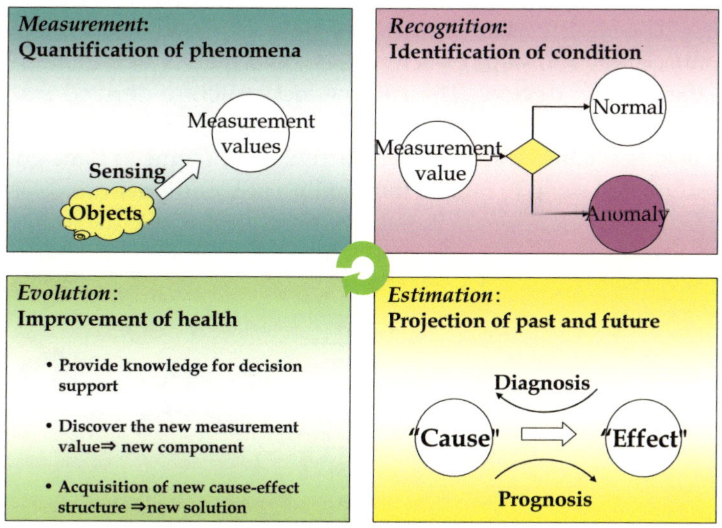

Fig. 3. Four functions of health management technology

- *Measurement* is to quantify of phenomena to arrive at a value from analyzing signals from sensors. The function is realized by the elemental technologies of feature extraction, feature selection, and feature evaluation.
- *Recognition* is to identify the condition of the target system using the measured value. The function is based on the pattern recognition technologies such as discrimination, classification, and identification.
- *Estimation* is to project the past and future status of the system. The functions of diagnosis and prognosis are realized by employing cause-effect structure. The elements of technology for realizing this function are probability graphs and causal models such as Bayesian network, structure equation model, etc.
- *Evolution* is to improve the target system and to update causality by the discovery of new events and make changes in the target system. The function should be realized by human-machine collaborative systems analysis and design.

It is important for us to manage our health by considering diet meal, sleep and rest, and exercise. There is important causality among these lifestyle habits and vital signals such as blood pressure, blood glucose, and blood adipose. Even though it has not been realized yet, the ideal example is shown in Fig.4.

The example of human health management is introduced for explaining effectiveness and efficiency of multivariate time series data and their cause-effect structure. The sensory data are used for composing the causality that can be applied to prevent diseases and to improve health. Among biological information, blood pressure is usually used as an important index of health condition because it is closely associated with cardiovascular events such as brain infarction, stroke, myocardial infarction, and heart failure. Besides other important factors such as total cholesterol, casual glucose, etc., blood pressure is easy to be measured at home and medical facilities. There are also easy and useful indices; body composition, active mass, and sleep condition. The composition of muscle and fat is measured by a body composition monitor. The indices could be used as one of alternative reference indices for quality and quantity of diet in our life. An active mass monitor or a pedometer could measure types, intensity, and quantity of exercises in daily life. A sleep monitor measures quality and quantity of sleep. The multivariate time series data of blood pressure, weight or body composition of muscle and fat, steps or active mass, and quality and quantity of sleep could be gathered by the sensing devices. The cause-effect structure derived from the data will provide important knowledge for diagnosis and prognosis of health condition optimized for individuals. For instance, continuous and well active mass seems to have good influence on the body composition and sleep to realize the stability of blood pressure.

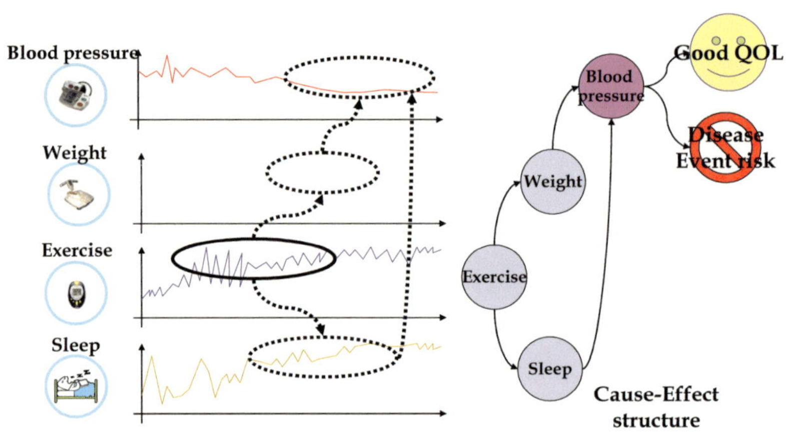

Fig. 4. Multivariate time series data and causal analysis for life style and vital signal

2.2 Discussions on invasion, intrusion, and consciousness

As long as the application domain in human health management, it is required for us to discuss and study on the relationship between human live body and instrumentation. In this section, invasion, intrusion, and consciousness in biomedical sensing are studied and discussed from the views of both human burden and technology performance. Invasion has been studied more so far than intrusion and consciousness. However, latter two issues are also important to provide different meanings and values from invasion.

2.2.1 Invasion

Invasion levels can be defined by distance between sensory head and sensing target or location of them (Yamagoe, 2000). There are five invasion level of biomedical sensing as follows;

1. A catheter is inserted into body to send transmitter to a sensor head.
2. A sensor head is implanted to send sensory signals via fixed line.
3. A sensor head is implanted to send sensory signals via wireless communication.
4. A sensor head is contacted on skin of the body to detect signals.
5. A sensor head is not contacted on skin of the body to detect signals.

As mentioned above, the invasion levels are defined by the positional relationship between sensory head and live body. Compared with invasion, intrusion and consciousness sensing are new ideas in biomedical but important for both of sensing accuracy and human comfort.

2.2.2 Intrusion

Nonintrusion is important idea for sensing daily life activity. Electrocardiogram (ECG) and blood pressure (BP) are very important physical indices used in medical and healthcare. The indices can be measured in just in hospital and clinic. It is strongly required to monitor for 24 hours to detect anomaly condition of body in daily life. However, it is impossible to monitor ECG in daily life in the case of using ordinary ECG equipment. A Holter electrocardiographic monitor has been realized for gathering the ECG signals and an ambulatory blood pressure monitor for accumulating blood pressure signals for 24 hours. Although the equipment could be used for sensing live body, it is far from non-intrusion. The user has to use contacted sensory head and to carry on the equipment.

2.2.3 Consciousness

Consciousness or realization to be sensed would have some influence to the sensing signals. White coat hypertension and masked hypertension (Messerli, 2005) are serious examples for understating the importance of unconsciousness sensing. Not just for these serious cases, other examples can be easily pointed out with considering consciousness such as video and image sensing. Long and continuous sensing for 24 hours requires unconsciousness. Besides them, unconsciousness helps for users not to forget the measurement.

Through these definitions and observations on invasion, intrusion, and unconsciousness, some discussions on influences to patients and live bodies and to measurements.

2.2.4 Consideration on humans and instrumentation ends

It is strong requirements to reduce and to eliminate burden, pain, and damage both physically and mentally to live bodies and patients. According to the definitions of invasion level, the level is decided by distance and location between sensor head and body. However, even though X-ray CT scan is non contact sensing, it gives serious impact of X-ray exposure on the live body. Implant sensing requires surgery whose invasion level is quite high, but intrusion is very low when the sensor could be used for a long time. Additionally, a patient who is implanted sensor into could feel unconscious with the sensor for long time usage. As these discussions, invasion is not the only perfect idea in biomedical sensing. Intrusion and consciousness should be also thought for realizing the effective and efficient bioinstrumentation.

Sensing performance would be generally good with high invasion level. However, invasion sometimes brings negative results in sensing. Contact with sensor head and live body each other makes energy exchange between them to cause instability in sensing. For example, huge sensor head of clinical thermometer realizes good fitting with body however it takes body temperature. Like the examples pointed out in intrusion section, it would be very hard to keep the ideal situation of the patient such as in daily life activities with high intrusion. Besides, unconscious sensing might bring good results with the sensing performance as discussed in consciousness section.

Realization of biomedical sensing without invasion, intrusion, and consciousness brings some uncertainty in the sensing mechanism. Sensor signals superimpose not just target but other kinds of signals. Besides extraction of target signal, it is also required to compose causal structures which explain sensing principles well.

2.3 Causal analysis

Causal analysis studies have covered wide and various areas from psychology and philosophy (Pearl, 2000; Gopnik 2007) to image processing and bioinformatics (Mittal, 2007). Theoretical basics were also deeply studied (Whittaker, 1990) and some studies covered wide areas (Pearl, 2000; Lucas, 2007; Spirtes 2000). In this article, the path analysis that is one of principle causal analysis methods is employed to realize HMT as a first step of the technology because of its simple but powerful solution nature. Besides introduction to the method, acquisition and improvement of cause-effect structure are discussed.

As one of cause-structure acquisition, the path analysis (Wright, 1923) or the structural equation model (Scheines, 1999) is introduced here. The cause-effect structure is described by a cause-effect diagram shown in Fig.4.

The cause-effect diagram is formulated by the structural equations (1)-(3). A causal relationship between variables is quantified by the coefficients α_{YZ} which are called causal effect or path coefficient. The paths from X_1 to X_4 are the direct effect of $X_1 \rightarrow X_4$, the indirect effects of $X_1 \rightarrow X_2 \rightarrow X_4$ and $X_1 \rightarrow X_2 \rightarrow X_3 \rightarrow X_4$. The sum of the direct and indirect effects is called total effect which is calculated by the equation (4). By using these effects, the cause-effect structure can be quantified. Sometimes for simplification, means and variances of variables used in the cause-effect structure are normalized to 0 and 1 respectively.

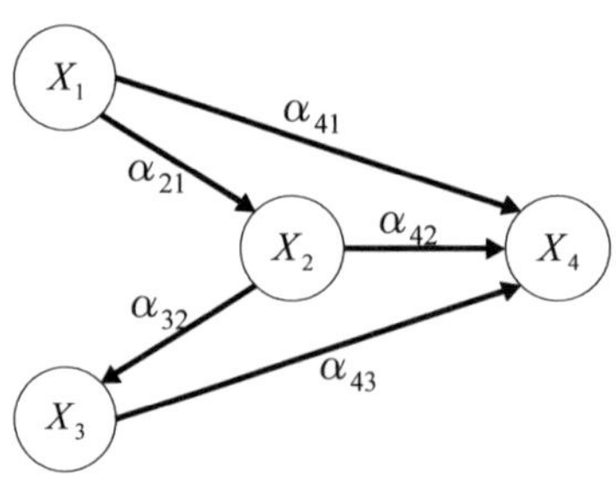

Fig. 5. Causality example

$$X_2 = \alpha_{21} X_1 + \varepsilon_1 \tag{1}$$

$$X_3 = \alpha_{32} X_2 + \varepsilon_2 \tag{2}$$

$$X_4 = \alpha_{41} X_1 + \alpha_{42} X_2 + \alpha_{43} X_3 + \varepsilon_3 \tag{3}$$

$$E_{T41} = \alpha_{41} + \alpha_{21}\alpha_{42} + \alpha_{21}\alpha_{32}\alpha_{43} + \varepsilon_4 \tag{4}$$

Besides model representations, causality acquisition methods have been studied. A Bayesian approach can be applied when data are categorical (Heckerman, 1999). Regarding sensing data, which are continuous values, a causality acquisition method using the data is studied for applying anomaly detection of a discrete manufacturing process (Endo, 2008). One of the reasons why cause-effect structure is employed as performable knowledge is its transparent nature for human machine collaboration. That is to say, the transparent aspect of causality would bring a more powerful solution to human machine collaborative improvement (Marutschke, 2008, 2009).

While a cause-effect structure has been acquired, progressive improvement of the structure is required according to the change of target systems. There are different directions of causality improvement. One is simplification or abstraction and the other complication or concretion. These ideas are useful to reduce the cost and to improve accuracy of health management. For instance, in the case of multiple sensors required for health management such as lifestyle habit monitoring which considers exercise, diet, and sleep, reduction of the number of sensors through updating cause-effect structure will work well for cost reduction of sensors and data management. On the other side, complication of causality would work for increasing estimation accuracy of target systems' condition. For adapting to the increase of system's complexity and preciseness, transformation of cause-effect structure is discussed from the viewpoint of a hierarchical modeling method (Tsuchiya, 2008, 2010).

3. Visceral fat estimation

In the medical profession, it has been realized that visceral fat (VF) is main cause of lifestyle diseases and metabolic syndrome. According to the trend, a medical instrument of VF measurement has been strongly required with low invasion, low cost, and ease of use. In this section, a visceral fat estimation method by bioelectrical impedance and causal analysis is proposed to realize the practical device with low invasion and low intrusion in the medical fields.

Metabolic syndrome is not just obesity disease but is associated with serious diseases such as diabetes mellitus and hypertension. They would cause complicating illness from diabetes and cardiovascular events to decrease quality of life. Even though the regulations in the countries might be slightly different, the indices of blood pressure, blood lipid, blood glucose, and visceral fat are mainly used for the criterion of medical diagnosis. First three criteria can be measured by a blood pressure meter and blood investigation with high accuracy. However, because VF of live body can not be measured directly, some other indices are generally used, such as body mass index, waist-hip ratio, and waist circumference. However, these indices are not accurate to estimate visceral fat volume. On the other hand, the cross sectional area at umbilicus level by using an X-ray computerized tomography (CT) scan or a magnetic resonance imaging (MRI) is the gold standard in medical fields for measurement of visceral adipose tissue (ECCODJ, 2002; Gomi, 2005). However, a CT scan causes X-ray exposure and requires difficulty of use and high cost. For solving these problems, a medical instrument is strongly required with non invasion, low intrusion, ease of use, and low cost. Besides these benefits, the instrument without X-ray exposure can be used for the follow-up measurement of visceral fat reduction after medical treatment for metabolic syndrome and obesity.

In response to the requirements, the visceral fat estimation method has been proposed by employing bioelectrical impedance analysis and causal analysis for realizing the medical device of VF measurement. Two kinds of impedance and information of body shape at umbilicus level are used as sensory data. The causal structure is designed by considering the measurement principle to be optimized based on statistical analysis to estimate visceral fat area as the dependent variable which is provided by a CT scan and image processing. The experiments were conducted to investigate the performance of the proposed method. The result was 0.88 coefficient of correlation value between the proposed instrument and a CT scan. The method works well to realize the practical instrument used in medical field. Besides the performance, the model brings understandability and transparency with the measurement nature of VF.

3.1 Analysis and design methods

In this section, the measurement principles are introduced and the related works are surveyed. Bioelectrical impedance analysis (BIA) and causal analysis (CA) follows the principles.

3.1.1 Measurement principles

Fig.6 shows a cross sectional area of the human body at umbilicus level provided by a CT scan and colored by image processing. There are three types of composition which are visceral fat, subcutaneous fat, and lean body. Lean body is not fat and internal organs, muscles, and bones. Each area can be calculated automatically by image processing technology applied to the image of cross sectional area gotten by a CT or an MRI. Visceral fat area can be calculated by the equation (5). It is the measurement principle of VF.

$$VFA = CSA - SFA - LBA \tag{5}$$

where VFA is visceral fat area, CSA all cross sectional area, SFA subcutaneous area, and LBA lean body area.

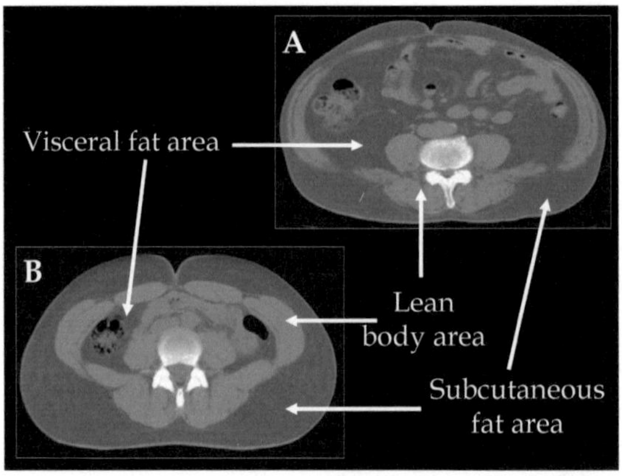

Fig. 6. Cross sectional area image by CT scan and Image Processing

Related studies to estimate visceral fat area have been done. All studies introduced here employ BIA because it is commonly and practically used for estimating body composition. Ryo et al. proposed the method which employs waist circumference and abdominal impedance which occurs at the flank to the flow of current between the umbilicus and the back (Ryo, 2005). They are used as the feature attributes in the equation (6).

$$\tilde{A}_{VF1} = \alpha_1 Vo Wc^3 + \varepsilon \tag{6}$$

where $\tilde{A}_{VF1}$ is the estimated VFA, Vo the impedance measured at the flank, Wc waist circumference, α_1 and ε regression coefficient and error term respectively.

Shiga et al. proposed the model to estimate VFA, which employed two types of impedance and will be described in Section 3.1.2. The model is given by the equation (7) (Shiga, 2007, 2009).

$$\tilde{A}_{VF2} = \alpha_1 Wc^2 + \alpha_2 WcZ_S + \alpha_3 / Z_T + \varepsilon \tag{7}$$

where $\tilde{A}_{VF2}$ is the estimated VFA, Z_S the surface abdominal impedance, Z_T the total abdominal impedance, $\alpha_i (i = 1,2,3)$ and ε regression coefficient and error term respectively. The model uses the only measured variables of waist circumference and the impedances. Some studies proposed the several models using the width and height of the cross sectional area of an abdomin (Shiga, 2009; Yoneda, 2007, 2008). Some of them also employ other variables such as gender and age besides them (Yoneda, 2007, 2008).
One of the models is given by the equation (8) which considers influence by gender and age.

$$\begin{aligned} \tilde{A}_{VF3} &= \alpha_1 a + \alpha_2 b + \alpha_3 / b + \alpha_4 a^2 + \alpha_5 b^2 \\ &+ \alpha_6 / b^2 + \alpha_7 / Z_T + \alpha_8 Z_S \sqrt{a^2 + b^2} \\ &+ \alpha_9 A + \alpha_{10} G + \varepsilon \end{aligned} \tag{8}$$

where a and b are the width and the height of a cross sectional area shown in Figure 2, Z_S the surface abdominal impedance, Z_T total abdominal impedance, A age, G gender, and $\alpha_i (i = 1,2,...,10)$ and ε regression coefficient and error term respectively.
The model denoted by the equation (7) is the most similar to the measurement principle given by the equation (5). However, the information of abdominal shape might be eliminated by using waist circumference. On the other side, height and width of the cross sectional area of abdomin would bring some information about it. The variables improved the estimation performance (Tsuchiya, 2010) but age and gender are not suitable for estimating VFA because they are not physical variables and not shown in the measurement principle given by the equation (5). The equation (8) seems to cause some problems of complexity and multicollinearity because it employed many variables and multiple appearances in different terms.

3.1.2 Bioelectrical impedance analysis

In order to extract visceral fat from the all composition of abdominal human body, two types of bioelectrical impedances named Dual Impedance (DI) are employed as shown in Fig.7. In the DI method, the electrodes are placed on the both hands' backs and the both feet's insteps with the subjects lying on the back. The surface abdominal impedance Z_S is measured by using the electrodes at the back. The electric currents are passed among the electrodes on the back. The total abdominal impedance Z_T is measured by using the electrodes placed on hands, feet, and abdomin. The currents are passed from both hands and feet to abdomin.
The surface abdominal impedance is highly correlated with the subcutaneous fat volume (Scharfetter, 2001) and the total one is inversely correlated with the lean body volume; that is fat-free mass (Lukaski, 1985). Thus, our strategy is to develop the estimation model which could explain well the measurement principle as shown in the equation (5) by using the DI method.

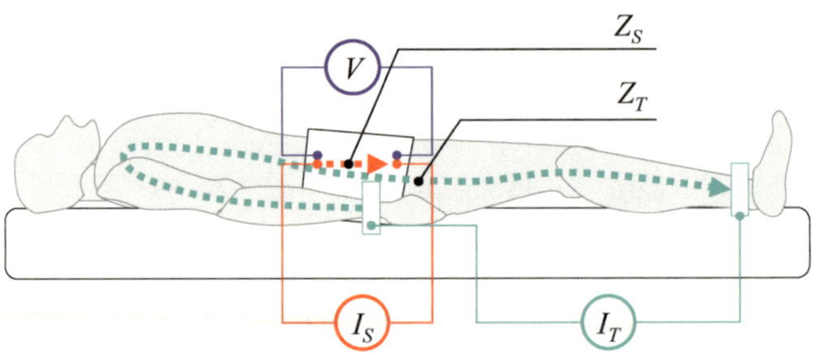

Fig. 7. Human body and the two types of impedances

3.1.3 Causal analysis

Fig.8 illustrates the causality of VFA estimation considering the relationship between the sensory variables and the measurement principle. The left and the right are the sensory variables and the principle measurement respectively. According to the causal structure, we prepare the variables which are the candidates for constructing the causality. By using the selected variables, multi linear regression was employed to acquire the estimation model. In this step, we carefully considered about nature of the model without over-fitting, multicollinearity, and some other difficulties; especially keeping the notion of the measurement principle. We finally derived the estimation model denoted by the equation (9).

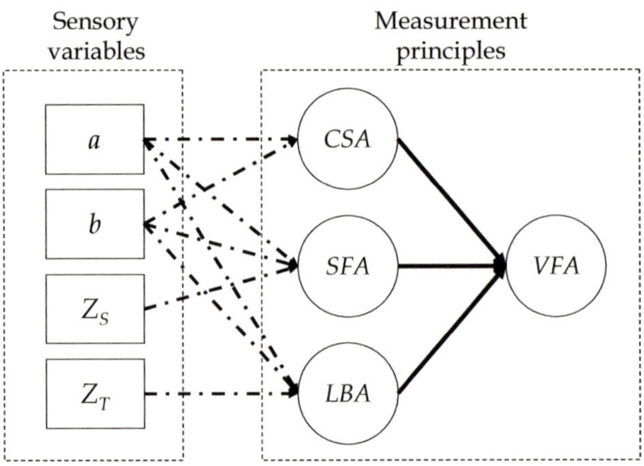

Fig. 8. Causality between the sensory variables and the measurement principle

$$\tilde{A}_{VF4} = \alpha_1 a + \alpha_2 b^2 + \alpha_3 Z_S \sqrt{a^2 + b^2} + \alpha_4 / Z_T + \varepsilon \tag{9}$$

In order to extract the causality for estimating VFA, we designed the following development steps;

1. Preparation of variables according to the measurement principles
2. Selection of the variables by applying AIC and VIF on the sample dataset

In the first step, we prepared the candidates of the variables as possible as used in the estimation equation. The idea here is that the candidates should bring some information about VFA estimation and be understandable from the point view of the measurement principles shown in the figure 8. The prepared variables are listed in Table 1.

Relations	Variables	Remarks
CSA	a , b	Primary measurement variables. a and b are width and height of a cross sectional area at umbilicus level as shown in Figure 2.
	a^2 , b^2	Extension of measurement values.
	ab	Correlation with a cross section.
	$\sqrt{a^2+b^2}$	Both size and shape information.
SFA	Z_S	A primary measurement variable of bioelectrical impedance. Z_S is surface abdominal impedance. It has high correlation with *SFA* (Scharfetter, 2001).
	aZ_S , bZ_S , a^2Z_S , b^2Z_S abZ_S , $\sqrt{a^2+b^2}Z_S$	The combination of the surface impedance and the shape and size information of the cross section.
LBA	Z_T	A primary measurement variable of bioelectrical impedance. Z_T is total abdominal impedance. It has high inverse correlation with *LBA* (Lukaski, 1985).
	a/Z_T , b/Z_T a^2/Z_T , b^2/Z_T ab/Z_T , $\sqrt{a^2+b^2}/Z_T$	The combination of inverse of the total impedance and the shape and size information of the cross section.

Table 1. Candidates of the variables used in the estimation equation

The second step is the suitable variables selection as a set of them named tuple. We employed two different criteria to realize the legitimate model for VFA estimation. Our consideration was to realize both performance guarantee and understandability. The first is the accuracy and simplification of the model without over-fitting to the sample dataset. The second is multicollinearity which causes some difficulties in the estimation results. The problem is caused by an almost linear relationship among independent variables in the regression model. Akaike Information Criterion (AIC) (Akaike, 1974) and Variance Inflation Factor (VIF) (Armitage, 2001) are the employed criteria for the former and later considerations. The criteria are given by the equation (10) and by equation (11) respectively.

$$AIC = n\log(2\pi\hat{\sigma}_e^{\,2}) + \frac{1}{\hat{\sigma}^2}\sum_{i=1}^{n}\{y-(\alpha_1 x_1+\cdots+\alpha_m x_m+\varepsilon)\}^2 + 2(m+2) \qquad (10)$$

where m and n is the numbers of independent variables and data respectively, y a dependent variable, $x_i(i=1,2,...,m)$ independent variables, $\alpha_i(i=1,2,...,m)$ coefficient terms, ε error term, $\hat{\sigma}_e$ the standard deviation of estimation errors.

$$VIF_i = 1/(1-R^2{}_i) \qquad (11)$$

where R_i is the multiple correlation coefficient between the independent variable $x_i(i=1,2,...n)$ and the rest of $(n-1)$ variables.

The variable sets were constructed by selecting the variables with the combination constraints given by the equations (11).

$$
\begin{aligned}
X_i &= [x_j, x_k, x_l] \\
x_j &= \{(a,b),(a^2,b^2),(a,b^2),(a^2,b),ab,\sqrt{a^2+b^2}\} \\
x_k &= \{Z_S, aZ_S, bZ_S, a^2Z_S, b^2Z_S, abZ_S, \sqrt{a^2+b^2}Z_S\} \\
x_l &= \{1/Z_T, a/Z_T, b/Z_T, a^2/Z_T, b^2/Z_T, ab/Z_T, \sqrt{a^2+b^2}/Z_T\}
\end{aligned}
\qquad (11)
$$

where X_i is a tuple of independent variables selected from the three categories of CSA, SFA, and LBA which consists of x_j $(j=1,2,...,6)$, x_k $(k=1,2,...,7)$, and x_l $(l=1,2,...,7)$. According to the equation (11), there are four or three variable combinations of the candidates. VIF and AIC were applied to all the tuples to select the top 10 according to the regulations of $VIF < 10$ and the ascending order of AIC. In this case, VIF values listed in the table are the maximum of all the combinations. A high value of the VIF indicates a multicollinearity problem and the value higher than 10 is of concern (Armitage, 2001). We applied these criteria to select the variable with using the sample dataset which consisted of 196 subjects; 95 females and 101 males of from 30 to 69 years old with 49.3 mean, and their VFA are from 8.1 to 213.4 cm^2 with 86.9 mean. The results are listed in Table 2.

No	Selected variables	VIF	AIC
1	a, b^2, $\sqrt{a^2+b^2}Z_S$, $1/Z_T$	7.494421	1202.845
2	a, b^2, aZ_S, $1/Z_T$	8.583536	1202.953
3	a, b^2, abZ_S, $1/Z_T$	9.680687	1203.16
4	a, b^2, bZ_S, $1/Z_T$	7.355794	1203.468
5	ab, a^2Z_S, $1/Z_T$	5.527161	1204.678
6	ab, aZ_S, $1/Z_T$	4.653251	1205.513
7	a^2, b^2, $\sqrt{a^2+b^2}Z_S$, $1/Z_T$	7.767823	1205.883
8	a^2, b^2, aZ_S, $1/Z_T$	8.961434	1206.023
9	a^2, b^2, bZ_S, $1/Z_T$	7.451921	1206.098
10	a, b^2, bZ_S, $\sqrt{a^2+b^2}/Z_T$	8.578534	1206.461

Table 2. Selected variables with VIF and AIC

3.1.4 Experimental results and discussions

We designed the experimental data set by using the three variables of gender, age, and waist circumference which is substituted to for VFA because it could not be used in the recruiting subjects phase. The number of subject is 180 (90 males + 90 females) who were 22 to 80 years old (the mean is 49.95) and had from 65.8 to 120 cm of their waist circumferences (the mean 90.09). All of the subjects are measured by both the proposed method and a CT scan.

The results were as follows; the correlation coefficient 0.88, the errors mean -1.38, and the errors standard deviation 27.28. The correlation coefficient between waist circumferences and CT scans is 0.77.

As the results, visceral fat areas estimated by the proposed method achieved high correlation with ones by the CT scan. Waist circumference which is used in a medical checkup works well but the estimation accuracy is lower than the proposed method. Besides, it cannot differentiate VF from subcutaneous one and lean body in principle.

4. Heart rate monitoring

Among vital signals, a heart rate (HR) is an important index for understanding and diagnosing human's health condition. Especially, heart rate variability includes much information on health condition, for example, symptoms of cardiac disease, and conditions of autonomic nerve system (Kitney, 1980; Kobayashi, 1999). HR is measured in medical checkups and clinical diagnosis by electrocardiograph (ECG) as the gold standard. Besides the medical field, continuous monitoring of HRs during daily life activities is also strongly required because HR depends on activity intensity and monitoring HR might bring its information. Considering with usage in daily life, the monitoring should be realized without burden of human side. Regarding the burden, non-invasive, low intrusive, and unconscious sensing should be desired. In this section, an HR monitoring on bed by using an air pressure sensor (APS) is proposed for considering the unconscious and low cost biomedical sensing.

Because an APS is low cost and has high sensitivity, it could realize non invasive, non intrusive, and unconscious sensing on a bed with low cost. However, it brings too much information other than heart rate. The signal analysis such as filtering noise is required to realize its stable performance of HR estimation.

4.1 Analysis domain

There are two main analysis directions for measuring HRs from sensory signals; i.e., frequency domain analysis and time one. As frequency domain analysis, short term fast Fourier transformation (SFFT) is commonly used. SFFT is capable of monitoring global variability of target waveform. Because FFT assumes constant frequency, it does not extract microscopic variability. As time domain analysis, there have been several methods for HR measurement; i.e., peak detection, pattern matching, etc. Especially, pattern matching based on autocorrelation is commonly used to estimate HR variability from signals obtained via ECG monitor. Because of its capability of sensing HR variability, it is recommended for extraction and sensing of microscopic variability of HR. As HR monitoring in daily life requires the microscopic variability, time domain analysis is much more suitable for the usage.

4.2 Causal analysis in biomedical sensing

Regarding the transparency of biomedical sensing, causal analysis is a powerful tool since the causality is easy to be visualized, and makes the measurement principle clear.

There have been many practical studies on causal analysis. For instance, Thang et al. proposed a medical diagnosis support system based on oriental diagnosis knowledge (Thang, 2006). In their approach, the causality among some subject's symptoms and their diagnostic outcome is described by using RBF neural network. Nakajima et al. proposed a

generic health management framework named Health Management Technology which is applied to not only human being but also manufacturing process, energy consumption management, and so forth (Nakajima, 2008a). Hata et al. suggested a concept named Human Health Care System of Systems which focus on health management, medical diagnosis, and surgical support (Hata, 2009). In the concept, the human health management technology is discussed from viewpoint of system of systems engineering. Marutschke et al. suggested that the causal analysis based on human-machine collaboration realizes transparent system model (Marutschke, 2009). From a viewpoint of theoretical development, lots of causal analysis theories have been proposed. Bayesian network describes statistical causality among phenomena observed from certain managed systems, and the statistical causality provides inference and reasoning functions (Pearl, 2001). Graphical model visualizes causality among components in complex systems (Miyagawa, 1991). Fuzzy logic helps intuitive representation of causality which is experts' implicit knowledge (Zadeh, 1996).
Through the discussions above, this section describes a transparent and accurate HR monitoring technology by employing an air pressure sensor and causal analysis among air pressure transit and HR.

4.3 Measurement principle and system architecture

4.3.1 System design

An HR monitoring equipment on a bed is implemented by using air pressure sensor (Hata, 2007). The equipment is not only capable of easy setup and application, but also unconscious and low intrusive. And the measurement principle is designed by employing causal analysis among air pressure and HR, and the cause-effect structure based on the designed causality is formed by using fuzzy logic (Zadeh, 1996; Tsuchiya, 2007; Tsuchiya, 2008).
Fig.9 shows the HR monitoring equipment. The human's body pressure is obtained via air pressure sensor, and the pressure is quantified into 1024 level (10bit) at 100 Hz by A/D converter. As a result, the HR transit is estimated from the quantified pressure. Fig.10 illustrates the principle of the measurement by using an air pressure sensor.

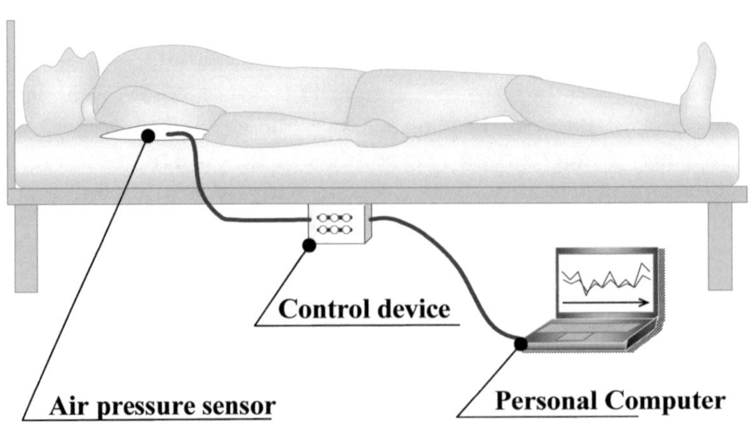

Fig. 9. Heart-rate monitoring equipment in sleep

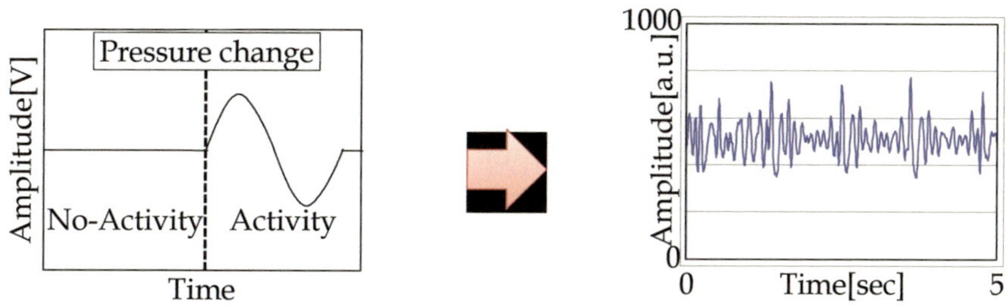

Fig. 10. Principle of the measurement by an air pressure sensor

4.3.2 Heart rate estimation and causal analysis

The basic idea of measuring HR monitoring is to extract heartbeats from pressure change of back in lying posture. The sensory signal superimposes not only heartbeat but also body movement and respiration. We need to extract the signal related to HR from the sensory source signal. In response to the requirement, causal analysis among air pressure and HR is employed to analysis and design the extraction method.

Firstly, the causality of heartbeat *HB*, body movement *BMV*, respiration *RSP*, and air pressure *APS* can be designed as the waveform analysis part as illustrated in Fig.11. Then, once R wave points τ_R could be extracted from *HB* signal, HR variability could be calculated from R-R interval τ_{RR} which is the time differences of R waves in the same manner as ECG.

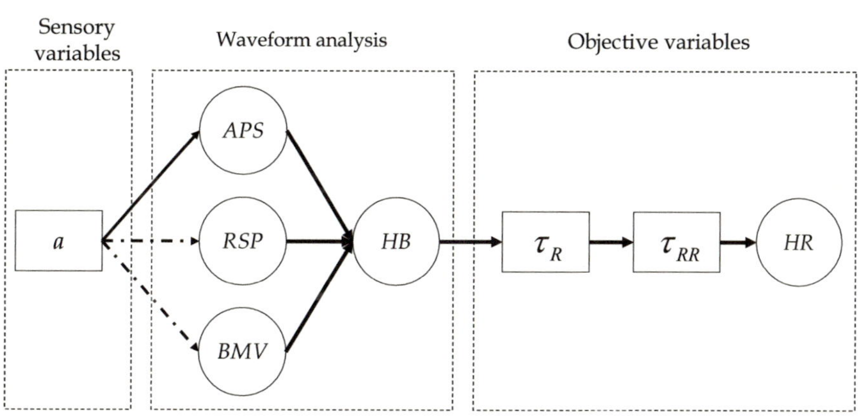

Fig. 11. Causality of heart rate estimation by using an air pressure sensor

As for τ_R extraction from pressure change, the pressure change involves not only heartbeat but also respiration and body movement. Because of the nature of the signals, it could be difficult to determine the precise position of R-waves τ_R by autocorrelation function and peak detection method. In this study, fuzzy logic is employed to formulate the knowledge about heartbeat.

Step 1. Firstly, full-wave rectification is applied to *APS*, and the pre-processed signal is determined as x_i .

Step 2. Then, the fuzzy logic based on the knowledge about τ_{RR} is applied to the pre-processed signal x_i . These fuzzy rules are described in the following.

Knowledge 1 : The large pressure change is caused by heartbeat.
Knowledge 2 : Heartbeat interval does not change significantly.

According to the knowledge on heartbeat characteristics, the fuzzy rules are denoted in the following.

Rule 1 : IF x_i is HIGH, THEN the degree of heartbeat point μ_{Amp} is HIGH.

Rule 2 : IF t_i is CLOSE to $\overline{T}$,THEN the degree of heartbeat point μ_{Int} is HIGH.

where μ_{Amp} is the membership function of Rule 1, x_i is pre-processed pressure change, t_i is the sampling point of obtained pressure change, $\overline{T}$ is the average of heartbeat intervals that calculated by using previous ten heartbeats, and μ_{Int} is the membership function of Rule 2. Then, the membership functions respond to the fuzzy rules are illustrated in Fig.12(a) and 12(b), and formulae are equations (12)–(14) and (15), (16).

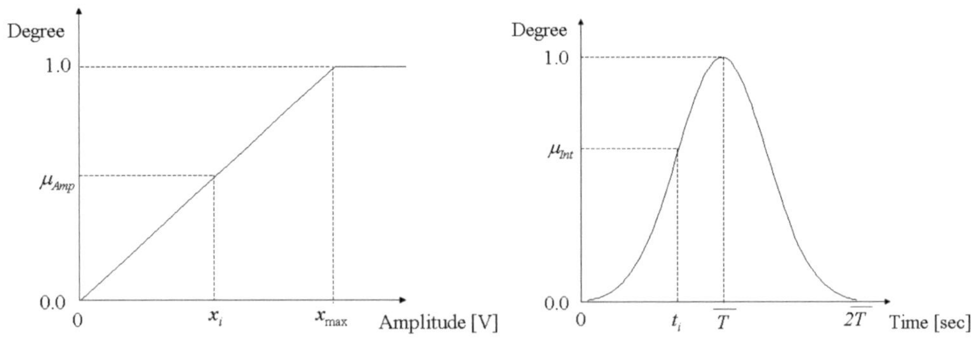

(a) Heartbeat amplitude (b) Heartbeat interval

Fig. 12. Membership functions

$$\mu_{Amp}(i) = \begin{cases} 0 & \text{if } x_i < x_{\min} \\ \dfrac{x_i - x_{\min}}{x_{\max} - x_{\min}} & \text{if } x_{\min} \le x_i \le x_{\max} \\ 1 & \text{if } x_i > x_{\max} \end{cases} \tag{12}$$

$$x_{\min} = \min(x_{APS}) \tag{13}$$

$$x_{\max} = \max(x_{APS}) \tag{14}$$

$$\mu_{Int}(i) = \exp\left(\frac{-(t_i - \overline{T})^2}{2\sigma^2}\right) \tag{15}$$

$$\sigma = \overline{T} / 3 \tag{16}$$

Step 3. Finally, μ_i is calculated by multiplying μ_{Amp} and μ_{Int} and the location with maximum μ_i is determined as heartbeat *HB* as formulated in equation (17).

$$\mu_i = \mu_{\mathrm{Amp}}(i) * \mu_{\mathrm{Int}}(i) \quad (17)$$

4.4 Experimental results

In this experiment, the developed HR monitoring is compared with conventional and typical method that is based on autocorrelation functions. Table 3 shows the profile of each subject, and their correlations between HR changes obtained from the ECG and those obtained from the HR monitoring equipment. The results indicate that the proposed method achieved higher performance for all of the subjects. In particular, the correlation to ECG for the subject A and E is over 0.97.

Subject	Attribute				Correlation coefficient	
	Age [yrs]	Gender	Height [cm]	Weight [kg]	Proposed	AC function
A	23	Male	175	76	0.973	0.703
B	23	Male	171	68	0.807	0.389
C	23	Male	165	50	0.754	0.621
D	25	Male	171	56	0.872	0.699
E	22	Male	180	92	0.972	0.658
F	22	Male	172	55	0.844	0.677
G	23	Male	170	62	0.737	0.346
Mean	23	-	172	65.6	0.851	0.585

Table 3. Experimental result on 7 males on a bed

Figure 13 shows an example of HR monitoring result for subject E. In the figure, the virtual axis is R-R interval (heartbeat interval), the horizontal axis is heartbeat count, the black line is R-R interval estimated by the proposed method, and the gray line is the one obtained by ECG. According the result around 200 beats, the proposed HR monitoring technology estimates the correct R-R intervals even if the significant change is occurred.

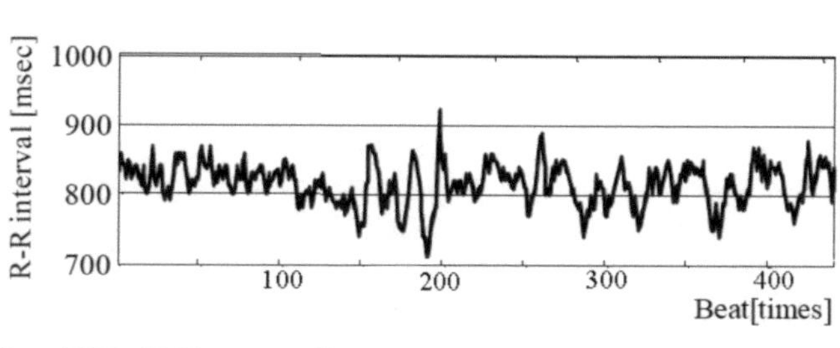

Fig. 13. An example of HR (R-R interval) monitoring result by using proposed method

5. Summaries and conclusions

In this chapter, the Smart Health Management Technology is proposed with introductions to its applications. The notion of the technology centers causality to realize the transparency and

the cyclic evolution of a target and its management system. It consists of four functions; i.e., *Measurement, Recognition, Estimation,* and *Evolution*. Each function plays an important role for realizing quantification, classification, diagnosis and prognosis, and solution providing respectively. The reason why causality is employed as an essential representation is that causality can be readable and improvable via interaction between human and machine and their collaboration brings powerful and developmental solution. In the applications, the expected benefits were verified. In the visceral fat estimation, the causality was used for both measurement principle and its relationship with sensory variables. Firstly, the causality was designed by human experts. Then, variable selection and parameter tunings followed to derive the final estimation model. In the heart rate estimation, the design of causality was from the view points of wave analysis and objective variables. According to the wave analysis causality, fuzzy logic was employed for filtering sensory signal related to heart beat. The experiments were conducted to evaluate efficiency and effectiveness of the proposed method in the applications. The visceral fat estimation worked well as the correlation coefficient was 0.88 with X-ray CT scan. The heart rate estimation resulted that the mean of the correlation coefficient was 0.85 with electrocardiograph.
According to the notion of SHMT, Fig. 4 illustrates the causality from multivariate time series data. The applications introduced here provide mainly the measurement functionality. In the future, the accumulation of sensory data will realize the notion of diagnosis and prognosis based on causalities.

6. References

Akaike, H., (1974), A new look at the statistical model identification, *IEEE Trans on Automatic Control*, AC-19, No. 6, pp. 716-723 (1974)

Armitage, P., Berry, G., & Matthews, J. N. S.,(2001), *Statistical Methods in Medical Research*, Wiley-Blackwell, 358-360 (2001)

Endo, M., Tsuruta, K., Kita, S., & Nakajima, H., (2008), A Study of Cause-Effect Structure Acquisition for Anomaly Diagnosis in Discrete Manufacturing Process, *Proceedings of 2008 IEEE International Conference on Systems, Man, and Cybernetics*, 2099-2104

Examination Committee of Criteria for 'Obesit Disease' in Japan (ECCODJ), (2002), Japan Society for Study of Obesity, "New Criteria for 'obesity disease' in Japan," Cric J 66 (11), 987-992 (2002)

Gomi, T., (2005), Measurement of Visceral Fat/Subcutaneous Fat Ratio by 0.3 Tesla MRI, *Radiation Medicine*, 23 (8), 584-587 (2005)

Gopnik, A., and Schulz, L., (2007), *Causal Learning - Psychology, Philosophy, and Computation*, OXFORD University Press, ISBN 978-019517680, USA.

Hata, Y., Kamozaki, Y., Sawayama, T., Taniguchi, K. & Nakajima, H., (2007), A heart pulse monitoring system by air pressure and ultrasonic sensor systems, Proceedings of IEEE System of Systems, 1-5 (2007).

Hata, Y., Kobashi, S. & Nakajima, H, (2009), Human health care system of systems, *IEEE System Journal*, Vol.3, No. 2, pp.231-238 (2009).

Heckerman, D., Meek, C., & Cooper, G., (1999), *A Bayesian Approach to Causal Discovery*, Chapter 4, Computation, Causation, and Discovery, AAAI PRESS/The MIT PRESS

Ho, K., Tsuchiya, N., Nakajima, H., Kuramoto, K., Kobashi, S., & Hata, Y., Fuzzy Logic Approach to Respiration Detection by Air Pressure Sensor, *Proceedings of 2009 IEEE International Conference on Fuzzy Systems*, August, 911-915 (2009)

Kitney, R.I. & Rompelman, O., (1980), The Study of Heart Rate Variability, Clarendon Press, Oxford (1980).

Kobayashi, H., Ishibashi, K. & Noguchi, H., (1999), Heart rate variability; an index for monitoring and analyzing human autonomic activities, AHS 18(2), 53-59 (1999).

Li, B.; Xu, Y. & Choi, J. (1996). Applying Machine Learning Techniques, *Proceedings of ASME 2010 4th International Conference on Energy Sustainability*, pp. 14-17, ISBN 842-6508-23-3, Phoenix, Arizona, USA, May 17-22, 2010

Lucas, P., Games, J. A., & Salmeron, A., (2007), *Advances in Probabilistic Graphical Models*, Springer,

Lukaski, H., Johnson, P., Bolonchuk, W., & Lykken, G., (1985), Assessment of fat-free mass using bioelectrical impedance measurements of the human body, *American Journal of Clinical Nutrition*, 41, 810-817 (1985)

Marutschke, D. M., Nakajima, H., Tsuchiya, N., Yoneda, M., & Iwami, T., (2008), Causality-Based Transparency And Accuracy In System Modeling with Human-Machine Collaboration, *Proceedings of World Automation Congress 2008*, pp. 1-6

Marutschke, D. M., Nakajima, H., Tsuchiya, N., Yoneda, M., & Iwami, T. and Kamei, K., (2009), Actualization of Causality-Based Transparency and Accuracy in System Modeling with Human-Machine Collaboration, *International Journal of Intelligent Computing in Medical Sciences and Image Processing*, Vol.3, No. 2, pp. 131-141 (2009)

Messerli, F. H., & Cotiga,D., (2005), Masked hypertension and white-coart hyptertension – Therapic navigation between Scylla and Charybdis, *Jouranal of the American College of Cardiology*, Vol.46, No.3, pp.516-517, 2005.

Mittal, A., & Kassim, A., (2007), *Bayesian Network Technologies - Applications and Graphical Models*, IGI Publishing,

Miyagawa, M., (1991), Statistical causal inference using graphical models, *JJSS*, Vol.29, No. 3, 327-356 (1991).

Nakajima, H., Hasegawa, Y., Tasaki, H., Iwami, T., & Tuchiya, N. (2008a). Health Management Technology as a General Solution Framework, *SICE Journal of Control, Measurement, and System Integration (SICE JCMSI)*, Vol.1, No.3, (May 2008), pp.257-264, ISBN 978-4-339-89203-1

Nakajima, H., Hasegawa, Y., Tasaki, H., & Kojitani, K., (2008b), SoS Aspects of Health Management Technology in Substrate Manufacturing Process, *Proceedings of IEEE SMC System of Systems Engineering*, 1-6, (2008)

Nakajima, H., Tasaki, H., Tsuchiya, N., Hamaguchi, T., & Shiga, T., (2011), Visceral fat estimation method by bioelectrical impedance analysis and causal analysis, *Proceedings of SPIE Defense, Security + Sensing*, to appear (2011)

Pearl, J., (2000), *Causality - Models, Reasoning, and Inference*, Cambridge University Press, ISBN 978-0521773621, New York, USA.

Pearl, J., (2001), *Models, Reasoning and Inference*, Cambridge University Press, Cambridge (2001).

Ryo, M., Maeda, K., Onda, T., Katashima, M., Okumiya, A., Nishida, M., Yamaguchi, T., Funahashi, T., Matsuzawa, Y., Nakamura, T., & Shimomura, I., (2005), A New Simple Method for the Measurement of Visceral Fat Accumulation by Bioelectrical Impedance, *Diabetes Care*, Vol. 28, No. 2, pp. 451-453 (2005)

Scharfetter, H., Schlager, T., Strollberger, R., Felsberger, R., Hutten, H., & Hinghofer-Szalkay, H., (2001), Assessing abdominal fatness with local bioimpedance analysis:

basics and experimental findings, *International Journal of Obesity,* Vol. 25, No. 4, 502-511 (2001)

Scheines, R., Spirtes, P., Glymour, C., Meek, C., & Richardson, T., (1999), Truth is among the Best Explanations : Finding Causal Explanations of Conditional Independence and Dependence, Chapter 5, *Computation, Causation, and Discovery,* AAAI PRESS/The MIT PRESS

Shiga, T., Oshima, Y., Kanai, H., Hirata, M., Hosoda, K., & Nakao, K., A Simple Measurement Method of Visceral Fat Accumulation by Bioelectrical Impedance Analysis, *Proceedings of ICEBI 2007,* IFMBE 17, 687 - 690 (2007)

Shiga, T., Hamaguchi, T., Oshima, Y., Kanai, H., Hirata, M., Hosoda, K., & Nakao, K., A new simple measurement system of visceral fat accumulation by bioelectrical impedance analysis, *Proceedings of WC 2009 IFMBE 25/VII,* pp. 338 – 341 (2009)

Spirtes, P., Glymour, C., & Scheines, R., (2000), *Causation, Prediction, and Search, second edition,* The MIT Press,

Thang, C., Cooper, E.W. & Hoshino, Y.,(2006), A proposed model of diagnosis and prescription in oriental medicine using RBF neural networks, *JACIII* 10(4), 458-464 (2006).

Tsuchiya, N., Yoneda, M., Nakajima, H., Hata, Y., Taniguchi, K., & Sawayama, T., (2007), Fuzzy Extraction Method of Heart Rate by Air-Pressure Sensor," *Proceedings of International Conference on Soft Computing and Human Sciences,* 2-5 (2007)

Tsuchiya, N., Yamamoto, K., Nakajima, H., & Hata, Y., (2008), A Comparative Study of Heart Rate Estimation via Air Pressure Sensor, *Proceedings of 2008 IEEE International Conference on Systems, Man, and Cybernetics,* 3077-3082 (2008)

Tsuchiya, N., Yoneda, M., & Nakajima, H., (2010), Causal-effect structure transformation based on hierarchical representation for biomedical sensing, World Review of Science, Technology and Sustainable Development 2010, 7(1/2) (2010)

Whittaker, J., (1990), *Graphical Models in Applied Multivariate Statistics,* John Wiley & Sons,

Wright, S., (1923), The method of path coefficients, *Annuals Mathematical Statistics,* 5, 161–215

Yamagoe, K. & Togawa, T., "1.4 Perticularity of Bioinstrumentation and Sensing Method," Biomedical Sensors and Instruments, Corona Publishing Co.,Ltd. 2000 (In Japanese)

Yamaguchi, H., Nakajima, H., Taniguchi, K., Kobashi, S., Kondo, K., & Hata, Y., (2007), Fuzzy Detection System of Behavior before Getting Out of Bed by Air Pressure and Ultrasonic Sensors, Proceedings of 2007 IEEE International Conference on Granular Computing, 114-119, (2007)

Yoneda, M., Tasaki, H., Tsuchiya, N., Nakajima, H., Hamaguchi, T., Oku, S., & Shiga,T., (2007), A Study of Bioelectrical Impedance Analysis Methods for Practical Visceral Fat, *Proceedings of 2007 IEEE International Conference on Granular Computing,* pp. 622-627, ISBN , Fremont, California, USA.

Yoneda, M., Tasaki, H., Tsuchiya, N., Nakajima, H., Hamaguchi, T., Oku, S., & Shiga,T., (2008), Development of Visceral Fat Estimation Method based on Bioelectrical Impedance Analysis Method, *Journal of SOFT,* Vol. 20, No. 1, pp. 90-99, ISSN 1347-7986, Japan, (In Japanese).

Zadeh, L.A., (1996), *Fuzzy Sets, Fuzzy Logic, Fuzzy System,* World Scientific Publishing, ISBN 978-9810224226, Singapore.

5

Association of Intimate Partner Physical and Sexual Violence with Childhood Morbidity in Bangladesh

Mosiur Rahman and Golam Mostofa
Department of Population Science and Human Resource Development, University of Rajshahi, Rajshahi Bangladesh

1. Introduction

Although Bangladesh is on track to achieve Millennium Development Goal 4 (MDG4: reduce child mortality, approximately less than 50 per 1000 live births by 2015) (International Center for Diarrheal Disease Research, Bangladesh [ICDDR, B], 2007), child mortality rate still remains very high in this country. In Bangladesh, the mortality rate of under-five children was 65 per 1000 live births in 2007 and diarrhea (20%), acute respiratory infections (ARI) (18%) accounted for 38 % of the under-five deaths (United Nations International Children's Emergency Fund [UNICEF], 2010). Fever, is another symptom of acute infections and malaria among children in Bangladesh and contributes to high levels of malnutrition and mortality (National Institute of Population Research and Training [NIPORT], 2009; Rayhan, Khan, & Shahidullah, 2007).

Although clinical (Haque et al., 2003), nutritional (Daniel et al., 2008; Tomkins, Dunn, & Hayes, 1989), household environmental (Gasana et al., 2002; Cairncross et al., 2010) and socio-demographic (Barros et al., 2010; Rayhan, Khan, & Shahidullah, 2007) risk factors of ARI, diarrhea, and fever are well documented, research has only begun to investigate the influence of other aspects of the social environment. Intimate partner violence (IPV) is defined as the range of sexually, psychologically, and physically coercive acts used against women by current or former male intimate partners (World Health Organization [WHO], 1997). Intimate partner violence is considered to be one of the psychosocial factors that might influence child morbidity status (Campbell 2002). It can affect child morbidity status through psychological stress of the child, resulting from observing IPV; stress in turn can exert an effect on immune reactivity and link to increase vulnerability to illness (Friedman & David, 2002). Besides, IPV can affect child health outcome through direct violence, injury, and mistreatment of children from fathers who abuse their female partners (Herrenkohl et al., 2008; Christian et al., 1997), or through physical or psychological maternal health outcomes such as stress and depression, suicidal thoughts and infectious diseases including HIV/AIDS (Ellsberg et al., 2008; Sutherland, Bybee, & Sullivan, 1998; Coker et al., 2002; Silverman et al., 2007; Silverman et al., 2008) or through diminishing mother's autonomy, social isolation, and lack of control over financial resources (Ellsberg et al., 2008; Smith & Martin, 1995; Forte et al., 1996), that can prevent proper care of the child.

Within and outside of South Asia, increasing evidence has shown a linkage between high rates of IPV among women (IPV; 18%-66%) (Bates et al., 2004; Bhuiya, Sharmin & Hanifi, 2003; Jain et al., 2004) and poor child health outcomes, such as miscarriage (Silverman et al., 2007; Bair-Merritt, Blackstone, & Feudtner, 2006), child under-nutrition (Ackerson & Subramanian, 2008; Hasselmann & Reichenheim, 2006), and infant and child mortality Jejeebhoy, 1998; Ahmed, Koenig, & Stephenson, 2006; Leland KA &Subramanian, 2009). However, the literature on consequences of IPV on young children's morbidity pattern is limited, and weaknesses in methodology. Within South Asia a recent investigation in India indicates an association between IPV and childhood asthma (Subramanian, Ackerson, & Subramanyam, 2007). Another study found that young children of Bangladeshi women abused by their husbands were more likely to be at risk of ARI and diarrhea diseases (Silverman et al., 2009). Outside the region of South Asia, a recent study in Uganda supports that the history of women subjected to IPV predicts the risk of diarrhea and overall illness of the infant (Karamagi et al., 2007). However, most of these studies have some methodological weaknesses such as based on community specific small samples or based on husband's report of IPV or measured only the physical type of IPV by using single global question. This lack has limited our understanding of the extent to which childhood morbidity may be affected by the physical and sexual IPV, using the multiple, behaviorally specific questions based on women's report of IPV. Thus, this study, aimed to examine the association of physical and sexual forms of IPV with childhood fever, ARI, and diarrheal morbidity in a nationally representative sample in Bangladesh.

2. Methods

2.1 Data sources

The present study used data from the 2007 Bangladesh Demographic Health Survey (BDHS), conducted by the National Institute for Population Research and Training of the Ministry of Health and Family Welfare of Bangladesh from March 24 to August 11, 2007. The BDHS sample was drawn from Bangladeshi adults residing in private dwellings. A stratified, multistage cluster sample of 361 primary sampling units was constructed (134 in urban areas and 227 in rural areas). The primary sampling units were sourced from a sampling frame created for the 2001 census of Bangladesh, in which they were termed "enumeration areas".

The 2007 BDHS used five questionnaires. Of the 11,178 women deemed eligible to participate in the women's questionnaire on maternal and child health behaviors and outcomes, 10,996 participated (98.4% response rate). One woman from each household was selected at random for the domestic violence module to answer an additional set of questions regarding IPV perpetrated by her husband. Out of 4,489 women eligible to respond to the domestic violence module, only seven had to be excluded due to lack of privacy. An additional 15 women were not interviewed for other reasons. The present analyses included only currently married women aged 15-49 years with at least one singleton child below five years of age living with the respondent (n=1851) **(Figure 1).**

2.2 Outcome measures

To provide an assessment of child morbidity outcomes we analyzed three common childhood illness: diarrhea, ARI and fever, assessed via responses to the BDHS questionnaire given to women. For each child under five years of age, women indicated whether the child had been ill with fever, experienced an episode of diarrhea, and ill with a cough accompanied by short, rapid breathing in the 2 weeks prior to the survey. A symptom of ARI was defined as report of cough accompanied by short, rapid breathing. Binary variables were created to define diarrhea, ARI and fever, which indicated the presence of each of these outcomes among the children in the past 2 weeks. A binary variable was also created to assess the overall level of illness in the child, which was dichotomized into "0" no illness and "1" as illness (combined fever, ARI and diarrhea).

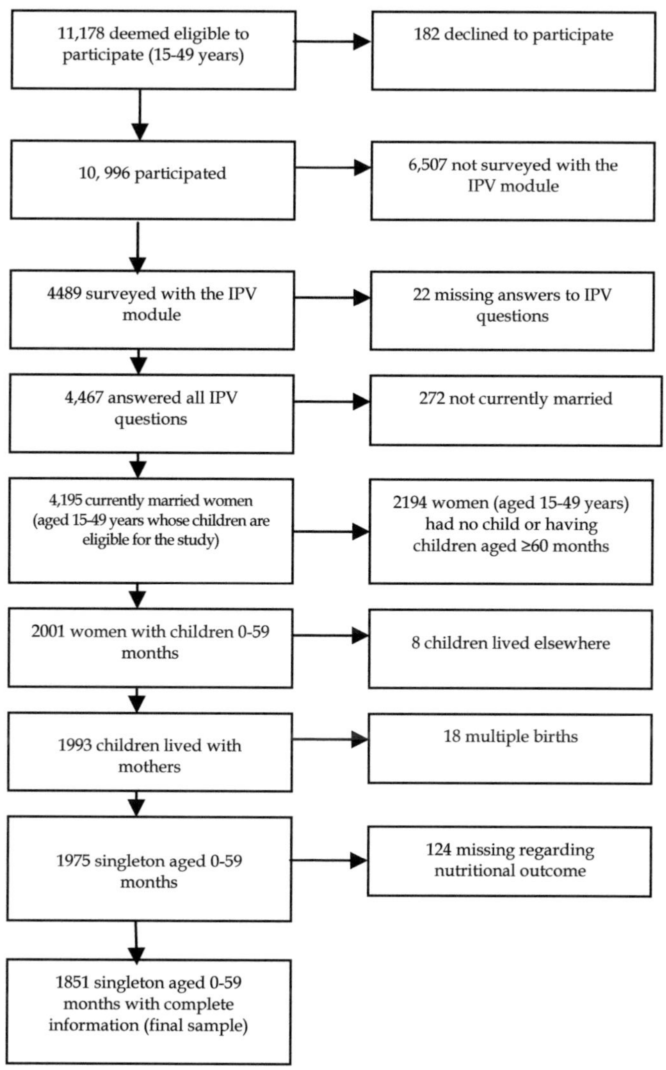

Fig. 1. Selection of sample

2.3 Exposures

Women's experience of IPV was the main exposure of interest in this study. The BDHS measured IPV using a shortened and modified Conflict Tactics Scale (CTS) (Straus, 1979;

Straus & Gelles, 1990). Perpetration of IPV by the husband in the year prior to the survey was assessed via 8 items included in the survey given to the women. A positive response to any one of the following behaviors indicated the perpetration of physical IPV: (1) pushing, shaking, or throwing an object; (2) slapping; (3) twisting her arm or pulling her hair; (4) punching or hitting with a fist or something harmful; (5) kicking or dragging; (6) choking or burning; or (7) threatening or attacking with a knife or gun. Perpetration of sexual IPV was indicated by a positive response to 'physically forcing her to have sexual intercourse even when she did not want to'. These assessments were recorded to create a four-level categorical variable reflecting the experiences of three categories of IPV: physical IPV only, sexual IPV only, and both physical and sexual IPV. The fourth category was a referent group of no IPV perpetration of either form. We also created a binary variable measuring whether a mother reported any form of IPV (physical, sexual or both); this was termed "any IPV". Though psychological violence is one of the important indicators of all IPV incidents (Leland & Subramanian, 2009) this information was not available in the current study, as it was not collected in the BDHS.

2.4 Covariates

We included several socio-demographic, environmental and nutritional variables theoretically and empirically linked to IPV (Uthman, Lawoko,& Moradi T, 2009; Bates et al., 2004) and common childhood illness (Rayhan, Khan, & Shahidullah, 2007; Daniel et al., 2008; Tomkins, Dunn, & Hayes, 1989; Gasana et al., 2002; Cairncross e al., 2010; Barros et al., 2010).These variables included: maternal age (15-24 years, 25-34 years or 35-49 years), maternal education (no education, primary or secondary and higher), maternal decision making autonomy, mother's occupation (unemployed or agriculture/non-manual or manual), mother's BMI (thin, normal or overweight), residence (rural or urban), household members (2-4, 5-6 or 7+), parity (1, 2 or 3+), wealth index, type of cooking fuel (biomass/charcoal or LPG/natural gas/biogas), child sex (male or female), child's age (0-11 months, 12-23 months, 24-35 months or 36-59 months), initiation of breastfeeding (early or late), and duration of breastfeeding (0-11 months, 12-23 months or ≥24 months). We used BDHS wealth index as a proxy indicator for socioeconomic position. The BDHS wealth index was constructed from data on household assets, including ownership of durable goods (such as televisions and bicycles) and dwelling characteristics (such as source of drinking water, sanitation facilities, and construction materials). Principal components analysis was used to assign individual household wealth scores. These weighted values were then summed and rescaled to range from 0 to 1, and each household was assigned to either the poorest, middle, or richest tertials.

2.5 Statistical analyses

We calculated descriptive statistics for socio-demographic, environmental, IPV, nutritional, and morbidity characteristics for our sample. Demographic and socio-economic differences of any physical or sexual IPV perpetration were assessed by $\chi 2$ analyses. The 2-tailed significance level for all analyses was $p < .05$. We created 2 fully adjusted models to analyze the appropriate binary for each morbidity outcome of diarrhea, ARI, fever, and any illness (any vs. no IPV; and the separate effects of physical only, sexual only and both physical and sexual IPV). We entered all covariates simultaneously in the multiple regression models. Adjusted odds rations (AOR) were estimated to understand the strength of the associations while 95% confidence intervals (95% CI) were estimated for significance testing. Multicolinearity in the logistic regression analyses was checked by examining the standard errors for the regression coefficients. A standard error larger than 2.0 indicates numerical problems, such as multicollinearity among the independent variables (Chan, 2004). In this study, all of the independent variables in the two models for each nutritional outcome had a standard error <0.90 indicating an absence of multicolinearity. Stata, version 9.0 (Stata Corp., College Station, TX, USA) with survey commands was used to account for stratification, clustered sampling, and weighing provided by the BDHS to reproduce the national population.

2.6 Ethical considerations

Data collection procedures for the BDHS were approved by the ORC Macro Institutional Review Board. Several specific protections based on WHO"s ethical and safety recommendations for research on domestic violence were built into the 2007 BDHS (Straus, 1979; WHO, 2001). For the domestic violence section, respondents were read an additional statement informing them that the questions to follow could be sensitive and reassuring them of the confidentiality of their responses (NIPORT, 2009). Interviews were conducted under the most private conditions afforded by the environments encountered. If privacy could not be ensured, the interviewer was instructed to skip the module.

3. Results

3.1 Descriptive statistics

Nearly half of the women (49.1%) were 15-24 years old, 29.2% were uneducated, and 78.5% lived in rural areas **(Table 1)**. About 11% of the respondents had no decision-making autonomy. Regarding nutritional status, 60.3% women were considered to have normal BMI; 32.0% were undernourished or thin (BMI less than 18.5); and 7.5% were overweight or obese (BMI 25 or higher). From the total sample population, 69.9% of children were below three years of age, nearly half were female and 42.8% of the children were breastfed for 24 months or more, and only 8.8% used LPG/natural gas/biogas as cooking fuel.

The prevalence of underweight, stunting, and wasting was 40.8%, 42.0%, and 19.0% respectively, while the prevalence of diarrhea, fever, and ARI was 10.1%, 38.7%, and 13.3% respectively. Overall, 45.6% children were suffering from any type of illness (diarrhea or ARI or fever) two weeks before the survey. Substantial numbers of mothers (29.0%) reported that they had suffered any IPV in the year prior to the survey; 15.5% of mothers indicated that they had experienced only physical IPV, 6.2% indicated that they had experienced only sexual IPV, and 7.3% indicated that they had experienced both types of IPV **(Table 1)**.

In bivariate analysis, several significant differences were observed in the prevalence of IPV perpetration across various socio-demographic groups **(Table 2)**. Specifically, significantly a higher prevalence of perpetration of any form of IPV, physical IPV only and both physical and sexual IPV was identified among younger women (aged 15-24 years) and women who used LPG/natural gas/biogas as cooking fuel compared with older women and women used Biomass/charcoal as cooking fuel. Regarding educational status, significantly a higher prevalence of any form of IPV and past-year perpetration of both physical and sexual IPV was identified among women having no education. Significantly a higher prevalence of any form of IPV and past-year perpetration of both physical and sexual IPV was also identified among women having children suffering from any types of recent illness.

Characteristics	n*	% (95% CI)†
Maternal age		
15-24 y	816	49.0 (46.2-51.9)
25-34 y	840	41.2 (38.5-44.1)
35-49 y	195	9.7 (8.2-11.4)
Maternal education		
No education	565	29.2 (26.7-31.9)
Primary	511	27.0 (24.6-29.6)
Secondary and higher	775	43.8 (41.0-46.6)
Maternal decision making autonomy (aspects)*		
0	223	11.0 (9.-13.0)
1	126	6.9 (5.5-8.4)
2	199	11.8 (9.9-14.1)
3	272	15.1 (12.9-17.4)
4	308	16.3 (14.4-18.5)
5	721	38.9 (36.0-41.9)
Missing data	2	
Mother's BMI		
Thin (BMI<18.5)	591	32.0 (29.3-34.9)
Normal (BMI 18.5-24.9)	1088	60.4 (57.7-63.2)
Overweight/obese	167	7.6 (6.2-9.8)
(BMI≥25)	5	
Missing data		
Residence		
Rural	1200	78.5 (76.3-80.6)
Urban	651	21.5 (19.4-23.7)
Household members (tertiles)		
2-4	627	30.4 (27.8-33.1)
5-6	716	36.6 (33.8-39.6)
7+	508	33.0 (30.1-35.9)
Parity		
1	546	33.7 (30.9-36.6)
2	556	28.7 (26.4-31.3)
3+	749	37.5 (35.1-40.1)
Occupation of respondents		
Unemployed	1322	69.6 (66.9-72.3)
Agriculture/non-manual	369	22.7 (20.4-25.2)
labor	157	7.7 (6.2-9.1)
Manual works	3	
Missing data		
Type of cooking fuel		
Biomass/charcoal	1621	91.2 (0.89-92.7)
LPG/natural gas/biogas	224	8.8 (7.3-10.6)
Missing data	6	
Wealth index		
Poor	812	46.0 (43.1-49.0)
Middle	317	16.7 (14.8-18.8)
Rich	722	37.3 (34.4-40.2)

Characteristics	n*	% (95% CI)†
Child age		
0-11 m	440	24.5 (22.1-27.1)
12-23 m	436	24.4 (22.0-26.9)
24-35 m	394	21.0 (18.9-23.3)
36-59 m	581	30.1 (27.6-32.8)
Child sex		
Female	931	49.9 (47.0-52.8)
Male	920	50.1 (47.2-53.0)
Initiation of breastfeeding¥		
Early	635	34.2 (31.6-36.8)
Late	1212	65.8 (63.2-68.4)
Missing data	4	
Duration of breastfeeding		
0-11 m	497	27.7 (25.2-30.2)
12-23 m	528	29.5 (27.0-32.2)
≥24 m	824	42.8 (40.2-45.5)
Missing data	2	
Diarrhea in the past 2 weeks		
No	1665	89.9 (88.2-91.4)
Yes	195	10.1 (8.6-11.8)
Fever in the past 2 weeks		
No	1140	61.3 (58.4-64.2)
Yes	711	38.7(35.8-41.6)
Symptoms of ARI		
No	592	86.7 (84.6-88.4)
Yes	259	13.3 (11.6-15.4)
Any illness		
No	1007	54.4 (51.3-57.3)
Yes	844	45.6 (42.7-48.9)
Stunting		
No	1081	58.0 (55.4-61.1)
Yes	770	42.0 (38.8-44.5)
Underweight		
No	1099	59.2 (56.3-62.2)
Yes	752	40.8 (38.0-43.7)
Wasting		
No	1504	81.0 (78.4-83.3)
Yes	347	19.0 (16.7-21.6)
Any physical or sexual IPV		
No	1290	71.0 (68.4-73.4)
Yes	559	29.0 (26.6-31.6)
Missing data	2	
Types of IPV		
None	1290	71.0 (68.4-73.4)
Physical only	315	15.5 (13.6-17.6)
Sexual only	106	6.2 (5.0-7.8)
Both physical and sexual	138	7.3 (5.9-8.9)
Missing data	2	

† Unweighted n's and † weighted percentages (%, 95% CI) presented

* Number of decisions in which women could participate: alone or jointly with husband/partner or other person

¥ Early: initiation of breastfeeding within one hour of birth

Table 1. Socio-demographic, Nutritional, and IPV Characteristics of Currently Married Mothers of Under-five Children (n=1851)

Across wealth categories, wealthier married women were less likely to report past-year perpetration of any form of IPV, physical IPV alone, sexual IPV alone, and past-year perpetration of both physical and sexual IPV. Significantly, a higher prevalence of any form of IPV and physical IPV alone was observed among women considered to have thin BMI and mothers with household"s member size 2-4. In addition, lower proportion of experiencing any form of IPV and sexual IPV alone was observed among unemployed women. A higher prevalence of perpetration of any form of IPV in the past year was identified among women having five aspects of decision-making autonomy, but these differences were not significant for the three mutually exclusive categories of violence assessed **(Table 2)**.

Characteristics	**Any form of IPV % (95% CI)**	**Physical IPV only % (95% CI)**	**Sexual IPV only % (95% CI)**	**Both physical and sexual % (95% CI)**
Maternal age				
15-24 y	33.8 (29.7-38.1)	18.0 (14.9-21.6)	6.9 (4.9-9.7)	8.9 (6.6-11.8)
25-34 y	24.6 (21.5-27.9)	14.0 (11.5-16.9)	5.6 (4.0-7.6)	5.1 (3.6-7.9)
35-49 y	24.1 (17.6-31.9)	9.5 (5.9-15.0)	5.8 (2.7-12.0)	8.7 (5.1-14.6)
p value	0.001	0.018	0.652	0.031
Maternal education				
No education	34.8 (30.5-39.4)	18.4 (15.1-22.2)	6.8 (4.6-9.9)	9.6 (6.9-13.2)
Primary	28.1 (23.5-33.2)	15.2 (11.6-19.7)	5.1 (3.2-8.1)	7.7 (5.3-11.2)
Secondary and higher	25.8 (22.0-30.0)	13.8 (11.0-17.1)	6.6 (4.6-9.4)	5.4 (3.6-8.1)
p value	0.014	0.17	0.635	0.048
Maternal decision making autonomy (aspects)				
0	29.9 (22.6-38.5)	13.8 (8.6-21.3)	8.0 (4.1-15.0)	8.1 (4.7-13.7)
1	38.9 (28.7-50.2)	17.8 (10.9-27.7)	11.7 (6.4-20.7)	9.4 (4.2-19.7)
2	28.0 (20.4-37.1)	16.7 (10.5-25.6)	2.9 (12.9-6.5)	8.3 (4.4-15.1)
3	31.2 (24.5-38.7)	15.6 (11.3-21.1)	6.4 (3.6-11.1)	9.1 (5.4-14.9)
4	34.6 (28.7-41.2)	18.9 (14.6-24.0)	8.3 (4.8-14.1)	7.5 (4.4-12.3)
5	24.2 (20.8-28.1)	13.8 (11.2-16.9)	4.9 (3.2-7.3)	5.6 (3.9-7.9)
p value	0.038	0.617	0.081	0.621
Mother's BMI				
Thin (BMI<18.5)	33.4 (29.1-37.9)	18.5 (15.4-22.0)	7.6 (5.3-10.7)	7.3 (5.2-10.2)
Normal (BMI 18.5-24.9)	28.5 (25.1-32.2)	14.9 (12.3-17.9)	5.8 (4.2-7.9)	7.9 (6.0-10.3)
Overweight/obese (BMI≥25)	15.1 (9.5-23.2)	8.4 (4.4-15.3)	4.7 (1.8-11.6)	2.1 (0.9-4.8)
p value	0.002	0.030	0.421	0.062
Residence				
Rural	30.1 (27.4-33.0)	16.0 (13.8-18.4)	6.7 (5.2-8.7)	7.4 (5.8-9.4)
Urban	25.1 (21.0-29.6)	13.8 (11.0-17.3)	4.4 (2.9-6.8)	6.8 (4.6-9.9)
p value	0.050	0.266	0.104	0.701
Household members				
(tertiles)	36.7 (31.9-41.8)	23.1 (19.1-27.5)	4.9 (3.2-7.5)	8.7 (6.3-12.0)
2-4	28.3 (24.5-32.3)	15.1 (12.4-18.4)	5.7 (4.0-8.0)	7.4 (5.3-10.4)
5-6	22.8 (18.3-27.9)	8.9 (6.4-12.4)	8.0 (5.3-12.1)	5.8 (3.6-9.1)
7+	<0.001	<0.001	0.208	0.336
p value				
Parity				
1	32.2 (27.3-37.6)	17.8 (14.0-22.4)	6.6 (4.2-10.3)	7.9 (5.6-10.9)
2	28.9 (24.6-33.6)	15.2 (12.0-19.1)	5.7 (3.8-8.5)	7.8 (5.1-11.6)
3+	26.3 (22.8-30.1)	13.6 (11.1-16.7)	6.3 (4.5-8.8)	6.4 (4.6-8.8)
p value	0.169	0.235	0.885	0.642
Occupation of respondents				
Unemployed	26.8 (24.1-29.7)	15.1 (12.8-17.7)	4.5 (3.2-6.2)	7..3 (5.7-9.2)
Agriculture/non-manual labor	35.8 (29.9-42.3)	18.6 (14.5-23.5)	9.7 (6.6-14.1)	7.5 (4.5-12.1)
Manual works	28.4 (20.1-37.9)	10.4 (6.6-15.8)	11.4 (6.4-19.7)	6.7 (2.3-14.6)
p value	0.018	0.083	0.001	0.970

Characteristics	Any form of IPV % (95% CI)	Physical IPV only % (95% CI)	Sexual IPV only % (95% CI)	Both physical and sexual % (95% CI)
Wealth index				
Poor	35.6 (31.9-39.5)	18.5 (15.8-21.5)	7.8 (5.9-10.4)	9.3 (7.0-12.2)
Middle	27.4 (22.1-33.4)	15.6 (11.6-20.7)	4.1 (2.2-7.8)	7.6 (4.7-12.3)
Rich	21.7 (17.9-26.1)	11.8 (9.1-15.3)	5.2 (3.3-8.1)	4.6 (2.9-7.2)
p value	<0.001	0.007	0.049	0.025
Type of cooking fuel				
Biomass/charcoal	30.8 (28.0-33.6)	17.3 (15.1-19.7)	5.2 (4.6-6.7)	8.3 (6.7-10.2)
LPG/natural gas/biogas	15.0 (9.7-22.5)	7.9 (4.8-12.7)	6.5 (2.9-14.2)	0.57 (0.08-3.9)
p value	<0.001	0.001	0.589	<0.001
Child sex				
Female	26.9 (23.7-30.4)	14.7 (12.2-17.7)	5.5 (3.9-7.7)	6.7 (5.0-9.0)
Male	31.1 (27.5-35.0)	16.3 (13.4-19.6)	7.0 (5.1-9.4)	7.8 (5.8-10.6)
p value	0.105	0.478	0.303	0.485
Child age				
0-11 m	27.3 (22.3-33.0)	13.4 (10.3-17.2)	8.0 (5.0.3-12.5)	6.0 (3.7-9.4)
12-23 m	33.6 (28.3-39.4)	18.1 (14.1-22.9)	6.7 (4.1-10.8)	8.8 (5.7-13.4)
24-35 m	26.6 (21.8-32.1)	17.8 (13.8-22.7)	3.2 (1.7-6.0)	5.6 (3.7-8.4)
36-49 m	28.4 (23.8-33.6)	13.6 (10.3-17.7)	6.6 (4.7-9.2)	8.2 (5.8-11.5)
p value	0.274	0.177	0.162	0.333
Initiation of breastfeeding				
Early	28.6 (25.6-31.7)	15.8 (12.5-19.7)	7.1 (5.1-9.8)	7.1 (5.0-9.9)
Late	30.0 (25.9-34.4)	15.3 (13.1-17.8)	5.8 (4.3-7.8)	7.4 (5.7-9.6)
p value	0.594	0.833	0.348	0.816
Duration of breastfeeding				
0-11 m	26.2 (21.6-31.5)	12.8 (9.9-16.3)	7.4 (4.7-11.5)	6.1 (3.9-9.4)
12-23 m	30.9 (26.2-36.0)	16.6 (13.2-20.7)	5.4 (3.3-8.7)	8.9 (6.1-12.7)
≥24 m	29.3 (25.5-33.4)	16.6 (13.6-20.1)	5.8 (4.3-7.9)	6.9 (5.0-9.5)
p value	0.429	0.227	0.579	0.398
Total	29.0 (26.6-31.6)	15.5 (13.6-17.6)	6.2 (5.0-7.8)	7.3 (5.9-8.9)

Table 2. Descriptive Statistics According to Different Forms of IPV of Currently Married Mothers of Under-five Children (n=1851)

4. Association between IPV and child morbidity

4.1 IPV and diarrheal morbidity

Maternal experience of any physical or sexual IPV (AOR: 1.50; 95% CI: 1.04–2.27) was associated childhood diarrheal morbidity; as were physical IPV only (AOR: 1.35; 95% CI: 1.01–2.30) and both physical and sexual IPV (AOR: 2.38; 95% CI: 1.32-4.31) **(Table 3).**

4.2 IPV and symptoms of ARI

Maternal experience of any physical or sexual IPV (AOR: 1.46; 95% CI: 1.02–2.12) was associated with ARI morbidity; as were physical IPV only (AOR: 1.72; 95% CI: 1.13-2.64) and both physical and sexual IPV (AOR: 1.83; 95% CI: 1.03-3.37) **(Table 3)**.

4.3 IPV and childhood fever

Maternal experience of any physical or sexual IPV (AOR: 1.30; 95% CI: 1.00–1.72) and both physical and sexual IPV (AOR: 1.90; 95% CI: 1.19-3.03) were associated with fever among children **(Table 3)**.

4.4 IPV and any childhood illness

Maternal experience of any physical or sexual IPV (AOR: 1.38; 95% CI: 1.05–1.80) and both physical and sexual IPV (AOR: 2.21; 95% CI: 1.37-3.60) were associated with any illness among children **(Table 3)**.

Measure of Maternal IPV	AOR (95% CI)			
	Diarrhea	**ARI**	**Fever**	**Any illness**
Types of IPV				
None (reference)	1.00	1.00	1.00	1.00
Any physical or sexual	1.50 (1.04-2.27)	1.46 (1.02-2.12)	1.30 (1.00-1.72)	1.38 (1.05-1.80)
Physical only	1.35 (1.01-2.30)	1.72 (1.13-2.64)	1.21 (0.87-1.68)	1.28 (0.93-1.77)
Sexual only	0.97 (0.43-2.20)	0.59 (0.28-1.25)	1.00 (0.57-1.76)	0.97 (0.56-1.66)
Both physical and sexual violence	2.38 (1.32-4.31)	1.83 (1.03-3.37)	1.90 (1.19-3.03)	2.21 (1.37-3.60)

Models were adjusted for maternal age, maternal education, maternal decision making autonomy, mother's occupation, mother's BMI, parity, residence, household members, child sex, child age, initiation of breastfeeding, duration of breastfeeding,, types of cooking fuel, stunting, underweight, wasting, and wealth index.

Table 3. Adjusted ORs and 95% CIs for Associations between Different Aspects of Maternal IPV and Morbidity Status for Children Under-five Years (n=1851)

5. Discussion

The findings of this study revealed that approximately one-third (29.0%) of currently married Bangladeshi women with children below the age of five years experienced any form of physical or sexual IPV in the past year. In Bangladesh, maternal experience of any physical or sexual IPV was associated with increased risk of diarrhea, ARI, fever, and any illness in children aged younger than five years. The findings of an increased risk of childhood diarrhea and ARI of abused women was in accordance with previous reports in Bangladesh (Silverman et al., 2009) of an association between physical or sexual partner violence and diarrhea and ARI of the child. Other study outside South Asia (Karamagi et al., 2007) found mixed evidence for an association between maternal lifetime IPV and common childhood illness. The current research expands on these previous two studies by using a large national sample from Bangladesh and added information on the association between maternal physical or sexual IPV and all common childhood illness.

Another important new finding was that a combination of both physical and sexual IPV appeared to have more profound consequences on the outcome measured. Previous studies found that experienced of both physical and sexual IPV are stronger predictors of long-term negative physical and mental health outcomes of mothers (Ferri et al., 2007; Peter, 2004; Cripe et al., 2008; Bizu et al., 2010). Its impact on mental health can be as serious as its physical impact, and may be equally long lasting. Evidence has shown that such negative physical and mental health outcomes reduce a mother's ability to cope with the everyday needs of a small child and diminish the quality of different care-giving behaviors; this in turn leads to the negative health consequences for her children (Marie, Carol, & Armar-Klemesu, 1999; Stewart, 2007). Our results, therefore, indicate that the prevention of both physical and sexual violence from husbands is important for the improvement of childhood morbidity status in Bangladesh.

Currently identified associations of any physical or sexual IPV with all common childhood illness provide a critical context for the elevated rates of infant and early childhood deaths demonstrated in prior work (Jejeebhoy, 1998; Ahmed, Koenig, Stephenson, 2006; Leland & Subramanian, 2009) among women who experience IPV (i.e., the currently documented increased rates of diarrhea, ARI and fever likely relate to increased risk of child death).

Some limitations should be considered when interpreting our findings. First, the current analyses are cross-sectional and, thus, do not allow for assessment of the chronology of the associated events or inferences regarding causality. Longitudinal research regarding the relations of IPV to childhood morbidity outcomes is needed to provide clarity regarding these concerns. Second, though psychological violence is an important fact of IPV (Leland & Subramanian, 2009), this information was not available in the current study. Finally, the possibility of underreporting must also be considered; because IPV is by nature a private phenomenon and one that is often stigmatized, women may be reluctant to reveal their abuse status. However, the personal interview method used in this study is widely used for this type of IPV research (Fried at al., 2006). In addition, to ascertain physical and sexual IPV, this study used multiple, behaviorally-specific questions, which are considered the best, methodologically, for eliciting correct responses (Leland & Subramanian, 2009; Straus, 1979).Moreover, according to the BDHS interviewers were provided training for implementing the domestic violence module based on a training manual specially developed to enable the field staff to collect violence data in a secure, confidential, and ethical manner, in order to create a safe atmosphere in which respondents would feel comfortable discussing this issue (NIPORT, 2009). In addition, the domestic violence module was administered at the end of the interview, so that both interviewers and respondents become well acquainted with each other by the time they reach the section on domestic violence.

6. Conclusion

In conclusion any physical or sexual IPV was associated with the increased risk of all common childhood illness namely, diarrhea, ARI and fever among children below five years of age in Bangladesh. In interventions aimed at improving child morbidity status, efforts are needed to protect women from the physical and sexual violence of their husbands. These findings may be relevant in other resource-limited settings as well where the prevalence of child morbidity is high and may be of interest to clinicians when assessing children with different problems related to morbidity status. Future longitudinal studies, however, are needed for assessment of the chronology of the associated child morbidity or inferences regard.

7. Financial disclosure

The authors have indicated they have no financial relationships relevant to this article to disclose.

8. Conflict of interest

None

9. Acknowledgements

We are grateful to the MEASURE DHS for providing us with the data set. In addition, we would like to acknowledge all individuals and institutions in Bangladesh involved in the implementation of the 2007 BDHS.

10. References

Ackerson, L.K., Subramanian. S.V. (2008). Domestic violence and chronic malnutrition among women and children in India. *Am J Epidemil,* 167, 1188-96.

Ahmed, S., Koenig, M.A., & Stephenson, R. (2006). Effects of domestic violence on perinatal and early-childhood mortality: evidence from north India. *Am J Public Health,* 96, 1423-1428.

Bair-Merritt, M.H., Blackstone, M., & Feudtner, C. (2006). Physical health outcomes of childhood exposure to intimate partner violence: a systematic review. *Pediatrics,* 117, e278-e290.

Barros, F.C., Victora, C.G., Scherpbier, R., Gwatkin, D. (2010). Socioeconomic inequities in the health and nutrition of children in low/middle income countries. *Rev Saúde Pública,* 44, 1-16.

Bates, L.M., Schuler, S.R., Islam, F., & Islam, M.K. (2004). Socioeconomic factors and processes associated with domestic violence in rural Bangladesh. *Int Fam Plan Perspect,* 30, 190-199.

Bhuiya, A., Sharmin, T., & Hanifi, S.M.A. (2003). Nature of domestic violence against women in a rural area of Bangladesh: implication for preventive interventions. *J Health Popul Nutr,* 21, 48-54.

Bizu, g., Nelly, L., Cripe, S.M., & Sanchez, S.E., Williams, M.A. (2010). Correlates of Violent Response Among Peruvian Women Abused by an Intimate Partner. *Interpers Violence,* 25, 136-151.

Cairncross, S., Hunt, C., Boisson, S., Bostoen, K., Curtis, V., Fung, CH., & Schmidt, W.P. (2010). Water, sanitation and hygiene for the prevention of diarrhea. *Int J Epidemiol*,39,193-205.

Campbell, J.C. (2002). Health consequences of intimate partner violence. *Lancet,* 359, 1331–1336.

Chan, Y.H. (2004). Biostatistics: logistic regression analysis. *Singapore Med J,* 45, 149.

Christian, C.W., Scribano, P., Seidl, T., & Pinto-Martin, J.A. (1997). Pediatric injury resulting from family violence. *Pediatrics,* 99, e8.

Coker, A.L., Davis, K.E., Arias, I., et al. (2002). Physical and mental health effects of intimate partner violence for men and women. *Am J Preventat Med,* 23, 260e8.

Cripe, S.M., Sanchez, S.E., Perales, M.T., Lam, N., Garcia, P., & Williams, M.A. (2008). Association of intimate partner physical and sexual violence with unintended pregnancy among pregnant women in Peru. *Int J Gynaecol Obstet*,100, 104-8.

Daniel, E.R., Laura, E.C., Ezzati, M., & Black, R.E. (2008). Acute lower respiratory infections in childhood: opportunities for reducing the global burden through nutritional interventions. *Bull World Health Organ,* 86, 321-416.

Ellsberg, M., Jansen, H.A., Heise, L., Watts, C.H., & Garcia-Moreno. C. (2008). WHO Multicountry Study on Women's Health and Domestic Violence Against Women Study Team. Intimate partner violence and women's physical and mental health in the WHO multi-country study on women's health and domestic violence: an observational study. *Lancet,* 371, 1165-1172.

Ferri, P.C., Sandro, S.M., Marina, C.M.B., Elisa, C., Guinsburg, R., Patel, V., Martin, P., & Ronaldo, L. (2007). The impact of maternal experience of violence and common mental disorders on neonatal outcomes: a survey of adolescent mothers in Sao Paulo, Brazil. *BMC Public Health,* 7, 209. doi: 10.1186/1471-2458-7-209.

Forte, J.A., Franks, D.D., Forte, J.A., & Rigsby, D. (1996). Asymmetric role-taking: comparing battered and non-battered women. *Soc Work,* 41, 59-73.

Fried, L.E., Aschengrau, A., Cabral, H., Amaro, H. (2006). Comparison of Maternal interview a medical record ascertainment of violence among women who has poor pregnancy outcomes. *Matern Chil Health J,* 10, 451-460.

Friedman, E.M., & David, A.L. (2002). Environmental stress mediates changes in neuroimmunological interactions. *Toxicol Sci,* 67, 4-10.

Gasana, J., Morin, J., Ndikuyeze, A., & Kamoso, P. (2002). Impact of water supply and sanitation on diarrheal morbidity among young children in the socioeconomic and cultural context of Rwanda (Africa). *Environ Res,* 90, 76-88.

Haque, R., Mondal, D., Beth, D., Akther, S., Farr, B.M., Sack, R.B., & Petri, W.A. (2003). Epidemiologic and clinical characteristics of acute diarrhea with emphasis on entamoeba histolytica infections in preschool children in an urban slum of Dhaka, Bangladesh. *Am. J. Trop. Med. Hyg,* 69, 398-405.

Hasselmann, M.H., & Reichenheim, M.E. (2006). Parental violence and the occurrence of severe and acute malnutrition in childhood. *Paediatr Perinat Epidemiol,* 20, 299-311.

Herrenkohl, T.I., Sousa, C., Tajima, E.A., Herrenkohl, R.C., & Moylan, C.A. (2008). Intersection of child abuse and children's exposure to domestic violence. *Trauma Violence Abuse,* 9, 84–99.

ICDDR, B (2007). *MDG 4 Reduce child mortality: annual report 2007.* ICDDRB: Center for Health and Population Research. Dhaka, Bangladesh.

Jain, D., Sanon, S., Sadowski, L., & Hunter, W. (2004). Violence against women in India: evidence from rural Maharashtra, India. *Rural Remote Health,* 4, 304.

Jejeebhoy, S.J. (1998). Associations between wife-beating and fetal and infant death: impressions from a survey in rural India. *Stud Fam Plann,* 29,300-308.

Karamagi, C.A., Tumwine, J.K., Tylleskar, T., Heggenhougen, K. (2007). Intimate partner violence and infant morbidity: evidence of an association from a population-based study in eastern Uganda in 2003. *BMC Pediatr,* 7; 7, 34. doi:10.1186/1471-2431-7-34.

Leland, K.A., & Subramanian, S.V. (2009). Intimate partner violence and death among infants and children in India. *Pediatrics,* 124, e878-e889.

Marie, T.R., Carol, E.L., & Armar-Klemesu, M. (1999). *Good care practices can mitigate the negative effects of poverty and low maternal schooling on children's nutritional status: evidence from Accra.* FCND Discussion paper, No.2. Food Consumption and Nutrition Division, New York, U.S.A; International Food Policy Research Institute.

NIPORT (2009). *Bangladesh Demographic and Health Survey 2007.* Dhaka, Bangladesh and Calverton, Maryland, USA: National Institute of Population Research and Training, Mitra and Associates, and Macro International.

Peter, B. (2004). Lone mothers' experience of physical and sexual violence: association with psychiatric disorders. *Br J Psychiatry,* 184, 21-27.

Rayhan, M.I., Khan, M.S.H., & Shahidullah, M. (2007). Impacts of bio-social factors on morbidity among children aged under-5 in Bangladesh. *Asia-Pacific Population Journal,* 22, 65-75.

Silverman, J.G., Decker, M.R., Kapur, N.A., Gupta, J., & Raj, A. (2007). Violence against wives, sexual risk and sexually transmitted infection among Bangladeshi men. *Sex Transm Infect,* 83, 211-215.

Silverman, J.G., Gupta, J., Decker, M.R., Kapur, N., & Raj, A. (2007). Intimate partner violence and unwanted pregnancy, miscarriage, induced abortion, and stillbirth among a national sample of Bangladeshi women. *BJOG,* 114, 1246-1252.

Silverman, J.G., Michele, R.D., Gupta, J., Kapur, N., Raj, A., & Naved, R.T. (2009). Maternal experiences of intimate partner violence and child morbidity in Bangladesh: evidence from a national Bangladeshi sample. *Arch Pediatr Adolesc Med,* 163, 700-705.

Silverman, J.G., Michele, R.D., Niranjan, S., et al. (2008). Married Indian Women Intimate Partner Violence and HIV Infection Among. *JAMA,* 300, 703-710.

Smith, M.D., Martin, F. (1995). Domestic violence: recognition, intervention, and prevention. *Med surg Nurs,* 4, 21-25.

Straus, M.A. (1979). Measuring intra family conflict and violence: The Conflict Tactics Scale. *J Marriage Fam,* 41, 75-88.

Straus, M.A., & Gelles, RJ. (1990). *Physical violence in American families: Risk factors and adaptations to violence in 8,145 families.* New Brunswick, NJ: Transaction Publications.

Subramanian, S.V., Ackerson, L.K., & Subramanyam, M.A., Wright, R.J. (2007). Domestic violence is associated with adult and childhood asthma prevalence in India. *Int J Epidemiol,* 36, 569- 79.

Sutherland, C., Bybee, D., & Sullivan, C. (1998). The long term effects of battering on women's health. *Women's Health Issues,* 4, 41-70.

Tomkins, A.M., Dunn, D.T., Hayes, R.J. (1989). Nutritional status and risk of morbidity among young Gambian children allowing for social and environmental factors. *Trans R Soc Trop Med Hg,* 589, 83, 282-7.

UNICEF (2010). *Child survival in Bangladesh.* Child Survival.docx. UNICEF, Dhaka, Bangladesh.

Uthman, O.A., Lawoko, S., & Moradi, T. (2009). Factors associated with attitudes towards intimate partner violence against women: a comparative analysis of 17 sub-Saharan countries. *BMC International Health and Human Rights,* 9,14. doi:10.1186/1472-698X-9-14.

WHO (1997). *World Report on Violence.* Geneva, Switzerland.

WHO (2001). *Putting women first: Ethical and safety recommendations for research on domestic violence against women.* Geneva: Department of Gender and Women"s Health.

6

Making a Healthy Living Space Through the Concept of Healthy Building of Building Medicine

Chih-Yuan Chang
Feng Chia University,
Taiwan

1. Introduction

Planning, diagnosis, and management of the healthy living space are crucial to human health management. Modern people spend at least half of the time indoor for their domestic lives, working lives, education, medical treatments or entertainment activities. Some of them even spend more than two-third of the time indoor, such as educators or health professionals. In terms of medical science, four categories affect the health of modern people—genetic inheritance, environment, life style, and health care. The environment category includes biological, physical and chemical factors, such as bacterium and excess funguses which influence indoor air quality (IAQ), radiation in buildings, and formaldehyde in harmful building materials. Furthermore, World Health Organization (WHO) also set forth a set of standards for healthy buildings, which lists fifteen recommendations for building planning. These standards are closely connected with the planning of healthy indoor environment.

This study aims to diagnose and manage healthy living space with the concept of healthy building in the field of Building Medicine. This subject can be divided into three parts: Physical Health of the Buildings, Environmental Health, and User's Safety and Health. More emphasis is placed on the aspect of the Users' Health. It is hoped that through the investigation of the interrelationship between problems in building environment with human heath, harmful elements which damage the health of building occupants can be discovered. Also, with the assistance of non-destructive testing technology, cases are diagnosed following WHO's standards on healthy buildings and health hazards hidden in the environment are pointed out to readers. These hazards include: harmful building materials, radiation emitted by steel bars, high frequency electromagnetic waves, electromagnetic fields (EMF), residual chlorine in drinking water, turbidity of drinking water, pH values in drinking water, noise, sunlight ratio, temperature and humidity, O_2 content, hazardous particles, total volatile organic compounds (TVOCs), formaldehyde, CO, CO_2, and O_3. Finally, following the concept of human medical science, this study suggests remedies and preventive measures for these problems so that the problems can be diagnosed and treated early, which is parallel to the secondary prevention stage of the disease prevention in medical science.

2. Building Medicine

Building Medicine is a new management perspective, which is mainly applied to the management of buildings' health (including home living environments.) In the field of engineering, the discussion on building health management used to be only limited to proposals of ideas that the engineering field should learn from health management practices of human medicine. In contrast with these general ideas, the discipline of Building Medicine not only fully defines how to apply the model of human health management analogously, but also develops application tools based on its theories, such as Building Diseases Classification (BDC), Building Medical Record (BMR), Building Doctor Navigation System (BDNS), Building Physiology Information System (BPIS) and Building Health Diagnosis (BHD).

2.1 The theory of Building Medicine

The management concept of Building Medicine is that the behaviours and management models of human health and building health are similar in terms of their structures, functions, life cycles, and service years. Theories, methodologies, mechanisms or roles played medical science can be applied analogously to building health management. The analogous application considers theories and practices of the building construction and maintenance, evaluates constraints and limitations in applying human medicine approaches to building health management. The goal of building health management is to uphold the health and safety of the buildings and their occupants or even to promote the sustainability, environment friendliness, artistry or economical benefits of the buildings. Furthermore, the study will further explore how the theories of medical science can be applied analogously to buildings at different stages of their life cycles, such as its health system, legal framework, health promotion activities, emergency treatments, diagnosis procedures, patient care, health administration, pathology or misdiagnosis (Chang, 2006).

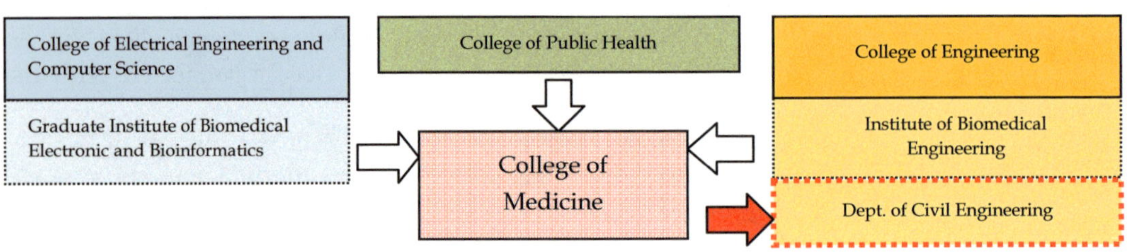

Fig. 1. Reverse thinking: Enhancing the research strength of technological and engineering fields by borrowing concepts from medical filed

As shown by Figure 1, except for the pubic health field, which has a close tie with the medical field, the currently available educational and technological applications are more oriented toward the field of electrical engineering, computer science, or civil engineering. Applying these technologies to medical treatment or research is part of the trend of cross-disciplinary collaboration, which can be also seen in the organization restructuring of academic institutions. For example, in National Taiwan University, the Institute of Biomedical Engineering was founded under the College of Engineering in 1988, and Graduate Institute of Biomedical Electronic and Bioinformatics was created under College of Electrical Engineering and Computer Science in 2006. The two institutes were established to enhance the research strength of the medical science field. In contrast with the support lent to the medical field by the engineering field, the concept of Building Medicine takes a reverse turn of thinking: In view of the speedy progress and thorough thinking of medical field, why not apply its well-developed health management mechanism and methods in the medical field analogously to building health management? In this way, architects or civil engineers who not only know how to design and construct buildings, they can also learn how to be building doctors and safeguard building safety and healthy living environments.

2.2 Roles played by Building Medicine

In medical science, cares and treatments are provided to humans from their birth and death. Based on its development trajectory, three roles are played by medical science. First, patients' pain is relieved and their health is restored through 'health care'. Second, through 'scientific researches,' causes and mechanisms of the diseases are investigated, and new treatments are discovered and developed. Third, through 'medical education,' knowledge of medical science and technology is passed down, and the bedrock of health care service and medical researches is constituted (Hsieh, 2003). The same principles are also applied to Building Medicine. Although the subject managed by Building Medicine is a building, Building Medicine also play similar roles as medical science does. It maintains a building's health through health care, scientific researches, and medical education of buildings. The safety and health of the occupants can only be safeguarded on the condition that the occupied buildings are in a healthy state. See Figure 2 for the roles played by Building Medicine. Pathology is one of the discipline under meidical education. Similarly, building pathology (Watt, 2007) is also devloped in the filed of civil engineering. Wang & Yau (2002) pointed out in their book, *Building Pathology*, building health can be compared analogously with human health. Therefore, a large amount of human pathology studies have been carried out to understand the essence of diseases and find their treatmeant and prevention methods.

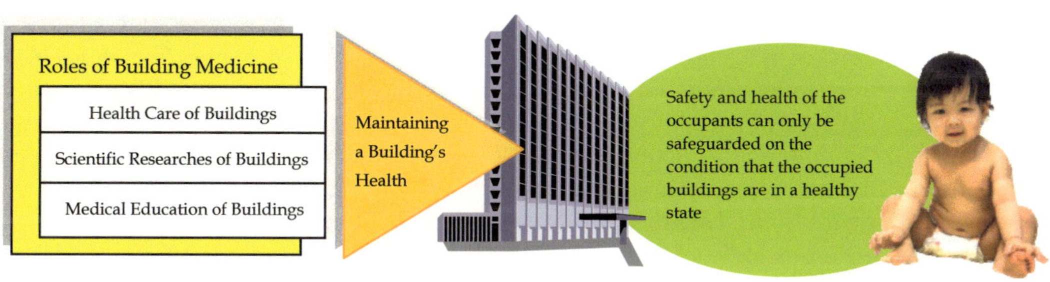

Fig. 2. Roles Played by Building Medicine

Building Medicine is not a discipline of pure theories. It has already been practiced on real cases. The author has already undertaken the three roles of Building Medicine outlined in Fig. 2. For the role of Health Care of Buildings, the previous position held by the author in the asset mangement industry was a consultant for household health diagnoses. Even though he is an assistant professor in Feng Chia University now, he teaches a service-learning course (Course Title: Building Diagnosis Technology) and leads students to provide test service of hazard factors in public environments of communities. For the role of Scientific Researches of Building, recent researches on application technologies are shown in Section 2.3 of this paper. The author also advised many master's theses which discuss diagnoses and solutions on health hazard factors in household environments, such as detection of EMF in living environments (Ma, 2010). As to Medical Education of Buildings, he opens many courses to teach students how to plan, make diagnoses, manage, and maintain a healthy living environment, including Building Medicine (post-graduate programs), Building Health Diagnosis (undergraduate program), Building Diagnosis Technology(undergraduate program), and Intelligent Living Space(undergraduate program).

2.3 Implements for Building Medicine

Until now, several analogous studies based on the concepts of Building Medicine have been conducted. For example, a Building Medical Record (BMR) is designed analogously to medical records used in medical science; a Building Diseases Classification (BDC) is designed analogously to WHO ICD-9-CM(The International Classification of Diseases, Ninth Revision, Clinical Modification) Codes; a Building Doctor Navigation System (BDNS) is designed analogously to electronic diagnosis systems used in hospitals; a Building Physiology Information System(BPIS) is designed analogously to measuring blood pressure, pulses and temperature of human bodies; and a Building Health Diagnosis (BHD) is designed analogously to regular health checks taken by people.

1. BMR: The problem-oriented medical record (POMR) which has been generally adopted in medical science was derived from the problem-oriented recording(POR) proposed by Dr. Laurence Weed in 1964. After 1968, the POMR was gradually formed (Chen, 2001). The problem-oriented medical record (POMR) is widely used in medical science. Cheng at al. (2007) adopts the concept of POMR analogously and develops Building Medical Record (BMR) in order to make diagnostic process for building health become more systematic and complete, similar to that for human health.
2. BDC: When doctors around the world make diagnoses and give treatments to patients, the classification coding of human diseases, ICD-9-CM, is an important common language for communication between them. ICD-9-CM also serves as a reference guide for governments to determine reimbursement rates for medical services, and it is also a universal basis for statistical analyses within medical database systems. Therefore, ICD-9-CM is crucial to research and practices in the medical field. Similarly, diagnoses and statistical analyses of building diseases require a common communication language. Chang (2008) follows the logic of ICD-9-CM and applies it to the development of Building Diseases Classification (BDC) suitable for diagnosing building diseases. BDC includes Disease Code, Treatment Code and Supplement Code.
3. BDNS: The design logic of medical records aims to make records more organized, cohesive, credible, and easier to track and verify. In operation/maintenance stage of building life cycle, maintenance records are important reference data for on-site building managers when diagnosing the condition of facilities and making treatment decisions. However, three common problems often arise in the use of maintenance records. First, the inputs and updates of maintenance records and knowledge from internal sources may be unorganized and they may not be verified by practices on actual cases. Second, data and knowledge obtained from external sources may lack credibility. Third, the large quantity of data may not be able to be processed. As a result, Building Doctor Navigation System (BDNS) has been developed based on the author's BMR research. Through knowledge extraction method that combined the semantic indexing and the clustering analysis technology, BDNS can make up for the shortcomings of the systems built by private property management companies and help on-site building managers to solve the aforementioned problems encountered when building database of maintenance records. Managers or users can look up information

in cloud database via mobile devices. By doing so, they can obtain real-time and correct information regarding to diagnoses on building diseases, treatment measures, and prevention strategies, etc. See the left picture of Fig. 3.

4. BPIS: Physiology signs of human bodies are a basis for human health checks. From the viewpoints of Building Medicine, physiology signs of buildings (temperature, humidity, stress, strain) hold the same importance to building health management. Since a significant amount of human power and time can be saved by using computer systems to maintain buildings' functions and performances and extend their service years, Chang (2010) built a computer system: BPIS. After smart humidity/temperature information materials being installed inside buildings, signals detected by the materials are sent to BPIS wirelessly. Then, building managers are able to consult the detection data through the user interface of BPIS, and quickly learn about the temperature and humidity values inside the building structures (just like temperature and blood pressure measurement of human bodies.) Therefore, BPIS makes buildings become smart buildings with self-detection ability. Furthermore, BPIS also provides auto-alert function which can help managers discover problems right when they arise (see the right picture on Fig. 3).

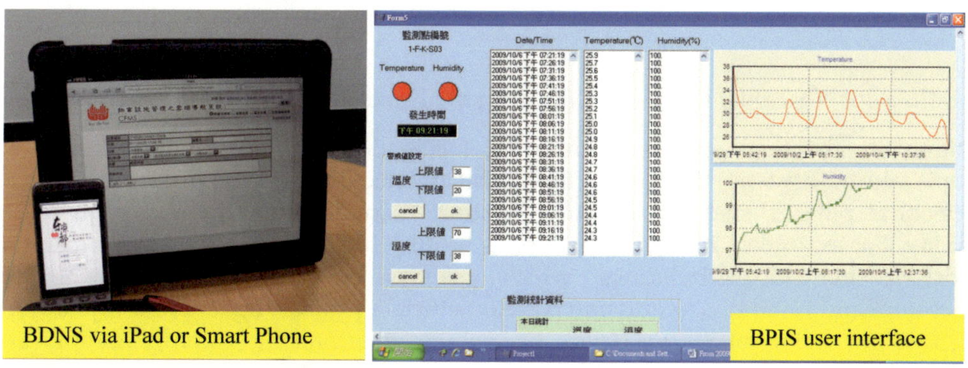

Fig. 3. User control panels of BDNS (left) and BPIS (right)

5. BHD: Building Health Diagnosis is one link of preventive maintenance management of Professional Maintenance Management (PMM). BHD is conducted by personnel with building diagnosis training background. Based on their knowledge and techniques, they make diagnoses periodically or sporadically on various aspects of building maintenance and management, such as safety, health, performance, environmental impacts, appearance, energy conservation, and sustainability, etc. When it is necessary, maintenance and renovation works are carried out to safeguard users' safety and health, maintain the proper function of the buildings, protect environments, conserve energy and improve the urban aesthetics (Chang et al., 2007). Due to these considerations, the author has opened two courses related to BHD-Building Health Diagnosis and Building Diagnosis Technology—in order to teach building diagnosis knowledge and technology under the concept of BHD and train students to equip with the fundamental knowledge for becoming building doctors in the future.

2.4 Healthy Building of Building Medicine

Healthy Building of Building Medicine is a concept which combines medical science, public health, civil engineering, architecture, environmental engineering, and it stresses on maintaining the physical health of buildings, including the health of their indoor environments, because healthy buildings are prerequisite for maintaining users' safety and health. Furthermore, from the point of view of sustainability, impact to the environment must be lessened as much as possible by current technology. See Fig. 4.

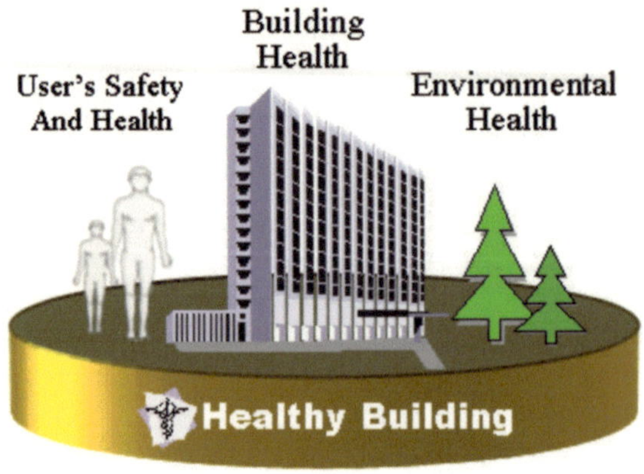

Fig. 4. Concept of Healthy Building in Building Medicine

Traditionally, the field of civil engineering focuses on buildings' physical health, for example, shock resistance of the structures. The architecture field emphasizes the aspect of architectural physics, such as acoustics, lighting, thermal environment, air quality, and humidity. For example, Chiang (2001) defines healthy buildings as 'A way of experiencing indoor environment of buildings, which includes physical measurements (such as temperature and humidity, ventilation aeration efficiency, noise, light, and air quality), and subjective psychological factors (such as layouts, environment colour, lighting, space, building materials, job satisfaction, and interpersonal relationship).' Furthermore, the field of green architecture has also discussed the subject of healthy buildings. For example, healthy buildings promoted by the Healthy Building Network (2011) also stressed the impact of hazardous building materials to environmental health. Health Care Without Harm is a medical organization concerned about issues of healthy buildings. Until 2010, 494 organizations in 53 countries have joined force to promote green hospital buildings and devote attention to the impact of hazardous materials to human health (Health Care Without Harm, 2010). Also, 15 planning standards are recommended by Healthy Household Guidelines of World Health Organization:

- Low concentration of chemicals which may trigger allergies
- In order to meet the requirement in the first point, avoid using ply-woods or wall renovation materials containing chemicals not easy to vaporize
- Install ventilation system of high ventilation function to emit indoor pollutants to outside. Central ventilation systems with air-supply ducts must be installed in spaces of air-tightness or thermal insulation design
- Local exhaust ventilation systems must be installed in kitchen or smoking areas
- The temperature of living rooms, bedrooms, kitchens, toilets, hallways, bathrooms must be kept at 17°C~27°C year-round
- Indoor humidity must be kept between 40%~70% year-round

- Concentration of CO_2 must be under 1,000 ppm
- Concentration of suspended particles must be under 0.15mg/m^2
- Noise volume must be under 50 dB (A)
- The house should be lit by the sun for at least 3 hours/per day
- Install lights of sufficient illumination
- Households must be equipped with sufficient ability to withstand natural disasters
- Sufficient floor area per capita, and ensure privacy of the occupants
- The household design must be suitable for nursing elderly and handicapped
- Since building materials contain toxic volatile organic compounds, so it is not inhabitable some time after completion of construction. During this period, the newly completed house must be ventilated

In contrast with the focuses and definition of the fields of traditional civil engineering, architecture, public health or medicine, Healthy Building of Building Medicine covers a wider range of issues. Except for the discussion of health management activities for protecting building users' health and safety, Building Medicine also concerns itself about management projects which prevent receptors from contracting diseases as a result of unhealthy buildings. Receptors which may be affected by unhealthy buildings include users, buildings, and the environments of the affected zone. The purpose of physical health management of buildings is to prevent building damages and concerns of user safety caused by building deterioration. Proper management of indoor environmental health can also prevent users from contracting environment-related diseases, such as Legionnaires' disease, allergy triggered by particles, or cancers induced by strong electromagnetic wave or radiation. Finally, Building Medicine is also dedicated to eradicate harmful environmental impacts caused by improper management or inappropriate choices of building materials (such breaking the sustainability of green buildings or adopting building materials of higher carbon footprints.)

3. Interrelationship between living space and health problems

Environmental impacts to human health have long been confirmed by the medical field. An epidemiological model that supports health policy analysis and decisiveness must be broad, comprehensive, and must include all matters affecting health. Consequently, four primary factors have been identified: (1) System of Health Care Organization; (2) Life Style (self-created risks); (3) Environment; and (4) Human Biology. Taking the analysis of cancer causes as an example, the impact degrees of the four factors are 10%, 37%, 24% and 29% (Dever, 1976). The impact degree of environment factor in cancers is 24%. People are highly concerned about cancer prevention when it comes to their health management. Many cancer insurance policies are on offer in the market. However, the possible health hazards caused by the environment factor have been often overlooked in the education and training of architects and civil engineers who design and construct physical structures and interior environments. Not only recently do the issues of green buildings and non-toxic building materials gradually become more and more important in the fields of civil engineering and architecture, and these fields start to take steps to build healthy environments for the general public.

Living space is closely related with human health problems. From the viewpoint of civil engineering field, the issue can be explored initially by looking into building materials, building physics, and building management and maintenance and searching which factor would result in users' health problems. By doing so, it can make architects and civil engineers aware the importance of building a healthy environment at the stage of design and construction. This concept can be seen as building eugenics promoted by Building Medicine. Since there are many factors which affect health, this study cannot cover all the health hazardous factors. Therefore, this study discusses hazardous factors which are covered by current teaching and research plans of non-destructive tests on buildings.

Common hazardous factors in the living space include:

1. Noise: Increased risk for long-lasting syndromal anxiety states (Generalized Anxiety Disorder and Anxiety Disorder NOS), thus supporting the hypothesis of a sustained central autonomic arousal due to chronic exposure to noise (Hardoy et al., 2005). Sound louder than 70 decibel (dB (A)) makes people uncomfortable. Their blood vessels would start to contract, and their blood pressure would rise. And their concentration would waver, become more nervous, and affect their learning performance. Spending a long time in an environment of 85 dB (A) cause hearing impairment, sometimes even severe hearing loss. Sound louder than 90 dB (A) may affect endocrine system, trigger mood swings, anxiety and headache, and cause people more prone to make mistakes. Sound louder than 130 dB (A) results in ear pain. Sound which register 140 dB (A) or more would make eardrum burst.
2. Illumination: Light suppresses melatonin (Boyce et al., 1987) and may cause serious sleeping problems. Either excessive or poor lighting would affect human bodies. Poor outdoor lighting may cause injuries or even death because people are easier to trip and fall. Excess indoor lighting may be harmful to vision. Therefore, both indoor and outdoor lighting should be at a proper level.
3. ELF-EMF: International Agency for Research on Cancer (IARC) classifies extremely low frequency (ELF) as a possible carcinogen (Kheifets et al., 2005). Allergic reaction may be shown in a small number of people when they are exposed to ELF. The symptoms include skin rash, itchy skin, skin burning sensation, nervous exhaustion and other unspecific symptoms, such as fatigue, vertigo, nausea, palpitation, and gastric disorder.
4. HF-EMF: Research shows high-frequency electromagnetic fields (HF-EMF) with a carrier frequency and modulation scheme typical of the GSM signal may affect the integrity of DNA (Franzellitti et al., 2010). Living in an environment of HF-EMF for a long time may cause eye diseases, lower resistance against disease, higher chance of cancer occurrence, affecting reproductive systems of both sexes with possible consequence of infertility, headaches, dizziness, nausea, loss of memory, sleeping difficulties, and hair loss. Long-term influences include higher chance of Alzheimer occurrence, tinnitus, loss of balance, skin diseases, irregular pulse, arrhythmia, labored breathing, joint pain, and sore muscle.
5. Radiation: If being exposed to high levels of ionizing radiation, infants and pregnant women have a higher chance of leukaemia and solid cancer (Lane et al., 2010). It may trigger gene mutation, infertility, cataract, nausea, blood cell deformation. If pregnant women are exposed to radiation, the babies they carry are prone to mental retardation, miscarriage, polydactyl, and Down syndrome.
6. PH level of water: The impact of pH level to human health is indirect. Only extreme pH level is harmful to human bodies. When pH level of water is too low, metal water pipes will be eroded, which will cause high level of lead, copper, and zinc in water. Related studies show copper would cause acute and chronic poisoning. In Germany, copper in tap water caused a series of severe disease (such as liver cirrhosis), and other

gastroenterology diseases (Eife et al., 1999). When pH level is over 8.0, water would be less disinfected, which would cause potential health threats. PH level of water exceeding 8.5 may cause bitter taste and produce pipe scale.

7. Water turbidity: Turbidity exceeding a certain level may result in gastroenterology diseases (Mann et al., 2007). Turbidity is one of the key indicators of drinking water quality. High turbidity means there might be micro-organisms in water particles and it would be harmful to human health. If turbidity is visible to naked eyes, the level of turbidity is usually over 5 NTU.
8. Chloride residues in water: Consumption of drinking water with high trihalomethane content may increase the risk of melanoma and possibly of hormone-dependent cancers such as neoplasm of the prostate, the breast, and the ovary. (Marco et al., 2004) Free chloride is added in water as a disinfectant. It may cause unpleasant smell, and it may be interacted with organic matters and form a hazardous by-product. Chloride residues remaining in water pipelines are not powerful enough to sterilize and may be harmful to human bodies. Chloride residues in tap water would damage hair and skin. After chloride is being absorbed by human bodies, it enters directly into blood, and is metabolized by the kidneys. However, if people absorb an amount too large or their kidney functions are low, they would show symptoms of chloride poisoning.
9. Temperature: High temperature may cause heatstroke, heat exhaustion, and heat cramps. Heat exhaustion means human body temperature exceeds 38.0℃. Its symptoms include profuse sweating, malaise, headache, dizziness, anorexia, nausea, vomiting, vertigo, chills, muscle or general weakness, tachycardia and hypotension, visual disturbances and cutaneous flushing. Heat stroke happens when body temperature reaches 40.5℃ or higher, and its symptom is neurologic impairment. Heat stroke is a medical emergency. Patients must be given cooling treatment and their temperature must be lowered to at least 38.8°C.
10. Humidity: Highly humid environment induce the growth of fungus, which would trigger respiratory tract irritation, allergies (Bornehag et al., 2004), rheumatism, athlete's foot, and mosquito infestation.
11. CO: Minor carbon monoxide poisoning results in higher blood pressure, rising heart rate, higher breathing frequency, rapid and shallow breathing, chest pain, dizziness, anxiety, nausea, and headaches. Severe carbon monoxide poisoning makes people slip into coma, twitching, cardiac arrest (Goldstein, 2008).
12. CO_2: When the density of carbon dioxide reaches 15,000 ppm or more, it would affect breathing function. When it exceeds 30,000 ppm, it would stimulate respiratory center and causes breathing difficulties (Jones, 1999), headaches, drowsiness, hyporeflexia, lethargy.
13. O_3: Absorption of O_3 of high density would reduce lung function, increase bronchial contraction, and raise the risk of asthma attack (D'Amato et al., 2005). When O_3 level exceeds the permissible exposure limit, it would causes coughing, short of breath, headache, decreasing lung function, respiratory inflammation, decrease the resistance of lungs against contagion and toxins. In the severe condition, it may result in pulmonary edema.
14. TVOCs: Among indoor air pollutants, total volatile organic compounds (TVOCs) are one type of common and hazardous pollutants. Many kinds of volatile organic gas are strong poison, which would suppress the central nervous system, irritate eyes and respiratory tracts, and trigger allergies in eyes, skin, and lungs (Jones, 1999). TVOCs

existing in the environment include formaldehyde, toluene, xylene, styrene, etc. Being exposed to high level of volatile organic compounds for a long time would inflict damages to the nervous system, liver, and kidneys.

15. Formaldehyde: United States Environmental Protection Agency classified formaldehyde as a carcinogen (Salthammer et al., 2010). Direct contact with formaldehyde causes skin allergies, eye irritation, allergic asthma, and other diseases of less pronounced symptoms (Wu et al., 2003). High level formaldehyde affects the nervous system, the immune system and the liver. Long-time contact with formaldehyde would result in chronic respiratory diseases, irregular menstrual period, decreasing resistance of babies, and even respiratory system cancers (such as nasopharyngeal cancer) and deformity.
16. O_2: When there is no sufficient oxygen, people would lose concentration, forgetful, worse vision, more difficult to lose fat, and prone to ageing. In the work environment, the level of oxygen in the air must be more than 18%. Anoxia would be triggered when oxygen level is lower than 18%. The symptoms of anoxia are nausea, vomiting, headache, drowsiness, and sleeping difficulties (Nilles et al., 2009).
17. Particles: The harmful effects of particles include respiratory diseases, cardio-vascular diseases, and allergies (D'Amato et al., 2005). People exposed to an environment of high concentration of particles for a long time usually can not detect any pronounced symptoms at first. However, when the condition is getting worse, they would start to have asthma and more phlegm. Their asthma may be so acute that they even feel hard of breathing and rapid heart beats when walking, which makes them unable to perform any work. This condition is called particles toxic syndromes.

The indoor air quality test taken by this study included all the general items except for bacteria and fungus because testing equipments are not yet acquired. For physical environment of the buildings, the levels of noise, illumination, humidity, and oxygen are tested, and the other tested items include radiation, ELF-EMF, HF-EMF, pH level of water, turbidity, and chloride residues. In total, 17 items are tested. Of course, environmental factors which affect health are more than 17 items. However, due to the restraints of time and budget, this study only discusses items which are covered by current teaching and testing practices.

4. Building health diagnosis for public health

The application of Building Medicine is a management project which prevents building occupants from becoming ills due to staying in an unhealthy building. It manages occupants, buildings, and environments of the affected areas. Illness caused by an unhealthy environment-such as Legionnaires' disease (caused by air-conditioning,) cancer (caused by excess electromagnetic wave, radiation or harmful building materials,) allergy (caused by poor indoor air quality) or Sick Building Syndrome (SBS)-can be prevented by proper management of the building health. How these health-hazardous factors can be eliminated? From the point of view of Building Medicine, building's health should be maintained by playing the three roles of Building Medicine (see 2.2 Roles Played by Building Medicine). Besides conducting scientific researches and medical education on buildings, when engineers engage in health care of buildings to protect public health and find out signs of diseases at the early stage, building health diagnosis (BHD) is a good strategy for maintaining and managing healthy buildings.

Diagnosis Items		Sources of Problems
01	Noise	Public facilities (such as motors or transformer boxes), modes of transport, events or activities, public address systems, construction works, airports, factories, railways
02	Illumination	LED advertisement board(too bright), insufficient natural light, poor lighting, no lighting equipment installed
03	ELF-EMF	Indoor air-conditioning, computers, speakers, television sets, refrigerators, electric water boilers, and other electrical appliances Outdoor electric boxes, machinery rooms, utility poles, cables
04	HF-EMF	Radio, mobile phone base stations, wireless handsets, wireless local area network (WLAN), blue tooth, radar, radio stations, and wireless TV signals
05	Radiation	Building materials polluted by radiation, laboratories, areas adjacent to hospital radiology rooms
06	PH level of water	Water supply piping, improper processing of raw water
07	Water turbidity	Pollution of water supply piping, improper processing of raw water
08	Chloride residues in water	Water supply piping is too long, improper processing of raw water
09	Temperature	Geography and climate, bad ventilation of the environments, improper design of air-conditioning
10	Humidity	Geography and climate, bad ventilation of the environments, improper design of air-conditioning
11	CO	Incomplete combustion of household heating system, incomplete combustion of vehicles or electricity generators in undergroud parking lots
12	CO_2	High occupant density, bad air exchange efficiency
13	O_3	Photocopiers, all-in-one printers, air cleaners
14	TVOCs	Solvent-based coating, adhesives for bonding plates and panels together in renovation
15	Formaldyhyde	New interior building materials or furniture, such as carpets, PVC tiles, plywood, new sofas, chairs, wardrobes, or system furniture
16	O_2	Basements, storage rooms, or closed and unventilated space
17	Particles	Damp walls and ceilings, synthetic fiber, asbestos, carpets, furniture, ill-maintained dehumidifiers, air-conditioning, bedding, pets

Table 1. Diagnosis items of BHD and source of problems

In order to promote BHD, the author has started to offer a class called Building Diagnosis Technology (BDT) in Feng Chia University. As the University was promoting the attitude of 'learning through community service', this class was designed as a long-term learning program of community service. The University agreed to allocate funds for purchasing building and environment test devices, so students not only fulfil their community service responsibility, they also can apply the knowledge of civil engineering they learned in class to health diagnosis cases in communities. The author taught students how to make use of the management concepts of Building Medicine and the diagnosing and management knowledge they had learned in the preparatory class (BHD). Then he taught them how to use test devices. Finally, students were sent to communities arranged by this community service program to perform environment health diagnosis and practice their testing skills. Because this was a large class, the number of students made it unfeasible for them to go into each household and perform their service. As a result, the environment health diagnosis provided by BDT class was usually carried out in public space. The diagnosis items include: radioactive house test, ELF-EMF level test (community utility facilities/utility poles/substations/power towers), HF-EMF level test (mobile phone base stations/ wireless internet), environment noise test, degree of illumination in the public space (following the CNS standard), water quality test (pH level, turbidity, pH colorimeter value), humidity in public environment, IAQ air quality standard ($CO/CO_2/O_3$/TVOC/formaldehyde/temper-ature/particles) recommended by Taiwan's Environmental Protection Administration, and the test of oxygen content. See Table 1 for diagnosis items and possible sources of problems for each item.

For the convenience of field instruction and on-site tests, the devices used in this study are all handheld readout devices. Some of the devices can also be used with software for visual interface management. Although they are not expensive (the price of each device is between 500 USD to 5,000 USD), they are sufficient for introducing students to environmental education or initial tests of hazardous environmental factors. The devices used are introduced briefly below:

1. Noise: Programmable Sound Level Meter (Model: TES-1352H) is used for testing. Its test range is 30~130 dB (A), and can be used with software. See Fig. 5.

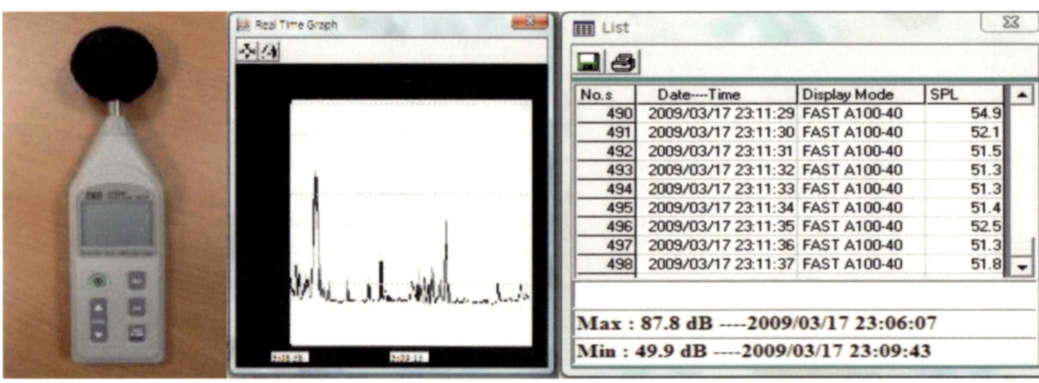

Fig. 5. Programmable Sound Level Meter and operation screen of its software

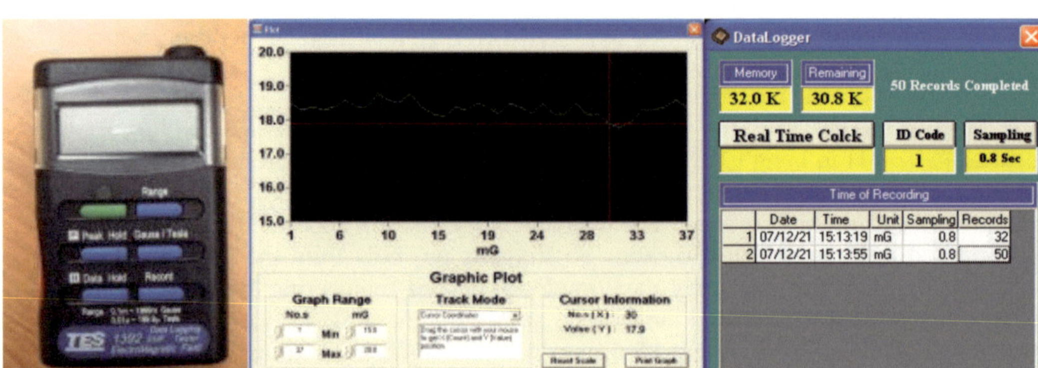

Fig. 6. EMF Tester and operation screen of its software

2. ELF-EMF: This is tested by EMF Tester (Model: TES-1392). Maximum detection limit is 2,000 mG, and its analytic precision can be as high as 0.1mG. The meter can be used with software. See Fig. 6.
3. HF-EMF: This is tested by ElectroSmog Meter (Model: TES-92). Its display resolution is 0.1mV/m, 0.1 μA/m and 0.01 μW/m2. See the left picture of Fig.7.
4. Temperature and humidity: These are measured by Data logging Humidity / Temperature Meter (Model: TES-1365). The meter can start measuring at pre-set time. The measurement range of temperature is between -20°C~+60°C, and the measurement range of humidity is 10%~95 % RH. See the middle picture on Fig. 7.
5. Illumination: This is measured by Data Logging Light Meter (Model: TES-1336A). The measurement range is 20, 200, 2,000 and 20,000 Lux/Fc (1Fc=10.76 Lux). Sample rate= 2.5 times/per second. See the right picture on Fig. 7.

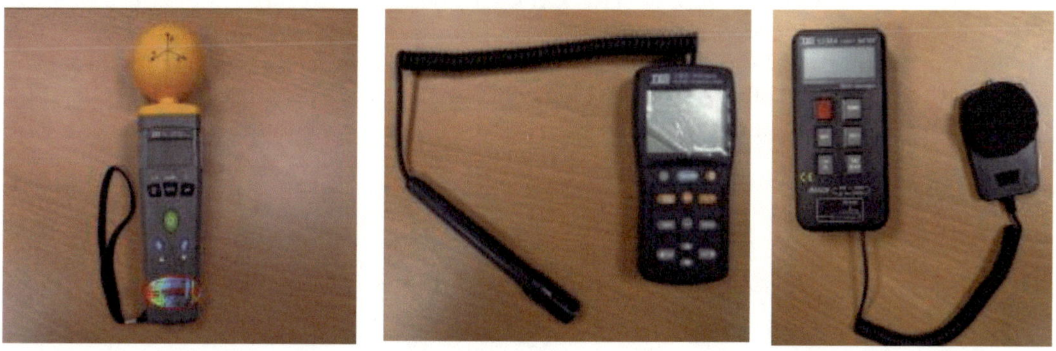

Fig. 7. ElectroSmog Meter (left)/ Humidity/Temperature Meter (middle)/ Light Meter (right)

6. Radiation: This is tested by Programmable Dosimeter (Model: PM1203M), which can detect gamma ray. The dose rate in the detection range is 0.1~2000μSv/h. See Fig. 8.
7. PH level and turbidity of water and chloride residues: PH level of water is tested by digital pH Meter (Model: PH-207). The measurement range of pH level is 0~14. See left picture of Fig. 9. The water turbidity is tested by Turbid Meter (Model: TN 100). The detection range is 00.00~19.99 / 20.0~99.9 / 100~1000 NTU. See the middle picture on Fig. 9. Chloride residues are tested by Portable Colorimeter (Model: C201). The detection range of chloride residue content is 0~1.99 ppm and the detection range of total chloride content is 2.0~6.0 ppm. See the right picture of Fig. 9.

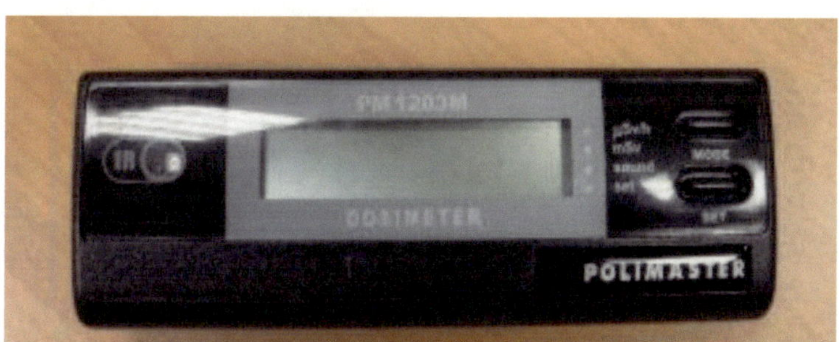

Fig. 8. Programmable Dosimeter

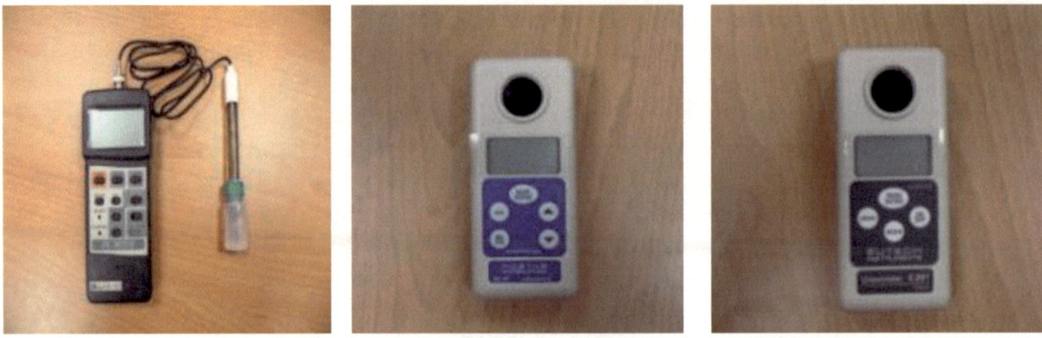

Fig. 9. PH Meter (left)/ Turbid meter (middle)/ Portable Colorimeter (right)

8. Content of CO, CO_2, TVOCs, HCHO, O_2, O_3 in the air: CO content is measured by CO Meter (Model: GCO-2008). See left picture of Fig. 10. The measurement range is 0~1,000 ppm and the resolution is 1ppm. The meter can be used with software. The measurement range of CO_2 Meter (Model: GCH-2018) is 0~4,000 ppm and the resolution is 1 ppm, and the meter can be used with software. See the right picture of Fig. 10.

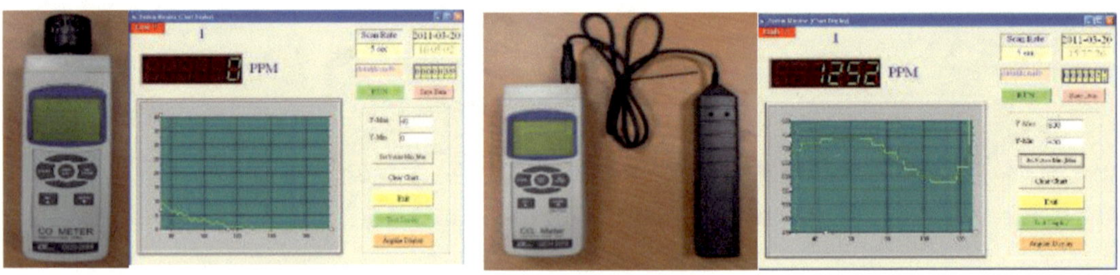

Fig. 10. CO Meter (left)/CO_2 Meter (right)

TVOCs content is measured by TVOCs Monitor (Model: Series 500). See the left picture of Fig. 11. The measurement range is 0~500 ppm, and the resolution is 1 ppm. The unit of concentration can be ppm or mg/m^3. The meter can be used with software. HCHO content is detected by HCHO Detector (Model: FP-30). See the right picture of Fig. 11. The measurement range is 0~0.4 ppm, and the meter can be used with software.

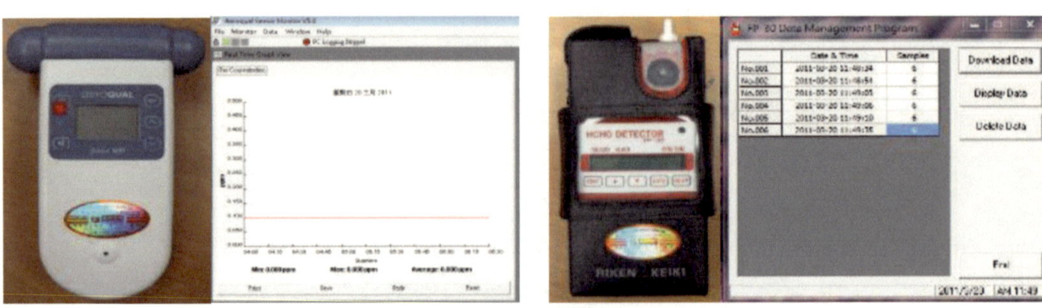

Fig. 11. TVOC Monitor (left)/HCHO Detector (right)

Oxygen content is measured by GMI-Portable Gas Detector, whose measurement range is 0%~25% Vol. See the left picture of Fig. 12. Ozone content is measured by O_3 Monitor

(Model: Series 200), whose measurement range is 0~50 ppm and resolution is 0.01 ppm. See the right picture of Fig. 12.

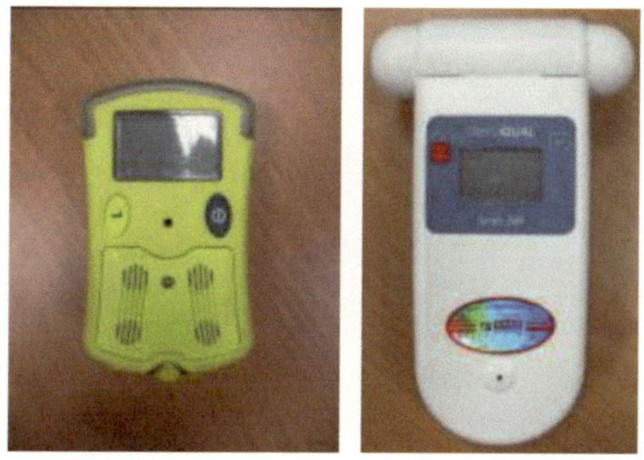

Fig. 12. GMI-Portable Gas Detector (left) / O_3 Monitor (right)

9. Particles: This is measured by Met One-Particle Mass Profiler & Counter (Model: AEROCET 531). The quantity of particles can be detected are PM_1, $PM_{2.5}$, PM_7, PM_{10}, and TSP. The measurement range is 0~1 mg/m^3. The number of particles which can be detected is 0.5 and 5.0μm. Its measurement range is 0~3,000,000 /ft^3, and it can be used with software. See Fig. 13.

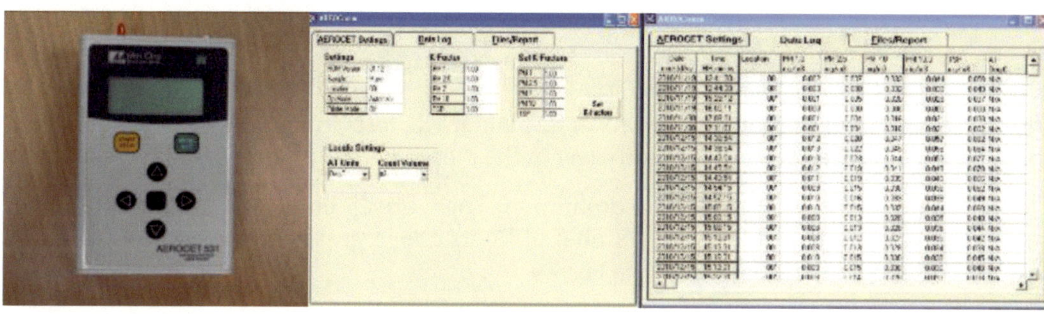

Fig. 13. Particle Mass Profiler & Counter

5. Case study

The cases presented here is the combined result of the service learning course, Building Diagnosis Technology (BDT), and Building Medicine. The teaching goal of BDT is to train students to be able to use technological meters to diagnose the health and safety hazardous factors hidden in the community environment, and are also able to describe the sources of the problems. Finally, they work in teams and perform health diagnosis service in the public environments of communities. Through this course, they can understand and experience the training and practice of building doctors, and they can also make presentation to residents to explain the hazardous factors which may be hidden in their environments. The tested items are the 17 items listed in Table 1.

From 2009 to 2010, the total number of students who took these two classes is 154, and the service was performed in 3 communities (public space) and 1 elderly day care center (indoor environment). The total number of the serviced buildings is 30, which are of RC structures. The total testing service time in each community is 12 hours. There are 3 buildings in Case 1 community. It is a condominium, and its buildings are 17-years-old with 13 floors above ground and 3 floors underground. See Fig. 14.

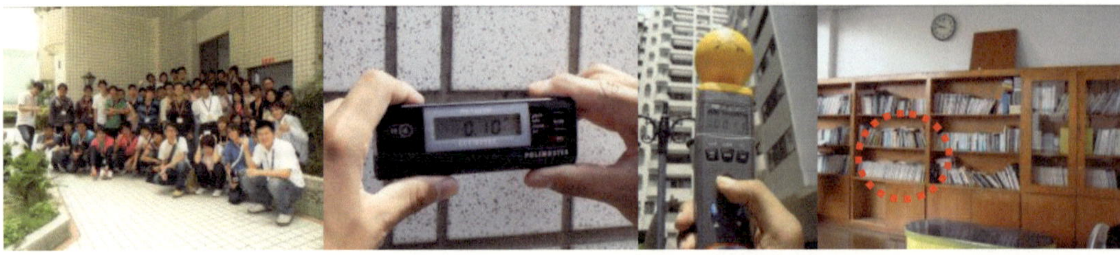

Fig. 14. The author led students to perform radiation tests on steel bars, electromagnetic waves tests in courtyards, and formaldehyde tests in the library room

Case 2 community only has one building. The building is a 2-years-old condominium with 26 floors above ground and 4 floors underground. See Fig. 15.

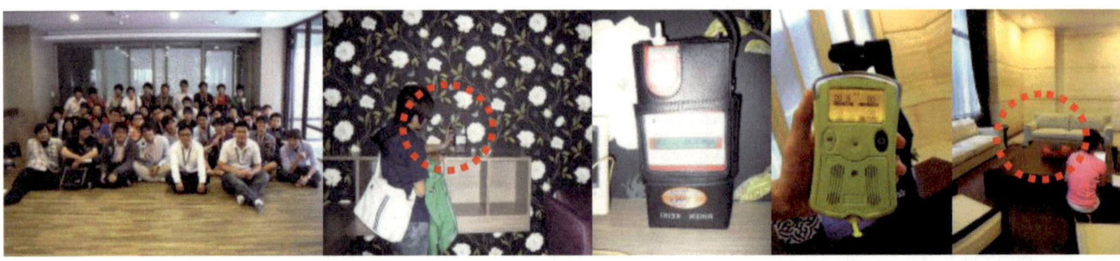

Fig. 15. The author led students to perform formaldehyde tests in the rest area of SPA center, and oxygen, temperature, and humidity test in the lobby

Case 3 community is a mega-size condominium. There are 25 buildings and the number of households is more than 1,200. The number of floors above ground is from 8 to 12, and the number of floors underground is 2. See Fig. 16.

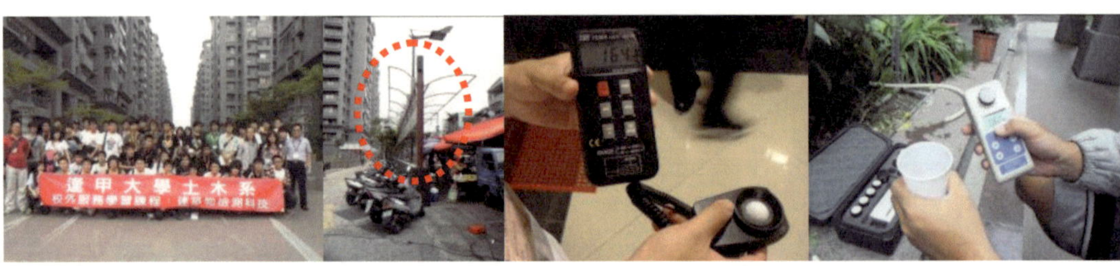

Fig. 16. The author led students to perform noise tests on sound-proof walls, illumination tests in stairways, and turbidity test on public use water

Case 4 is a case of diagnosis service performed on an elderly day care center. The center is located on the ground floor of one building. The space is divided into a rest area, a dining area, an activity area, and two bathrooms. See Fig. 17.

In the field of medical health, not all the items are tested in a health check. Health check items for each patient are recommended based on the patient's sex, age, symptoms, or living condition. Building health checks should be done this way. However, the health check cases discussed in this study are community services performed by students. Therefore, instead of customizing the number of health check items based on the conditions of each building, all the items are performed. Students are also taught that some of the problems are less likely to happen in certain conditions. For example, the interior fitting and decoration of the Case 1 buildings have been installed for more than 10 years, which makes the problem of high formaldehyde level unlikely to happen. Nevertheless, the author still wanted students to do all the tests to verify this hypothesis, and the result can also be compared to the formaldehyde levels of new buildings' interior fitting.

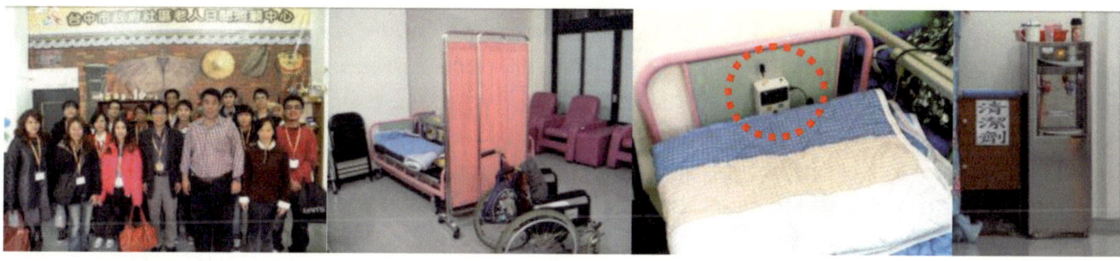

Fig. 17. The author led students to perform particle test in the rest area of elderly residents and water quality tests on drinking fountains

As it is discussed above, each building's conditions vary just like every human patient's health is affected by various conditions. As a result, when making a health check plan for buildings, building doctors should consider each diagnosed subject's condition. For example, the building age of Case 1 is higher, as a result; the tests on public area should focus on water quality (the pH level), basement ventilation (CO and O_2 level), and whether indoor lighting is insufficient because of lack of maintenance. Case 2 building is younger, and it is a luxury housing project with a lot of interior decoration works. Therefore, Indoor Air Quality (IAQ) should be the focus of building health checks, such as the tests of formaldehyde and TVOCs. Case 3 buildings are located next to a night-market. The noise during the nights is louder, so the night noise test is important. As to the elderly day care center of Case 4, since the occupants are the elderly, particles which may trigger allergies or lung diseases are the focus of the test. Furthermore, the water quality test on drinking water and TVOCs test on bathroom detergents are also important.

The tests performed in these four cases have produced many valuable experience and information. However, this study follows the non-disclosure policy of medical records, and do not disclose and discuss the test result of each case (the results of most items are in the safe range). Therefore, in the following discussion, the author shares common problems and their solutions based on his 'clinical experience.'

1. Noise: The common causes of the noise level which exceeds the standard are ambulance siren, engine sounds of motorcycles, construction works, religious events held by temples, and engine sounds of ventilation fans in basements. Ambulance sirens and engine sounds of motorcycles are transient noises. Because they only last for a very short time, they wouldn't affect hearing. To lower down the noise of construction works and religious events, the occupants may report to local environmental protection bureaus and have the noise sources keep their noise down to the legal standard. If the recurring noises have constituted a psychological anxiety to occupants, it is suggested that occupants should install acoustic windows, which usually can reduce noise level up to 30 dB (A). Furthermore, the noise of the ventilation fans in basements can be reduced by installing vibration reduction devices or improving the motor's

performance. However, if occupants would not listen to the noise for a long time, they do not need to worry about the problem.

2. Temperature and humidity: High indoor temperature would only cause discomfort of occupants. Opening windows or turning on air-conditioners would alleviate the hotness and stuffiness inside a room. The high temperature and humidity problem of underground parking lots can be solved by increasing the operation times and length of ventilation fans. Humidity measurements taken on raining days are usually higher. However, building managers still need to check if the indoor ventilation planning is adequate, and they should find air-conditioning professionals to do a close evaluation. If the water which evaporates from swimming pools spread to the entire indoor public space or households, the higher humidity tends to make mildew grow on the surface of interior fitting and decoration. When the fungus of mildew spread in the air, occupants may be prone to develop respiratory diseases or allergies.
3. High CO content: The students once detected a value of CO content slightly higher than the standard recommended by the Taiwan government (9 ppm) in a basement. The recommendation given to the occupants was not to stay in the basement for a long time. If people need to work in the basement such as cleaning, they should turn on ventilation fans to emit carbon monoxide. However, if the air quality is still not improved after frequency of ventilation has been increased after another test by a CO content meter; the manager must check if it is due to bad planning of ventilation systems or malfunction of ventilation fans. If that is the case, they must change the planning or replace the ventilation fans. Furthermore, the news reports of CO poisoning incidents shows that CO poisoning usually happens at home in the winter, which can be explained by people tend to close windows in the winter, which results in bad ventilation, and they also do not install forced exhaust ventilation device on their gas stoves or water heaters. As a result, even if CO content measurements are normal, if the indoor ventilation is bad, it is still necessary to advise occupants to improve the ventilation.
4. High CO_2 problem: If a crowd stay in an indoor space for a long time, the content of CO_2 tends to rise higher than the normal value. If space size is the limiting factor, the number of occupants or staying time should be lowered. If the number of occupants and staying time are both the limiting factors, it is advised to improve the efficiency and power of the ventilation systems.
5. Illumination: Due to the consideration of energy saving or the close distance from the neighbouring buildings, the degree of illumination in some lobbies' seating areas tends to be low (for example, one is as low as 67 Lux). If the area is simply used for resting instead of reading, low lighting would not cause any inconvenience. In the daytime tests, some of the insufficient lighting areas are stairways and driveways of underground parking lots. It is suggested to install more lights. If the managers want to avoid unnecessary energy costs, they can install motion sensor lights. For the driveways of underground parking lots, the lights in some areas are often blocked by fire protection or water supply piping, so its degree of illumination does not meet CNS recommendation values. Under the circumstance, the lights can be changed to hanging lights (or adjust the location of lights slightly).
6. Problem of TVOCs: The figures measured inside new system furniture closets tended to be higher, but the closets are usually closed so it is not a serious problem. As it is easier for TVOCs to vaporize during the summer time, building managers may use electric fans or other means of ventilation to let TVOCs flow out. High level of TVOCs was also

found in stairways, elevators, and underground parking lots, which may be caused by fresh paints or new interior fitting and decoration. Building managers should consider choosing green building materials for future renovation. If the circumstance allows, building mangers may consider growing some plants which can absorb TVOCs, such as aglaonema, pleomele, dracaena, chrysanthemum, peace lily.

7. Problems of chloride residues in the water: Some of the drinking water was detected insufficient chloride residues (lower than 0.2 mg/L), which can result in improper disinfection, higher bacteria, and possible contraction of typhoid, dysentery, and cholera. Excess chloride residues in the swimming pool were also detected in some cases. Building managers should review the chloride adding process and amount, and hire professionals to test water quality regularly.
8. Problem of electro-magnetic field: Some of the indoor entertainment and exercise equipments have bigger motors. When people use these equipments, the EMF figures measured near the motors would be higher (180mG, for example). The measured figures are still lower than Taiwan government's legal standards (833mG), but the legal standard is transient exposure value, so it is not suitable to be used as a long-term safety standard. As a result, it is recommended the users should avoid using the equipments too long or keep their heads away from the motors.

6. Discussion and suggestion

As the influence of indoor air quality and indoor environment quality are so significant to human health, the knowledge of BHD is also crucial to architects and civil engineers. In 2010, an incident of carbon monoxide killed several people in an apartment building. Architects and civil engineers who had built the building faced criminal charge and were sentenced jail time because the improper design and construction of the building caused carbon monoxide flowed to different floor levels. Although the higher court is still deliberating on the appeal, it also showed the training and education of healthy environment planning, construction, and inspection are still insufficient or have been long ignored in the traditional architecture and civil engineering fields. Thus, in the future, cross-disciplinary knowledge, such as medicine, public health, and environmental protection, should be integrated to form a discipline of healthy environment planning and management which would be taught, studied and applied to the field practices of architecture and construction. In this way, architects and civil engineers are able to make sure future building users are protected from any health hazards. Furthermore, at the later stage of building lifecycle, property managers must be able to apply their management and maintenance expertise to eliminating any health hazard problems hidden in the environment or hardware of the buildings for 50 or more years of building use and management period.

There are many potential health hazard factors existing in household environments, including: hazardous gas, poor air quality, bad water quality, EMF, radiation, over-bright or insufficient lighting, noise, temperature, and humidity. Particular space, building materials, facilities, or inappropriate use habits can become the direct or indirect source of pollution. For example, bad ventilation plan (especially close or underground space), hazardous building materials (such as vaporized formaldehyde or high concentration of TVOCs), unsatisfying building material performance (such as bad sound proof performance of windows or doors), using electrical appliances for a long time and in close distance (for example, long-time use of an electric blanket), decreasing facility performance (such as brightness of fluorescent lights reduced because they are covered by dust). In conclusion, when occupants show signs of discomfort during the indoor activities, building managers may need to check if the discomfort is caused by building environments. The association chart of building health check items, symptoms, and possible disease above (see Fig. 18) can be used as a reference. If it is necessary, professional test agencies or experts can also be brought in to maintain the health and safety of our own living environments.

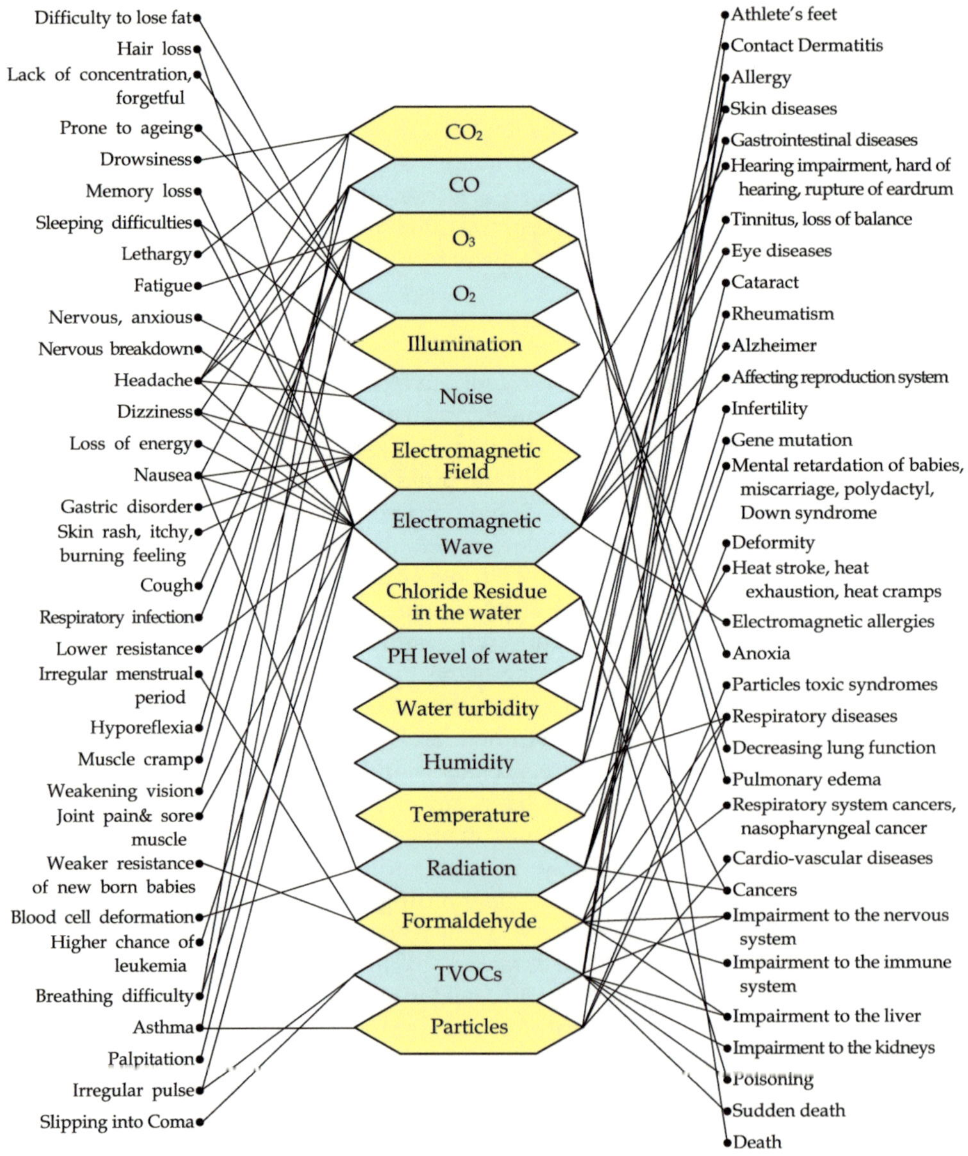

Fig. 18. The association chart of building health check items, symptoms, and possible disease

A few things must be noted when using the test devices. Before using test devices, inspectors must check if the devices are calibrated (or calibrating the devices regularly), and must make sure consumable sensor parts are within their expiratory dates (such as HCHO sensing strips) to avoid inaccurate measurements. Furthermore, when performing tests with devices, inspectors also need to choose an appropriate testing location and testing time. For the choice of location, taking EMF test as an example, if inspectors perform the test in the area of electrical facilities, they will get a higher figure (see Fig. 19). However, people usually do not spend a lot time in this area. Even if the figure is higher, as long as it is lower than the standard value, it does not need to feel concerned, and the test report based on this result is not very meaningful. Therefore, inspectors should find the locations frequented by occupants, for example, the activity areas of elderly and children (such as the children playground in Fig. 19). Furthermore, Fig.20 shows that test of CO_2 level in the library room should be done when there are people inside so that the result would be closer to the reality. It is also more appropriate to perform the test of CO level during the peak hours because cars come in and out frequently. Tests on photocopiers should be done when the photocopiers are being operated to gather a more precise and reasonable figures.

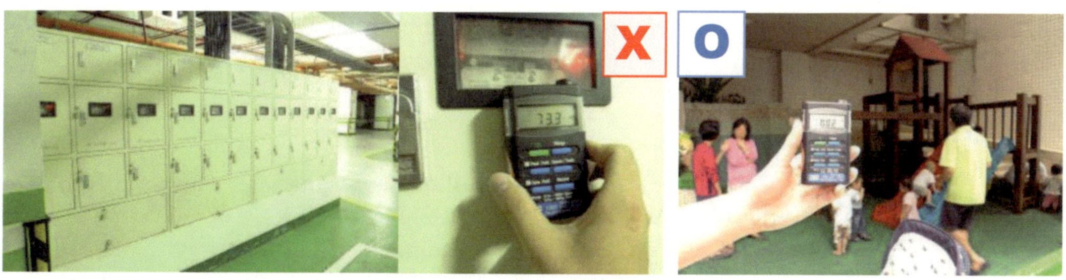

Fig. 19. EMF tests in the electric facility area (left) and the children playground (right)

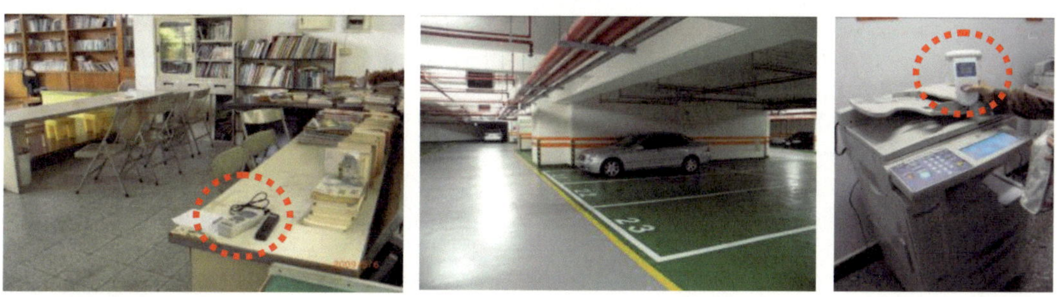

Fig. 20. CO_2 level test in the library (left) / CO level test in the basement(middle) / O_3 level test on a photocopier(right)

7. Conclusion

Undoubtedly, healthy building is a very important research subject. However, no matter how many studies on the correlation between indoor environment and health of occupants have been done to stress the importance of this subject, if there is no participation on the part of building designers, construction engineers, and managers, the importance of the issue would not be fully recognized. Therefore, architects, civil engineers and property managers play an important role in promoting healthy buildings. Furthermore, from the viewpoint of Building Medicine, the field of construction can learn from the field of medical medicine. As a result, the model of medical field which aims to train physicians to possess the expertise of 'Holistic Care' is a feasible model for the education and training of future building doctors. By following this model, architects, civil engineers or property managers can also learn how to be a building doctor.

Based on the idea of building lifecycle, Building Medicine promotes the concept of building eugenics. If architects and civil engineers starts to evaluate how to construct a healthy building at the design and construction stage of building lifecycle, such as using green building materials or non-toxic building materials, eliminating noise problems, illumination and lighting, ventilation, EMF problems, and water supply problems, they can provide a healthy living and work environment for the public. Unfortunately, beautiful exteriors, low costs, maximum investment benefits are goals which most building developers pursue. Therefore, architects and civil engineers must develop their expertise in planning and management of healthy environment, and use their expertise to influence developers or government owners gradually. At the operation and maintenance stage of building life cycle, property managers can continuously monitor, manage, and eliminate health hazard factors in the living and working environment through regular Building Health Diagnosis (BHD) to make building occupants enjoy a healthy living space forever.

8. References

Barrow, MW. & Clark, KA. (1998). Heat-related illnesses. American Family Physician, Vol.58, No.3, (September 1998), pp. 749-756, ISSN 0002-838X

Bornehag, CG.; Blomquist, G.; Gyntelberg, F.; Jarvholm, B.; Malmberg, P.; Nordvall, L.; Nielsen, A.; Pershagen, G. & Sundell, J. (2001). Dampness in buildings and health - Nordic interdisciplinary review of the scientific evidence on associations between exposure to 'dampness' in buildings and health effects (NORDDAMP). *Indoor Air*, Vol.11, No.2, (January 2001), pp. 72-86, ISSN 0905-6947

Bornehag, CG.; Sundell, J.; Bonini, S.; Custovic, A.; Malmberg, P.; Skerfving, S.; Sigsgaard, T. & Verhoeff, A. (2004). Dampness in buildings as a risk factor for health effects, EUROEXPO: a multidisciplinary review of the literature (1998-2000) on dampness and mite exposure inbuildings and health effects. *Indoor Air*, Vol.14, No.4, (August 2004), pp. 243-257, ISSN 0905-6947

Boyce, P. & Kennaway, DJ. (1987). Effects of light on melatonin production. *Biological Psychiatry*, Vol.22, No.4, (April 1987), pp. 473-438

Chang, Chih-Yuan. (2006). The Concept and Implements for Building Medicine, Doctoral dissertation, National Taiwan University, Taiwan

Chang, Chih-Yuan.; Huang, Shyh-Meng. & Guo, Sy-Jye. (2007). Medical Records for Building Health Management. *Journal of Architectural Engineering*, Vol.13, No.3, (September 2007), pp. 162-171, ISSN 1076-0431

Chang, Chih-Yuan. (2008). International Classification of Building Diseases for Prolonging Life Management, Academic Research of National Science Council, Taiwan

Chang, Chih-Yuan. (2010). Surveying and diagnosing leakage problems automatically : to put smart humidity chip in RC structure for building health management, Academic Research of National Science Council, Taiwan

Chen, Chu-Chi. (2001). *Health information management* (2nd Ed.), Hong-Han Press, ISBN 957-8676-06-9, Taipei, Taiwan

Chiang, Che-Ming. (2001). Development of « Taiwan, Sustainability, Architeture » in the next one hundred years-Applying Nature-friendly Construction Strategy to Maintain a Sustainable Environment, Taiwan Architect Magazine, No. 320, pp. 98-105

D'Amato, G.; Liccardi, G.; D'Amato, M. & Holgate, S. (2005). Environmental risk factors and allergic bronchial asthma. *Clinical and Experimental Allergy,* Vol.35, No.9, (September 2005), pp. 1113–1124, ISSN 0954-7894

Dever, G. E. Alan. (1976). An epidemiological model for health policy analysis, *Social Indicators Research 2,* pp. 453-466, D. Reidel Publishing Company, Dordrecht-Holland

Eife, R.; Weiss, M.; Barros, V.; Sigmund, B.; Goriup, U.; Komb, D.; Wolf, W.; Kittel, J.; Schramel, P. & Reiter, K. (1999). Chronic poisoning by copper in tap water: I. Copper intoxications with predominantly gastointestinal symptoms. Vol.4, No.6, (January 1999), pp. 219-223

Franzellitti, Silvia.; Valbonesi, Paola.; Ciancaglini, Nicola.; Biondi, Carla.; Contin, Andrea.; Bersani, Ferdinando. & Fabbri, Elena. (2010). Transient DNA damage induced by high-frequency electromagnetic fields (GSM 1.8 GHz) in the human trophoblast HTR-8/SVneo cell line evaluated with the alkaline comet assay. *Mutation Research-Fundamental and Molecular Mechanisms of Mutagenesis,* Vol.683, No.1-2, (January 2010), pp. 35-42, ISSN 0027-5107

Goldstein, Mark. (2008). Carbon Monoxide Poisoning. *Journal of Emergency Nursing,* Vol.34, No.6, (December 2008), pp. 538–542, ISSN 0099-1767

Hardoy, MC.; Carta, MG.; Marci, AR.; Carbone, F.; Cadeddu, M.; Kovess, V.; Dell'Osso, L. & Carpiniello, B. (2005). Exposure to aircraft noise and risk of psychiatric disorders: the Elmas survey. *Social Psychiatry And Psychiatric Epidemiology,* Vol.40, No.1, (January 2005), pp. 663-672, ISSN 0933-7954

HBN The Healthy Building Network, 19.03.2011, Available from http://www.healthybuilding.net/

Health Care Without Harm, 07.04.2011, Available from http://www.noharm.org/

Hsieh, Po-Sheng. (2003). *Introduction to Medicine,* National Taiwan University College of Medicine, ISBN 957-01-5639, Taipei, Taiwan

Jones, AP. (1999). Indoor air quality and health. *Atmospheric Environment,* Vol.33, No.28, (December 1999), pp. 4535–4564, ISSN 1352-2310

Kheifets, L. & Shimkhada, R. (2005). Childhood Leukemia and EMF: eview of the Epidemiologic Evidence. *Bioelectromagnetics,* (2005), pp.51-59, ISSN 0197-8462

Lane, Rachel.; Reinhardt, Pascale. & Thompson, Patsy. (2010). Evidence of children's vulnerability to radiation in the context of radiological/nuclear events and considerations for emergency response. *Radiation Protection Dosimetry,* Vol.142, No.1, (November 2010), pp. 36-39, ISSN 0144-8420

Ma, Shao-jing. (2010). A Strategic Research on Effects and Improvement Measuresof Extremely Low Frequency Electromagnetic Fields in Households andWorkplaces, Doctoral dissertation, Feng Chia University, Taiwan

Mann, Andrea G.; Tam, Clarence C.; Higgins, Craig D. & Rodrigues, Laura C. (2007). The association between drinking water turbidity and gastrointestinal illness: a systematic review. Bmcpublic Health, Vol.7, No.256, (September 2007), ISSN 1471-2458

Marco, Vinceti.; Guglielmina, Fantuzzi.; Lucia, Monici.; Mariateresa, Cassinadri.; Guerrino, Predieri. & Gabriella, Aggazzotti. (2004). A retrospective cohort study of trihalomethane exposure through drinking water and cancer mortality in northern Italy. Science of The Total Environment, Vol.330, No.1-3, (September 2004), pp. 47-53, ISSN 0048-9697

Nilles, E.; Sayward, H. & D'Onofrio, G. (2009). Vascular endothelial growth factor and acute mountain sickness, Journal of Emergencies Trauma Shock , pp. 6–9

Tunga, Salthammer.; Sibel, Mentese. & Rainer, Marutzky. (2010). Formaldehyde in the Indoor Environment. *Chemical Reviews*, Vol.110, No.4, (April 2010), pp. 2536–2572, ISSN 0009-2665

Wang, JL. & Yau, SC. (2002). Building Pathology, China Electric Power Press, Beijing, China

Watt, David S. (2007). *Building Pathology* (2nd Ed.), Blackwell publishing, ISBN 978-1-4051-6103-9, UK

Wu, PC.; Li, YY.; Lee, CC.; Chiang, CM. & Su, HJJ. (2003). Risk assessment of formaldehyde in typical office buildings in Taiwan, *Indoor Air*, Vol.13, No.4, (December 2003), pp. 359-363, ISSN 0905-6947

7

Mycotoxins: Quality Management, Prevention, Metabolism, Toxicity and Biomonitoring

C. N. Fokunang et al.*
Faculty of Medicine and Biomedical Sciences, University of Yaoundé 1, Republic of Cameroon

1. Introduction

When fungi grow on a living organism or on stored food material that we consume, they may produce harmful metabolites that diffuse into their food (Garcia et al., 2009; Kabak and Dobson, 2009). It is believed that fungi evolved these metabolites as a means of protecting their food supply by preventing other organisms from eating it. These metabolites are referred to as mycotoxins, which literally mean "fungus poisons". Fungi that produce mycotoxins do not have to be present to do harm. When a fungus grows grains in storage, the environment may become unsuitable for the fungus and it dies. Although the fungus dies, during the growth stage, if it produces mycotoxins, this can poison the grains (Fokunang et al., 2006). The effects of poisoning by mycotoxin are referred to as mycotoxicoses. The knowledge that mycotoxicoses is the result of fungal actions was a relatively, recent discovery (Lackner et al., 2009). This is understandable since illnesses in this case are due to consumption of mycotoxins that has been released by the fungus and is not directly caused by the fungus (Coppock and Jacobsen, 2009).

1.1 The mycotoxin system

The mycotoxin system as shown in figure 1 may be considered in terms of four interacting subsystems namely; toxicology, metabolism, health, productivity and wealth. After exposure through ingestion, inhalation or skin contact, the toxicity of a mycotoxin is determined by a sequence of events such as metabolism, involving the administration, absorption, transformation, pharmacokinetics, molecular interactions, distribution, and excretion of the toxin and its metabolites (Fokunang et al., 2006). In turn, the toxicity of the mycotoxin will be manifested by its effect on the health and productivity of crops, human efforts and agricultural and livestock products.

* O. Y. Tabi[1], V. N. Ndikum[1], E. A. Tembe-Fokunang[1], F. A. Kechia[1], B. Ngameni[1], N. Guedje[1], R. B. Jiofack[1], J. Ngoupayo[1], E. A. Asongalem[1], J. N. Torimiro[1], H. K. Gonsu[1], S. Barkwan[2], P. Tomkins[2], B. T. Ngadjui[1], J. Y. Ngogang[1], T. Asonganyi[1] and O. M. T. Abena[1]
1 Faculty of Medicine and Biomedical Sciences, University of Yaoundé 1, Republic of Cameroon,
2 Centre for Biopolymer and Biomolecular Research, Athlone Institute of Technology, Republic of Ireland.

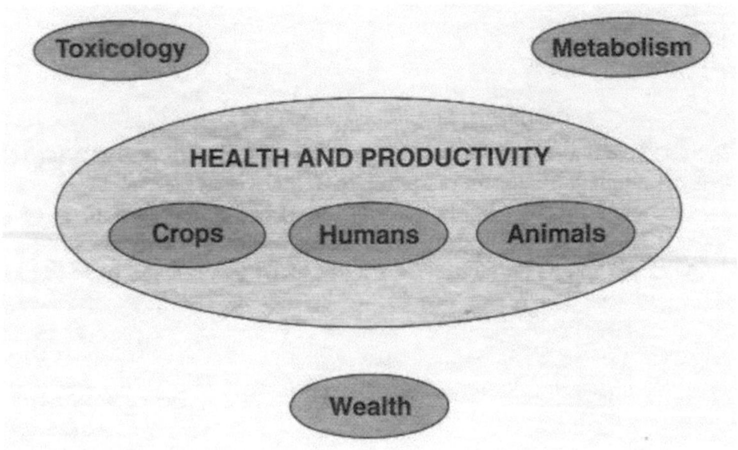

Fig. 1. The Mycotoxins system

1.2 The spoilage system

Biodeterioration is the net result of many interacting spoilage agents which may be widely described as biological, chemical, physical, micro-environmental and macro-environmental (Figure 2). However, the relative impact of these agents will often be mainly determined by the nature and extent of human intervention, occurring within the socio-economic system (Coker 1998). The factors that contribute to bio deterioration within an ecosystem are mainly moisture, temperature and pests status (Christensen, 1975; Hussein and Brasel 2001).

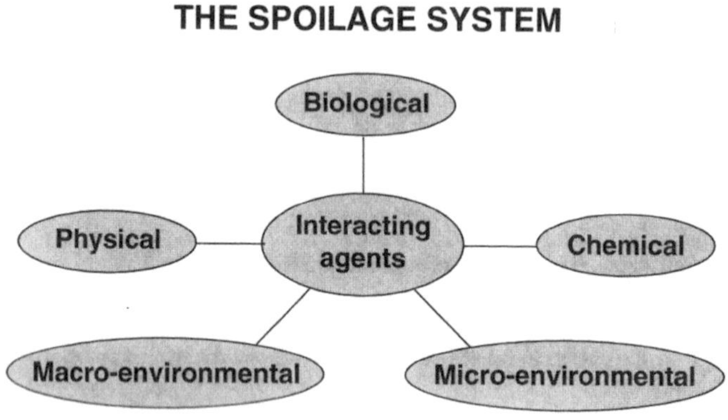

Fig. 2. The mycotoxin spoilage system

1.3 Mycotoxins of economic importance

The moulds and mycotoxins which are now considered to be of world-wide importance are shown in figure 3. Some mycotoxins are however of regional importance as illustrated in table 1. Regional myxcotoxins are specific to certain regions and the occurrence is link to climatic changes. The important mycotoxins have shown the capacity to have a significant impact upon human health and animal productivity in a wider distribution in a number of countries, most especially in the warm humid countries in sub-saharan Africa and Asia (Fokunang et al., 2006; Khlangwiset and Wu 2010).

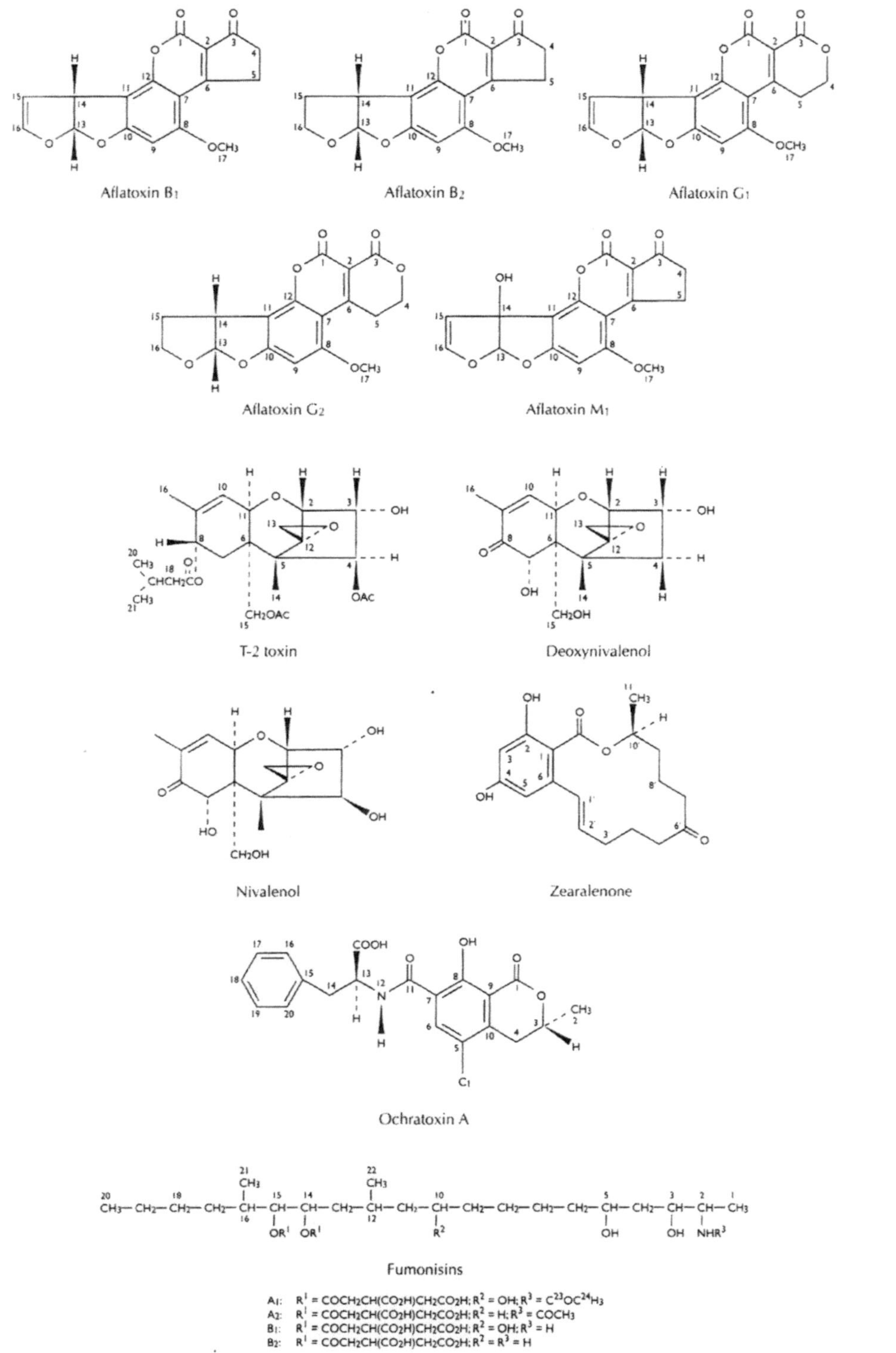

Fig. 3. Mycotoxins of worldwide importance (Coker, 1999)

Fungal species	Mycotoxin products	Mycotoxicosis	Reference
Claviceps fusiformis	clavinet alkaloids	Ergotism	Cocker, 1999, Ding et al., 2006
C. purpurea	Ergotamine alkaloids	Ergotism	Anderson, & Conning, 1993
C. paspali	paspalinine	Paspalum staggers	Van Egmond. 1989 ; Fokunang et al., 2006
Diplodia maydis	diplodiatoxin	Diplodiosis	Desjardins et al 1997 ; Friesen et al., 2008
Phomopsis leptostromiformis	phomopsin	Lupinosis	Takayuki, and Bjeldanes, 1993; Hussein et al., 2001
Balasia spp	alkaloids	Fescue foot	Bowman, & Rand. 1990; Kiso et al., 2004
Stachybotrys atra	satratoxins	Stachybotryotoxicosis	Bresinky and Besl, 1990; Purzycki & Shain 2010.
Rhizoctonia legumicola	slaframine	Slobber syndrome	Pitt 1996; Wu et al., 2008.
Acremonium loliae	lolitrem	Ryegrass staggers	Cocker et al. 1999
Pithomyces chartarum	sporidesmin	Facial eczema	Lacey, 1991; O'Brian et al 2007

Table 1. Fungi species and mycotoxins of regional importance (Fokunang et al., 2006

2. Mycotoxin fungi

2.1 *Aspergillus flavus*

A. flavus is not a single species, but a "species complex", made up of eleven species that are known to occur in many kinds of plant materials, including stored grains (Christensen, 1975; Meggs, 2009). One of the species in the complex, *A. oryzae* has long been used in the Orient to prepare various kinds of food products, such as sake, tofu and soy sauce, which in turn are used in the United States (Pitt & Miscamble, 1995; Shuaib at al., 2010).

What was determined in early research of aflatoxins is that the condition which allows for growth of *A. flavus* and aflatoxins is very narrow (Klich, 2009). *A. flavus* hardly invades stored grains alone, that is as a pure culture (Purzcki and Shain 2010). Various other species of fungi will normally grow on a substrate prior to invasion by *A. flavus*, such as. *A. glaucus* and *Candida pseudotropicalis (Khlangwiset and Wu, 2010)*. In a preinvaded substrate, regardless of how dense the *A. flavus* invasion may be, aflatoxin will not form. Thus, in order for aflatoxin formation to occur in say a storage bin full of peanuts, *A. flavus* must be growing alone and the peanuts cannot have been previously or simultaneously invaded by other fungi, an occurrence that is rare (Lugauskas and Stakeniene; Magan et al., 2010). In the case of the Turkey-X disease, the peanuts that were responsible for the aflatoxin poisoning were from South America, where the process used to harvest and dry the peanuts was responsible for providing an environment that allowed for growth of *A. flavus* and aflatoxin (Edlayne et al., 2009). *Aspergillus flavus* does not normally contaminate grains and other crops while they are still in the field. It is only after the grains are harvested and stored does *A. flavus*, as well as other so-called "storage fungi" that have a low moisture requirement, can the grain be invaded (He and Zhou, 2008). Although conditions favourable for growth of the *A. flavus* and production of aflatoxin is narrow, the fungus is common and widespread in nature. Under warm humid condition *A flavus* can invade stored gains such as corn as shown in figure 4. It can be found growing on various decaying vegetation where it may heat up the substrate to as high as 113-122°F as it consumes the material (Hedyati et al., 2007; Lee, 2009).

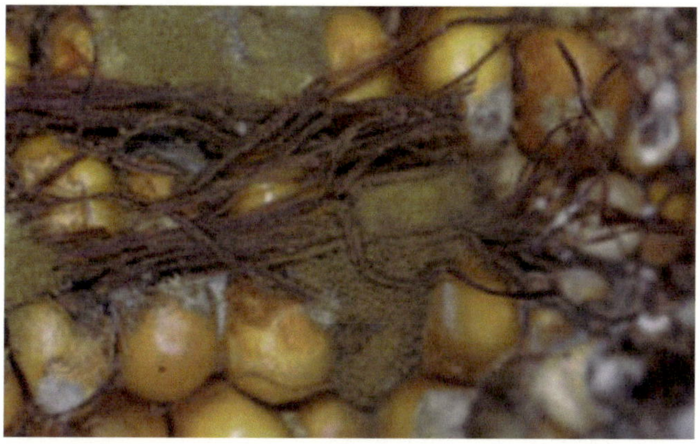

Fig. 4. *Aspergillus flavus* infestation on corn *Zea mays* (Hedyati et al., 2007)

The term aflatoxins was derived in the early 1960s when the death of thousands of turkeys (Turkey X' disease) ducklings and other domestic animals was attributed to the presence of *A. flavus* toxins in groundnut meals imported from South America (Nageswara et al., 2002). The amount of aflatoxin formed differs as to the substrate on which it is growing. Although the mycelial mass may be the same in each substrate, the aflatoxin produced would be far greater in peanuts than in say soybeans, where relatively very little would be produced. The growth of A. flavus producing aflatoxin in peanuts is shown in figure 5.

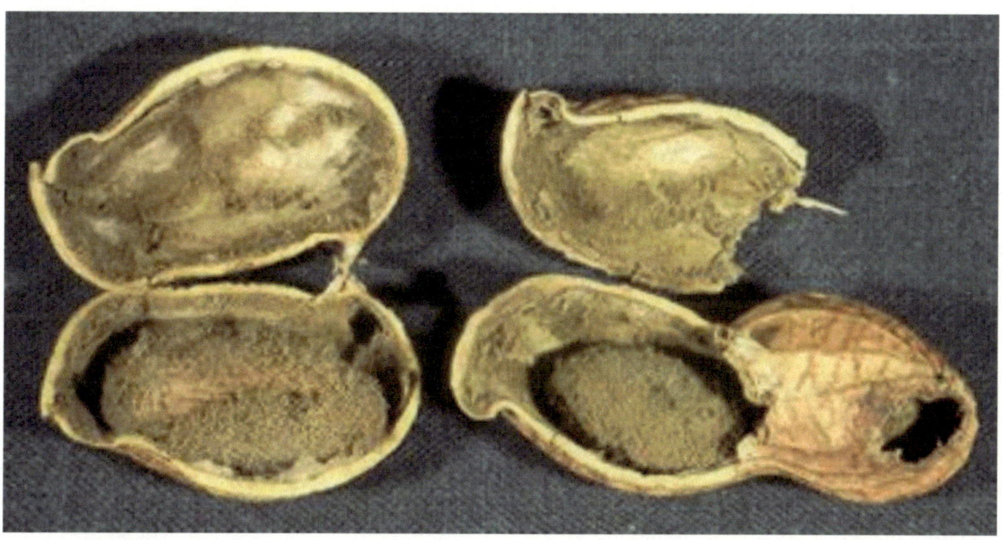

Fig. 5. Stored peanuts infected by *A flavus* producing aflatoxin (Kios et al., 2004)

Other seeds of cereal crops, wheat, corn, barley, oats and sorghum are also generally of low-aflatoxin-risk (Nageswararao et al 2002). Weather and climate were also contributing factors. The amount of toxin produced vary with the isolate of *A. flavus*. That is different sources of *A. flavus* will produce different amounts of aflatoxins. Some isolates of *A. flavus* may not even form aflatoxin (Fuchs et al., 1991; Awad et al., 2010). Although the aflatoxins are the major toxins associated with mycotoxicosis, another mycotoxin called cyclopiazonic acid (figure 6), has been associated in the aetiology of Turkey X disease (Bradburn et al., 1994; Kios et al., 2004).

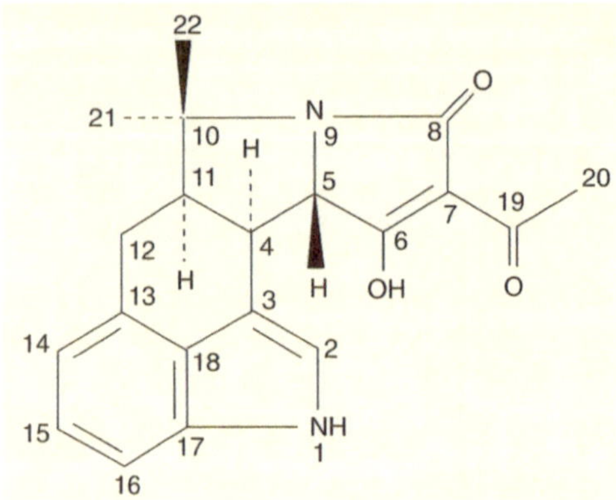

Fig. 6. Cyclopiazonic acid associated in the aetiology of Turkey X disease (Bradburn et al., 1994)

2.1.1 Aflatoxin toxic effects

Studies by Christensen (1975), over a period of several years, examined 100 different samples of black pepper from all over the world. In dilution cultures of these samples, the number of fungus colonies in whole or ground black pepper averaged 52,000 per gram/black pepper and the upper range was over half a million per gram (Coker, 1998). These colonies were mostly of *A. flavus*, *A. ochraceus* and *A. versicolor*. All three species are known to be aflatoxin producers. Some samples of ground pepper were caked lightly with fungus mycelium when first opened in the laboratory and with time, a number of these became solidly caked with mycelium (Jalili et al., 2011).

How heavily contaminated is 52,000 to 500,000 colonies of fungi, per gram? Let's make a comparison for what is acceptable levels of fungal colonies isolated in other food products at the time Christensen published his results. Wheat, for example, that is intended for milling into flour seldom contains any more than a few thousand colonies of fungi per gram of grain. If barley has as many as 10,000 colonies of the same kind of fungi per gram as in black pepper, it would be rejected for malting in beer making. If breakfast cereals or bread were as contaminated as black peppers, they would have so musty an odour and taste that they would be too revolting to eat. Apparently, the natural spicy odour and flavour of black, as well as white pepper are potent enough to conceal the taste and odour of these fungi.

2.1.2 Mycotoxins of other fungal species of *Aspergillus*, *Penicillium* and *Fusarium*

2.1.2.1 *Aspergillus ochraceus* and ochratoxin

Aspergillus ochraceus is also a species complex, and consist of nine species. These species are common in soil, decaying vegetation, and in stored seeds and grains undergoing microbial deterioration. However, this fungus is seldom isolated from more than a small percentage of seeds or grains that are undergoing microbiological deterioration in storage because it is evidently not a good competitor, as is also the case with *A. flavus*. This is a general rule, but *A. ochraceus* has been isolated from 40% or more of surface-disinfected kernels of corns from bins in which deterioration was in progress. It has also been the major organism in some lots of whole black pepper (Desjardins and Hohm, 1997; Chang et al., 2011).

Production of ochratoxin, by *A. ochraceus*, was first described in South Africa (Christensen 1975), where it was isolated along with a number of other fungi. In experiments done with this isolate, the LD50 (the single dose that will kill 50 percent of the individual animals tested) of ochratoxin for rats is 22mg/kg (= 22 milligrams of the toxin per kilogram of body weight of the rat), but a lesser amount will result in severe liver damage. A single dose of 12.5 mg/kg (=12.5 milligrams of the toxin per kilogram of body weight of the rat) was administered to pregnant rats on the tenth day of gestation, and of the 88 foetuses involved, 72, or 81.8% died or were resorbed (Coker 1998; He & Zhou 2010). Ducklings seem to be equally sensitive to ochratoxin as they are to aflatoxin (Ates et al., 2011).

Another fungus, *Penicillium viridicatum*, can also produce ochratoxin, and is relatively common in stored corn and is a more common producer of ochratoxin than *A. ochraceus (Blumenthal, 2004).*

2.1.2.2 *Aspergillus versicolor* and sterigmatocystin

This species is another storage fungus. However, it is never found as the only fungus or as the predominating fungus in deteriorating cereals. Normally, by the time a grain sample has become very mouldy, *A. versicolor*, along with other *Aspergillus* species and usually other filamentous fungi and yeasts as well. Some of the black pepper mentioned earlier, as being decayed by fungi, was very heavily invaded by *A. versicolor*, but not by this fungus exclusively. This species, under the right conditions, produces sterigmatocystin, a toxic compound given the name because the fungus once was called *Sterigmatocystis*. The toxin is known to cause lung, liver and kidney tumours in laboratory animals and has been implicated as the cause of disease in calves that have consumed feed heavily invaded by *A. versicolor (Ben-Ami et al., 2011)*.. Experiments carried out in which the fungus were grown, on feed that was fed to calves, produced symptoms of the disease in the calves. However, tests were not done to detect the toxin in the calves. The toxin has also been detected in mouldy coffee beans in Africa, but no evidence indicates that even if these beans were used to brew coffee that the toxin would be in the drink.

2.1.2.3 *Aspergillus fumigatus* and fumagillin

This particular species is known to be an animal pathogen. Infection occurs through inhalation of spores and affects the lungs. Infection may also occur in eggs and the foetuses of cows. However, it also produces a metabolic product that may be considered a toxin or an antibiotic. This species differs from the others that we have discussed in that it is said to be thermophilic, that is, it is found in substrate where there are extremely high temperatures, up to 122°F (=50°C). This species is usually found on material that is in the advanced stages of decomposition in which the substrate temperature has been significantly raised by microbial decomposition (Edward, 2009). Under the proper conditions, *A. fumigatus* produces fumagillin. This compound is used as an amoebicide that is, as a means to rid the body of amoebae that are human pathogens and has been used effectively in honey bees as well. However, the correct dosage of this compound is critical. A little bit more than you need to get rid of the amoebae and you will be getting rid of the patient as well (Fokunang et al., 2006).

2.2 The genus *Fusarium*

Species of Fusarium are widespread in nature as saprobes in decaying vegetation and as parasites on all parts of plants (Harris et al., 1999; Walters et al., 2010). Many cause diseases of economically important plants. For this reason, there has been a great deal of research carried out in this genus by both plant pathologist and mycologist. However, there are a number of species that produce mycotoxins, mostly trichothecenes and zearalenone. We will discuss a few common examples.

2.2.1 *Fusarium tricinctum*

The effects of the first trichothecene toxin, T-2, documented was in the 1940s where it was associated with an outbreak of alimentary toxic aleukia (ATA). At its peak, in 1944, the population in the Orenbury District and other districts of the then USSR suffered enormous casualties, more than 10 percent of the population was affected and many fatalities occurred. The term *alimentary toxic* refers to the toxin being consumed in foods and *aleukia* refers to the reduced number of leucocytes or white blood cells in the affected person. Other symptoms included bleeding from nose and throat, multiple, subcutaneous haemorrhages (IARC, 1993; Bily et al., 2004).

The infected food in this case was millet, which made up a great part of the diet of the people in the region, and at times, during WWII, it was not uncommon to allow the millet to be left standing in the fields over winter because bad weather in the fall prevented its harvest at the proper time. During the late winter and early spring the millet would become infected with a variety of fungi, including *F. tricinctum*, and when the people gathered and ate this fungus, many came down with what was diagnosed as ATA. Thousands were affected, and many died. Locally, Joffe, a plant pathologist determined the outbreak of ATA was caused by consumption of a toxin, present in the millet, which had been contaminated by *F. tricinctum* (Biley et al., 2004). This was a remarkable conclusion since this was 20 years before aflatoxin was discovered. However, Joffe did not isolate or identify the toxin involved and as a result his work remained unknown until about 1965 when he presented a summary of his research at a symposium on mycotoxins. The mycotoxin involved was later given the common name T-2, and classified as one of several trichothecenes. Fed orally to rats, it has an LD50 of 3.8mg/kg, which is lower than that of aflatoxin, but still toxic enough.

2.2.2 *Fusarium graminearum* production

Corn is a stable in many countries and is used as a major ingredient in preparation of food for pigs and other domestic animals. Like many other grains, the kernels can be infected with fungi before and after harvest, and can affect the nutritional value of corn as food or feed. If the weather is rainy and the ears of corn are maturing in late summer and early fall, *F. graminearum* may infect only a few to a third of the kernels (Bennett et al., 1988; Cheng et al., 2011). Whatever amount of the ear is infected, all the kernels in that portion becomes heavily infected and decayed by the fungus. This fungus-infected corn is unattractive to pigs, as well as other animals, and they refuse to it. For this reason, this phenomenon has been called a *refusal factor*.

Regardless of what the composition of the rest of the feed, if it contains more than 5 percent of kernels with this refusal factor, the pigs will not eat it and weight loss will occur. They will starve rather than consume it. The infected corn contains an emetic compound produced by the fungus, and if this corn is consumed by pigs, they suffer prolonged

vomiting, after which they sensibly refuse to eat more of the corn. The toxin involved is deoxynivalenol (DON), also known as vomitoxin. The isolation and identification of this toxin has occurred only within the last 25 years (Bhat 2008).
Various methods have been tried to make the vomitoxin contaminated corn more acceptable to pigs. Among some of the means that have been tried are adding molasses to the feed to conceal whatever flavour or odour makes it unacceptable to the pigs, heating the feed, in hopes of destroying or inactivating whatever it is that is making the pig refuse to eat it, and composting it so that the heat will break down the toxin. However, none of these treatments have made the corn acceptable to pigs and are impractical (Bluhm et al., 2004).
The detection of infected corn or feed is also a problem. Since we are talking about mycotoxin here, the inability to isolate the causal agent, *F. graminearum*, is not evidence that the mycotoxin is absent. Long after a fungus has died off, mycotoxin secreted into the substrate, will still be present. The refusal of pigs to eat feed or corn is an indication that the refusal factor is present, but not necessarily conclusive. There are a number of reasons as to why pigs will refuse to eat. Pigs may be traumatized by being moved to a new pen, strange surroundings or even being offered different food. The only way that the toxin can be detected is to isolate, purify and identify it by spectrographic or other analysis (Taranu et al., 2011).

2.2.3 Importance of Trichothecenes as a biological weapon

2.2.3.1 Yellow rain

During the mid 1970s, when Vietnam was invading Laos, there were stories of "yellow rain" in areas where entire villages were killed. One eye witness account of such an event was told by a Hmong refugee, in Thailand. While tending his poppies, outside of his village, he and his family witnessed the bombing of their village by the Vietnamese, with a yellow powder that came down like yellow rain. Returning to the village, he found all of the animals and most of the people were dead. The bodies were bleeding from the nose and ears and their skin were blistered and yellowed. The few people left alive, when he arrived, were "jerking like fish when you take them out of the water". These people also eventually died. The witness took his family away from the village, but as they left they felt shortness of breath and sick to their stomach. This story is similar to other stories that were heard concerning yellow rain (Coppock and Jacobsen, 2009).
It was believed by the United States at that time that the Soviet Union was somehow involved in what occurred in the Hmong village, and medical teams were sent to investigate. However, because of the remoteness of these villages, news of such attacks normally took 4 to 6 weeks to reach someone who could notify the medical teams. By the time investigators reached a village, there was no evidence as to what happened. It would not be until 1980 that a Defense Department chemist recognized the symptoms described by victims of the bombing as similar to trichothecene mycotoxicosis. Samples from victims and from vegetation in the areas were tested and some were found to contain trichothecenes. With this information, President Ronald Reagan accused the Soviet Union of violating the Geneva Convention and Biological Weapons Convention, which of course they denied. However, these accusations would continue for three more years (Sudakin, 2003).
While the accusations and denials were aired, the media and scientific community gave a more critical examination of the yellow rain story. The analysis that demonstrated

Trichothecenes were being used was initially based on a single leaf, collected where one of the chemical attacks occurred. Subsequent specimens were collected later that also showed Trichothecenes were present, but the ratio of trichothecenes differed where it was found and was entirely absent in some samples. In addition, little fanfare was given to the over one hundred samples analyzed by the United States Army, which *did not find any indication of trichothecenes.* The eye witness accounts also came into question. Although it was implied that many villages were attacked with yellow rain, all of the witnesses were from a single refugee camp in Thailand, and even these accounts were thought to be unreliable (Kankunen et al., 2009). For example in relating a story of the bombing, one villager had initially said that 213 villagers were killed, but in a later retelling, there were only thirteen people killed and then forty.

Further erosion of the government's yellow rain story came about when a Yale University entomologist, whose expertise was in Southeast Asian bees, examined yellow rain samples and observed that they contained pollen from the native plants in the area. Based on the appearance of these samples, it was concluded that they were faeces of bees. In one species of bees, present in the area, there is a tendency for the bees to swarm when they defecated, as a cleansing ritual, which could give the appearance of yellow rain falling. News of such chemical attacks soon stopped and many civilian scientists were convinced that the entire yellow rain incident was a hoax that was carried out by the military to increase funding for defensive chemical and biological weapons. While a plausible alternative was given as to the cause of the yellow rain, the eye witness accounts while questionable, contradicted this theory. To date, the question as to what caused the yellow rain has still not been satisfactorily resolved and may never be (Hsueh et al., 1999).

2.3 Zearalenone

Zearalenone is a widely distributed oestrogenic mycotoxin occurring mainly in Maize, in low concentrations, in the developing countries, Europe, Japan, and North America (Hussein and Brasel, 2001). The concentrations in developing countries can be very high, especially when maize is grown in highland regions, under more temperate conditions. Zearalenone is co-produced with deoxynivalenol by *F. graminearum* and has been implicated with DON, in outbreaks of acute human mycotoxicoses (Prelusky et al., 1989). The exposure to zearalenone-contaminated maize has caused hyperoestrogenism in livestock, especially pigs, characterized by vulvar and mammary swelling and infertility (Bennett et al., 1988). There is limited evidence in experimental animals for the carcinogenicity of zearalenone (Kuiper-Goodman, 1991; Ding et al., 2006).

2.3.1 The fumonisins

The fumonisins are group of recently characterized mycotoxins produced by *F. moniliforme,* a mould that occurs world-wide and is frequently found in maize. Fumonisin B_1 has been reported in maize and maize products from a variety of agroclimatic regions including Brazil, Canada, USA, Austria, Italy, France and South Africa (Ding et al., 2006). The toxins especially occur when maize is grown under warm, dry conditions. Exposure to fumonisin B_1 (FB_1) in maize causes leuko-encephalmalacia (LEM) in horses and pulmonary oedema in pigs (Nair, 1998). LEM has been reported in many countries such as Argentina, Brazil, China, Egypt, South Africa and USA. FB1 is also toxic to the central nervous system, liver, pancreas, kidney and lungs of a number of animal species. The presence of fumonisins in maize has been linked with the occurrence of human oesophageal cancer in the Transkei, southern Africa and China (Rheeder et al., 1992). There is however, sufficient evidence in experimental animals for the carcinogenicity of cultures of *F. moniliforme* that contain significant amounts of the fumonisins, whereas there is limited evidence, in experimental animals, for the carcinogenicity of fumonisin B_1 (Naiker and Odhav, 2004).

2.4 Ochratoxin A

Ochratoxin A (OA) is caused by the fungi *Aspergillus ochraceous, A. parasiticus, A. niger* and *Penicillium verrucosum,* (Kuiper-Goodman, 1991; Blumenthal, 2004). This toxin is produced within the temperature range of 15-37°C, with an optimal production at 25-28°C. The exposure to ochratoxin A occur mainly in wheat and barley growing areas in temperate zones of the northern hemisphere (Abarca et al., 2001). The levels of ochratoxin A reported in these products ranges from trace amounts to 600μg/kg, in Canadian wheat. In the United Kingdom, reported levels have included 5000 and 2700μg/kg in barley and wheat respectively (Anderson & Conning, 1993). It also occurs in maize, rice, peas, beans and cowpeas; developing country origins of ochratoxin A include Brazil, Egypt, Chile, Senegal, Tunisia, Nigeria, India and Indonesia (Wild and Hall, 2000). The ability of OA to transfer from animal feeds to animal products has been demonstrated by the occurrence of this toxin in retail pork products, and the blood of pigs in Europe (Fazekas et al., 2001; Friensen et al., 2008). It has been suggested that pork products are a significant human dietary source of OA which has been found in blood (and milk) from individuals in a variety of European countries, such as France, Italy, Germany, Dewnmark, Sweden, Poland the former Yugoslavia, and Bulgaria (Abarca et al., 2001)). One of the highest reported levels is 100ng/ml OA in blood from the former Yugoslavia (Fuch et al., 1991), while a level of 6.6 ng/ml OA in milk has been reported in Italy (Micco et al., 1991; Huffman et al., 2010).

The existing or proposed regulations for OA are in place in about eleven countries, the permitted levels ranging from 1 to 50 μg/kg in foods and from 100 to 1000 μg/kg in feeds. In Denmark, for example, the acceptability of pork products from a specific carcass is determined by analysis of the OA content of the kidney. The pork meat and certain organs can be consumed as food if the OA content of the kidney is no more than 25 and 10 μg/kg respectively (van Egmond, 1989; Wild & Hall 2000).

The WHO/FAO Joint Expert Committee of Food Additives has recommended a provisional tolerable weekly intake of 112ng/kg body weight of OA (WHO, 1991). The ochratoxin A has been linked with the human disease Balkan endemic nephropathy, which is a fatal chronic renal disease, reported in limited regions of the former Yugoslavia, Romania and Bulgaria (Cocker, 1999). OA causes renal toxicity, nephropathy and immunosuppression in several animal species and it is carcinogenic in experimental animals (Abarca et al., 2001; Yoshinari et al., 2007).

3. The metabolism of mycotoxins

Examination of the metabolic fate of aflatoxin B_1 can be used to illustrate the importance of the metabolic process in determining toxicity, and as a means of determining exposure to mycotoxins, by measuring; mycotoxin-macromolecular conjugates, the parent mycotoxin and a biochemical change initiated by the mycotoxin, respectively (Coker 1999).

3.1 Metabolism of aflatoxin

Many animal studies in order to study the metabolic fate of aflatoxins, *in vivo* and *in vitro* studies using animal tissues have been conducted mainly on aflatoxin B_1. Limited studies have also been performed on humans involving the measurement of aflatoxin B_1, and its metabolites, in blood, urine, milk and isolated tissues. Metabolism has been studied in many species and under many different conditions (Dalezios et al., 1973, Yunus et al., 2010).

The metabolic fate of aflatoxins may be considered under the headings of administration, absorption, transformation (activation and detoxification), distribution and excretion.

3.1.1 Administration

Under natural conditions, exposure to the aflatoxins may occur orally (by food ingestion) and by tracheal and bronchial absorption (by the inhalation of contaminated dust particle). In addition to these natural routes, intraperitoneal (ip), intravenous (iv) and dermatitis administration have been used under experimental conditions.

3.1.2 Absorption

Studies using radiolabelled aflatoxin B_1 in rats and monkeys have demonstrated little difference in the distribution and excretion of the toxin after either oral or intraperitoneal administration, therefore implying that absorption after oral exposure is complete (Dalezios et al., 1973; Wilson et al., 2002).

Aflatoxin B_1 can also be absorbed rapidly, by passive diffusion, from the small intestines (especially the duodenum) into the mesenteric venous blood. Given the lipophilic nature of aflatoxin B_1, the composition of the intestinal epithelium is an important criterion. Although the liver is regarded as the main site of aflatoxin transformation, gastrointestinal metabolism will reduce the exposure of the liver to aflatoxin B_1 and, in terms of hepatic toxicity, is an important means of detoxification (Hsieh & Wong, 1994; Avantaggiato et al., 2004).

3.1.3 Transformation

The transformation of aflatoxin B_1 results in both the activation and the detoxification of the toxin and may be considered as occurring in two phases (Ben-Ami et al., 2010). Firstly, the transformation of the toxin to a selection of metabolites and, secondly, the conversion of some of these metabolites to either water soluble conjugates or macromolecular adducts (Huffman and Gerber, 2010). The transformation process will be modulated by numerous factors including the genetic make-up of the species, nutritional and health status, and exposure to metabolic modifiers in foodstuffs (Meggs, 2009)

The major metabolites of aflatoxin B_1 includes aflatoxin B_1 -8,9-epoxide, -8,9-dihydro-8,9-diol;the aflatoxins-B2a, -P_1 , M_1 -Q_1; aflatoxicol, aflatoxicol H_1 and aflatoxicol M_1 (Essigmann et al., 1982; Klich, 2009)(Figure 7). However, not all metabolites have been identified in all species.

3.1.4 Activation

In the liver, aflatoxin B_1 may interact with both DNA and proteinto elicit the carcinogenic and acutely toxic effects of aflatoxin, respectively. Initially, aflatoxin B_1 is converted, by cytochrome P450, to the highly reactive aflatoxin B_1 -8,9-epoxide which in turn may be converted to aflatoxin B_1 -dihydrodiol (Figure 8) (Baertschi et al., 1989; Coker, 1999; Kremer et al., 2007)

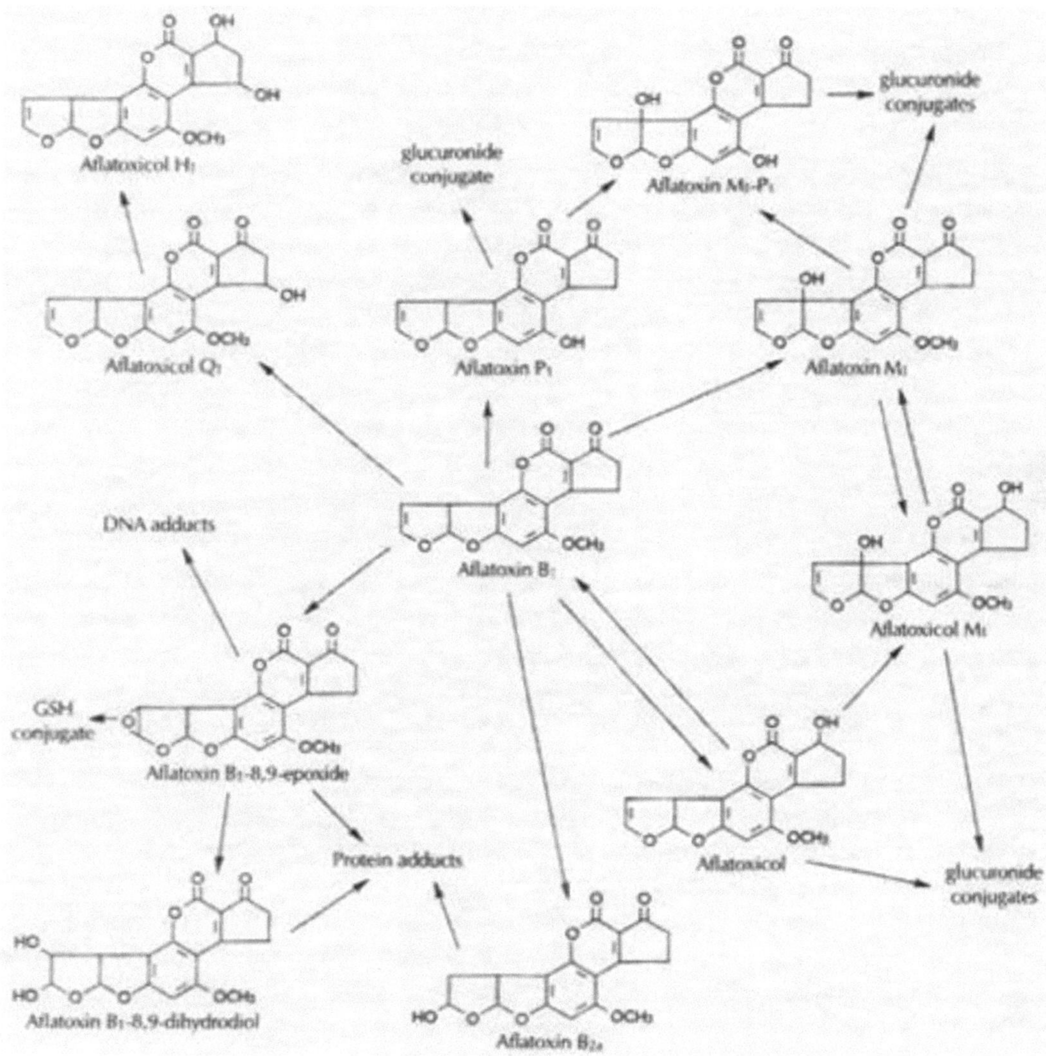

Fig. 7. The biotransformation of aflatoxin B_1 (Baertschi et al., 1998)

Aflatoxin B_1 is converted to at least seven metabolites, including a proposed unstable metabolite, the aflatoxin B_1 -8,9-epoxide, which is the so called ultimate carcinogenic form (Hsieh and Wong, 1994; Magan et al., 2010). Aflatoxin M_1 occurs in milk of cows fed on aflatoxin B_1-containing feeds. This metabolite is found in the liver, kidneys and urine of sheep and in the livers of rats treated with aflatoxin B_1 (Appleton et al., 1982; Micco et al., 1991). The carcinogenicity of aflatoxin B_1 arises from interaction with guanine moiety of DNA, to produce the aflatoxin-N^7-guanine adduct (Baerstchi et al., 1989), whereas the acute toxicity of aflatoxin B_1 is believed to stem from interaction between the dihydrodiol and protein amino groups to produce Schiff base adduct (Autrup et al., 1987).

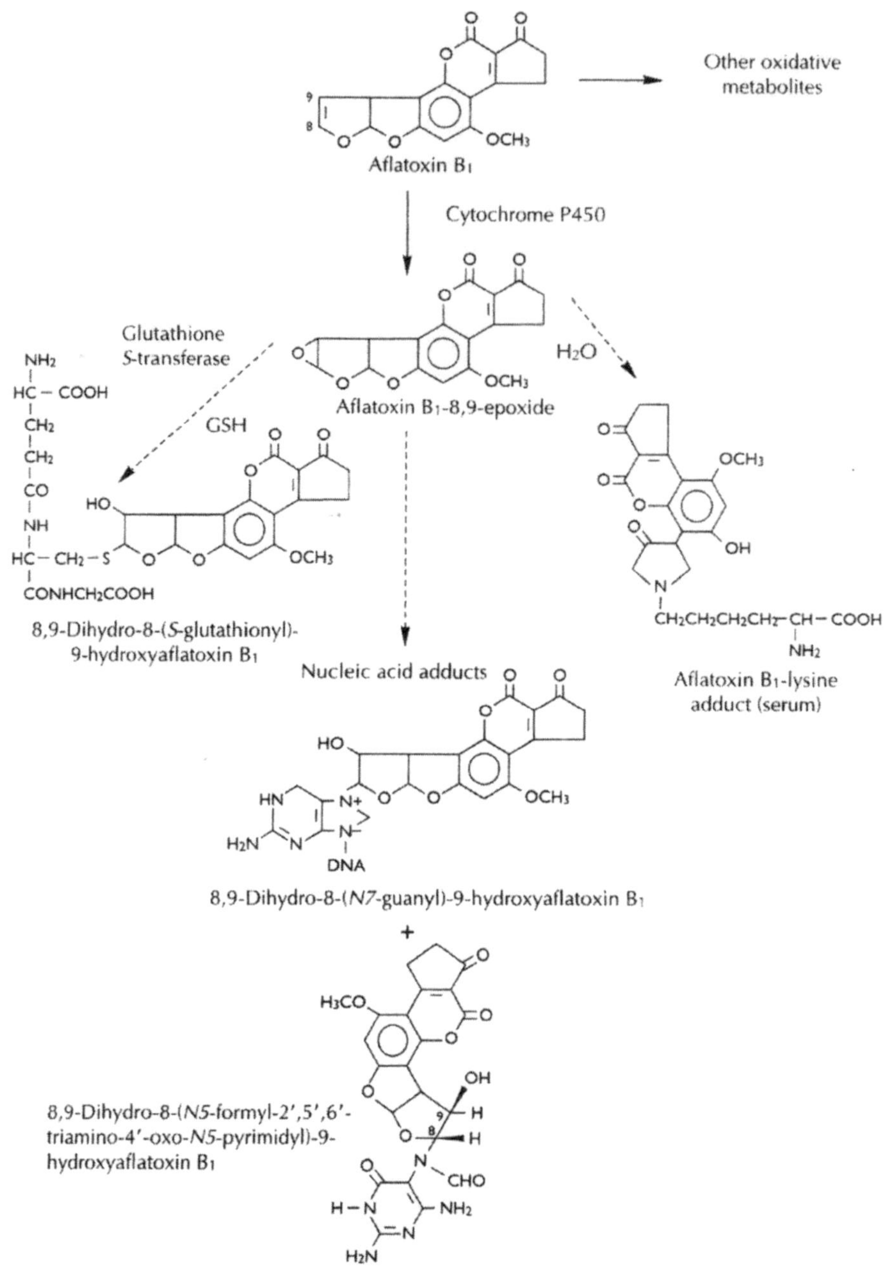

Fig. 8. Biotransformation process of aflatoxin B_1 (Parker et al., 1998)

The major metabolites of aflatoxin B_1 includes B_1-8, 9-dihydro-8-9-diol; the aflatoxins $-B_2a$,-P_1, M_1, -Q_1; aflatoxicol, aflatoxicol H_1 and aflatoxicol M_1 (Essigmann et al., 1982; Smith et al., 2007). However, not all metabolites have been identified in all species. Aflatoxicol is a major aflatoxin B_1 in rat plasma (Wong and Hsieh, 1978; Pestka & Bondy 1990). It is reported as having equivalent carcinogenic potency as aflatoxin B_1 (Schoenhard et al., 1981; Pasquali et al 2010), and about 70% the mutagenicity (Coulombe et al., 1982Porbst et al., 2007). Since aflatoxicol can be readily converted back to aflatoxin B_1, it has been proposed that aflatoxicol may act as a reservoir for aflatoxin B_1, *in vivo,* thereby prolonging the lifetime of the toxin in the body (Wong and Hsieh, 1978).

Total conversion of aflatoxin B_1 to M_1 in cow's milk is estimated to be about 1%. In comparing carcinogenic activity in rats, aflatoxin M_1 is less than one-tenth as active as aflatoxin B_1. However, the acute toxicities of these substances are almost similar. The aflatoxin metabolites M_1 and P_1 can also form DNA adduct (Essigmann et al., 1983). Similarly, there is evidence that aflatoxin G_1 can bind to DNA (Garner et al., 1979; O'brian et al., 2007).

3.2 Detoxification

Many methods have been used in an effort to detoxify contaminated feeds. Physical separation of obviously contaminated materials has proven successful in controlling aflatoxin contamination in peanuts. *Aspergillus flavus* and several other fungi emit a bright yellow-green fluorescence under ultraviolet light (Takayuki and Bjeldanes, 1993; Wilson et al., 2002). This telltale signal of fungal contamination has been useful in the physical separation of contaminated peanuts and corn as well as a few other crop samples.

Heat treatment of contaminated crops has also been used to detoxify food or feed material. Generally, under dry conditions the aflatoxins are quite heat stable. Normal roasting conditions can reduce the aflatoxin B_1 content in peanuts by 80% after an hour. Heating under conditions similar to the moist conditions used for autoclaving is much more effective in reducing aflatoxin content than dry heating (Park et al., 1988; Pitt & Miscamble, 1995).

Several chemicals such as hydrogen peroxide, ozone, and chlorine have been used to destroy aflatoxins. These substances react readily with aflatoxins in food as well as with many desired substances, including vitamins. A more useful method of chemical detoxification of contaminated feed is treatment with ammonia.

3.2.1 Ammonia detoxification

Ammonia was first used for the detoxification of aflatoxin-contaminated cottonseed meal, in the USA in the late 1960s (Park et al., 1988). The use of ammonia to detoxify corn meal and cotton meal increases the nutritional value of the feed.

The detoxified feed supports the growth of trout, cows, and other animals without apparent ill effects. An ammoniation process developed in Arizona involves placing a mixture of aqueous ammonia and cottonseed in large plastic bags used for silage (Cocker, 1999; Wu & Munkvold, 2008). The bags are sealed and allowed to stand in the sun for several weeks. The process has been shown to be effective in reducing the levels of aflatoxin in highly contaminated cottonseed (800ppb) to less than the 100 ppb action levels set by the FDA (Pepplinski et al., 1983).

Detoxication process involves numerous oxidising agents, aldehydes,acids and bases (inorganic and organic) that have been reported as potential chemical detoxification agents (Wild and Hall, 2000).

3.2.2 Chemistry of ammoniazation

The nature of the reaction products produced by the ammoniation of aflatoxin is still poorly defined. Most studies have focused on the reaction products of aflatoxin B_1 produced under a variety of conditions including the treatment in vitro, of pure toxin or of pure toxin on an inert carrier. The ammoniazation process of aflatoxin B_1 is illustrated in figure 8. Ammoniation, *in vitro*, of pure aflatoxin B_1 has afforded four compounds of molecular weights (MW) 286, 256, 236 and 206, together with many unidentified compounds of MW less than 200. The compound of MW 286 has been characterized as the decarboxylated derivative (aflatoxin D1) of aflatoxin B1, whereas the compound of MW 206 lacks the cyclopentenone ring of aflatoxin D1. The loss of the methoxy group from aflatoxin D_1 affords the compound of MW 256. The reaction product of molecular weight 236 is still to be identified

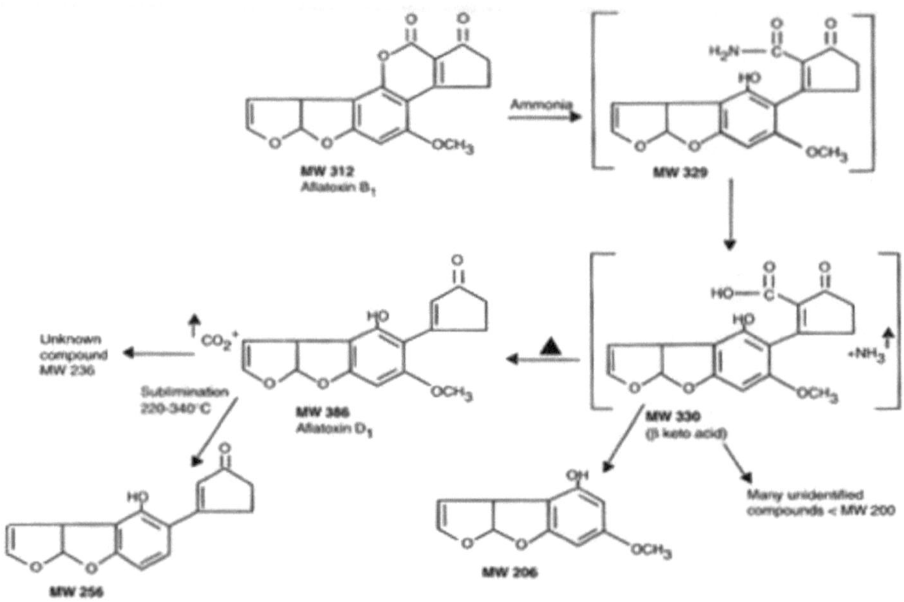

Fig. 9. Ammoniazation process of aflatoxin B1 (Parker et al., 1998)

3.2.3 Ammoniation and feed toxicity

The interaction of ammonia with both aflatoxin and nutritional components of feedstuffs has been. The resultant composition of these reaction products will determine the effect of ammoniation on both the nutritional and toxicological properties of treated commodity. These properties in turn, will determine the productivity of animals fed ammoniated feeds, together with the acceptability of animal products (milk, meat and eggs) used as human food.

3.2.4 Toxicity of ammonization reaction products

The toxicity of the reaction product, aflatoxin D_1, has been compared to that of the aflatoxin B_1 using a) the Ames test (Salmonella mutagenicity), b) the DNA covalent binding index CBI and c) the chick embryo bioassay as indicators of toxicity. Aflatoxin B_1 was reported (Lee et al., 1981; Yunus et al., 2010), as representing a 450-fold decrease in mutagenic potential, a 300-fold decrease, at least, in the DNA CBI (46), and (c) a 20-fold decrease, in toxicity to check the embryo (Lee et al., 1981; Kisoh et al., 2004). The reaction product MW 206, was over 600 times less mutagenic than aflatoxin B_1 (Hawarth et al., 1989; Faisal et al., 2008).

3.3 Distribution

After absorption from the intestine, aflatoxin B_1 rapidly enters the liver through the hepatic portal vein. The toxin is heavily concentrated in the liver after orla, ip and iv administration;much less aflatoxin accumulated in the kidney. The ip administration of radiolabelled aflatoxin B1 to rats resulted in the presence of approximately 17% of the label in the liver within 30 minutes. The kidneys and the eviscerated carcass contained about 5 and 27% respectively; traces (< 0.5%) of labelled material were present in the adrenal glands, brain, heart, pancreas, spleen, thymus and testes (Wogan et al, 1967). The radioactivity reduces rapidly, only 10% remaining in the liver after 2 hours.

3.4 Excretion

The excretion of aflatoxin B_1 occurs mainly through biliary pathway and, to a lesser extent, by the urinary pathway, and by excretion into milk of lactating animals.

3.4.1 Biliary excretion

Studies show that when radiolabelled aflatoxin B_1 was feed to rats, the reported plasma half-life for radioactivity was 91.8 hours. Twenty-three days after dosing, 70% of the radioactivity had been excreted; 55% was present in the faeces compared to 15% in the urine (Coulombe and Sharma, 1985; Herwaarden et al., 2006).

3.4.2 Urinary excretion

Urinary excretion shows that approximately 15% of radiolabelled aflatoxin B_1 was excreted in rats' urine 20-24 hours after ip administration. The major metabolites were the aflatoxin M1 (45% radioactivity) and P1 (<10%), and aflatoxin B_1 -N7-guanine (16%). The later is the major degradation product of hepatic B1-DNA adducts (Groopman, 1994).Eighty percent of the excreted B_1 -guanine occurred in the urine during the 48-hour period after dosing (Essigmann et al,1982); a dose-dependent correlation between B_1 and B_1 -guanine has been observed in male rats (Bennett et al., 1981; Baerschi et al., 1989).

3.4.3 Excretion through cow milk

Aflatoxin B1 in dairy feed can be metabolised and transferred to cow's milk in the form of aflatoxin M_1. The percentage carry-over rate typically lies within the range of 1-5% depending upon, for example, the level of aflatoxin within the feed and the productivity of the cow. Generally, the carry-over rate increases as the feed contamination level decreases and as the productivity increases. However, the carry over rate varies significantly from cow to cow and on an individual cow basis.

3.4.4 Excretion through human milk

The aflatoxins have also been reported in human breast milk. In Africa (Sudan, Ghana, Kenya and Nigeria), for example, the aflatoxin M_1, B_1, B_2, G_1 and G_2 have all been found in breast milk (Maxwell et al 1989). Aflatoxin M_1 was the major metabolite, occurring at concentrations ranging from 20 to 1800ng/L, in Ghana.

4. Biomonitoring of mycotoxins

4.1 Biomonitoring of aflatoxins

The introduction of methods for biomonitoring individual members of the population is a major development which will make a significant contribution towards confirming the perceived linkage between mycotoxin exposure and human diseases. Biomarkers for the aflatoxin, in humans, will now be discussed in terms of their role as markers of internal dose, biologically affective dose, early biological effect and susceptibility.

4.2 Markers of internal dose

4.2.1 Markers in urine

Aflatoxin M1 is a predominant metabolite in human urine. The presence of aflatoxin M_1 in urine may be detected by TLC, HPLC and ELIZA methods. Immunoaffinity columns have also been used to clean-up the samples prior to quantification.

Zhu et al. (1987) have compared dietary exposure to the aflatoxins with the urinary excretion of aflatoxin M_1, over a 3-day period, by analysing 252 urine samples in Guangxi Region of China. Between 1.2 and 2.2% of the dietary aflatoxin B_1 appeared in the urine as aflatoxin M_1, with a good correlation between the ingestion and excreted toxins.

4.2.2 Markers in milk

The occurrence of aflatoxin M1 in human breast milk is both an indicator of exposure of individual mothers to aflatoxin in food, and of the exposure of their infants to this toxin. However, no studies have reported a good correlation between levels of ingested aflatoxin B_1 and levels of aflatoxin M_1 in human breast milk. The occurrence of aflatoxin M_1 in human breast milk has been studied in Zimbabwe and France (Wild et al., 1987). In Zimbabwe , 11% of 54 samples of milk contained up to 0.05ug/L) aflatoxin M_1, whereas none of the 42 samples collected in France was contaminated.

4.2.3 Markers in blood

Unmetabolised aflatoxin B_1 in human blood serum has been used as an indicator of recent exposure to aflatoxins in food. Aflatoxin B1 has been detected (Tsuboi et al., 1984; Denning et al., 1988), for examples, in serum samples collected in Japan, Nigeria and Sudan. The detection methods used were ELIZA and HPLC; up to 3ug/kg B_1 were detected.

The aflatoxin M_1, B_1, B_2, G_1 and G_2 have been detected in cord sera from Ghana (34% of 188 samples); and aflatoxin M_1, M_2 and in B_2 cord sera collected in Nigeria (12% of 78 samples) (Lamplugh et al., 1988).

4.2.4 Markers of biologically effective dose

Two biomarkers of biologically effective dose have been developed. The first marker is a urinary aflatoxin B_1 -DNA adduct whereas the second is an adduct between aflatoxin B_1 and serum protein.

4.2.5 Aflatoxin B1-DNA adduct in urine

Studies in rats have examined the urinary excretion kinetics of specific metabolites after a single exposure to aflatoxin B1-N7-guanine (the primary B1-DNA adduct (Figure 8) accounted for 7.5% of the total detectable aflatoxins, whereas the aflatoxins P1, Q1, M1 and B_1 accounted for 31.5, 3,0, 2.2 and 0.3% of total aflatoxins, respectively (Groopman et al., 1992). Over the 24 hours after exposure, an excellent correlation existed between the oral dose of aflatoxin B_1 and the urinary aflatoxin-N7-guanine adduct. The other metabolites showed no such relationship.

The use of the aflatoxin-albumin adduct as a marker of the biologically effective does offers two advantages over the measurement of the aflatoxin-DNA adduct. Firstly, whereas the aflatoxin-DNA adduct reflects exposure to aflatoxin on the previous day, the level of aflatoxin-albumin adduct is a measure of chronic exposure to aflatoxin, over the previous 2-3 months (Hall and Wild, 1994). Secondly, the collection of fingerprick samples of peripheral blood is a far more convenient operation than the collected urine.

4.2.6 Aflatoxin-albumin adduct in blood serum

The aflatoxin-albumin adduct has been measured in children and adults from a variety of African, and other countries. In Africa, between 12 and 100% of the samples contained the adduct, whereas samples from Thailand were contaminated at lower levels and incidence. An estimate of the average daily intake of aflatoxin B_1 was performed by determining the aflatoxin-albumin adduct in blood samples collected from population of 100 persons attending health screening at the Bangladesh Institute of Research and Rehabillitation in Diabetes, Endocrine and Metabolic Disorders, BIRDEM) and United Kingdom. A comprehensive studies of the major foods showed that the main staples such as rice, pulses and wheat, were relatively free of mycotoxin contamination, whereas maize and groundnuts were significantly contaminated. Over 60% of the groundnut samples contained aflatoxin, with some samples containing levels of toxin which were 40 times greater than the maximal level permitted in the European Union, EU. About 70% of maize were contaminated, and 17% of these contained more than one mycotoxin; one sample contained five different mycotoxins. Since the use of maize, both as an animal feed and as human food, is being activiely encourage in Bangladesh, it is essential that every effort is made to alleviate the occurrence of mycotoxin in this commodity.

4.3 Markers of early biological effect

4.3.1 Measures of mutation spectra

Studies in the field of molecular biology have led to a better understanding of the generic alterations which occur during the progression from initiation to tumour formation, and to the development of sensitivity tests for the diagnosis of tumours.

The p53 tumour suppression gene is mutated in more than 50% of all human tumours (Hollstein et al., 1991). The number and type of mutations in this gene (the mutation spectrum) are not equally distributed, but occur in specific hot-spots which vary with the etiology of tumour formation.

In vitro studies using the human p53 gene have shown that codon 249 is the preferential site for the formation of aflatoxin-N7-guanine adducts (Pusieux et al., 1991). Exposure of cultured human liver cells to aflatoxin B_1 has produced codon 249 mutations. Although the link between aflatoxin exposure and specific p53 gene mutations in human populations has still to be confirmed, the gene mutation spectrum has considerable potential as a marker for exposure to, and damage from, the aflatoxins.

4.4 Markers of susceptibility

4.4.1 Measures of genetic variation in metabolism

Susceptibility to a particular agent will be influenced by the ability of individuals to absorb, distribute and metabolize the agent, and the nature of the metabolic process. The ability of individuals to repair damage inflicted by the agent will also contribute to the level of susceptibility. Studies with human liver microsomes have shown that the cytochrome P450s involved in the activation (epoxidation) of aflatoxin B_1 vary with the level of exposure. The activation of high levels of aflatoxin B_1, for example, is performed by cytochrome P450 3A4

(CYP3A4), with the simultaneous production of aflatoxin Q_1. Conversely, low levels of aflatoxin B_1 are activated by cytochrome CYP 1A2, with the simultaneous formation of aflatoxin M_1.

5. Conclusion

The problem posed by mycotoxin contamination of foodstuff especially in warm humid tropical environment has call for great interest in research in this area. For a better control and alleviation of mycotoxin problems in food it is important that importing nation adapts policies that ensures that the permitted levels of mycotoxin is maintained to an acceptable level of consumer protection. Efforts are in progress to implement these techniques in areas of high aflatoxin contamination in the hope of reducing the incidence of liver cancer. Developing nation needs to work on prevention strategies from mycotoxin through a partnership scheme. This can be achieved through a better knowledge of the role of mycotoxins in the epidemiology of human disease; a better understanding of the metabolism and toxicity of mycotoxins in animals and humans. There is also the need to understand the aetiology of mould and mycotoxin production in the field and the development of detoxification procedures which afford a safe product. In order to foster and intensify research in mycotoxin there is the need for continuous studies in developing a rapid simple, cost effective mycotoxin analysis method which can be used in sub-saharan and developing countries. There is also the need to put in place simple in vitro test for both acute and chronic toxicity and biomarkers for the detection of the exposure of individuals to mycotoxins and for the detection of immunotoxicity.
Continuous analyses of the combined epidemiological data from such studies indicate that high-level intake of aflatoxin in combination with such other diseases as hepatitis is associated with an increased rate of liver cancer. Despite these uncertainties about the role of aflatoxins in human cancer, efforts to minimize human exposures continue. There are well-established methods for harvesting, drying, and storing crops that are effective in the control of fungal contamination and aflatoxin production.

6. Acknowledgement

We wish to acknowledge travel grant support from the Athlone Institute of Technology, Republic of Ireland, technical and financial research grant from the Ministry of Higher Education of Cameroon. The CABI-United Kingdom is also acknowledged for literature material support and training programme.

7. References

Abarca, M.L., Accensi, F., Bragulat, M.R & Cabanes, F.J. (2001), 'Current importance of ochratoxin A-producing *Aspergillus spp'*, *Journal Food Protection*, vol 64, pp 903-906.
Anderson, D., and Conning, D.M. (1993), *'Experimental Toxicology', The Basis Issues*, 2 eds. *Royal Society of Chemistry*,UK, pp, 566.
Ates I, Ulker OC, Akdemir C, & Karakaya G (2011). Correlation of ochratoxin a exposure to urinary levels of S-hydroxydeoxyguanosin and malondialdehyde in a Turkish population. Bulletin of Environmental Contamination and Toxicology. 86(3):258-62. Epub 2011 Feb 19.

Autrup, H., Essigmann, J.M., Croy, R.G., Trump, B.F., Wogan, G.N., & Harris, C.C. (1979), 'Metabolism of aflatoxin B_1-guanine adduct and hepatitis B virus infection in areas with different liver cancer incidence in Kenya', *Cancer Research*, vol 47, pp 3430-3433.

Avantaggiato, G., Havenaar, R., & Visconti, A. (2004), 'Evaluation of the intestinal absorption of deoxynivalenol and nivalenol by an in vitro gastrointestinal model, and the binding efficacy of activated carbon and other adsorbent materials', *Food Chemistry and Toxicology*, 42, pp 817-824.

Awad WA, Ghareeb K, Bohm J, & Zentek J (2010). Decontamination and detoxification strategies for the Fusarium mycotoxin deoxynivalenol in animal feed and the effectiveness of microbial biodegradation. Food Addit Contam Part A Chem Anal Control Expo Risk Assess. 27(4):510-20.

Baertschi, S.W., Raney, K.D., Shimada, T., Harris, T.M & Guengerich, F.P. (1989), 'Comparison of rates of enzymatic oxidation of aflatoxin B_1, aflatoxin G_1, and sterigmatocystin and activities of the epoxides in forming guanyl-N^7 adducts and inducing different genetic responses', *Chemical Research and Toxicology*, vol 2, pp114-122.

Ben-Ami R, Lewis RE, & Kontoyiannis DP (2010). Enemy of the (immunosuppressed) state: an update on the pathogenesis of Aspergillus fumigatus infection.British Journal of Haematology. Aug;150(4):406-17

Bennett, G.A., Wicklow, D.T., Caldwell, R.W., & Smalley, E.B. (1988). 'Distribution of trichothecenes and Zearelenone in *Fusarium graminearum*: Rotted corn ears grown in a controlled environment', *Journal of Agriculture and Food Chemistry*, vol 36, pp 639-642.

Bhat RV.(2008). Human health problems associated with current agricultural food production. Asia Pacific Journal of Clinical Nutrition. 17 Suppl 1:91-4.

Bhat, R.V., Beedu, S.R., Ramakrihna, Y., & Munshi, K.L. (1989), 'Outbreak of trichothecene mycotoxicosis associated with consumption of mould-damaged wheat products in Kashmir Valley, India', *Lancet*, vol 1, pp 35-37.

Bily, A.C., Reid, L.M., Savard, M.E., Reddy, R., Blackwell, B.A., Campbell, C.M., Arnason, J.T., & Regnault, C. (2004), 'Analysis of *Fusarium graminearum* mycotoxins in different biological matrices by LC/MC', *Mycopathologia*, vol 157, pp 117-126.

Bluhm, B.H., Cousin, M.A., &Woloshuk, C.P. (2004), 'Multiplex real-time PCR detection of fumonisin-producing and trichothecenes in grains using gas chromatography-mass spectrometry', *Journal of Food Protection*, vol 67, pp 536-543.

Blumenthal, C.Z. (2004). 'Production of toxic metabolites in *Aspergillus niger, Aspergillus oryzae* and *Trichoderma reesei*: justification of mycotoxin testing in food grade enzyme preparations derived from the three fungi', Regulatory Toxicology and *Pharmacology*, vol 39, pp 214-228.

Bowman, W.C., & Rand, M.J. (1990), '*Textbook of Pharmacology* (2 Eds)'. Blackwell Scientific Publications London, pp. 1.85.

Bradburn, N., Coker, R.D., & Blunden, G. (1994). 'The aetiology of turkey X disease', *Phytochemistry*, vol 35, pp 817.

Chang, C.-H., Yu, F.-Y., Wu, T.-S., Wang, L.-T & Liu, B.-H. (2011). Mycotoxin Citrinin Induced Cell Cycle G2/M Arrest and Numerical Chromosomal Aberration Associated with Disruption of Microtubule Formation in Human Cells. *Toxicological Sciences,* 119: 84-92.

Bresinsky, A., & Besl, H. (1990), 'A colour Atlas of Poisonous Fungi': A Handbook for Pharmacists, Doctors." Woolfe, London

Chen F, Zhang J, Song X, Yang J, Li H, Tang H, & Liao YC (2011). Combined Metabonomic and Quantitative Real-Time PCR analysis Reveal Systems Metabolic Changes of Fusarium graminearum Induced by Tris Gene deletion. Journal of Proteome Research; 17:214-237.

Christensen, C.M. (1975). Molds, Mushrooms, and Mycotoxins. University of Minnesota Press, Minneapolis.USA, 264 pp.

Coker, R.D. (1998), 'The design of sampling plans for the determination of mycotoxins in foods and feeds. In: Mycotoxins in agriculture and food safety'. K.K. Sinha and Bhatnagar (eds). New York: Marcelll Dekker.

Coker, R.D. (1999), 'Aflatoxin: past, present and future', *Tropical Science*, vol 21, pp 143-162.

Coppock RW, & Jacobsen BJ (2009). Mycotoxins in animal and human patients,,Toxicology of Industrial Health. 2009 Oct-Nov;25(9-10):637-55.

Coulomb, R.A., Shelton, D.W., Sinnhuber, R.O & Nixon, J.E. (1982), 'Comparative mutagenicity of aflatoxins using a *Samonella*/trout hepatic enzyme activation system', *Carcinogenesis*, vol 3, pp 1261-1264.

Coulombe R.A, & Sharma RP. (1985). Clearance and excretion of intratracheally and orally administered aflatoxin B1 in the rat. Food Chemistry and Toxicology 23, 827-830.

Dalezios, J.L., Hsieh, D.P.H., & Wogan, G.N. (1973), 'Excretion and metabolism of orally administered aflatoxin B_1 by rhesus monkeys', *Food and Cosmetic Toxicology*, vol 11, pp 605-616.

Denning DW. Allen R, Wilkinson AP & Morgan MR (1990). Transplacental transfer of aflatoxin in humans. Carcinogenesis 11, 1033-1035.

Desjardins, A. E., & Hohm, T.M. (1997). 'Mycotoxins in plant pathogenesis', *Moecular Plant-Microbe Interaction,* vol 10, pp 147-152.

Ding, X., Lichti, K., Staudinger, J. L. (2006). The Mycoestrogen Zearalenone Induces CYP3A through Activation of the Pregnane X Receptor. *Toxicological Science,* 91: 448-455.

Ding, Y., Bojja, R.S., & Du, L. (2004). 'Fum3p, a 2-Ketoglutarate-Dependent Dioxygenase Required for C-5 Hydroxylation of Fuminisins in *Fusarium verticillioides'*, *Applied Environmental Microbiology*, 70, pp 1931-1943.

Edlayne G, Simone A, & Felicio JD (2009).. Chemical and biological approaches for mycotoxin control: a review. Food and Nutritional Agriculture. Jun;1(2):155-61.

Eduard W.(2009). Fungal spores: a critical review of the toxicological and epidemiological evidence as a basis for occupational exposure limit setting.Critical Review of Toxicology, 39(10):799-864.

Essigmann, J.M., Croy, R.G., Bennett, R.A., & Wogan, G.N. (1982). 'Metabolic activation of aflatoxin B_1: patterns of DNA adduct formation, removal, and excretion in relation to carcinogenesis', *Drug Metabolism Review*, vol 13, pp 581-602.

Faisal, K, Periasamy, V S, Sahabudeen, S, Radha, A, Anandhi, R, & Akbarsha, M A (2008). Spermatotoxic effect of aflatoxin B1 in rat: extrusion of outer dense fibres and associated axonemal microtubule doublets of sperm flagellum. *Reproduction* 135: 303-310 .

Fazekas, B., Tar, AK., & Zomborszky-Kovacs, M. (2001), 'Ochratoxin a contamination of cereal grains and coffee in Hungary in the year 2001', *Acta Veterenia Hungaria*, vol 50, pp177-188.

Fokunang CN, Tembe-Fokunang EA, Tomkins P & Barkwan S. (2006). Global impact of mycotoxins on human and animal health management. Outlook on Agriculture Vol 35, No 4 , pp 247–253.

Friesen TL, Faris JD, Solomon PS, & Oliver RP (2008). Host-specific toxins: effectors of necrotrophic pathogenicity.Cell Microbiology. Jul;10(7):1421-8.

Fuchs, R., Radie, B., Ceovic, S., Sostaric, B., & Hult, K. (1991), 'Human exposure to ochratoxin A. In Mycotoxins, endemic nephropathy and urinary tract tumours' Castegnaro, M., Plestina, R., and Bartsch, H (eds), pp 131-134, IARC Scientific Publications No. 115, Lyon: International Agency for Research on Cancer.

Garcia D, Ramos AJ, Sanchis V, & Marín S. (2009). Predicting mycotoxins in foods. Reviews Food Microbiology. 26(8):757-69.

Garner, R.C., Martin, C.N., Smith, J.R.L., Coles, B.F., & Tolson, M.R. (1979), 'Comparison of aflatoxin B_1 and aflatoxin G_1 binding to cellular macromolecules in vitro, in vivo and after peracid oxidation: Characterization of the major nucleic acid adducts', *Chemical and Biological Interactions*, vol 26, pp 57-73.

Groopman JD. (1994). Molecular dosimetry methods for assessing human aflatoxin exposures. In: toxicology of aflatoxins: human health, veterinary and agricultural significance, D.L. Eaton & J.D Groopman, (eds), 259-279. New York: Academic Press.

Hall AJ, & Wild CP (1994). Epidemiology of aflatoxin related diseases. In: toxicology of aflatoxins: human health, veterinary and agricultural significance, D.L. Eaton & J.D Groopman, (eds), 233-258. New York: Academic Press.

Harris, L.J., Desjardsins, A.E., Plattner, R.D., Nicholson, P., Butler, G., Young, J.C., Weston, G., Proctor, H.R., & Hohn, M.T. 1999, 'Possible Role of Trichothecene Mycotoxins in Virulence of *Fusarium graminearum* on maize', *Plant Disease*, vol 56, pp 954-961.

He J, & Zhou T (2010). Patented techniques for detoxification of mycotoxins in feeds and food matrices.Recent Pat Food Nutr Agric; 2(2):96-104

Hedayati, M. T., Pasqualotto, A. C., Warn, P. A., Bowyer, P., & Denning, D. W. (2007). Aspergillus flavus: human pathogen, allergen and mycotoxin producer. *Microbiology* 153: 1677-1692.

Herwaarden, A. E.v., Wagenaar, E., Karnekamp, B., Merino, G., Jonker, J. W., & Schinkel, A. H. (2006). Breast cancer resistance protein (Bcrp1/Abcg2) reduces systemic exposure of the dietary carcinogens aflatoxin B1, IQ and Trp-P-1 but also mediates their secretion into breast milk. *Carcinogenesis* 27: 123-130 .

Hollstein M., Sidransky D., Vogelstein B & Harris CC (1991). P 53 mutations in human cancers. Science 253, 49-53.

Hsieh, D.P.H., & Wong, J.J. (1994), 'Pharmacokinetics and excretion of aflatoxins. In: The toxicology of aflatoxins: human health, veterinary and agricultural significance, Eaton, D.L., and Groopman, J.D', (eds), pp73-88, New York: Academic Press.

Hsueh, C.C., Liu, Y., & Freund, M.S. (1999), 'Indirect electrochemical detection of type-B trichothecene mycotoxins', *Annal of Chemistry*, vol 71, pp 4070-4080.

Huffman J, Gerber R, & Du L (2010).Recent advancements in the biosynthetic mechanisms for polyketide-derived mycotoxins.Biopolymers; 93(9):764-76

Hussein, H.S., & Brasel, J.M. (2001), 'Toxicity, metabolism and impact of mycotoxins on humans and animals', Toxicology, vol 167, pp 101-134.

IARC. (1993), 'Toxins derived from *Fusarium moniliforme*. Fumonisins B_1 and B_2 and Fusarin C'. In: IARC monographs on the evaluation of carcinogenic risks to humans, International Agency for Research on Cancer Lyon:.vol 56, 445-446.

Jalili M, Jinap S, & Son R. (2011). The effect of chemical treatment on reduction of aflatoxins and ochratoxin A in black and white pepper during washing.Food Additive Contamination Part A Chemical Analysis Control Exposure Risk Assessment; 28(4):485-93.

Kabak B, & Dobson AD (2009). Biological strategies to counteract the effects of mycotoxins. J Food Prot. 2009 Sep; 72(9):2006-16.

Kankkunen, P., Rintahaka, J., Aalto, A., Leino, M., Majuri, M.-L., Alenius, H., Wolff, H., & Matikainen, S. (2009). Trichothecene Mycotoxins Activate Inflammatory Response in Human Macrophages. *Jurnal of. Immunology.* 182: 6418-6425.

Khlangwiset P, & Wu F (2010).Costs and efficacy of public health interventions to reduce aflatoxin-induced human disease. Food Addit Contam Part A Chem Anal Control Expo Risk Assess. 27(7):998-1014.

Kiso, T., Fujita, K.-I., Ping, X., Tanaka, T., & Taniguchi, M. (2004). Screening for Microtubule-Disrupting Antifungal Agents by Using a Mitotic-Arrest Mutant of Aspergillus nidulans and Novel Action of Phenylalanine Derivatives Accompanying Tubulin Loss. *Antimicrobial. Agents Chemotherapy.* 48: 1739-1748 .

Klich MA (2009). Health effects of Aspergillus in food and air. Toxicology in Industrial Health. 25(9-10):657-67.

Kremer, A., Westrich, L., & Li, S.-M. (2007). A 7-dimethylallyltryptophan synthase from Aspergillus fumigatus: overproduction, purification and biochemical characterization. *Microbiology* 153: 3409-3416.

Kuiper-Goodman, T. (1991), 'Risk assessment to humans of mycotoxins in animal-derived food products', *Veterinary and Human toxicology,* vol 33,pp 325-332.

Lacey J. (1991). Natural occurrence of mycotoxins in growing and conserved forage crops. In:Mycotoxins and animal foods, Smith JE, & Hendersen RS, (eds), London CRC Press.

Lackner G, Partida-Martinez LP, & Hertweck C (2009). Endofungal bacteria as producers of mycotoxins.Trends in Microbiology. 17(12):570-6.

Lamplugh SM., Hendrickse RG, Apeagyei F, & Mwanmut DD (1988). Aflatoxins in breast milk, neonatal cord blood, and serum of pregnant women. British Journal of Medicine 295, 968.

Lee TG (2009). Mold remediation in a hospital.Toxicol of Industrial Health. 25(9-10):723-30.

Lugauskas, A., & Stakeniene, J. (2002), 'Toxin producing micromycetes on fruit, berries, and vegetables', Annals of Agriculture and Environmental Medicine, vol 9, pp 183-187.

Magan N, Aldred D, Mylona K, & Lambert RJ (2010). Limiting mycotoxins in stored wheat.Food Addit Contam Part A Chem Anal Control Expo Risk Assess. 27(5):644-50.

Maxwell SM., Apeagyei F, de Vries HR, Mwanmut DD, & Hendricks RG. (1989). Aflatoxins in breast milk, neonatal cord blood and sera of pregnant women. Journal of Toxicology; Toxin Reviews 8, 19-29.

Meggs WJ (2009). Epidemics of mold poisoning past and present. Toxicol of Industrial Health. 25(9-10):571-6.

Micco, C., Ambruzzi, M.A., Miraglia, M., & Benelli, L. (1991), 'Contamination of human milk with ochratoxin A'. In: Mycotoxins, endemic nephropathy and urinary tract tumours. Castegnaro, M., Plestina, R and Bartsch, (eds), pp 105-108. IARC Scientific Publication No.115. Lyon: International Agency for Research on Cancer.

NageswaraRao Rachaputi, Wright, G.C., & Krosch, S. (2002). Management practices to minimise pre-harvest aflatoxin contamination in Australian Peanuts. Australian Journal of Experimental Agriculture 42:595-605 .

Naiker, S., & Odhav, B. (2004), 'Mycotic keratitis: profile of Fusarium species and their mycotoxins', *Mycoses,* vol 47, pp50-56.

Nair, M.G. (1998), 'Fumonisins and human health', *Annals of Tropical Paediatrics,* vol 18, pp 47-52.

OBrian, G.R., Georgianna, D.R., Wilkinson, J.R., Yu, J., Abbas, H.K., Bhatnagar, D., Cleveland, T.E., Nierman, W., & Payne, G.A. (2007). The effect of elevated temperature on gene transcription and aflatoxin biosynthesis. *Mycologia* 99: 232-239.

Pasquali M, Giraud F, Lasserre JP, Planchon S, Hoffmann L, Bohn T, & Renaut J (2010). Toxin induction and protein extraction from *Fusarium* spp. cultures for proteomic studies. Journal of in vitro Experiments. 16; (36).

Park, D.l., Lee, L.S., Price, R.L., & Pohland, A.E. (1988), 'Review of the decontamination of aflatoxins by ammoniation: current status and regulation'. *Journal of Association of Official Analytical Chemistry.*

Peplinski, A.I., Eckhoff, S.R., Warner, K & Anderson, R.A. (1983), 'Physical testing and dry milling of high-moisture corn preserved with ammonia while drying in ambient air', *Cereal Chemistry*, vol 60, pp 442-445.

Pestka, J.J., & Bondy, G.S. (1990), Alteration of immune function following dietary mycotoxin exposure, *Canadian Journal of Physiology and Pharmacology*, vol, 68, pp1009-1016.

Pitt, J.L (1996). What are mycotoxins? Australia Mycotoxins Newletter, 7 (4):1-3.

Pitt, J.L & Miscamble, B.F. (1995), 'Water relations of *Aspergillus flavus* and closely related species', *Journal of Food Protection*, vol 58, pp86-90.

Probst, C., Njapau, H., & Cotty, P. J. (2007). Outbreak of an Acute Aflatoxicosis in Kenya in 2004: Identification of the Causal Agent. *Applied Environmental Microbiology.* 73: 2762-2764.

Prelusky, D.B., Hamilton, R.M., & Trenholm, H.l. (1989), 'Transmission of residues to eggs following long-term administration of 14C labelled deoxynivalenol to laying hens', *Poultry Science*, 68, pp, 744-748.

Puisieux A., Lim S, Groopman J & Ozturk M (1991). Selective targeting of p53 gene mutational hotspots in human cancers by etiologically defined carcinogens. Cancer Research 51, 6185-6189.

Purzycki CB, & Shain DH. (2010). Fungal toxins and multiple sclerosis: a compelling connection. Brain Research Bulletin. 29;82(1-2):4-6.

Rheeder, J.P., Marasas, W.F.O., Thiel, P.G., Sydenham, E.W., & van Schalkwyk, D.J. (1992), '*Fusarium moniliforme* and fumonisins in corn in relation to human esophageal cancer in Transkei', *Phytopathology*, vol 82, pp 353-357.

Schoenhard, G.L., Hendricks, J.D., Nixon, J.E., Lee, D.J., Wales, J.H., Sinhuber, R.O & Pawlowski, N.E. (1981),' Aflatoxicol-induced hepatocellular carcinoma in rainbow trout (*Salmo gairdneri*) and synergistic effects of cyclopropenoid fatty acids', *Cancer Research*, vol 41, pp 1011-1014.

Shuaib FM, Ehiri J, Abdullahi A, Williams JH, Jolly PE. (2010). Reproductive health effects of aflatoxins: a review of the literature.Reproductive Toxicology. 2010 Jun; 29(3):262-70

Smith, C. A., Woloshuk, C. P., Robertson, D., & Payne, G. A. (2007). Silencing of the Aflatoxin Gene Cluster in a Diploid Strain of Aspergillus flavus Is Suppressed by Ectopic aflR Expression. *Genetics* 176: 2077-2086.

Sudakin, D.L. (2003), Trichothecenes in the environment: relevance to human health, *Toxicology Letter*, vol143, pp 97-107.

Taranu I, Marin DE, Manda G, Motiu M, Neagoe I, Tabuc C, Stancu M, & Olteanu M (2011). Assessment of the potential of a boron-fructose additive counteracting the toxic effect of Fusarium mycotoxins. British Journal of Nutrition, 14:1-11

Takayuki, S., & Bjeldanes, L.F. (1993), *'Introduction to Food Toxicology'*, Academic Press. Inc, San Diego, California, pp 213.

Van Egmond, H.P. (1989). 'Current situation on regulation for mycotoxins. Overview of tolerances and status of standard methods of sampling and analysis', *Food Additive Contaminants*. 6: 139-188.

Walter S, Nicholson P, & Doohan FM. (2010). Action and reaction of host and pathogen during Fusarium head blight disease. New Phytolology. 185(1):54-66.

Wogan GN., Edwards GS. & Shank RC. (1967). Excretion and tissue distribution of radioactivity from aflatoxin B1-14C in rats. Cancer Research 27, 1729-1739.

World Health Organization WHO. (1991), 'Evaluation of certain food additives and contaminants. In: 37th Report of the Joint FAO/WHO Expert Committee on Food Additives', WHO Technical Report Series No. 806, 28-31. Geneva: World Health Organization.

Wild, C.P., & Hall, A.J. (2000), 'Primary prevention of hepatocellular carcinoma in developing countries', *Mutation Research*, vol 462, pp381-393.

Wilson, D.M., Mubatanhema, W., & Jurjevic, Z. (2002), 'Biology and ecology of mycotoxicogeni *Aspergillus* species as related to economic and health concerns', *Advances in Experimental Medical Biology*, vol 504, pp 3-17.

Wu F, & Munkvold GP (2008). Mycotoxins in ethanol co-products: modeling economic impacts on the livestock industry and management strategies. J Agric Food Chem. 11;56(11):3900-11.

Yegani, M., Smith, T. K., Leeson, S., & Boermans, H. J. (2006). Effects of feeding grains naturally contaminated with Fusarium mycotoxins on performance and metabolism of broiler breeders.. *Poultry. Science.* 85: 1541-1549.

Yoshinari, T., Akiyama, T., Nakamura, K., Kondo, T., Takahashi, Y., Muraoka, Y., Nonomura, Y., Nagasawa, H.,& Sakuda, S. (2007). Dioctatin A is a strong inhibitor of aflatoxin production by *Aspergillus parasiticus*. *Microbiology* 153: 2774-2780.

Yunus, A. W., Awad, W. A., Kroger, S., Zentek, J., & Bohm, J. (2010). *In vitro* aflatoxin B1 exposure decreases response to carbamylcholine in the jejunal epithelium of broilers. *Poultry. Science.* 89: 1372-1378.

Zhu JQ., Zang LS, Hu X, Xiao Y, Chen JS, Fremy J & Chu FS (1987). Correlation of dietary aflatoxin B1 levels with excretion of aflatoxin M1 in human urine. Cancer Research 47, 1848-1852.

8

Non-Invasive Methods for Monitoring Individual Bioresponses in Relation to Health Management

Vasileios Exadaktylos, Daniel Berckmans and Jean-Marie Aerts
Measure, Model and Manage Bioresponses (M3-BIORES), Department of Biosystems, Katholieke Universiteit Leuven, Heverlee Belgium

1. Introduction

New technology offers more and more possibilities to measure variables on the human body and mind in a non-invasive way as a basis for health management. By using miniaturized sensors (implanted, injected, wearing on or attached to the body), several variables can be measured such as heart rate, skin temperature, movements etc. Several sensing techniques (image analyses, sound analyses,...) allow to measure other variables (such as posture, movements, facial expression,...) and sound production. Also at the other end of the scale, new technologies (e.g. remote sensing technology) in combination with smart algorithms offer possibilities for monitoring human health.

By applying this technology several easy measurable variables can be monitored continuously in a fully automated way. Data are transferred in a wireless way and more sophisticated algorithms can be applied to calculate several parameters from these data. In this way parameters of physical condition or components of mental status can be monitored.

An important element is that these measurements can now be done in a continuous way for the different individuals and that the algorithms can be adapted for individuals. This is a big difference with what has happened so far in most of the medical applications where mainly population models are used in the scientific literature and in the treatments. By applying individual algorithms in a continuous way it becomes possible to monitor living organisms as complex, individually different and time varying dynamic systems.

Next, examples are given where this technique has been used in a number of different applications.

2. Applications

This section presents a number of applications of non-invasive monitoring methods for individuals.

2.1 Monitoring health status of patients in the intensive care unit on the basis of real-time measured physiological variables and advanced modelling technology

In cardiac surgery it would be very helpful to have a system that provides an early alert if there is a high probability that a patient will be disconnected from ventilation during the next day since this would lead to a more optimal planning in the Intensive Care Unit (ICU). It was shown that alterations in vital signals are relevant to patient management (Rivera-Fernandez et al., 2007), so we wanted to use the trends of some of those vital signals during the first hours of ICU stay to predict a short or prolonged length of stay from early on. All living organisms are characterised by the fact that they are complex, individually different time-variant and dynamic (so called CITD systems) (Quanten et al., 2006). Consequently, it is expected that taking these characteristics into account will lead to better models of the physiological signals of intensive care patients. So far, univariate and multivariate autoregressive analyses as well as the calculation of the cepstrum of physiological variables have been applied in several medical studies (Wada et al., 1988; Curcie and Craelius, 1997) to analyze individual patients. For making classifications using many variables at the same time, several data mining techniques are available. However, in most cases no dynamic information about the patients is taken into account when applying the data mining approach. Several attempts on temporal feature extraction for time series classification have been made (Verduijn et al., 2007). We describe here a study in which information of patients' dynamics was used to predict the timeframe when the conditions to start weaning of mechanical ventilation are reached.

2.1.1 Analysis of time series of patient data

Physiological variables, such as heart rate (bpm), systolic arterial blood pressure (mmHg), systolic pulmonary pressure (mmHg), blood temperature (°C) and oxygen saturation are routinely monitored in these patients and can be sampled frequently when Patient Data Management System are used. In this example, we show results of a total of 203 patients that were followed in the Intensive Care unit of the University Hospital of Leuven. More information can be found in the work of Van Loon et al. (2010).

Besides the mean and standard deviations of the signals (Avgstd), more advanced time series models can be applied that allow quantifying the dynamics of these physiological variables such as univariate and multivariate autoregressive (AR) models.

Dynamic features that are extracted from time series of patient data, can be used in a next step to determine the status of individual patients when applying them to machine learning techniques such as Support Vector Machines or Gaussian Processes.

Gaussian processes (GP), a type of kernel method, are a machine learning technique that has been successfully used to model and forecast real dynamic systems. In probabilistic binary classification the task is to determine for an unlabeled test input vector the probability of belonging to a given class when a training set is given. The training set is comprised of training input vectors and their corresponding binary class labels (+1 if the input vector belongs to the class, -1 otherwise).

The considered task in the presented example can be restated as follows: Predict the probability that the patient will begin to satisfy the stability criteria within each of the following time frames (classes): class 1: earlier than nine hours after admission; class 2: later than nine hours after admission. This nine hour threshold was chosen such that the resulting classes contained roughly the same amount of patients. This division also conforms to an intuitive classification used by intensivists into patients that recover quickly and those that require prolonged ICU stays. Data from each patient, collected during the first four hours ICU stay, were used to generate the different time-series models, the parameters of which were used as the features of the examples. One of the two possible class labels was assigned to each example. Training examples for each classifier were labelled positive (+1) if the moment when the patient became stable started within the first nine hours after admission and were labelled negative (-1) otherwise. The classification performance can be calculated by the aROC (area under the receiver operating characteristic curve) for each classifier.

Table 1 gives the obtained aROCs for each experiment with the GP. The middle column contains the results obtained when using a logistic regression (LOGREG) model, included here as a baseline for performance. The increase in performance for all GP models versus the LOGREG models was found to be significant, except for the model based on admission. So, although logistic regression techniques are commonly used in medical applications, other classifiers might lead to better results. This was, among others, also concluded by Sakai et al. (2007) and Erol et al. (2005). It is also shown that the approach including dynamic information (MAR) performs better than the model purely based on admission information (in terms of the aROC).

aROC	LOGREG	GP
Avgstd (20)	0.628	0.713
MAR	0.591	0.708

Table 1. Classification results

This application shows that taking into account dynamic information in analysing time series of patients can be of added value when monitoring the health status of individual patients.

2.2 Dynamic algorithms of biomarkers for monitoring infection/inflammation processes

Disease management is becoming increasingly important in our current society, especially considering the growing population of elderly and immune compromised people. There is a general agreement that sepsis and the systemic inflammatory response syndrome (SIRS) are characterized by an inability to regulate the inflammatory response. The cause of this perturbation is still unknown. So far research did not result in a dramatic reduction of the high mortality rates which for critically ill patients in intensive care units where sepsis and SIRS remain major causes of death.

As strategies for the early treatment of sepsis mostly failed, this fully justifies the development of a novel biosensor array at the heart of an on line early warning monitoring system for prediction of disease evolution and subsequent adaptation of life saving therapy.

Complex biological processes are involved in these phenomena and therefore it is a challenge to quantify infection and inflammation processes in real-time. It is expected however that the use of biosensors in combination with real-time signal analysis allows monitoring infection/inflammation processes in real-time.

Developing such new sensing techniques requires an interdisciplinary approach between engineers, immunologists, medical experts and sensor developers. In a first step, we aimed at demonstrating the proof of principle in animal experiments (pigs). In a next step, the developed methodologies might be transferred to human patients.

2.2.1 Data generation

The aim of the experiments was to quantify the dynamics of 3 cytokines and 4 acute-phase proteins (APP) before and after infection by *Actinobacillus pleuropneumoniae* in pigs. More specific, the cytokines, tumor necrosis factor-alpha (TNF-α), interleukin-6 (IL-6) and interleukin-10 (IL-10), and the acute-phase proteins, C-reactive protein (CRP), haptoglobin (Hp), major acute phase protein (MAP) and serum-amyloid A (SAA), were analysed. In total, 22 pigs were infected. The blood sampling frequency that was used for the experiments was as follows: 1 sample/day: before infection, 1 sample/2 hours: starting from 2 hours before infection to end. The higher sampling frequency after infection was necessary to determine the dynamics of the response on the infection and to measure the entire course of the biomarker response. Due to the measuring frequencies, the focus of the modelling analysis was on the period starting with the infection of the pigs until the end of the experiment.

2.2.2 Modelling of biomarker responses to infection

In this example, the dynamics of all biomarkers were modelled using univariate autoregressive (AR) models. These time series models were defined as follows (Taylor et al., 2007):

$$y(k)A(z^{-1}) = e(k) \tag{1}$$

Where $y(k)$ is the considered biomarker, $A(z^{-1})$ is the polynomial of the model parameters and $e(k)$ is additive noise, a serially uncorrelated sequence of random variables with variance σ^2 that accounts for measurement noise, modelling errors and effects of unmeasured inputs to the process (assumed to be a zero mean). For the modelling the order of the AR models were ranged from 1 to 2, resulting in 2 possible AR models per biomarker for every pig. Since no significant results were found for second order AR models, all AR models described in this report are simple first order models which can be written in the time series form:

$$y(k) = -a_1 y(k-1) + e(k) \tag{2}$$

As the results of SAA and IL-6 were most significant, we will focus in this example on these two biomarkers. In a first step, models were developed for each individual pig. In a second step, the individual models of the pigs were compared to develop model-based criteria for the early detection of survival/non-survival.

2.2.3 Monitoring criteria

All the modelling results described below will focus on the prediction of disease outcome (survival vs. non-survival). Since many pigs died shortly after the infection, only the data of a short period after infection were used for the development of the TF- and AR-models. To obtain comparable models, samples of the same time interval were used for the calculation of these models. More specifically, for all pigs data were used starting from the moment of infection until 16 hours after infection.

For the biomarker SAA a significant difference between survivors (S) and non-survivors (NS) was found for the a-parameters of the AR models (mean S = -0.7915, mean NS = -1.3204, $p = 0.04$). Fig. 1 shows a scatter plot of the a-parameters of the different pigs.

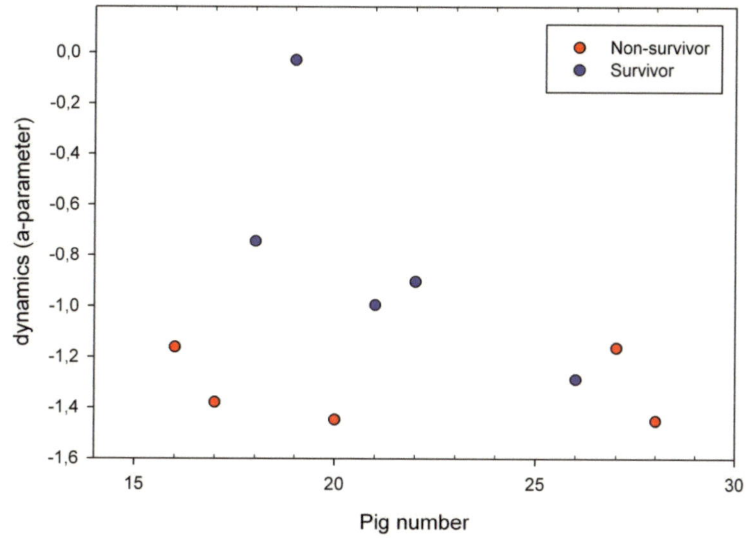

Fig. 1. Criterion for early detection of survival/non-survival based on SAA: stability of model. Overview of a-parameters of AR-models for all surviving (blue) and non-surviving (red) pigs

Also for the biomarker IL-6, there was a significant difference in a-parameters between survivors and non-survivors (mean S = -0.1272, mean NS = -0.5751, p=0.0085). Fig. 2 shows a scatter plot of the a-parameters for all pigs.

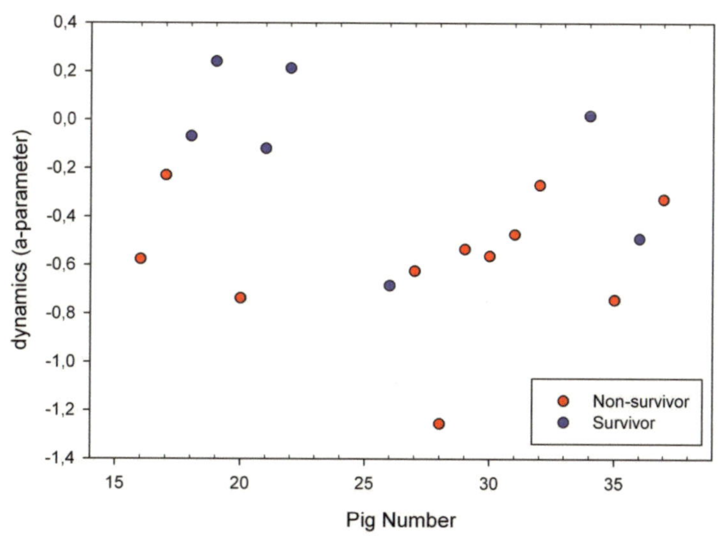

Fig. 2. Criterion for early detection of survival/non-survival based on IL-6: trend vs noise. Overview of a-parameters of AR-models for all surviving (blue) and non-surviving (red) pigs

These results show that there tend to be differences in dynamics of biomaekers between surviving and non-surviving pigs after infection. Although many more experiments are needed in order to confirm the actual findings, it is expected that the modelling results could be the first steps towards the development of an objective individualised method for a sensor-based early detection of sepsis and inflammation in animals and later on in humans. Combining the modelling approach with novel biosensors should allow monitoring the health status of animals and human patients in real-time and could form the basis of health management systems.

2.3 Pain management in elderly suffering from dementia

Pain in elderly at the latest stages of dementia is an underestimated factor for discomfort and quality of living. Being able to objectively measure pain allows caregivers to adjust the treatment of these patients with limited communication skils. In this regard, a big number of pen-paper observational pain scales have been developed by various researchers. However, data handling from these scales is not very easy and their use is limited by the amount of time that a caregiver can spend on a patient. To account for this, the Painvision (www.painvision.be) consortium has developed an electronic version of three popular observational pain scales (see section 2.3.1 below) that is currently sold by BioRICS nv (a K.U.Leuven spin-off, www.biorics.com).

The overall objective of the Painvision consortium was to develop an automatic pain detection system based on cameras. Since facial expression is a well-known and reliable indicator of pain, the algorithms of the system exploit this relationship and estimate the pain level of the observed patient. Continuous information about the pain level of a patient can subsequently be used to evaluate the medical as well as the physical treatment that the patient is receiving, their comfort level throughout the day and eventually their quality of life.

2.3.1 Electronic pain observational scales (assessment scales)

Pen-paper observational scales have proven to be useful to assess pain in severely demented elderly, but also have a lot of disadvantages. Their usability is often limited, they are time-consuming because of their length, difficulties in calculating scores, and post processing required to evaluate the pain evolution. Also the timing and timing patterns of the indicators could be very valuable to pain assessment, but cannot be grasped using pen-paper assessment instruments. The American Pain Society has indicated the importance of the pain assessment and suggested the guidelines for improving its quality (Max et al., 1995). In case a patient is not able to report his/her pain experience verbally, it is recommended to measure the pain-related behaviours (e.g., grimacing, restlessness, vocalisation, etc.). Demented elderly have limited ability to communicate verbally, as a result of which self report of pain is difficult. Therefore, different observational pain assessment scales have been developed and validated for this group of patients (Herr et al., 2006). Despite the introduction of new technologies in healthcare, to the authors' knowledge, the scores for all pain scales for severely demented elderly are still obtained manually on the paper.

Computerized technologies are already introduced in home care (Koch, 2006) and gaining high satisfaction response among patients (Chae et al., 2001; Lind et al., 2008) . The computerized-assisted decision systems are utilized in clinical practice (Mikulich, et al. 2001). The information systems are reducing costs and improving quality in managing diagnostic tests (Bates et al., 1999). The nurses have stated their expectations of Personal Digital Assistant (PDA) devices in the nursing practice (Nilsson et al., 2007). The computerized versions of the pain scales and questionnaires have lately been introduced successfully in pain assessment practice (Wincent et al. 2003). It has been reported in the literature that the computerized version of the self-report pain questionnaires is not altering the response of the patients (Caro et al., 2001). It is also decreasing the number of the missing responses by obligating the patients to answer before proceeding to the next question (Caro et al., 2001). Compared to the paper versions, the electronic pain self-report questionnaires and electronic diaries are offering considerable advantages: 1) completeness of data (Hanscom et al., 2002); 2) entered data are date and time stamped (Burton et al., 2007); 3) saving of time and reduction of errors from entering written data manually to the database for the analysis Ryan et al., 2002.

During the Painvision project (www.painvision.be), a digital scale was developed for data collection. This project took place in a specific geriatric centre, and was approved by a medical ethical committee. In this pilot study facial images of a bedside two-camera system were linked to the pain scores of the digital device (a tablet PC with a touch screen, Fig. 3, a commercial version has been introduced to the market by BioRICS nv. more details can be found on www.assessmentscales.com) carried out at the bedside by a nurse.

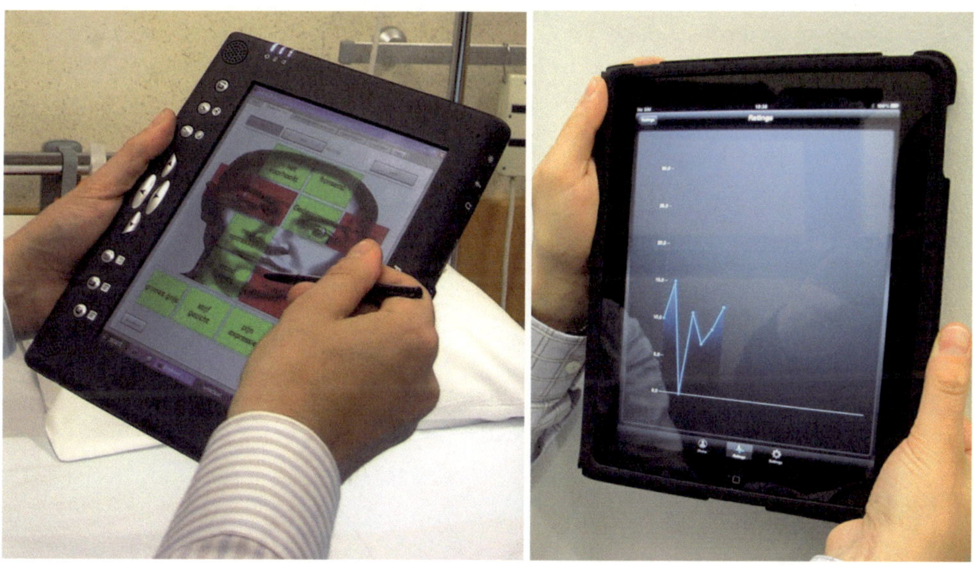

Fig. 3. Two implementations of the assessment scales (pictures courtesy of BioRICS nv (www.biorics.com)

As input for the digital device, 3 valid and reliable scales were chosen: the Pain Assessment Checklist for Seniors with Limited Ability to Communicate (PACSLAC), the Discomfort Scale - Dementia of Alzheimer Type, and the Faces Pain Scale Revised. After an informed consent was signed by a relative, two nurses tracked nineteen bedridden patients, with limited ability to communicate, for 6 random days, in which 6 assessment sessions were performed at clinically interesting moments (before - during - after care, before - after manipulation, and at rest). The usability was more concretely evaluated by ten other professional caregivers of this geriatric centre, via the 'think aloud method' and a

questionnaire. They performed a digital pain assessment twice, with an interval of four weeks, on two patients with severe dementia. Usability criteria were learnability, efficiency of use, number of manipulation errors and satisfaction.
The digital device allows the nurse to record facial indicator events, such as frequency and duration, as they occur in real time. Subsequently, the scores are calculated automatically. The digital information is stored in a database, improving administration and allowing database applications. The ten professional caregivers stated that the tool was easy to learn. After the second measurement their assessment time was reduced with approximately 50%, the number of detected manipulation errors was up to four times lower, and the general satisfaction has significantly increased ($p = 0.04$).
The Digital Pain Labelling Tool provides data completeness, reduces errors from the manual pen paper pain scores and offers easier and faster analysis of the patient's current condition. These findings illuminate the potential of implementing the computerized observational pain scale in nursing practice.

2.3.2 Automatic pain identification using a two-camera system

The Painvision project focused on the development of an algorithm for automatic estimation of the pain levels of elderly suffering from dementia by use of a two-camera system. The cameras are directed to the face of the patient that is bedridden. Initially, the face of the person is detected in both videos and, subsequently, pain indicators are automatically extracted. This procedure is presented in Fig. 4 and the different steps are explained in more detail in the following.

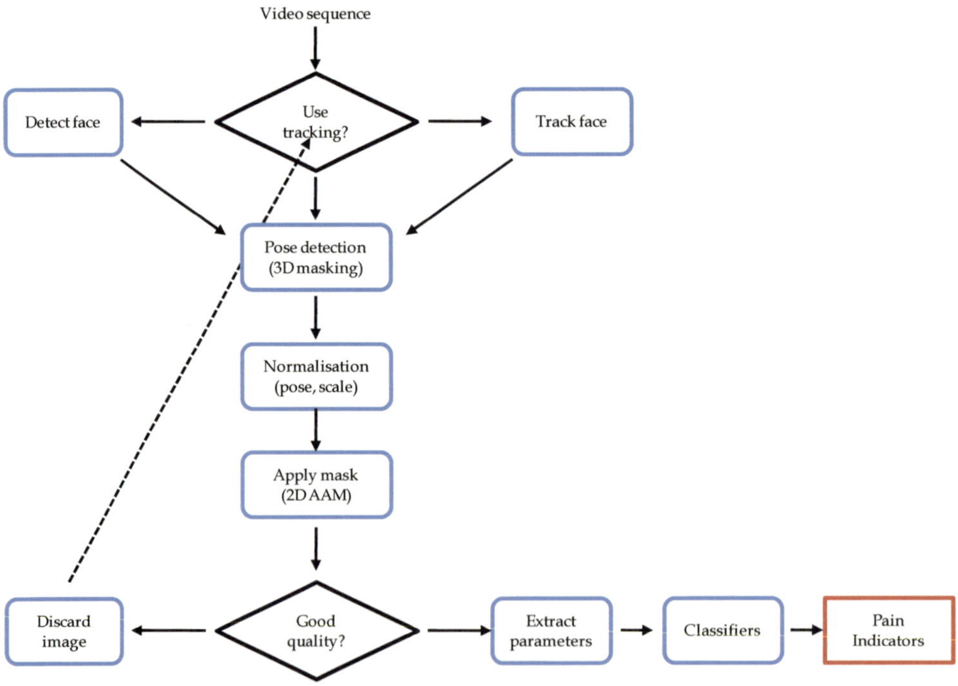

Fig. 4. Block diagram of the video processing algorithm for automatic estimation of pain in demented elderly based on visual information

Initially the incoming frame is passed to the face detector if the previous image in the sequence didn't contain a face. On the other hand when the previous frame did contain a face, a tracker will be used to relocate faces. At this stage it is known if the frame contains face(s) and their location. After detecting/tracking the face a rough 3D position of the head is known. However the normalization step requires an accurate estimation of the pose. Therefore the normalization step is headed by the pose estimation step. This step will iteratively estimate a more accurate pose. Once the pose in the incoming frame is known a normalization step can be preformed to bring the face to a frontal and fixed scale face. Next a 2D active appearance model (AAM) will be fitted. The parameters of this adaptive model describe both texture and shape information of the face. Now AAM parameters, the normalized face image, landmarks in the original and normalized image can be used in extracting pain related information.
It should be noted that the normalized texture is a forward warp of the original image pixels rather than a synthetic AAM instance. Although the warp could be deformed and incomplete, detailed texture features are preserved since the original texture is used. For instance wrinkles and person specific spots remain visible in the normalized image. These clues could be crucial in classification problems. Next, Fig. 5 is presenting the algorithm result for the detection of an 'open mouth' that is a pain indicator for demented elderly.

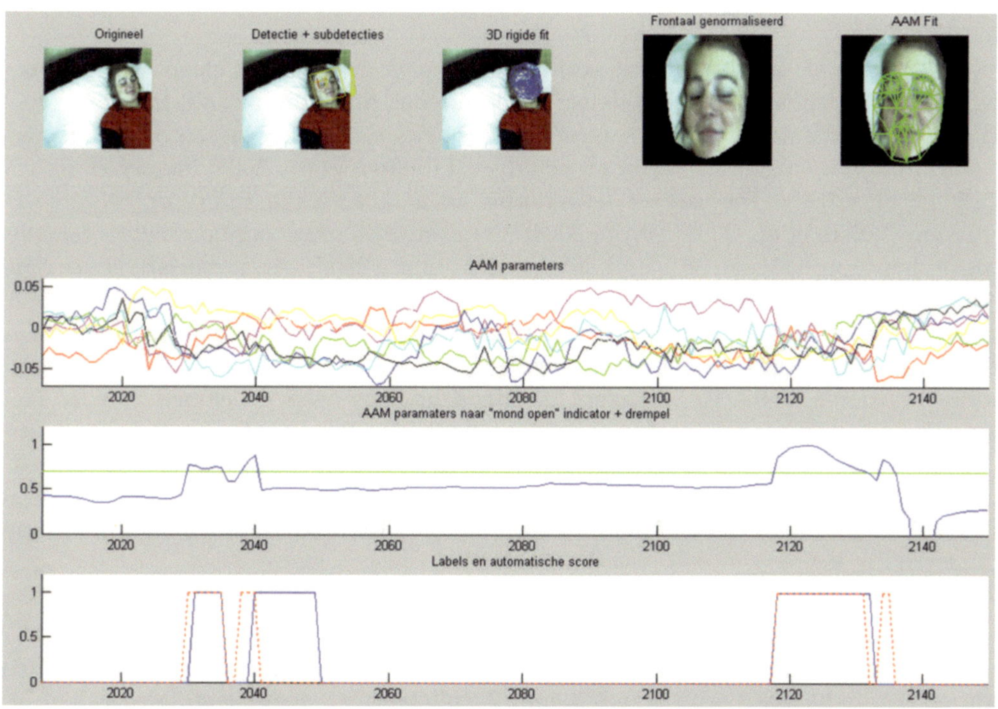

Fig. 5. Example of the different algorithm steps (i.e. face detection, 3D rigid fit, pose normalisation, AAM mask fit). From the different AAM parameters (top plot), an index is extracted (middle plot) that results in the detection of an open mouth (bottom plot)

2.4 Sleep monitoring as a tool for health management

Sleep loss, whether acute or chronic, poses significant risks in the performance of many ordinary tasks (e.g. driving, performing mental tasks, etc.) and has a substantial impact on social welfare. Studies have shown that people with lack of sleep constitute a major health risk for themselves and their surroundings. In light of this, the EASI (Enhancing Activity Through Sleep Improvement) project that consists of a multidisciplinary consortium is focusing on the monitoring and management of the sleep quality.

Algorithms have been developed that can automatically estimate parameters related to sleep quality of individuals such as sleep fragmentation and sleep stages. This information can be used in order to identify impaired sleep and with the use of environmental and bed variables sleep quality can be improved. Improved sleep quality will not only have positive effect on the individual's performance but also on the number of health problems related to sleep. In the commercial stage, the algorithms can be integrated in wearable devices that can provide visual feedback in relation to sleep quality and advice on actions that can improve sleep.

2.4.1 Automatic detection of awakenings

It has been presented in the literature that there exists a negative link between sleep fragmentation on daytime performance. Not only sleep duration, but also sleep continuity is an important factor in the recuperative sleep process. Sleep disturbances of only a few seconds contribute to the development of daytime sleepiness (Bonnet, 1985; Carrington & Trinder, 2008).

A popular method to monitor the number of awakenings during sleep is by using an actigraph. Actigraphs are used to detect body movements using a build-in accelerometer and give indices of awakenings. A number of studies have been presented that focus on the detection of awakenings based on activity (Lotjonen et al., 2003; Paquet et al., 2007; Sitnick et al., 2008). The use of actigraphy as a sleep-wake indicator is subject to discussion (Pollak et al., 2001; Tryon, 2004). Some studies using accelerometers have lead to wake detection between 35% and 50% (Paquet et al., 2007). An important shortcoming of these methods is their failure to detect an awakening when a person lies immobile in bed. In some extreme cases even a transition from supine to sitting position can sometimes be undetected (Sitnick et al., 2008).

During the course of the EASI project, an algorithm has been developed that is able to automatically detect every time the user is awake during the sleeping period (Bulckaert et al., 2010). Additionally, the algorithm is able to detect awakenings that are not scored as such according to the Rechschaffen & Kales (1968) criteria (i.e. awakenings that are shorter than 15s) and are referred to as 'short awakenings'. A visualisation of the algorithm output is shown in Fig. 6.

2.4.2 Detection of REM sleep

A normal sleep night consists of 5 distinct sleep stages, that occur in a structured sequence starting with light sleep with stages 1 and 2, followed by deep sleep, also called slow wave sleep with stages 3 and 4, and then followed by REM sleep. On average, light sleep occurs during 50-60% of sleep time, deep sleep during 15-20% of sleep time, REM sleep during 20-25% of sleep time and 5% or less is spent in wakefulness (Carskadon & Dement, 2000). Although REM is not the dominant part of the sleep time, most of sleep research focuses on REM sleep because this state resembles most to wakefulness and is being linked to dreaming and memory consolidation (Karni et al., 1994; Tilley & Empson, 1978; Takahara et al., 2008). In the same direction, during the course of the EASI project, an algorithm was developed that is automatically detecting periods of REM sleep. Additionally, the algorithm is contributing to the discussion of whether dreams occur only during REM sleep or not, by exploiting the concept of Additional Heart Rate and its link to emotions (Myrtek, 2004) during sleep. An example of the algorithm output is presented in Fig. 7.

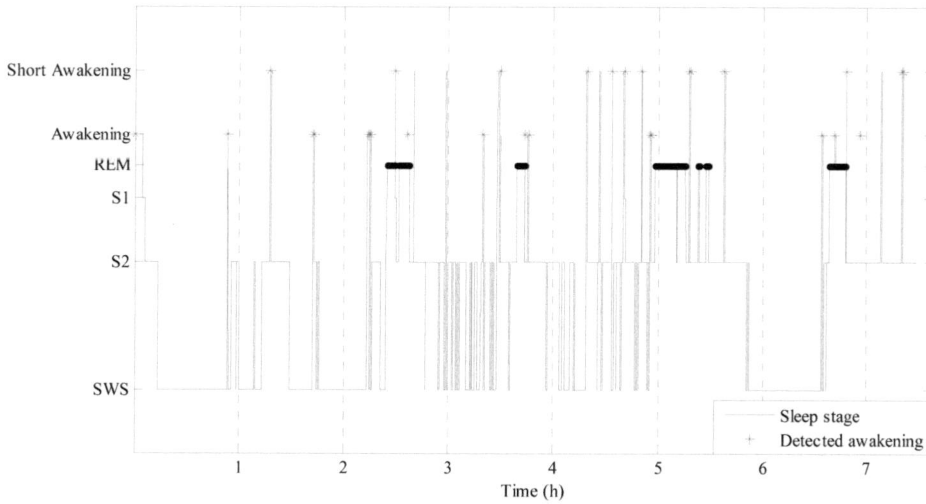

Fig. 6. Manual scoring of the sleep stages and the output of the developed algorithm for awakening detection

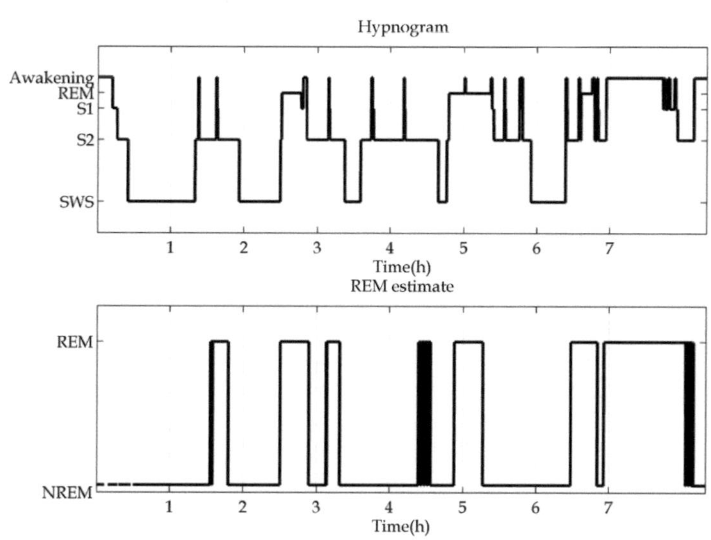

Fig. 7. Example of the algorithm output for the REM detection algorithm

The algorithm was tested on 11 subjects (mean age 23+3 years) and resulted in an average true positive classification of 75.8% and an average false positive classification rate of 21.1%.

2.5 Monitoring and predicting hanta viruses and Lyme infectious disease outbreaks by integrating remote sensing and climatic data with biophysical models

In the industrialized world with an intensive service sector, professional activities in agriculture, forestry and natural resources industry has been declining for decades. As such fewer professionals directly come into contact with the land. On the other hand, since people now spend more time for leisure, more outdoor recreational activities have been observed. Hiking, outdoor sports, picnicking, hunting etc has now enlarged the human exposure to the land. This increase has led to more contacts of humans with environmental related diseases such as Lyme Borreliosis (LB) and Nephropathia Epidemica (NE).

LB is a tick borne disease caused by the species of bacteria belonging to the genus Borrelia, whereas in Western Europe NE is caused by Pumuula viruses. Although different of nature, they share a common host, the bank vole. This small rodent is reservoir for both the bacteria as the viruses. For NE, the bank vole is also the vector species, whereas for LB ticks are the vector.

Since the abundance of ticks and bank voles depends on habitat characteristics for food supply and shelter among others, remote sensing techniques can be used to monitor vegetative systems that create habitats for these species. By integrating earth observation data from MODIS, LANDSAT, NOAA/AVHRR sensors with meteorological data of precipitation, temperature, relative humidity and estimates of bank vole and tick populations in data driven biophysical models, an expert based system is being developed to monitor and predict infection disease outbreaks of LB and NE for Belgium.

Hantaviruses are rodent or insectivore borne viruses and some of them are recognized as causes of human hemorrhagic fever with renal syndrome (HFRS). In western and central Europe and in western Russia one of the most important Hantavirus is *Puumala virus* (PUUV), which is transmitted to humans by infected red bank voles (*Myodes glareolus*). PUUV causes a general mild form of hemorrhagic fever with renal syndrome called nephropathia epidemica (NE) (Clement et al., 2006).

In general, only 13% of all PUUV infections are serodiagnosed, the other being interpreted as 'a bad flu' (Brummer-Korvenkontio et al., 1999; Clement et al., 2007) or remaining unnoticed. HFRS, including NE, is now the most underestimated cause of infectious acute renal failure worldwide, so the officially registered NE is only the top of the iceberg.

Because of the dynamic nature of the bank vole's population, a dynamic systems approach might also be the basis for the development of monitor applications. In this research we combine a data-based modelling approach with a mechanistic model (Sauvage et al., 2007) that allows modelling the dynamics of the NE cases with a compact model structure that takes into account climatological data. More specifically, we aimed at building a multiple-input, single-output (MISO) transfer function to model the incidence of NE cases in Belgium from 1996 till 2003 as a function of: measured average monthly air temperature (°C), monthly precipitation (mm) and carrying capacity (vole ha^{-1}) estimated from the mechanistic model described by Sauvage et al. (2007).

2.5.1 Available data

The Scientific Institute of Public Health (IPH, Brussels) in Belgium provided Nephropathia epidemica (NE) data. In Belgium, the weekly numbers of NE case per postal code (a spatial entity smaller than the municipality) were available from 1994 until 2008.

The Royal Meteorological Institute of Belgium (RMI, Ukkel) which is located at the centre of Belgium, provided daily data on air temperature (°C) and precipitation (mm) from 1996 to 2008. To be capable of catching the dynamics of the NE cases, we calculated monthly averages precipitation (mm) and average temperatures (°C) based on the daily reported climate data of Ukkel.

The Tree Seed Centre of the Ministry of the Walloon Region supplied categories of seed production of beech and native oak species (*Quercus robur, Quercus petraea*). Tree seed production for each tree species is divided into four categories: "very good years" (the species is fruiting throughout the Walloon territory and practically all trees are bearing seed in high quantities), "good years" (the species is fruiting throughout the territory, but the trees are bearing much less seed and some trees do not fruit), "moderate years" (there is a reduced number of trees bearing seeds and sometimes only located in a portion of the territory) and "low years" (years without fructification in significant quantities).

2.5.2 Modelling of NE outbreaks

The mehanistic population model used in this study was based on the equations proposed by Sauvage et al. (2007). Their model consists of two sub models. The first sub model (Bank vole's population model) describes the bank vole's demography and infection and the second sub model (Human population sub model) describes the access of human to the forest and the dynamics of the subsequent human infections. In the model the bank voles contaminated the environment that spread the virus into the human population. For a more detailed description of the model we refer to the work of Sauvage et al. (2007).

By combining the mechanistic model of Sauvage et al. (2007) and the transfer function model, the incidence of NE cases per year could be modelled accurately. The modelling results for the period 1996 - 2003 are shown in Fig. 8.

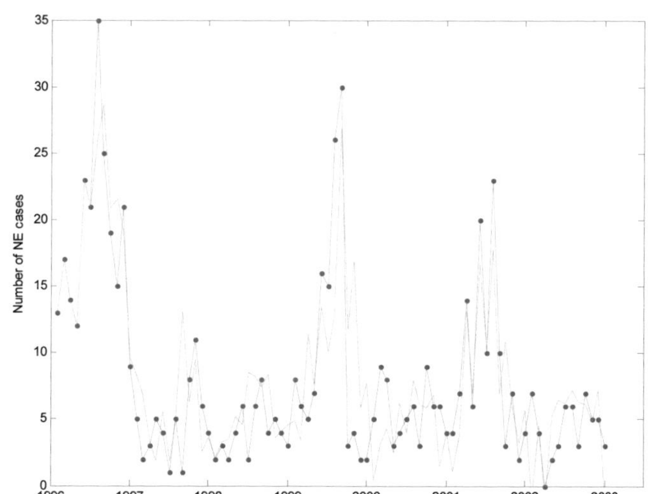

Fig. 8. The result (—) of the data-based MISO model with 3 inputs (average monthly temperature, precipitation and estimated carrying capacity) versus measured (-•-) incidence of NE in Belgium from January 1996 till January 2003 (R_T^2 of 0.68)

In future work the modelling approach may be improved by integration of estimated bank vole population dynamics measured in the field. This could give us the possibility to quantify the carrying capacity based on the field measurements instead of epidemiological models. More details on this application can be found in the work of Amirpour Haredasht et al. (2011).

2.5.3 Conclusion

The outbreaks and spread of Hantavirus have been questioned and studied for many years. An important added value of modelling NE cases is that it can be used in future as a tool to study the mechanism by which the virus spreads, to predict the future course of an occurrence and to evaluate strategies to control the epidemics.
The results of the current study furthermore help to define significant environmental factors on the spread of the disease. Determining a dynamic data-based model for NE which includes factors such as vegetation coverage and abundance of food for bank voles' may provide us with an expert tool to predict and prevent regional incidences of NE cases by making use of remote sensing tools for measuring broad leaves forest phenology and monitoring the vegetation dynamics together with climatological data.

3. Conclusion

With the above examples we would like to demonstrate how new technology can help in health monitoring and health management. Different aspects of health have been considered to demonstrate that the conceptual approach does not need to be very different from application to application. In all the above examples we have used mathematical modelling in order to identify and isolate the aspects of the 'system' (i.e. the living organism) that are of interest in every particular application. This way we have developed real-time and automatic algorithms for monitoring and management of health related issues.
At the moment, technology and sensors can still be bulky and not very comfortable for use in everyday applications, but it is expected that in the near future this situation will change. Sensors integrated in clothing and energy harvesting from the body pose two candidates to boost wearable device markets and provide solutions for health monitoring and management applications.

4. Acknowledgement

We would like to thank the IWT (agentschap voor Innovatie door Wetenschap en Technologie) in Flanders and the Katholieke Universiteit Leuven for funding the projects. We would also like to thank all the researchers involved in the projects and have contributed considerably to the results.

5. References

Amirpour Haredasht, S.; Barrios, J.M.; Maes, P.; Verstraeten, W.W.; Clement, J.; Ducoffre, G.; Lagrou, K.; Van Ranst, M.; Coppin, P.; Berckmans, D. & Aerts J.-M. (2011). A dynamic data-based model describing nephropathia epidemica in Belgium *Biosystems Engineering*, Vol. 109, No. 1 (May 2011) pp. 77-89, ISSN: 1537-5110.

Bates, D.W.; Pappius, E.; Kuperman, G.J.; Sittig, D.; Burstin, H.; Fairchild, D.; Brennan, T.A. & Teich, J.M. (1999). Using information systems to measure and improve quality. *International Journal of Medical Informatics*, Vol. 53, No. 2-3 (February-March 1999), pp. 115-124, ISSN: 1386-5056.

Bonnet, M.H. (1985). Effect of sleep disruption on sleep, performance, and mood. *Sleep*, Vol. 8, No. 1 (1985), pp. 11-19, ISSN: 0161-8105.

Brummer-Korvenkontio, M.; Vapalahti, O.; Henttonen, H.; Koskela, P. & Vaheri, A. (1999). Epidemiological study of nephropathia epidemica in Finland 1989-96. *Scandinavian Journal of Infectious Diseases*, Vol. 31, No. 5 (January 1999), pp. 427-435, ISSN: 0036-5548.

Bulckaert, A.; Exadaktylos, V.; De Bruyne, G.; Haex, B.; De Valck, E.; Wuyts, J.; Verbraecken, J. & Berckmans, D. (2010). Heart rate-based nighttime awakening detection. *European Journal of Applied Physiology*, Vol. 109, No. 2 (May 2010), pp. 317-322, ISSN: 1439-6319.

Burton, C.; Weller, D. & Sharpe, M. (2007). Are electronic diaries useful for symptoms research? A systematic review. *Journal of Psychosomatic Research*, Vol. 62, No. 5 (May 2007), pp. 553-561, ISSN: 0022-3999.

Caro, J.J.; Caro, I.; Caro, J.; Wouters F. & Juniper, E.F. (2001). Does electronic implementation of questionnaires used in asthma alter responses compared to paper implementation ? *Quality of Life Research*, Vol. 10, No. 8 (September 2001), pp. 683-691, ISSN: 0962-9343.

Carrington, M.J. & Trinder, J. (2008). Blood Pressure and Heart Rate During Continuous Experimental Sleep Fragmentation in Healthy Adults. *Sleep*, Vol. 31, No. 12 (December 2008), pp. 1701-1712, ISSN: 0161-8105.

Carskadon, M. & Dement, W.C. (2000). Normal human sleep: an overview, In: *Principles and Practive of Sleep Medicine*, Kryger, M.H.; Roth, T.; Dement, W.C. (Eds.) 3rd Edition, pp. 15-25 W.B. Saunders Co, ISBN: 0-72167-670-7, Philadelphia.

Chae, Y.M.; Lee, J.H.; Ho, S.H.; Kim, H.J.; Jun, K.H. & Won, J.U. (2001). Patient satisfaction with telemedicine in home health services for the elderly. *International Journal of Medical Informatics*, Vol. 61, No. 2-3 (May 2001), pp. 167-173, ISSN: 1386-5056.

Clement, J., Maes, P., & Van Ranst, M. (2006). Hantaviruses in the old and new world. *Perspectives in Medical Virology*, Vol. 16 (Emerging viruses in human populations.), pp. 161-177, ISBN: 978-0-444-52074-6

Clement, J.; Maes, P. & Van Ranst, M. (2007). Acute kidney injury in emerging, non-tropical infections. *Acta clinica belgica*, Vol. 62, No. 6 (2007), pp. 387-395, ISSN: 0001-5512.

Curcie, D. J. & Craelius, W. (1997). Recognition of Individual Heart Rate Patterns With Cepstral Vectors. *Biological Cybernetics*, Vol. 77, No. 2 (August 1997), pp. 103-109, ISSN: 0340-1200.

Erol, F.S.; Uysal, H.; Ergun, U.; Barisci, N.; Serhathoglu, S. & Hardalac, F. (2005). Prediction of Minor Head Injured Patients Using Logistic Regression and MLP Neural

Network. *Journal of Medical Systems*, Vol. 29, No. 3 (June 2005), pp. 205-215, ISSN: 0148-5598.

Hanscom, B.; Lurie, J.D.; Homa, K. & Weinstein, J.N. (2002). Computerized questionnaires and the quality of survey data. *Spine*, Vol. 27, No. 16 (August 2002), pp. 1797-1801, ISSN: 0362-2436.

Herr, K.; Bjoro, K. & Decker, S. (2006). Tools for assessment of pain in nonverbal older adults with dementia: A state-of-the-science review. *Journal of Pain and Symptom Management*, Vol. 31, No. 2 (February 2006), pp. 170-192, ISSN: 0885-3924.

Karni, A.; Tanne, D.; Rubenstein, B.S.; Askenasy, J.J. & Sagi, D. (1994). Dependence on REM sleep of overnight improvement of a perceptual skill. *Science*, Vol. 265 No. 5172 (July 1994), pp. 679-682, ISSN: 0036-8075.

Koch, S. (2006). Home telehealth-Current state and future trends. *International Journal of Medical Informatics*, Vol. 75, No. 8 (August 2006), pp. 565-576, ISSN: 1386-5056.

Lind, L.; Karlsson, D. & Fridlund, B. (2008). Patients' use of digital pens for pain assessment in advanced palliative home healthcare. *International Journal of Medical Informatics*, Vol. 77, No. 2 (February 2008), pp. 129-136, ISSN: 1386-5056.

Lotjonen, J.; Korhonen, I.; Hirvonen, K.; Eskelinen, T.; Myllymaki, M. & Partinen, M. (2003) Automatic sleep-wake and nap analysis with a new wrist worn Online activity monitoring device Vivago WristCare (R). *Sleep*, Vol. 26 No. 1 (February 2003), pp. 86-90, ISSN: 0161-8105.

Max, M.B.; Donovan, M.; Miaskowski, C.A.; Ward, S.E.; Gordon, D.; Bookbinder, M.; Cleeland, C.S.; Coyle, N.; Kiss, M.; Thaler, H.T.; Janjan, N.; Weinstein, S. & Edwards, T. (1995). Quality improvement guidelines for the treatment of acute pain and cancer pain. *Journal of the American Medical Association*, Vol. 274, No. 23 (December 1995), pp. 1874-1880, ISSN: 0095-7484.

Mikulich ,V.J.; Liu, Y.C.A.; Steinfeldt, J. & Schriger, D.L. (2001) Implementation of clinical guidelines through an electronic medical record: physician usage, satisfaction and assessment. *International Journal of Medical Informatics*, Vol. 63, No. 3 (October 2001), pp. 169-178, ISSN: 1386-5056.

Myrtek, M. (2004). *Heart and Emotion: ambulatory monitoring studies in everyday life*, Hogrefe & Huber Publishers, ISBN: 0-88937-286-1, Toronto, Canada.

Nilsson, G.; Berglund, M.; Nilsson, C.; Revay, P. & Petersson, G. (2007). Nurses' and nurse students' demands of functions and usability in a PDA. *International Journal of Medical Informatics*, Vol. 76, No. 7 (July 2007), pp. 530-537, ISSN: 1386-5056.

Paquet, J.; Kawinska, A. & Carrier, J. (2007). Wake detection capacity of actigraphy during sleep. *Sleep*, Vol. 30, No. 10 (October 2007), pp. 1362-1369, ISSN: 0161-8105.

Pollak, C.P.; Tryon, W.W.; Nagaraja, H. & Dzwonczyk, R. (2001). How accurately does wrist actigraphy identify the states of sleep and wakefulness? *Sleep*, Vol. 24, No. 8 (December 2001), pp. 957-965, ISSN: 0161-8105.

Quanten, S.; De Valck, E.; Mairesse, O.; Cluydts, R. & Berckmans D. (2006) Individual and Time-Varying Model Between Sleep and Thermoregulation. *Journal of Sleep Research*, Vol. 15, no. s1 (September 2006), pp. 243-244, ISSN: 0962-1105.

Rechtschaffen. A. & Kales, A. (Eds.). (1968). *A manual of standardized terminology, techniques and scoring system for sleep stages of human subjects*, US Government Printing Office, Washington DC.

Rivera-Fernandez, R.; Nap, R.; Vazquez-Mata, G. & Miranda, D.R. (2007). Analysis of Physiologic Alterations in Intensive Care Unit Patients and Their Relationship With Mortality. *Journal of Critical Care*, Vol. 22, No. 2 (June 2007), pp. 120-128, ISSN: 0883-9441.

Ryan, J.M.; Corry, J.R.; Attewell, R. & Smithson, M.J. (2002). A comparison of an electronic version of the SF-36 General Health Questionnaire to the standard paper version. *Quality of Life Research*, Vol. 11, No. 1 (February 2002), pp. 19-26, ISSN: 0962-9343.

Sakai, S.; Kobayashi, K.; Toyabe, S.I.; Mandai, N.; Kanda, T. & Akazawa, K. (2007). Comparison of the Levels of Accuracy of an Artificial Neural Network Model and a Logistic Regression Model for the Diagnosis of Acute Appendicitis. *Journal of Medical Systems*, Vol. 31, No. 5 (October 2007), pp. 357-364, ISSN: 0148-5598.

Sauvage, F.; Langlais, M.; & Pontier, D. (2007). Predicting the emergence of human hantavirus disease using a combination of viral dynamics and rodent demographic patterns. *Epidemiology and Infection*, Vol. 135, No. 1 (January 2007), pp. 46-56, ISSN: 0950-2688.

Sitnick, S.L.; Goodlin-Jones, B.L. & Anders, T.F. (2008). The use of actigraphy to study sleep disorders in preschoolers: Some concerns about detection of nighttime awakenings. *Sleep*, Vol. 31, No. 3 (March 2008), pp. 395-401, ISSN: 0161-8105.

Takahara, M.; Nittono, H.; Shirakawa, S.; Hori, T.; Onozuka, M. & Sato, S. (2008). Effect of voluntary attention on EEG activity during REM sleep. *Journal of Sleep Research*, Vol. 17, No. s1 (December 2008), pp. 238-239, ISSN: 0962-1105.

Tilley, A. & Empson, J.A. (1978). REM sleep and memory consolidation. *Biological Psychology*, Vol. 6, No. 4 (June 1978), pp. 293-300, ISSN: 0301-0511.

Tryon, W.W. (2004). Issues of validity in actigraphic sleep assessment. *Sleep*, Vol. 27, No. 1 (February 2004), 158-165, ISSN: 0161-8105.

Van Loon, K.; Guiza, F.; Meyfroidt, G.; Aerts, J.-M.; Ramon, J.; Blockeel, H.; Bruynooghe, M.; Van den Berghe, G. & Berckmans, D. (2010). Prediction of clinical conditions after coronary bypass surgery using dynamic data analysis. *Journal of Medical Systems*, Vol. 34, No. 3 (June 2010), pp. 229-239, ISSN: 0148-5598.

Verduijn, M.; Sacchi, L.; Peek, N.; Bellazzi, R.; de Jonge, E. & de Mol, B.A.J.M. (2007). Temporal abstraction for feature extraction: a comparative case study in prediction from intensive care monitoring data. *Artificial Intelligence in Medicine*, Vol. 41, No. 1 (September 2007), pp. 1-12, ISSN: 0933-3657.

Wada, T.; Akaike, H.; Yamada, Y. & Udagawa, E. (1988). Application of Multivariate Autoregressive Modeling for Analysis of Immunological Networks in Man. *Computers & Mathematics with Applications*, Vol. 15, No. 9 (1988), pp. 713-722, ISSN: 0898-1221.

Wincent, A.; Liden, Y. & Arner, S. (2003). Pain questionnaires in the analysis of long lasting (chronic) pain conditions. *European Journal of Pain*, Vol. 7, No. 4 (August 2003), pp. 311-321, ISSN: 1090-3801.

9

Environmental Pollution and Chronic Disease Management – A Prognostics Approach

Bernard Fong[1] and A. C. M. Fong[2]
[1]*Prognostics and Health Management Centre, City University of Hong Kong*
[2]*Faculty of Design and Creative Technology, Auckland University of Technology*
[1]*Hong Kong*
[2]*New Zealand*

1. Introduction

In many metropolitan cities, environmental pollution has a substantial impact on social and cultural well being. Statistically provable direct heath effects may require further studies to establish the influence on the community and the public healthcare system. The combined effects of fossil fuel burning and economic growth have negative impacts on health and financial costs in many areas. The main research objective aims at exploring the links between environmental pollution and health related problems. The inherently slow and reactive response over generations has repeatedly made corrective actions after an incident but not before and sometimes becomes too late. Also, health and safety precautions are often not properly exercised in a pre-emptive manner. Any proactive measure through proper early warning and environmental control methodologies would certainly yield a reduction in preventable illnesses as well as health degradation that result from improper care and environmental pollution.

Pollution is not only a problem in the community as a whole. Even at home, indoor air pollution causes a wide range of health-related issues (Bruce, 2000). The impacts of pollution on human health must therefore be assessed both for indoor and the broader outdoor environment. Since the industrial revolution of the 19th century, health hazards related to discharge of toxic chemicals and heavy metals from manufacturing plants has also become a more serious health issue. Air pollutants can travel hundreds of miles causing respiratory problems and chronic diseases. Heavy metal and toxic chemical deposits enter the food chain through the food chain and water supply (Nasreddinea, 2002). As health of the general population degrades, more people require medical attention that will eventually stretch healthcare resources to their limits.

Work on reducing health problems directly or indirectly caused by environmental pollution is urgently needed because demand on public health services is expected to grow substantially over the next two decades as a direct consequence of population aging in most developed countries (Christensen, 2009). In many cases, chronic disease is avoidable if appropriate actions are taken especially among senior citizens given access to the appropriate assistive technologies.

The environment has a substantial impact on both chronic and infectious disease (Hall-Stoodley, 2004). Take, for example, water contamination that was caused by massive flooding in Queensland, Australia, during summer 2011. The sewer system was overwhelmed by a sudden influx of water within a relatively short period of time that led to contamination of the region's water supply system. A soaring number of cases of ascariasis and giardia were reported soon after the floods. Pathogens such as bacteria, parasites and viruses responsible for spreading a range of infectious waterborne diseases across vast distances, can affect both drinking and recreational water (Colford, 2007). While a clear relationship exists between water contamination and infectious disease, the impacts on chronic diseases may not be obvious although the long-term health hazards are thought to be even more serious with a higher risk of fatality as a direct result of bladder cancer and chronic ingestion of arsenic in drinking water (Cantor, 1997).

Industrial processes such as mining, manufacturing and petroleum distillation discharge a vast amount of toxic chemicals. Even a small amount of highly toxic organic compounds can cause genetic disorders that lead to cancers and birth defects. The problem associated with an imbalance of aquatic ecosystems due to environmental pollution must therefore be thoroughly addressed. The process of managing industrial waste and pollution relates to both direct impact on human health and a broader scope of food contamination as animals along the food chain accumulate toxins in their fat and flesh from their food. The extent of contamination in the food chain increases as the toxin accumulates while propagating further up the food chain (Pereira, 2004). In an example of paralytic shellfish toxins, where the toxins first enter the food chain through waste discharged from a factory into the water eco-system. The chemicals are soaked up by shellfish that in turn becomes food of other animals that are ultimately consumed by humans. A range of other hazardous problems are also observed during this process, for example, some chemicals can cause genetic mutation that leads to cancer (Landrigan, 2002). The impacts of both microbiological and chemical contamination across the food chain must therefore be closely examined.

Water contamination is only one of the many examples of pollution-induced chronic disease contributor. Another classic example is the close relationship between second hand cigarette smoking and lung cancer (Arden Pope III, 2002). Essentially everything that we take, from the air we inhale to the water we drink and the food we eat, can potentially pose serious health risk. The primary objective of this chapter is to thoroughly investigate the relationship between environmental pollution and chronic disease in the perspective of health management and prevention by first taking a look at why health management is more difficult to address in some countries than others. Although this is generally a more serious problem in developing countries with inadequate sanitation infrastructures and policies, it may not necessarily be true that industrialized nations are less prone to pollution-induced health risks.

All these entail the collection and subsequent analysis of data from different sources; these include environmental pollution, disease prevalence, demographic variables, climatology and historical weather data analysis. To analyze such data for health management and planning, an efficient system such as prognostics and health management (PHM) is needed. PHM is a methodology widely used in different sectors of electronics for accurate prediction and computation modelling of system health degradation and maintenance (Lau, 2011). The term 'prognostics' simply means prediction of what is likely going to happen, as in medical science where prognostics has been used in the forecast of global pandemics (Wong, 2006). To understand how this puts into the context of health management for environmental health and chronic disease, we first take a look at the definition of PHM in engineering from *wiki*:

Prognostics is an engineering discipline focused on predicting the time at which a component will no longer perform a particular function. Lack of performance is most often component failure. The predicted time becomes then the remaining useful life (RUL). The science of prognostics is based on the analysis of failure modes, detection of early signs of wear and aging, and fault conditions. These signs are then correlated with a damage propagation model. Potential uses for prognostics is in condition-based maintenance. The discipline that links studies of failure mechanisms to system lifecycle management is often referred to as prognostics and health management (PHM), sometimes also system health management (SHM) or - in transportation applications - vehicle health management (VHM). Technical approaches to building models in prognostics can be categorized broadly into data-driven approaches, model-based approaches, and hybrid approaches.

From this definition, prognostics and health management (PHM) methodology has been used in the electronics industry to predict the system's *health* degradation thereby determining a product's remaining useful life. The word *health* here refers to a product's operational state, very similar in the context of a person's health and well-being. Putting these into the context of a human body as a *system*, which consists of sub-systems such as immune system and digestive system. Under certain circumstances, the health of a sub-system can degrade. Think of the case where predominant bacteria is accumulated in the stomach resulting in the reduction of nitrate and nitrite (Sobkoa, 2005), the bacteria will continue to grow while the environmental conditions remain unchanged and before they run out of space or nutrients. In this particular example, PHM can be used to model the growth of bacteria inside the stomach and how digestion is affected such that a number of corrective actions can be taken before the situation worsens. Put it quite simply, PHM as implemented in electronics, can also be applied to healthcare management in very much the same way. One of the key focus of this chapter is to discuss how PHM can assist with health management for environmental health and chronic disease. We shall look at the relationship between environmental pollution and chronic disease by exploring a number of different attributes. We shall commence by taking a look at the broader scope of public health.

2. Cultural and environmental impacts on public health

This section addresses the link between culture and environment that causes health concerns. For example, numerous mishaps have been reported in various developing countries as a direct result of excessive coal mining over the past decade. Business decision makers have put the sale of coal above the safety of miners and environmental damage. Such sentiment may ultimately lead to irreversible health consequences which far exceed that of the momentary financial gains. This is best demonstrated by the consequential healthcare costs and potential legal compensations that result from these incidents. In many cases, the remedy cost far exceeds that of prevention.

In response to these social and cultural factors that will almost certainly affect the health and well-being of millions of people, this section will concentrate on exploring how proper health management can provide a remedy and improve public health.

2.1 Perception, general health awareness and education

The link between health and general education, personal hygiene and habits has been comprehensively studied at the turn of the millennium (Lorig, 1996). (Kickbusch, 2001) suggests that there is a significant gap between developing countries and industrialized nations of which literacy is becoming increasingly important for social, economic and health development. Perception and awareness plays a vital role in disease control. In the case of infectious disease spread, pathogens can easily be spread from one person to another without any precautions. As a person coughs, air-borne disease spread by droplet infection can reach surrounding human traffic such that anyone who walks past can be caught off guard. Common sense may tell us that there are certain precautionary measures that can be taken to minimize the risk of disease spread. However, the threat must first be realized for an action to be taken, like a person will cover the mouth before coughing only with the knowledge that communicable diseases such as influenza can be spread through dispersion of air-borne transmission by droplets (Roy, 2004). The person should also understand the need of disposing of the tissue properly after use. This simple example reminds us the importance of general health awareness for disease prevention.

The issue of disease prevention, particularly for chronic diseases where some symptoms may not exhibit themselves for months or even years, delayed diagnosis may lead to premature mortality. Health degradation is sometimes gradual without any pain or discomfort until a series of other complications are developed. Although regular medical check-ups can detect or prevent illnesses and diseases, this also requires general awareness and the perception of needs. To elaborate on the details of chronic disease problems related to health education, the next section will look at a case study of coal mining and the nearby inhabitants.

2.2 Environmental health and energy supply

Soaring energy costs put tremendous pressure on the coal mining industry as coal is widely used for power generation as well as conversion into liquid biofuel. The impact of coal mining on health can affect both miners and nearby inhabitants. Health management policies are required to address different environmental circumstances for everyone concerned.

The primary health concern is air pollution. The air quality of an underground coal mine is usually regulated by a gas drainage line where toxic gases are pumped out and neutralized. Exposure to volatile organic compounds (VOCs) is one of the major toxic chemical risks on the human respiratory system (Manuel, 1999). It is estimated that as much as 4.23 g of methane is released per 1 kg of underground-mined coal (Spath, 1999). The idea of utilizing prognostics for the investigation into cumulative coal-mine-dust exposure of coal miners was proposed in (Bourgkard, 1998) such that a PHM system such as that illustrated in Fig. 1 can collect air samples from various parts of the mine shaft and to regulate the air quality as well as triggering an alarm when toxic gas concentration reaches a predetermined threshold specific to the gas measured.

This monitoring system consists of three key components, namely gas sampling sensor network for data acquisition, prognostics module for system monitoring with data analysis module for statistical modelling. The analyzed data is used to regulate the mine shaft ventilation and to trigger an alarm should an evacuation due to dangerous level of gas become necessary. Gas sampling is accomplished by analysis of solid particles and chemicals for the presence of a range of VOCs.

Gas concentration surveillance methods can be classified into three regression classes, namely linear regression, Poisson regression and regression with ARIMA (Autoregressive Integrated Moving Average) error structures (Jiang, 2007). Covariates such as miners' work shift indicators, seasonal trends with harmonic terms, and coal export indicators are often included in the regression models. By applying fuzzy ontology for assessment (Tho, 2006), ventilation control can be activated by using prospective estimation for the modeling of pollutant flow within the mine shaft. Known information is used to estimate the VOC spread and the change in concentration over time.

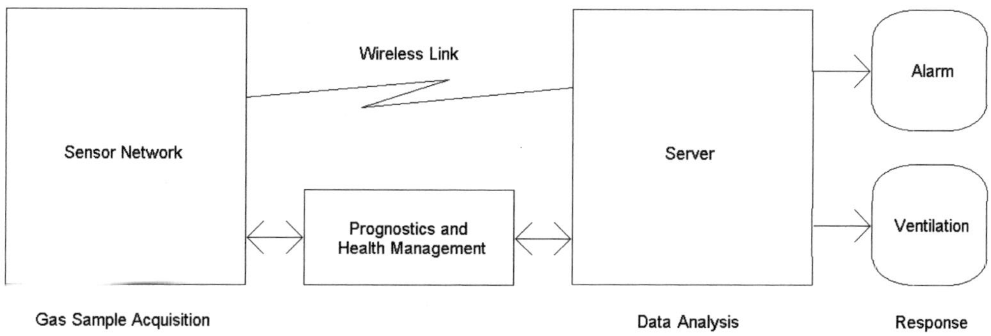

Fig. 1. A prognostics and health management system for air quality monitoring

Coal dust can also affect local residents surrounding a mining site. While we discuss issues related to indoor air quality and health in the next section in more detail, it is important to address the link between health management and those living nearby. Policies related to safe mining is therefore an important issue to look at. For example, the decision between opencast and underground mine development would, among various economic and practicality factors, have an implication on compromising between the hazards to miners working in the mine and the extent of environmental pollution to the surrounding areas. In adition to coal dust, opencast mining also produces a large amount of toxic gases such as methane and sulphur dioxide which can cause acid rain (Heinberg, 2009). Further, soot emission is also known to cause climate change (Karl, 2003). Coal pollution dust can also enter the food chain in areas where argricultral activities exist and toxic waste water can be discharged into rivers and underground without undergoing proper treatment. The discharged water combined with runoff from mine tailings can cause pollution to surface water and groundwater in mine areas resulting in soil contamination. Excessive discharge of water can also cause land to subsidence, such risk is even more prominant around coastal mines since water being pumped out from the mines can be combined with sea water that consequently leads to contamination of surrounding water sources.

The health risks posed to miners and their associated costs also need to be addressed. Among a long list of complications that can be developed including hearing impairment, neuromuscular disorders, rheumatism, chronic obstructive pulmonary disease (COPD) and acute respiratory infection (ARI) (Hnizdo, 2003); pneumonia caused by coal dust inhalation is perhaps the most serious fatal occupational diseases to hit coal miners. The cost of treating these diseass and compensation can be staggering.

Different energy sources may be responsible for different kinds of environmental pollution with varying degree of negative impacts on human health and how far the effects can be felt. Even so-called clean energy may not be totally free from causing pollution. For example, wind energy may be widely regarded as a clean energy source. Rotating wind turbines causes pollution in the form of noise although most of them may be installed far away from residential zones (Pedersen, 2004). Elevated level of noise produced from a wind turbine is often resulted from deficiency linked to lubrication and component wear (Gray, 2010), pollution control through noise control can be accomplished using the following prognostics approach: A prognostics system typically consists of a variety of onboard sensors, data acquisition systems, and signal processing and analysis algorithm. Application of prognostics based maintenance technology to wind turbine has the potential to significantly reduce induced noise and increase turbine reliability by enabling condition-based maintenance (CBM) thus enabling advance detection of dry lubricants as well as component tear and wear. Detection of faults in their early stages provides an opportunity to carry out necessary maintenance work prior to a turbine degradation that may generate excessive noise.

Among various energy sources commonly used over the past decade or more, nuclear energy is perhaps the deadiest that can kill many people over a long period of time spanning across decades due to radioactive pollution as a direct cause of many acute and chronic conditions (Andia, 1998). Although excessive discharge of radioactive pollutants does not occur often, once it happens the situation can be critical as radiation is released into the environment that can travel for thousands of miles across the world. Well-known accidents include the 1986 Chernobyl reactor meltdown in the former Soviet Union, Three Mile Island incident in the USA and more recently Fukushima nuclear plant in Japan overheated after an earthquake triggered tsunami damaged the plant's power supply to the cooling system. Note that the word 'meltdown' is appropriately used in a nuclear reactor disaster to describe the blast. This is because commercial nuclear reactor fuel is not enriched to the radioactive materials used in nuclear weapons intended to cause massive explosions. In the case of a meltdown, the core temperature inside the nuclear fuel rods casues the solid rod to melt, turning in liquid. As the happens the molten radioactive materials of the fuel rods would react with ground water (Caldicott, 2006). The wide range of fatal health problems will be seen for the decades to come as there is currently no known cure to radioactive poisoning as the damage to human tissue is irreversible.

2.3 Health management, policies and public reactions

Earlier in the section we have discussed the health management issues related to perception and general awareness. The role of health management and policies can differ significantly from country to country. While this chapter will not touch on politics, there are a number of issues that should be addressed. Take the table salt snatching example in March 2011 following the Fukushima nuclear incident in Japan, rumours triggered panic buying of table salt around the Greater China region (Pierson, 2011). Fear was sparked by internet rumours that salt consumption can ward off radiation exposure. Further panic was also driven by the theory that salt in future may be produced from radiation-contaminated sea water. Without citing any references, it should be obvious to readers that common table salt as a remedy and that production of salt by radioactive-pollution affected sea water cannot possibly be true.

Sometimes rumours are not totally unfounded. There are perhaps some related facts, such as in this particular example, iodine salt can yield a lower absorption of certain radioactive exposure (Mettler Jr., 2002). People with no knowledge on how radiation may affect human health can be driven to respond to rumours in an inappropriate way. Further, no effort has been made on finding out whether table salt sold on the market is iodized and they lack the knowledge of understanding the difference between iodine tablets and iodized salt. This is a classic example of an overreaction by people to rumours.

Whether people are willing to learn from past experience is another issue that health management needs to addressed. By recalling the SARS (Severe Acute Respiratory Syndrome) epidemic was initially erupted in China's Guangdong province in 2003, rumours claimed vinegar could be used as a disinfectant and kill the SARS virus (Rosling, 2003). Like stockpiling table salt in 2011, people responded in exactly the same way when they stocked up excessive quantities of vinegar some eight years earlier.
These examples, showing how people react to rumours, provide an insight into the importance of carefully planned policies in anticipation of public reactions. Certain clues may be made available to policy makers for prediction of how general perception will be driven.

3. Environmental monitoring technology

To assist with health management for prevention and control of environmentally related diseases, a general understanding of methodologies in monitoring environmental pollutions that cause a range of chronic diseases and premature death is vitally important. Environmental monitoring relies heavily on sensors and wireless networks that connect the sensors together. Wireless sensor networks provide a range of solutions for monitoring different sources of pollutions from the air we breathe to the water we drink. Different sensors exist for different applications.

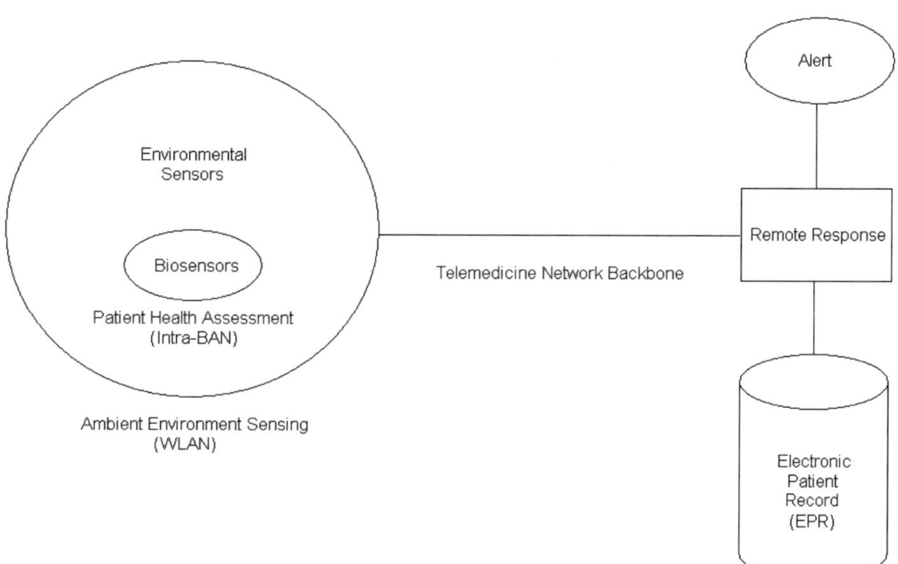

Fig. 2. Environmental health monitoring system

A wide range of sensors are deployed in different locations to monitor different parameters. These cover both human health and the surround environment

3.1 Sensors

A sensor is defined by (Carstens, 1992) as a device that provides a usable output signal in response to a specified measurement parameter, for example, methane gas concentration, or humidity. A sensor generally operates by translating physical, chemical, or biological phenomena into an electrical signal utilizing physical or chemical effects that corresponds to the measured value or through energy conversion from one form into another. To make any meaningful use of the measurement obtained from a sensor, it is necessary to have some means to connect the sensor to an electronic circuitry so that the raw measured value can be interpreted in a meaningful way. For example, by measuring the relative humidity of air, it would be necessary to have some kind of electronics that reads what the sensor picks up and translate it into an output such as an LCD (liquid crystal display) panel to be read. This is essentially to say that an interface, such as an electronic device, is necessary to connect a sensor to the outside world. In the case of serving environmental health management applications, sensors are broadly classified into three major groups, namely physical, chemical, and biological.

The types of sensors used in environmental monitoring are listed in Table I. Thermal sensors are resistance thermal detectors (RTDs), thermistors, thermocouples, or semiconductor junction diodes. The signals generated by most sensors are in electrical form with an output generated either as a voltage or a current that corresponds to the reading. Four major types of electrical sensor commonly used are inductive, thermal, capacitive, and Hall effect sensors; and these parameters can be used to represent different attributes. Mechanical sensors usually take a direct measurement of a change in property of a certain parameter and convert it into another energy domain. Humidity refers to the water vapour content in the air, usually measured with capacitive, resistive, or thermal conductivity humidity sensor. Absolute humidity is the ratio of the mass of water vapour to the volume of air whereas relative humidity (RH) to the ratio expressed in percentage of the moisture content of air compared to the saturated moisture level at the given ambient temperature and pressure. Biosensor makes use of biological materials or biologically derived materials to detect analyte that combines a biological component with a physicochemical detector component. Different types of biosensors include electrochemical, optical and piezoelectric sensors with enzymatic catalysis, electrodes, or biological receptor elements. Chemical sensors detect composition and concentrations of a substance to be measured. They make use of electrochemical, mass humidity or thermochemical sensors.

Type	Parameter
Thermal	Temperature, heat flux, heat dissipation
Electrical	Voltage, current, resistance, inductance, capacitance, impedance
Mechanical	Length, acceleration, flow, force, torque, stress, strain, density, strength pressure, acoustic power
Humidity	Relative humidity, absolute humidity
Biological	pH, molecular concentration
Chemical	Chemical concentration, molecular mass, reactivity
Optical	Intensity, phase, wavelength, polarization, transmittance, refractive index
Magnetic	Magnetic field, flux density, permeability, direction, flow

Table 1. Types of Environmental Sensors

In most sensor networks that are set up for environmental health applications, they typically consist of a combination of different sensor types. Management of different type of disease has different requirements on what and where to measure. Each sensor collects its reading and communicates with a console in a polling system such that all sensors are individually and sequentially addressed one after another. In theory, sensors irrespective of types can be polled together, for example, chemical sensors sensing the presence of gaseous hydrocarbon substances can be connected in the same network as a humidity sensor that senses water vapour. However, each of these sensors requires its own electrical interface in order to convert the reading into a form that is suitable for transmission to the console.

Optical sensors can take the form of photoconductors, photoemissive, photovoltaic, and fibre optic variants. All they have in common is that they all produce an electrical output based on the intensity of light that reaches a photocell. Finally, magnetic sensors respond to the change of a certain effect such as:

- Galvanomagnetic effect, manifested as a Hall field and carrier deflection
- Magnetooptic effect, which is any one of a number of phenomena in which an electromagnetic wave propagates through a medium that has been altered by the presence of a quasistatic magnetic field
- Magnetoresistance, which is the property of some materials to change the value of their electrical resistance when an external magnetic field is applied
- Magnetostrictive effect, where the imposed magnetic field causes strain on a certain material

The parameters which are to be monitored in the environment as well as human health can be selected based on their relationship to functions that are vital to the operating conditions, where it is possible to be implicated in an elevated risk of developing a health problem or trigger a symptom of an existing condition. Selection criteria are usually based on knowledge of the critical parameters established by the ambient environment and medical history of the patient. Sensing of multiple parameters can be accomplished using one single sensor system that can measure multiple types of parameters such as temperature, humidity, air pollution, and toxins. Systems that can realize multiple sensing include a sensor array which contains several different sensing elements internally; a sensor system can also include external ports for additional sensors to be attached such that it can support a combination of various sensor nodes.

Physical attributes of a sensor includes its physical size, form factor, weight, case or housing, as well as how it is mounted according to their operating environment. In a body area network (BAN), the sensor's physical size and weight may become the most important selection criterion since limitations of movement for attaching the sensor or due to the inaccessibility of locations to be sensed can affect its wireless communication capability.

3.2 Communication networks

A communication network can be either wired or wireless. The former uses conducting wires and the latter relies on electromagnetic waves. Their common task is to convey information from one point to another (point-to-point). A transmitter that sends information from the source to two or more receivers is said to be point-to-multipoint. Generally speaking, the choice between wired and wireless depends on the trade-off between security and reliability versus mobility and flexibility (Varshney, 2002). In particular, the saving in terms of implementation and material costs without wires in point-to-multipoint communications can sometimes be very significant. In environmental monitoring, an array of sensors is interconnected across different areas, making wireless communications the best option.

Fixed WiMAX networks provide broadband distribution services in urban environments as last mile access for a diverse range of applications with carrier frequencies in excess of 10 GHz (Stamatelos, 1996). There are a number of issues that have to be considered when designing a WiMAX system in the frequency range spanning from 10 to 66 GHz. At these frequencies, multipath does not have any significant impact since high gain antennas with narrow beamwidth can be used for short paths (Fong, 2003). System performance is greatly affected by link availability under various atmospheric conditions. Also, line-of-sight (LOS) or near line-of-sight is normally necessary between antennas. The selection of carrier frequency depends primarily on spectrum allocation by local authorities and operational conditions; the choice of operating frequency is also determined by population density and rainfall statistics.

Although WiMAX offers a more economical alternative to wired networks in many point-to-multipoint scenarios making it particularly suited for environmentally-related chronic disease monitoring, in some areas a WiMAX network may share the same portion of the spectrum with other nearby communication networks and systems. Moreover, data transfer is carried out in a very harsh environment subject to numerous causes of signal degradation and atmospheric phenomena; these include interference, rain-induced attenuation, and depolarization. Frequency planning for an allocated spectrum uses multiple sector systems with each sector supported by a base station of the access service network (ASN) serving a cell site. Uncontrollable factors such as rain-induced attenuation and depolarization must be considered to ensure adequate network availability.

The concept of the Fresnel zone is central to virtually any outdoor environmental monitoring network. The dimensions of the Fresnel Zone can be calculated by simple geometry and the Fresnel zone distance is obtained the difference between the direct path and the indirect path.

Height restriction is often imposed in urban areas where maintaining an unobstructed path for LOS may be virtually impossible. Fig. 3 shows the variation in radio hub distance for first Fresnal zone clearance where the demand for foliage clearance increases as the carrier frequency increases; at least 10 m of clearance is necessary to avoid disproportionate loss. This is a very important consideration for environmental monitoring because any signal that is blocked by physical obstacles would mean the information gathered for a given location is simply lost. Ensuring network reliability and availability entails thorough understanding of the network structure. Similar to passive optical networks (PONs), fixed WiMAX exhibit the same characteristics of the point-to-multipoint topology (Lu, 2007). In this context, network optimization can be realized through deployment of scheme comparable to cascaded arrayed waveguide gratings (AWGs) due to their cyclic property (Zhang, 2009). Both WiMAX and PON share the same topology given a fixed routing such that the position and placement of communicating nodes can be optimized in much the same way as the cascaded AWG structure in PONs so as to optimize how much bandwidth each communicating node can receive. Redundancy is often required in a tree topology to combat the occurrence of link outage that can be addressed by the reliable scheme (Ansari, 2004). Network deployment considerations therefore require careful planning of where each sensor is mounted.

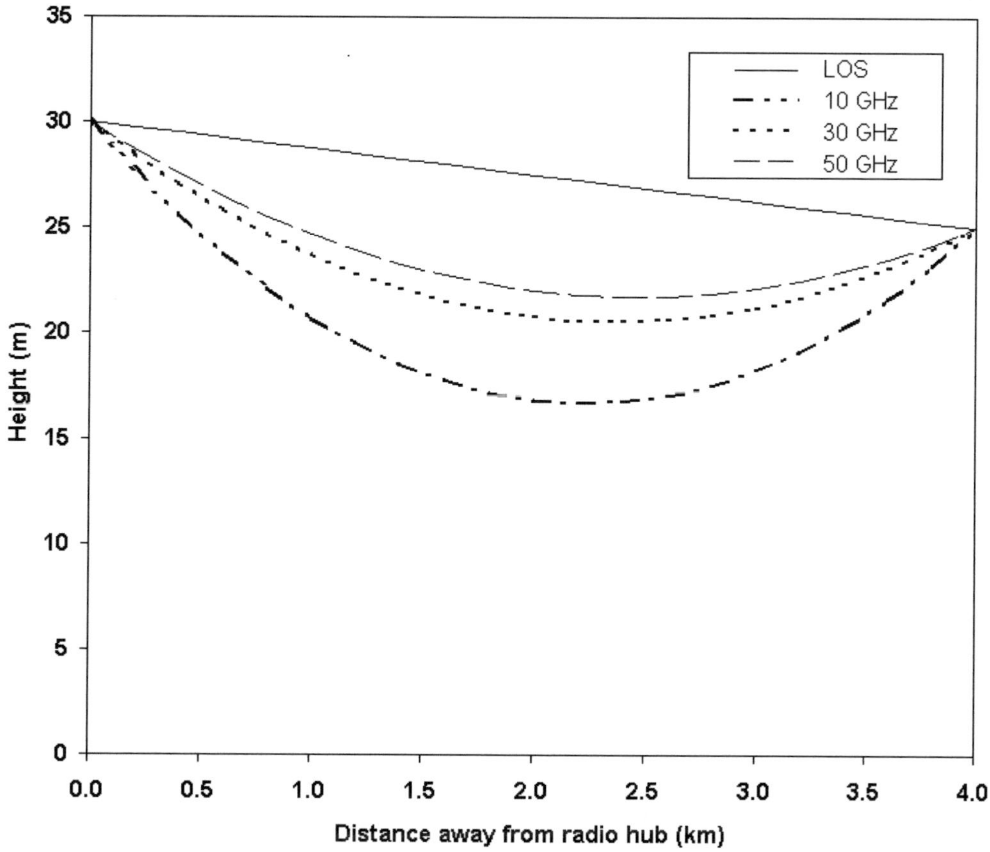

Fig. 3. Fresnel zone clearance for wireless environmental monitoring systems

Wireless communication systems play a significant role in the monitoring and prevention of environmentally related chronic disease. In addition to pollution monitoring, health monitoring provides information technology (IT) solutions for both passive and active prevention with wireless telehealth technology (Fong, 2011). We shall illustrate this by following through an example with asthma patient care, which is known to be a chronic disease closely associated with both indoor and outdoor air pollution (Koenig, 2005).

3.3 Environmental monitoring for asthma patients: A case study

Environmental monitoring for asthma patients is an important topic since some ten percent of Americans are reported to be asthma sufferers according to the US Centers for Disease Control and Prevention (CDC) statistics. Air pollution is a well-known trigger for asthma symptoms. Indoor air pollution is becoming a serious health issue as a range of chemicals found in many homes such as acid aerosols and volatile organic compounds (VOCs) can trigger asthma symptoms (Koutrakis, 1992). The biosensors need to measure and record a patient's peak flow breathing for refractory asthma management. Improving indoor air quality by reducing indoor particulate pollutant concentrations will provide a vital means of improving asthma patients' health. Reduction of respiratory health risk to asthma patients through ubiquitous healthcare entails a series of longitudinal health data to be coupled with detailed monitoring of personal exposure is necessary such that an accurate estimation of the exposure-response relation for air pollutants from various sources can be established.

Among a number of environmentally-linked chronic diseases, asthma alone contributes to over 13 million ambulatory care cases annually for outpatients with asthma as primary diagnosis and hospitalization of almost half a million cases with an average length of stay of three and a half days according to the figures published by the US CDC in its report entitled 'Asthma Prevalence, Health Care Use, and Mortality: United States, 2005–2009'. Many of these cases would have been avoidable if appropriate actions were made to prevent asthma symptoms from being triggered. A healthier living environment to reduce asthma symptoms can be provided by ubiquitous healthcare solutions in monitoring environmental pollutions. Wireless sensor networks provide a range of solutions for monitoring different sources of pollutions in the patient's home by monitoring any changes in concentration of various pollutants.

To thoroughly address this problem for patients living in rural areas, the first necessary step is to provide swift response to a patient when the disease symptoms are triggered. This issue is particular important in the context of rural areas where a lack of skilled healthcare professionals can cause substantial delay in getting medical attention. Telemedicine system that supports remote camera control with a stethoscope for remote auscultation implemented for this purpose. The stethoscope installed at the patient's home would allow a remote respiratory therapist to hear the heart tones and oscillations while simultaneously controlling the camera to see the patient. Through technological advances in telecommunications, many people who require special attention can live alone with the assurance that help is always available and they are taken good care of. Wireless telemedicine is particularly suitable for rural areas and people with limited mobility such that support can be provided to those who live alone with the assurance that they are well looked after. For example, a comprehensive system may be installed at an elderly home with features such as fall detection, smoke and flood warning system.

To address the issue of indoor air pollution that affects asthma patients, spatial and spatio-temporal models used to investigate pollutant distribution, so that information about both space (location) and time will be utilized. Pollutant prediction at unmeasured sites, and pollutant prediction over time. One major challenge is to achieve a comprehensive view of air quality by combining time series of multiple pollutants at different rooms, spatio-temporal measurements with different instruments, and different level summary statistics. To integrate multiple data streams and capitalize the complex dependence across time and space, it is of both theoretical and practical importance to develop a hierarchical model with conditional sub-models defined hierarchically at different levels. The uncertainty is apportioned to different levels and propagated through the hierarchy, which also provides a formal way to borrow strength between various components and improve the precision of statistical inference.

4. Pollution-induced diseases: Challenges for policy makers, medical professionals, and the general public

Having looked at various issues surrounding general education and perception, this section will look at how policy makers can strike an optimal balance between business interests and community well-being. These also have impacts on driving down public healthcare demands and reduce avoidable hospitalization. In a major catastrophe, the risk of causing panic and chaos can further complicate any recovery efforts. Authorities often face the challenges of censoring what kind of information should be released to the media (Massey, 2006). Numerous mismaps throughout the world in recent years have shown that what to release at which stage is vital during a significant event, be it a major disease outbreak or environment disaster. Any inappropriate action can lead to mass hysteria. While the general public usually relies heavily on the media that usually obtain updates from government press releases (Adam, 1999) even though the authorities and the media soemtimes have opposing views regarding sharing and disseminating information to be released to the public. How and when information should be released is therefore an important issue to be addressed in response to a crisis.

Any situation that may lead to problems related to environment-induced diseases has further implications than the link between authorities and the general public. For example, any disclosure delay may lead to treatment postponement. Sometimes, symptoms may not be detected for a long time, such as the case of short term explosure to a dose of very high energy Gamma-ray radiation (Veenema, 2003). The announcement of any radiation leakage may spark mass evacuation and panic. The legacy may well continue for a long time due to contamination of the food chain (Salunkhe, 1961). The impact on any swift action taken by policy makers can greatly increase the chance of survival for many and health professionals require up-to-date information in anticipation of an influx of patients for urgent treatment. Analysis of disease transmission and control often entails mathematical modelling for integration into the process of public health decision making (Keeling, 2007).

4.1 An overview on air pollution and prediction methods

Air pollution is one of the major environmental factors in chronic disease. Main sources of air pollution include manufacturing industry, fossil fuel power generation and motor vehicles (Mayer, 1999), this is a far more severe problem in metropolitan cities where roads are crowded with frequent lengthy traffic jams. Over 200 vehicles can be queued up in a kilometer of road that keep releasing contaminants in the exhaust gas emissions like carbon monoxide, toxic hydrocarbons and nitrogen oxides (Zhang, 1995). Rapid industrialisation and urbanisation of many developing countries over the past decades also accelerate the air pollutin problem with pollutants emissions from electricity generation, petrochemical industry and a growing number of motor vehicles. Although individuals can help by reducing the amount of energy usage with a bit of common sense; monitoring, detecting, and, control of urban air pollution, as well as to improve decision making and creation of sustainable air quality strategies are all necessary actions for air quality improvement. This would entail identification of correlations and casual relationships among different social, geographic, networks and environmental factors through data mining and statistical learning models and algorithms. A fuzzy ontology framework with multiple data sources of global satellite aerosols and pollutants data would be necessary to predict impacts on human health in different areas.

Monitoring air quality requires handling multiple data sources of pollutants-related data. Within each data source there are usually multiple series. Directly applying existing surveillance algorithms into those multiple datasets will reduce computational complexity.

Complexity reduction is particularly important in situations where rapid successive measurement is necessary so that any adrupt change can be detected.

4.2 Disease transmission and the environment: Infectious vs. chronic

Infectious disease requires three elements to spread from one person to another as illustrateed in Fig. 4. The pathogen is carried by some kind of medium, such as air and fluid, as in the case of droplet transmission. Once it settles down on a host, it can also travel across the world via airplane passengers or even wild birds as the infected host (Li, 2004). The environmental plays an important part in how quickly a disease is carried over a medium. For example, (Woo, 2006) studied the transmission of infectious disease in a wet market. Regulations governing operation and hygene of places such as markets and restaurants would prevent the transmission of diseases from animals to a human host.

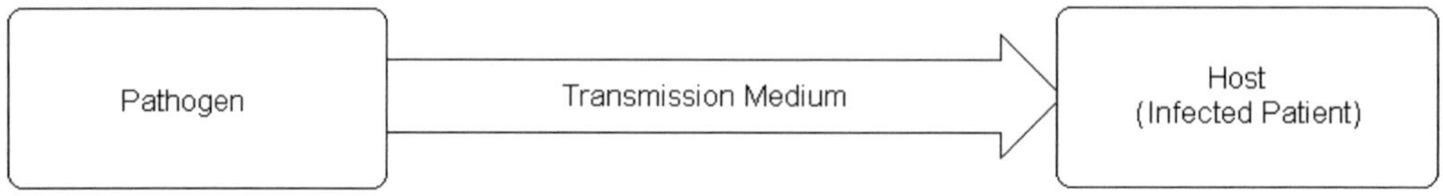

Fig. 4. Infectious disease transmission

A person is prone to infection when all these three elements are present. While it is impossible to eliminate the host, certain measures can control the environment to prevent the pathogen from growing. The transmission medium can also be disrupted if appropriate measures are taken. For example, a person uses alcohol-based hand sanitizer can make the environment, i.e. the hands, safe from bateria. Likewise, when the bateria is subdued the likelihood of the hands being the transmission medium for the bateria is significantly reduced.

The transmission of pathogen from a source can be either direct or indirect. The former is usually through close contact with another host whereas the latter often entails a contaminated fomite such as gastrointestinal pathogens. When the pathogen reaches a host via the medium, it needs a portal of entry, usually the respiratory or gastrointestinal tracts, to enter the host in order to cause an infection. Environmental control and policies can. To some extent, reduce the reduce the spread of an infectious disease, these include disinfection or sterilization, and immunization for people who are particularly vunlerable, like small children and chronically ill patients.

Environment and policies also play a significant role in the control and prevention of chronic disease. Section 2.2 briefly discussed a number of occupational hazards related to the coal mining and nuclear power industry. Occupational health and safety is an important topic to prevent environmentally induced chronic diseases. Measures such as prognostics would be able to predict the development of certain chronic diseases related to work activities. Generally, environmental monitoring for infectious diseases require close surveillance of the breeding grounds of pathogens as well as the transmission media. In chronic disease management the concentration of certain pollutants relevant to the particular condition of interest as well as around the patient's body are of primary interest. The ambient environment needs to be safegarded prevention surveillance in chronic disease just as important as providing a safe place to minimize the risk of an injury. People who need to routinely perform certain tasks are more prone to chronic diseases, such as the case of chronic back pain reported by many health professionals especially among dentists (Andersson, 1999). Ensuring a safe and healthy work environment remains an important aspect of reducing the risk of chronic diseases.

4.3 Laboratory vs. real-life chronic disease management

When conducting experiments in a laboratory environment, observation of activities usually include three steps, namely symptom identification through prognosis, detection through diagnosis, and providing subsequent remedies. In carrying out each of these steps and manipulating the captured data, their time values are collected in segments. The treatment time can be defined as the summation of these three time values. Statistically, the probability distribution of the treatment time cannot be defined as a certain known distribution, and how to utilize segmental information for treatment effectiveness verification may differ in a controlled environment so that the result can be far less effective in real-life situations. The observations from laboratory experiments usually do not take into consideration any changes in the ambient environment can commonly occur in real-life, and the symptoms identified in the verification stage are naturally produced during experiment. The two sets of data captured from different environments, that is, the laboratory data verses the field data in real-life situations, do not have a direct relation due to the differences in the experimental environment. In order to make use of laboratory data for chronic disease management in the real-world, data fusion is a necessary step before conducting integrative verification. This is primarily performed to integrate different sources of data in order to yield improved information than can be derived from each single data source. The simplest method of fusion is to take a weighted average of redundant information obtained from multiple data sources.

The Bootstrap method is used in statistics as a computer-based method for used for uncertainty analysis that does not require any a prior assumptions for the unknown distribution of experimentally observed data. This is an important feature for disease management since the actual environment surrounding a patient cannot be known. It makes use of the given patient's health information and simulate the unknown distribution through resampling of the available data. Resampling creates an ensemble of data sets, where each set is replicated from the original samples (MacKinnon, 2004) and creates new data sets by sampling with replacement. Given that the laboratory data and the actual field data are two different characterizations from the same sample under two different environments and due to the random nature of the data, these two different data sets can be considered as two evidences from different information sources within the same time frame.

5. Prognostics and health management for disease control

We shall conclude this chapter by covering condition-based monitoring techniques on health deterioration. Prognostics techniques have been proven for effectively predict the remaining useful life of a given system. Similar methodologies can be applied to monitoring the state of human health subject to different environmental impacts, such as chronic diseases caused by contaminated water supplies and acid rain.

The most common existing methods for detection of an outbreak include temporal and spatial surveillance. In reality, the disease incident data are likely to be heterogeneous, correlated, and often exhibit seasonal patterns over time. Efficient detection and prognostics methods under these situations are lacking. Effective mitigation strategies and resource management require new scientific theory and approaches that are needed for disease spread simulation, diagnostics, prognostics, and forecasting methods. The public healthcare infrastructure needs a mechanism for comprehensive real time infectious disease data collection, monitoring and management during the early stage of an outbreak. Accomplishing this will require data mining and forecasting approach for diagnostics and prognostics of real time monitoring and acquisition of infectious disease data collected during outbreaks. Besides, for timely outbreak detection, bio-surveillance and syndromic surveillance approaches will also be needed for prompt detection by monitoring disease symptoms or correlated indicators to effectively gather and analyze suspected cases through use of small-world-like model which has been widely reported in Europe in recent years (Lee, 2009). In addition to monitoring confirmed incidents, efficient spatio-temporal surveillance algorithms will be part of the key infrastructural elements for monitoring multiple streams of data including disease symptoms, correlated indicators, and confirmed incidents.

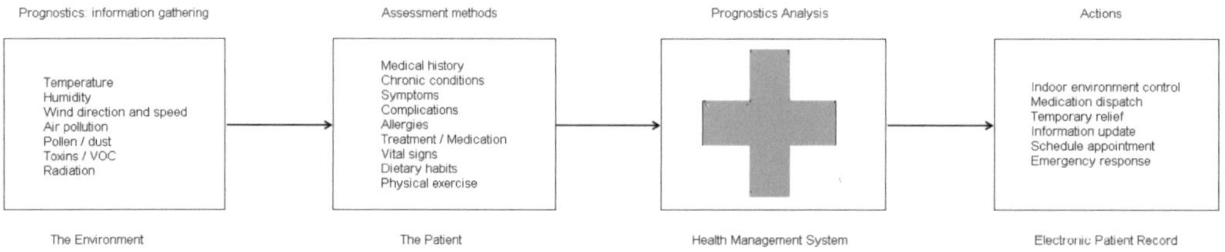

Fig. 5. A prognostics framework for managing chronic disease

The first step involves an overall environmental assessment, where environmental condition, patient's health, vital signs, current medications taken, and any symptoms exhibited are the inputs to perform an assessment. Based on the assessment results, it is possible to prioritize the necessary actions to take and the potential health risks. The existing sensor data (both ambient environment and patient's health), recent monitored data, and medical history and electronic patient record can also be used to identify the health condition. Based on this information, the monitoring parameters and sensor locations for PHM can be determined.

Chronic Disease management entails an active approach that tackles any signs of symptom at the early stage of the disease cycle to minimize the impact of disease progression and potential health complications. PHM makes use of early warning of health degradation to provide early treatment thereby improving the health of patient diagnosed with certain conditions so to avoid the risk of further complications and interventions at a later stage. Fig. 5 shows the framework for prognostics for managing environmentally linked chronic diseases. Environmental data obtained from various locations of different pollutants can be monitored and analyzed using prognostic methodology. Different implementation approaches can be adopted individually or in combination. The principle of PHM is to utilize current information and forecast the future condition. Information about the patient's current health can be used for prediction of any further complication. Chronic disease management involves the monitoring of environmental conditions that may trigger a symptom and to alert all registered patients who have been diagnosed with chronic disease.

Further, prognostics can be used to identify patients with elevated risk of developing a chronic condition. For example, by monitoring the health condition of an obese patient who is known to be prone to developing diabetes, necessary precautionary actions can be proactively taken to reduce such risk. The patient can be of different stage from free of disease to early stage of disease without exhibiting any signs or symptoms. PHM is particularly suited for managing patients with multiple chronic conditions and special health needs. Based on the definition of data driven prognostics, we can intepretate Fig. 5 as utilizing monitored current environmental conditions and assessment data related to patient health. The principal advantage to data driven prognostics is that it can often be deployed quicker and cheaper compared to other approaches, and that it can provide comprehensive coverage of symptoms and signs; making it particularly suited to managing the fluctuating nature of illness. To the patient, information obtained can also be used for assisting with adjustments of lifestyles based on changes to health condition. Disease management with environmental monitoring technology serves as a means of caring for patients with chronic conditions. Prognostics and health management methodology provides an assistive option for decision support and condition-based monitoring for active prevention.

6. References

Adam B (1999). Environmental Risks and the Media, Taylor & Francis, Inc. ISBN: 0203164997.

Andersson GBJ (1999). Epidemiological features of chronic low-back pain, The Lancet, 354(9178):581-585.

Ansari N, Cheng G and Krishran RN (2004). Efficient and reliable link state information dissemination", IEEE Communications Letters, 8(5): 317-319.

Anden Pope III C, et. Al. (2002). Lung cancer, cardiopulmonary mortality, and long-term exposure to fine particulate air pollution, JAMA 287(9):1132-1141.

Andia JSD (1998). Radiation Situation and Health Statistics of the People in the Tula Region of Russia after the Chernobyl Catastrophe, KURRI-KR-21:157-164.

Bourgkard E, et. Al. (1998). Can the Evolution to Pneumoconiosis Be Suspected in Coal Miners?, American Journal of Respiratory and Critical Care Medicine, 158(2):504-509.

Bruce N, Perez-Padilla R and Albalak R (2000). Indoor air pollution in developing countries: a major environmental and public health challenge, Bulletin of the World Health Organization, 78(9).

Caldicott H (2006). Nuclear Power Is Not the Answer to Global Warming or Anything Else, New Press, ISBN: 9781595580672.

Cantor KP (1997). Drinking water and cancer, Cancer Causes and Control, 8(3):292-308.

Carstens J (1992). Electrical Sensors and Transducers, Prentice-Hall, ASIN (Amazon Standard Identification Number): B0034DFEV0.

Christensen K, Doblhammer G, Rau R and Vaupel JW (2009). Ageing populations: the challenges ahead, The Lancet, 374(9696):1196-1208.

Colford JM et. Al. (2007). Water Quality Indicators and the Risk of Illness at Beaches, Epidemiology, 18(1):27-35.

Fong B, Rapajic PB, Hong GY, and Fong ACM (2003). Factors Causing Uncertainties in Outdoor Wearable Wireless Communications, IEEE Pervasive Computing, 2(2):16-19.

Fong B, Fong ACM and Li CK (2011). Telemedicine Technologies: Information Technologies for Medicine and Telehealth, Wiley.

Gray CS and Watson SJ (2010). Physics of Failure approach to wind turbine condition based maintenance, Wind Energy, 13(6):395-405.

Hall-Stoodley L, Costerton W and Stoodley P (2004). Bacterial biofilms: from the Natural environment to infectious diseases, Nature Reviews Microbiology 2:95-108.

Heinberg R (2009). Blackout: coal, climate and the last energy crisis, New Society Publishers, ISBN: 9780865716568.

Hnizdoand E and Vallyathan V (2003). Chronic obstructive pulmonary disease due to occupational exposure to silica dust: a review of epidemiological and pathological evidence, Occupational and Environmental Medicine, 60(4):237-243.

Jiang W, Au T and Tsui KL (2007). A statistical process control approach to business activity monitoring, IIE Transactions, 39(3):235-249.

Karl TR and Trenberth KE (2003). Modern global climate change, Science, 302(5651):1719-1723.

Keeling MJ and Rohani P (2007). Modeling Infectious Diseases in Humans and Animals, Princeton University Press, ISBN: 9780691116174.

Kickbusch IS (2001), Health literacy: addressing the health and education divide, Health Promotion International, 16(3):289-297.

Koenig JQ et. Al. (2005), Pulmonary Effects of Indoor- and Outdoor-Generated Particles in Children with Asthma, Children's Health, 113(4):499–503.

Koutrakis P, Briggs SLK and Leaderer BP (1992). Heaters using kerosene can also produce acid aerosols, Environmental Science and Technology, 26(3):521-527.

Landrigan PJ, Schechter CB, Lipton JM, Fahs MC and Schwartz J (2002). Environmental pollutants and disease in American children: Estimates of morbidity, mortality, and costs for lead poisoning, asthma, cancer, and developmental disabilities, Environmental Health Perspectives, 110(7):721-728.

Lau D and Fong B (2011), Special Issue on Prognostics and Health Management. Microelectronics Reliability 51(2):253-254

Lee VJ, Lye DC and Wilder-Smith A (2009). Combination strategies for pandemic influenza response - a systematic review of mathematical modeling studies, BMC Medicine, 7:76(1-8).

Li KS, et. Al. (2004). Genesis of a highly pathogenic and potentially pandemic H5N1 influenza virus in eastern Asia, Nature, 430:209-213.

Lorig K, et. Al. (1996). Outcome measures for health education and other health care interventions, Sage Publications, Inc., ISBN: 0761900675.

Lu K, Qian Y and Chen HH (2007). Wireless broadband access: WiMAX and beyond, IEEE Communications Magazine, 45(5):124-130.

MacKinnon DP, Lockwood CM and Williams J (2004). Confidence Limits for the Indirect Effect: Distribution of the Product and Resampling Methods, Multivariate Behavioral Research, 39(1):99-123.

Manuel J (1999). A healthy home environment?, Environmental Health Perspectives; 107(7): A352–A357.

Massey JE and Larsen JP (2006). Crisis management in real time: How to successfully plan for and respond to a crisis, Journal of Promotion Management, 12(3):63-97.

Mayer H (1999). Air pollution in cities, Atmospheric Environment, 33(24):4029-4037.

Mettler Jr. FA and Voelz GL (2002). Major radiation exposure—what to expect and how to respond, New England Journal of Medicine, 346:1554-1561.

Nasreddinea L and Parent-Massin D (2002). Food contamination by metals and pesticides in the European Union. Should we worry?, Toxicology Letters, 127(1):29-41.

Pedersen E and Waye KP (2004). Perception and annoyance due to wind turbine noise—a dose–response relationship, Journal of Acoustical Society of America, 116(6): 3460-3470.

Pereira P, et. Al. (2004). Accumulation and depuration of cyanobacterial paralytic shellfish toxins by the freshwater mussel Anodonta cygnea, Aquatic Toxicology, 69(4): 339-350.

Pierson D (2011). Japan radiation fears spark panic salt-buying in China, Los Angeles Times March 18, 2011.

Rosling L and Rosling M (2003). Pneumonia causes panic in Guangdong province, British Medical Journal, February 22; 326(7386): 416.

Roy CJ and Milton DK (2004). Airborne transmission of communicable infection--the elusive pathway, New England Journal of Medicine, 350:1710-1712.

Salunkhe DK (1961). Gamma radiation effects on fruits and vegetables, Economic Botany, 15(1):28-56.

Sobkoa T et. Al. (2005). Gastrointestinal bacteria generate nitric oxide from nitrate and nitrite, Nitric Oxide, 13(4):272-278.

Spath PL, Mann MK and Kerr DR (1999). Life Cycle Analysis of Coal-Fired Power Production, National Renewable Energy Laboratory, A U.S. Department of Commerce publication.

Stamatelos GM and Falconer DD (1996). Millimeter radio access to multimedia services via LMDS, Proc. IEEE Globecom Conf., London U.K., pp. 1603-1607.

Tho QT, Hui SC and Fong ACM (2006). Automatic fuzzy ontology generation for semantic Web, IEEE Transactions on Knowledge and Data Engineering; 18(6):842-856.

Varshney U (2002). Multicast over wireless networks, Communications of the ACM, 45(12):31-37.

Veenema TG and Andrew KP (2003). Radiation: Clinical responses to radiologic incidents and emergencies, American Journal of Nursing, 103(5):32-40.

Wong SSY and Yuen KY (2006). Avian influenza virus infections in humans, Chest, 129(1):156-168.

Woo PCY, Lau SKP and Yuen KY (2006). Infectious diseases emerging from Chinese wet-markets: zoonotic origins of severe respiratory viral infections, Current Opinion in Infectious Diseases, 19(5):401-407.

Zhang J and Ansari N (2009). On Minimizing the AWG Cost and the Optical Cable Cost in Deploying WDM PONs, IEEE/OSA Journal of Optical Communications and Networking, 1(5):352-365.

Zhang Y et. Al. (1995). Worldwide On-Road Vehicle Exhaust Emissions Study by Remote Sensing, Environmental Science and Technology, 29(9):2286-2294.

10

Epidemiology and Prevention of Traffic Accidents in Cuba

Humberto Guanche Garcell and Carlos Martinez Quesada
University Hospital Joaquín Albarrán, La Habana, Cuba

1. Introduction

At the beginning of the XX century, Cuba's economy was not diversified or developed. The main source of income was sugar cane production, a technology which, seen from nowadays, could be considered almost artisanal. It involved an ox-driven mill which squeezed the juice out of the cane, first step in order to obtain sugar.

We must tie the development of the sugar cane, rum and the tobacco industries to the progressive increment of the number of vehicles, as they were also instrumental to that development. The first automobile that circulated in our country made it for the Havana streets in 1898, and it is said that the first accident reported in Cuba was in 1906, in which a pedestrian was implied. That brought along the fact that car accidents began to be considered the eighth cause of death in 1958, from being almost nonexistent (Dirección Nacional de Registros Médicos y Estadísticas de Salud [DNE], 2011).

CAUSES OF DEATH	Deaths	
	No.	rate
Cardiovascular	9 996	147,8
Malignant Tumor	5 327	78,8
Gastritis, enteritis, duodenitis and colitis	2 784	41,2
Newborn related diseases	2 302	34,0
Vascular lesions affecting the Central Nervous System	2 245	33,2
Pneumonia and flu	1 943	28,7
War injuries	1 635	24,2
Accidents	1 266	18,7
Tuberculosis	1 076	15,9
Nephritis and nephrosis	984	14,5

Source: DNE, 2011.

Table 1. Deaths and mortality rate (by 100 000 inhabitants). Cuba 1958.

To the first clunker cars manufactured in North America, more vehicles were added predominantly from the United States, which in turn dictated the characteristics of the vehicle inventory. After 1959 vehicles coming from the extinct Soviet Union and others European countries were added to the stock. Starting 1990, there is an economical crisis the country must face against, resulting in important changes in the Cuban society, which in turn changed the way vehicles were employed due to fuel shortages. As an alternative transportation mean, bicycles are started to be used massively by the population to run their usual chores as well as to go to workplaces. At the same time animal-hauled vehicles, especially those using horses are starting to show up in cities throughout the country, less often in the nation's capital.

To remedy the shortcomings of the capital city's public transportation system, alternatives are sought as well, basically employing trucks and tractors without the required safety standards. Along this period, due to the same financial crisis which affected the public transportation system, the pavement of the city's thoroughfares began to deteriorate as well, along with the transit signals. All these factors increase the risks of car crashes and the injuries and casualties' toll.

Regarding the increased use of bicycles it should be stated that the modifications needed in the traffic system in order to protect bicycle riders -- as dedicated lanes or mandatory use of helmets -- were not immediately adopted.

However since the beginnings of the XXI century, the number of bicycles has dwindled significantly, which today circulates simultaneously to old built vehicles in North America in the fifties (e.g. Chevrolet, Chrisler), with others of European origin built in seventies (e.g. Lada, Moskvichs, Polski) and other more modern vehicles (e.g. Peugeot, Mercedes Benz, Toyota).

2. Incidence, mortality and economic impact of traffic accidents

Before 1970, there are recorded health statistics only from 1958. And they recorded all accidental fatalities together regardless the cause, although the vast majority comes from road traffic accidents (table 1).

According to official reports, there are 10,000 car accidents a year in Cuba (Graph 1). Most of them happen in Havana, followed in descending order by Santiago de Cuba and Holguin (Graph 2), which happens to be the more populated cities in the country with population of 2 147 539, 1 048 377 and 1 036 504 respectively (Oficina Nacional de Estadísticas [ONE], 2010; DNE, 2010).

Each year, injuries account for more than 1.3 million deaths globally, and more than 90 per cent of these deaths occurred in low and middles income countries. The Word Health Statistics 2008 Report predicts that road traffic injuries will be one of the most rapidly growing public health concerns over the next 25 years, primarily owing to increased motor vehicle ownership and use associated with economic growth in low and middle income countries (WHO, 2008). According to this report, in 2004 traffic accidents constituted the ninth cause of death of the world population. In 2030 it is expected that it would be the fifth cause of death, displacing infectious and tumor diseases, with countries with low-to-middle income rates having the bigger share (Peden et al., 2002; WHO, 2010).

In Cuba, from seventies of last century, accidents in general have constituted between the fourth and fifth cause of mortality, preceded by the cardiovascular disease, stroke, cancer and influenza and pneumonia. The traffic accidents together with the accidental falls constitute a fundamental cause of deaths for accidents. (DNE, 2010).

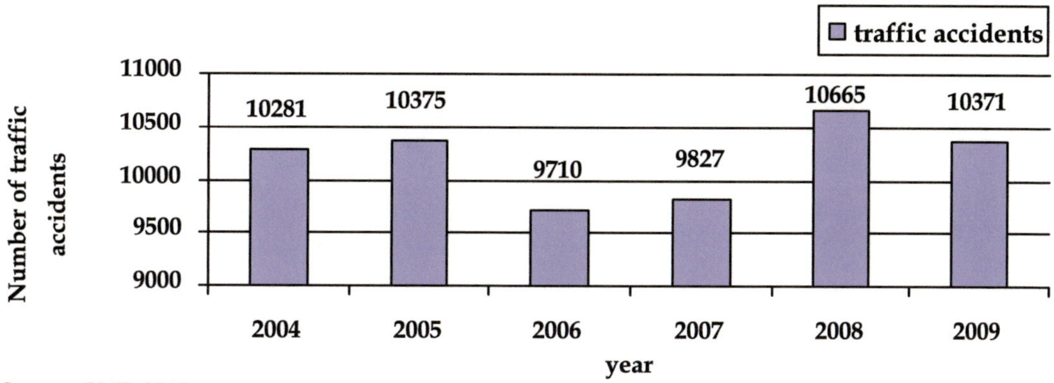

Source: ONE, 2010.

Fig. 1. Traffic accidents. Cuba 2004-2009

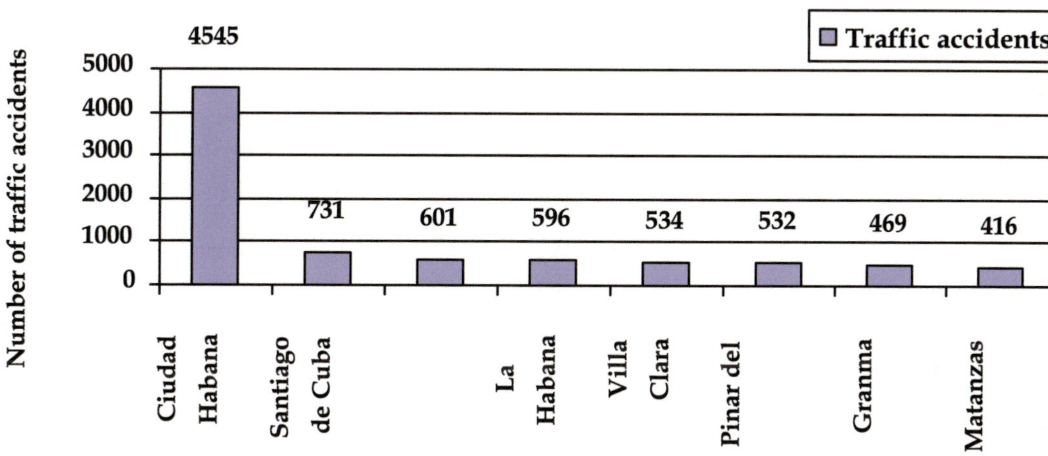

Source: ONE, 2010

Fig. 2. Traffic accidents in cuban counties (2009)

Traffic accidents mortality had an increasing trend in the 1970 to 1989 period as can be seen in fig.3, in which it soared up to 24.1 deaths by 100,000 habitants (Asamblea Nacional del Poder Popular, 1987; Ministerio de Salud Pública, 2010). Afterward it became evident its decrease down to 7.8 in 2008, which is related to changes in the national prevention strategy as it is reflected in the 60 Act, which includes:

1. Mandatory use of helmets in motorbikes.
2. Mandatory use of safety belts.
3. Increased measures to avoid driving under influence (DUI) of alcoholic beverages.
4. Strengthening of the medical emergency system, increasing the number of ambulances and skilled medical personnel.
5. Public education throughout the broadcasting of many factors concurring in traffic accidents.
6. Mandatory technical supervision of motor vehicles, especially those involved in the public transportation system (Ministerio del Transporte, 1999).

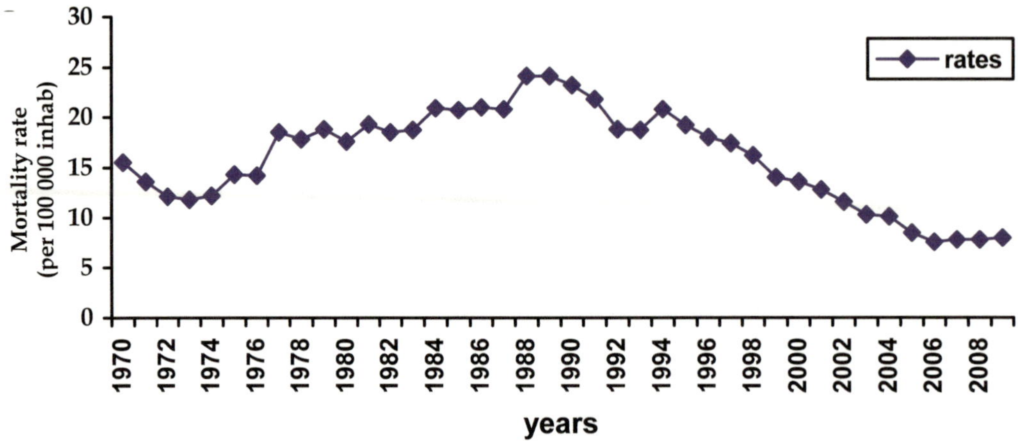

Source: Dirección Nacional de Registros Médicos y Estadísticas de Salud, 2010.

Fig. 3. Traffic accidents adjusted mortality rate (by 100 000 hab), Cuba, 1970 -2009.

An element strongly related to traffic accidents mortality's incidence, starting from the 90 decade, was the massive introduction of bicycles on the streets as a mean of transportation. This related with economic problems that reduced in an important way the use of vehicles that use fuel. Although the number of bicycles have since decreased significantly, in 2009 the bicycle related accidents accounted for the 6.5% of the traffic fatalities.

To the death casualties should be added, as an additional burden, the lesions and injuries, with figures that, as a whole, soar to a staggering 7000 a year. According to Graph 4 there is a dominance of male individuals at productive age (fig 4) (DNE 2010). In 2009 the accident mortality rate in Cuba was 14.5 by 100,000 habitants (male) and 3.4 by 100,000 habitants (female) (ONE, 2010). Similar outcome was observed at the Villa Clara Project, where 65% of fatalities and 70% of injuries were male individuals (Guanche, 2008).

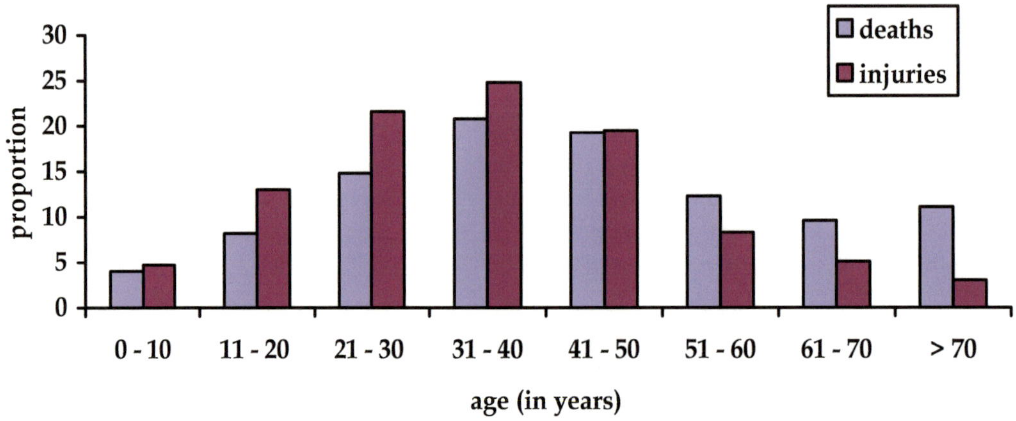

Source: ONE, 2010

Fig. 4. Proportional distribution of deaths and injuries in traffic accidents according age. Cuba 2009.

In national reports there is no evidence of the relative impact of the employment of bicycles as a mean of transportation in the traffic accident's mortality notwithstanding the primary role this vehicle had as such. In 2009 bicycle related accidents yielded the 6.5% of all fatalities (DNE, 2010). A study conducted in Cienfuegos, province located amid Island, the mortality rate related to bicycles was 6.44 by 100,000 habitants, mainly from the 15 - 44 age groups, males (Jorge et al., 2010). Vulnerability of bicycle-riders circulating in thoroughfares is a world class problem (WHO, 2004).

Traumatism due to traffic accidents occupied the ninth place in the 2009 worldwide as morbidity and lesions agents, considering their share in years of life potentially lost due to incapacity. It forecast for 2020 is the third place, getting the lion share countries among low-to-middle GDP (WHO 2009).

In Cuba, traffic accidents were the fourth cause of years of life potentially lost, behind cardiovascular diseases, stroke and cancer, which should be considered when it comes to evaluate its impact on society (DNE, 2010). According to evaluations in Villa Clara, in 2003, the years-of-life potentially lost rate was 11.58 by 1000 habitants, with males yielding 14.46 and females 8.35.

The impact of traffic accidents in healthcare system could be evaluated be means of use of emergency services for healthcare of injuries, admission in hospital and rehabilitation of patients to survive. Detailed information about this it is not included in the official statistics in Cuba and few published articles in national biomedical journal and in Infomed, the national medical web, refers to this topic. A descriptive study of patients admitted in the main rehabilitation center in Cuba, Hospital Julio Díaz, show that neurologic injured and amputated patient, as consequence of traffic accidents, are the major cause of admission, displacing other previous causes of disability as infectious diseases (Berbes VL, no date).

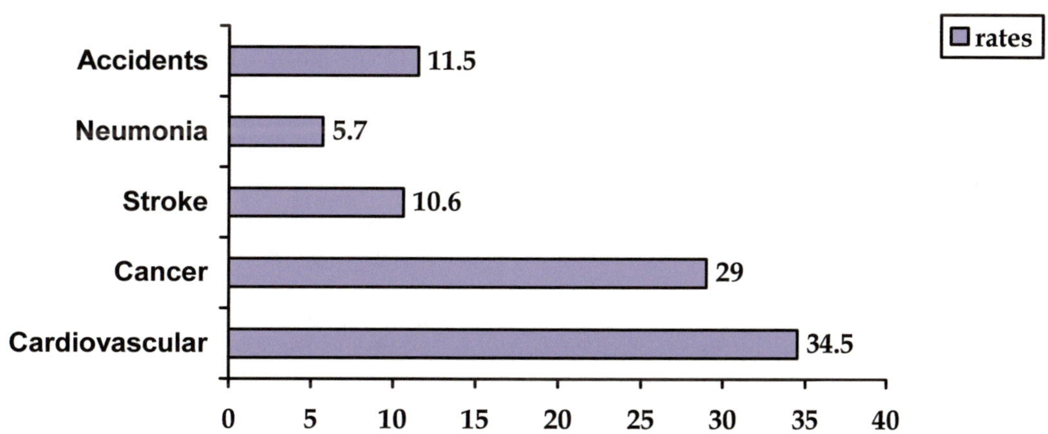

Source: DNE, 2010

Fig. 5. Rates of potential life years lost (per 1000 habitants) according selectec causes of death. Cuba 2009.

Studies dealing with the economic impact of traffic accidents are scarce in Cuban literature, and the existing ones do not analyze the problem integrally, as they do not account the direct and indirect costs involved, as should be considered medical assistance and rehabilitation. Main biomedical publications deal fundamentally with clinical aspects, centering on the description of injuries (Scielo Cuba, 2011). A study in the province of Villa Clara which is one with a high incidence of traffic accidents, first semester of 2009, described the use of hospital services by traffic injuries patient (Guanche, 2008). About 25% of patients were admitted to critical care units, 30% underwent major surgery and 31.3% were prescribed antibiotics. Rough estimates using the abovementioned information give that traffic accidents in Cuba account for some 50 million pesos a year.

According to the National Statistic Office (ONE, 2010), damages caused by traffic accidents to public or private property amounted to 5 978,2 million of pesos in 2008 and 4 390,4 million of pesos in 2009. The global economic loses due to road traffic injuries are estimated to be US$ 518 billion with a particular impact in low and middle income countries (WHO, 2009).

3. Risk factors of traffic accidents

An integral vision of risk factors for traffic accidents and its consequences should consider those related with the man (drivers or pedestrian), the vehicle and the roads (WHO, 2009). Classically it has been postulated that an important proportion of the risk is contributed by the man, basically drivers, with smaller participation of other factors. Researchers have indicated that only one of them is the cause of each traffic accident, although it would be necessary to consider the influence of several factors in their genesis.

Among more importance factors they are those related with technical deficiencies of vehicles (for example, controls, tires, suspension), atmospheric factors (darkness, fog, rain, hail, snow, ice, others), the design and conservation of roads, but it is the human factor the one that explains most of the accidentality.

In Cuba most of companies vehicles are government's property, about which the information that we present information in Tabla 2 (ONE, 2010). Bus and passengers transported in these they possess very similar values in the period 2004 - 2007, with an increment in the years 2008 and 2009. Bus constitutes the main way of the population's transport as much in the cities as in rural areas, in which is reflected an important variability of makers and years of construction, modern (Ej. Yuton, China) and old (Girón, built in Cuba with Soviet Union components), being able to observe in the roads of the Havana a Leylan Bus built in the United Kingdom in the seventies. In a similar way it happens to the trucks and taxis.

The technological variability of vehicles determines the frequent observation of vehicles without good conditions for its roads circulations, in relation to the natural deterioration of its components, the difficulties of purchase replacement pieces adapted for their repair, with the frequent adaptation of components of other classes of vehicles to maintain their operation (fig 6).

In rural areas is more frequent to observe the massive transportation of passengers in trucks or in vehicles of animal traction, where it is equally more frequent the use of bicycles as a fundamental way of population's and goods transport, example agricultural products and little animals. In the Cuban cities, including the capital of the country, the bicycles are used as rent vehicles, calls in Castilian "bicitaxis", being able to be used in the transport of goods for small business.

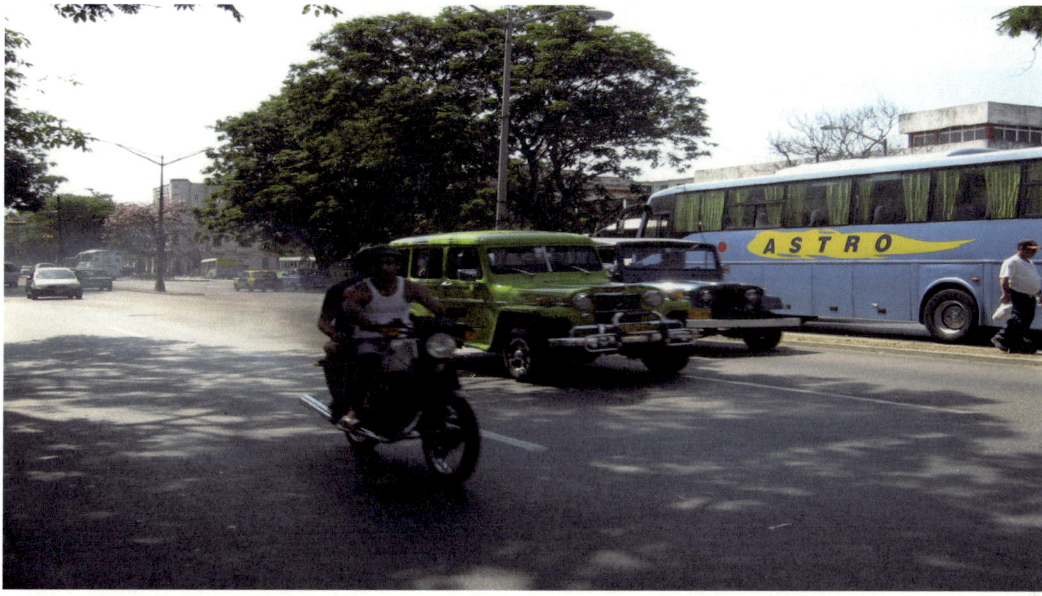

Fig. 6. Antique and modern vehicles in urban roads and risk of accidents

variables	2004	2005	2006	2007	2008	2009
Goverment vehicles						
Ómnibus	11.491	10.561	11.319	10.460	11.979	12.194
Taxi	3.306	3.544	4.280	4.243	4.310	3.015
Trucks	12.510	15.014	11.658	11.893	10.249	11.326
Passenger transported (million of passenger)						
Ómnibus	647,5	679,5	697,9	755,6	898,1	922,6
Taxi	40,4	41,3	40,2	43,7	45,6	46,7

Source: ONE, 2010

Table 2. Government vehicles and passengers transported. Cuba 2004 - 2009.

Related with quality of road infrastructure, was evident an important deterioration in the nineties, that included physical damage of roads and deficiencies in signalings (horizontal and vertical). The construction activities and maintenance of roads net is responsibility of state entities. Recently, in correspondence with the economic recovery, a program of improvement of roads has been developed, included the construction of asphalt factories and solutions to signaling deficiencies (Salgado, 2010).

Is important consider that in national road infrastructure they are few alternatives to protect pedestrians, elevated bridges for traffic of vehicles in the cities and others, partly determined by financial possibilities for their implementation. Also, the employment of exclusive roads for the circulation of bicycles that was used during the nineties, has decreased in a significant way, although its circulations continues in urban and rural roads, which increased vulnerability to occurrence of traffic accidents. WHO Report of Road Safety (WHO, 2009) define as vulnerable road user to pedestrians, cyclist and user of motorized of two wheelers.

According to National Highway Traffic Safety Administration (USA), the human factor is implied between the 71 and 93% of the cases, the roads factors 12 and 34%, and those related to vehicles between the 4,5 and 13% (NHTSA, 2010).

At the present time they are recognized a series of risk factors of the driver that affect capacity to drive motor vehicles. Among these they are diseases or conditions that can affect the conscience, for example myiocardial infaction and other acute coronary syndromes, high blood pressure, cerebrovascular disease, rupture of the aorta, vasovagal syncope, epilepsy and hypoglycemia. Also known the transitory influences of alcohol, certain medications, the drugs and the fatigue. Other factors are related with the training level and style in driving, the knowledge and fulfillment of regulations and laws, psychophysical condictions (sensorial, physical and mental), the disposition to act (attitudes and motivation) and the efficiency, capacity, know-how, psycomotor coordination , and skills to overcome situations during driving.

Among man related factors, we wish highlighting the existence of diseases and psycophysical, as well as the effect of alcohol and drugs (legal or not) that can interfere in driving capacity. Non communicable diseases or chronic conditions as diabetes mellitus, hypertension and ischaemic hearth diseases, bronchial asthma, chronic obstructive pulmonary disease and stroke are frequent in Cuban population (DNE, 2010).

Diabetes mellitus is estimate to be affects 8% of Cuban population's , alone 50% has been diagnosed, and constitutes the eighth cause of death (Dominguez, 2008). In relation with accident risks depends on the effect of the variability glycaemia in neurological system, including the increased risk of hypoglicemya, conditioned by antidiabetic drugs and non adherence to the treatment. Also it should be considered the adverse effects of retinopathy in visual acuity, neuropathy in sensibility and strength in extremities, and mascrovascular complications and the risk of cerebral or heart ischaemia (Ministerio del Interior, 2004).

High blood pressure affects 30% of Cuban population, more frequent in adults, and is associated to the incidence and mortality of iscahemic hearth disease and cerebrovascular diseases, which constitute the first and third cause of the Cuban population's death (DNE, 2010; Buergo, 2008). The possibilities of ischaemic symtoms and signs n this diseases and its effect on the level of conscience and the degree of attention constitute elements compactly associated with risk of accidents (Ministry of the Interior, 2004).

Also cancer, that constitutes the second cause of the population's death, has demonstrated growing incidence in the last decades, in correspondence with the world tendencies (DNE, 2010). Its relationship with risk accidents associated with this health problems, not depends alone of the own clinical manifestations but of the effects of the treatments. Should be considered the increment of its survival of current therapeutic resources. (Ministry of the Interior, 2004).

It is estimate that 2,5 million people die worldwide from harmful use of alcohol a year standing out deaths related with traffic accidents (WHO, 2011). Numerous studied carried out have been demonstrated the important paper of alcohol in traffic accidents. In this investigations it has been evidenced that accidents related with alcohol, are of more prejudicial results, what increases the risk of suffering mortal lesions, partly to the reduction of answer to trauma, besides other circumstances that surround him (Hingson, 2003). According to studies carried out in USA, of the population of drivers 32% are abstemious, 45% moderate social drinkers, and 23% strong social drinkers, frequent drinkers or alcoholic (Korelitz, 1993). In Cuba it has been considered that at least 5% of the population's with more than 15 years old are alcoholic (abuse or alcoholic dependence), not including in these those with non advisable consumption patterns (Gonzalez, 2008).

The main studies on drink and driving in Cuba were carried out between 2001 and 2006, which were published by our team in national biomedical journals (Scielo Cuba,2011) and in Gaceta Sanitaria (Gaceta Sanitaria, Elsevier, 2005 - 2008). We demonstrate that drinking and driving constitutes an important and frequent risk factor for traffic accidents, wich is underestimate in official statistics. In these the main violations are not assist the vehicles control and not respect the right of road circulation identified in 29% of accidents, while alone in 3% of drivers was found under the effect (ONE, 2010). The results above mentioned related with the systems and procedures of detection of drivers under the effect of alcohol.

For decades they are known in Cuba the equipment for mensuration of alcohol in exhaled air, initially equipment of qualitative mensuration as knows as ¨globitos¨, and in recent years more modern have been used that allow to quantify the amount of alcohol present in exhaled air. However the use of these technologies has been for short periods, given its low readiness, not existing in our country a methodology of surveillance of drivers under the effect of alcohol, and still to certify if a driver ingested alcohol the testimonial of a doctor is demanded, by means of a legal written document (Ministerio de Salud Pública, no date).

An important proportion of population drive vehicles take medications, some of which can alter driving capacity. Important to mention between this drugs those that generate bigger risk like those used for treatment of psiquiatric disorders, hypoglicemians, antiallergic with depressor effects in central nervous system. Due to it is essential that healhtcare professionals know the effects of drugs commonly used and its effects in driving capacity and they can make recommendations to diminish the risk of occurrence of traffic accidents.

In Cuba the illicit drugs are little consumed, being those most used marijuana and cocaine. Their deleterious influence is known in conduction capacity by its effects on central nervous system. (Ministry of the Interior, 2004). Equally it should be considered the mixture of medications with alcohol, especially in young population, which produces stimulating or depressors effects in central nervous system.

4. National prevention program and activities for prevention of traffic accidents

Traffic accidents prevention activities constitutes a world priority, with special focus in those countries where they constitute fundamental cause of morbilidity and mortality, and produce an important economic impact. Many have been strategies applied in prevention activities, that in general pretend to act on their potential causes: man, roads and vehicles (OMS, 2004), that includes activities for the prevention of accidents and its consequences.

In 1987 the Law 60, Code of Traffic, was approved (Asamblea Nacional del Poder Popular, 1987) that established the main regulations related with the prevention of traffic accidents. This law was modified in 2010 by means of the Law 109, which introduced as novel elements the definition of *beginner driver's* to refers to those with less than two years experiences in driving, and of *pedestrian with disability* to refers to those with any type of disability (motor, visual, other), also valuable modifications focus on risk controls like drinking and driving, use of drugs or substances that alter capacity to drive, the employment of cycles or animal traction vehicles, the massive transportation of passengers, passengers' of vehicles procedures and pedestrians. It highlights the recommendations for the technical revision of the vehicles and for population education in this topic.

Next we will comment important aspects included national strategic plan for traffic accidents prevention.

1. Drinking and driving (article No. 93 and 95 of Law 60)
    a. Professional drivers cannot drive under the effect of alcohol. Similar restrictions should fulfil the beginner drivers and applicants during the period of learning, elements of new introduction in the law.
    b. In non professional drivers are accepted a low level of alcohol as permissible. This level are not defined in the law, assigning to the Ministry of Public Health the responsibility of determining the levels of concentration of alcohol in blood, exhaled air or in other corporal fluids incompatible with driving.
    c. Also, constitutes a novel element in law, the prohibition of ingestion of alcoholic drinks inside vehicles or their transportation in the compartments dedicated to the driver and the passengers
2. Regulations about the circulation of cycles (article 112). Prohibits the conduction of cycles to individuals smaller than 12 years old, not being clearly defined the obligatory use of the protective helmet for their drivers.
3. For massive transportation of people (article 135). Consider the frequent use of massive transportation of people in load vehicles (ex. Trucks) is established that these they should circulate to inferior speeds with security conditions for the passengers.
4. Technical vehicles revision (article 211). The technical revision of vehicles using specialized equipment is carried out by Ministry of Transport as a requirement for determination of state of security systems and other excellent aspects as emission of combustion gases. Bigger emphasis must be attributes to vehicles dedicated to passenger's transport or those driven by professionals, which should carry out revision every two years.
5. Education related to prevention of traffic accidents.
    a. The education and promotion program constitute an essential component in the preventive strategies, being reflected in the articles 239 - 248 of the Law 109.
    b. Prevention program focus in children and adolescents includes the use of massive means of diffusion (television, radio, newspapers) and scholars programs address to the population's sensitization about the topic , offering information on risk factors, consequences and accidents prevention (Comisión Nacional de Prevención de Accidentes, 2010).
    c. Related with the conduction under the effect of alcohol. National promotion programs have demonstrated to be very effective for the confrontation of other health problems, measures have been applied as: control of prices of beverages containing alcohol, actions on localization, schedules of opening and density of places of distribution of drinks, control of the social readiness, community education in general and to drivers.
6. School for drivers. These entities are made responsible of preparing the applicants to driver's licenses, and the training of professional drivers, as well as of promoting preventive strategies in the population.
7. Animal traction vehicles (fig 7). Drivers of vehicles of animal traction should have more than 16 years old, and these they won't be able to traffic for roads of quick circulation (e.g. Freeways), neither in night hours. They will also possess measures of security for its restrain.

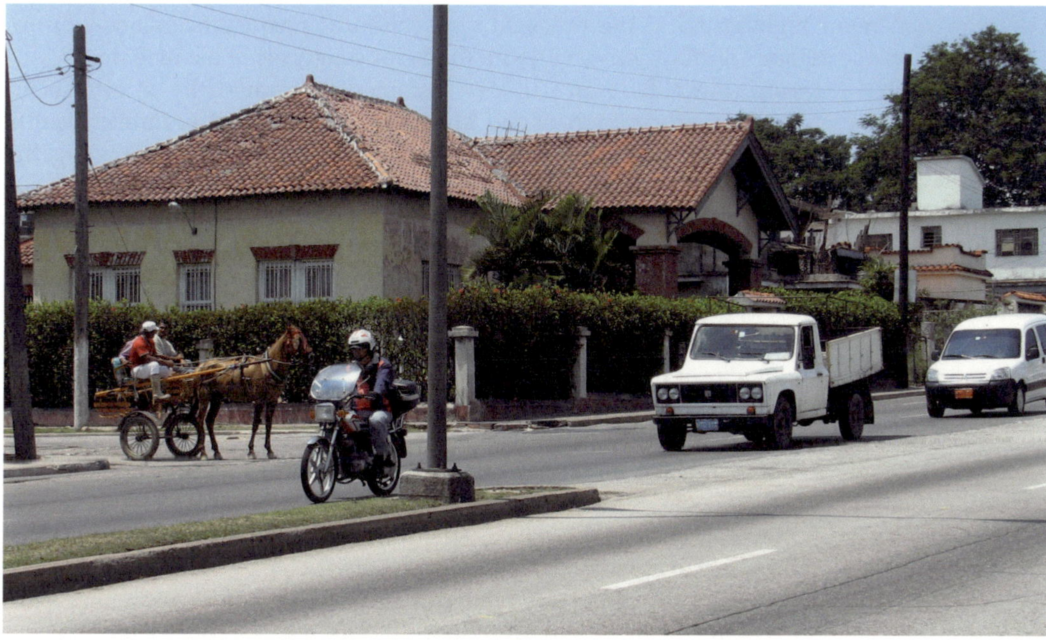

Fig. 7. Vehicles of animal traction in urban roads

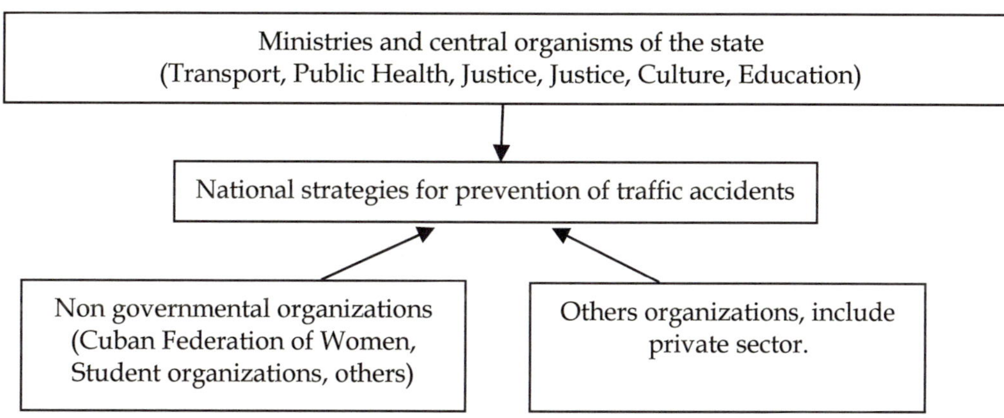

Fig. 8. Intersector system in prevention of traffic accidents in Cuba.

8. Medical evaluation of drivers (Ministerio de Salud Pública, no date)
   a. The current methodology for medical exams of drivers, edited by the Ministry of Public Health possesses more than two decades of having approved.
   b. The medical exams to obtain or renovate the conduction license in carried out in communitarian healthcare services by a team of professionals that included general practitioner, specialists in ophthalmology, psychology and others.
   c. Considering current knowledge on this topic is evident, that this methodology has several limitations due that includes health problem that at the moment are not considered that interfere with driving capacity, example hiperinsulinism, renal disease, epilepsy. Equally they are not defined differences in the requirements to drive vehicles for professional and non professional's drivers.

d. An element highlighted in the practical application of medical exams constitutes the non systematic application of valid methods for diagnosis of alcoholism.

9. The national program of accidents in Cuba is sustained fundamentally in intersector actions by means of the participation of the Ministries of the Interior, Public Health, Transport, Culture and other non government organization and state organisms (fig. 8).

5. Future research and development activities

1. Precise information about this health problem, obtained by means of scientific research and analysis of information, is essential to define the priorities of these problems for their prevention and control. (Borse & Hyder, 2009). Still when is included in the strategies and national programs of prevention, research published on the topic in biomedical journals, included peer review journals, could be considered insufficient. Also, like we mention previously, they approach clinical aspects related with those injured during traffic accidents, while investigations focused to identification of risks and to demonstrate the effectiveness of prevention practices were scarce.
2. Methodology of medical evaluation of drivers. It is required a revision of this methodology and bring up to date in correspondence with the new evidences.
3. Prevention and control of traffic accidents related with drinking and driving. Since this constitutes a relevance factor related with accidents and its severity, bigger emphasis is required in its control by means of the application of procedures that have demonstrated its effectiveness (e.g. Sobriety Checkpoint) (Shults RA, 2001)
4. Strengthen the intersector actions directed in a national strategic plan for prevention of traffic accidents.

6. Conclusion

Still when traffic accidents have had in Cuba a tendency to decrease in recent years, they continue being a major health problem when constituting the fourth cause of years of potential life lost, besides an impact in healthcare in relation to the attention of those injured and the disabilities, that which additionally generates important economic lost for society. Evident potentialities exist for the prevention of traffic accidents, superior to the main causes of Cuban population's death, that which can be achieved by means of the consolidation of prevention program prevention with the introduction of more recent evidence about this topic.

7. Acknowledgment

I would like to acknowledge to the Engineer Tomás Suárez Enriquez by their teaching and dedication to road traffic prevention activities. Dr. Francisco Gutierrez García and RN Rosa Peña Sandoval for their cooperation in research during the conduction of Villa Clara project. Lic. Adolfo Gomez Calá for their assistance in translation and correction of this paper.

8. References

Asamblea Nacional del Poder Popular (2010). Ley No. 109 Código de Seguridad Vial. *Gaceta Oficial de la República de Cuba. Edición Ordinaria* , No. 40, (17 de septiembre de 2010), ISSN 1682-7511.

Asamblea Nacional del Poder Popular (1987) .Ley 60. Código de vialidad y transito. *Gaceta Oficial de la República de Cuba. Edición Especial*, Miércoles 21 de noviembre de 1987, ISSN 0864-0792.

Berbes VL, Villanueva MM & Martínez SH (no date). *Accidentes del tránsito y discapacidad*. Disponible en http://www.sld.cu/print.php?idv=6267.

Borse, NN & Hyder, AA (2009). Call for more research on injury from the developing world: results of a bibliometric analysis. *Indian Journal Medical Research*, No. 129, 321 - 326, ISSN 0971-5916.

Buergo Zuaznábar MA, Fernández Concepción O, Coutín Marre G & Torres Vidal RM (2008). Epidemiology of Cerebrovascular Diseases in Cuba, 1970 to 2006. *MEDICC Review*, Vol 10, No 2, (Spring 2008) 33 - 38, ISSN 1527-3172.

Comisión Nacional de Prevención de Accidentes (2010). *Programa para la prevención de los accidentes en menores de 20 años*. Disponible en http://www.sld.cu/galerias/doc/sitios/puericultura/programa_para_la_prevencion__(rev_)de_los_accidentes_en_menores_de_20_anos.doc.

Dirección Nacional de Registros Médicos y Estadísticas de Salud (2011). Principales causas de mortalidad en Cuba (1958). Ministerio de Salud Pública, República de Cuba.

Dirección Nacional de Registros Médicos y Estadísticas de Salud (2010). *Anuario estadístico de salud 2009*. Ministerio de Salud Pública. República de Cuba. Available from http://files.sld.cu/dne/files/2010/04/anuario-2009e3.pdf.

Domínguez Alonso Emma, Seuc Jo Armando H, Díaz Díaz Oscar, Aldana Padilla Deysi (2008).La carga de la diabetes en Cuba, período 1990-2005.. Revista Cubana Endocrinol, Vol.19, No.2, (agosto), ISSN 1561-2953

González Menéndez, Ricardo (2008). Atención integral al alcoholismo. La atención integral al alcoholismo: experiencia cubana. *Rev Cubana Medicina*, Vol. 47, No. 2, (junio). Disponible en http://scielo.sld.cu/pdf/med/v47n2/med12208.pdf, ISSN 0034-7523.

Guanche Garcell Humberto, Martínez Quesada Carlos, Peña Sandoval Rosa, Gutiérrez García Francisco, González López José & Sánchez Villalobo Jesús (2008). Hospitalizaciones por accidentes de tráfico en Villa Clara (enero a junio de 2003). *Revista Cubana Cirugía*, Vol. 47, No. 3, (diciembre). Disponible en: http://scielo.sld.cu/scielo.php?script=sci_arttext&pid=S0034-74932008000300007&lng=es, ISSN 0034-7493.

Guanche Garcell H, Suárez Enríquez T, Gutiérrez García F, Martínez Quesada C, Peña Sandoval R & Sánchez Villalobos J (2008). Impact of a drink-driving detection program to prevent traffic accidents (Villa Clara Province, Cuba). *Gaceta Sanitaria* ; Vol. 22, No. 4, (Jul - Aug), pp. 344-7, ISSN 0213-9111.

Hingson R & Winter M (2003). Epidemiology and consequences of drinking and driving. *Alcohol Research Health, Vol* 27, No. 1, pp. 63-78, Available from http://pubs.niaaa.nih.gov/publications/arh27-1/63-78.pdf, ISSN 1535-7414.

Jorge Miguez Angela, Godoy del Sol Haray & Ortis Sagasta Mavis (2010). Caracterización de la mortalidad por accidentes del tránsito con participación de ciclos: un problema sociomédico. *MediSur*, vol 8, No 4, (agosto), 57-62. Disponible en: http://scielo.sld.cu/scielo.php?script=sci_arttext&pid=S1727-897X2010000400009&lng=es, ISSN 1727-897X.

Korelitz JJ, Fernandez AA, Uyeda VJ, Spivey GH, Browdy BL & Schmidt RT (1993). Health habits and risk factors among truck drivers visiting a health booth curing a trucker trade show. *American Journal Health Promotion* , Vol. 8, No. 2 , (Nov-Dec) , pp. 117-123, ISSN 0890-1171.

Ministerio del Interior (2004). *Manual sobre aspectos médicos relacionados con la ccapacidad de conducción de vehículos. Segunda Edición*. Ediciones Doyma, S.L., ISBN 84 7592 724 6, Barcelona, España,.

Ministerio de Salud Pública (2006). *Guía cubana para la prevención, diagnóstico y tratamiento de la hipertensión arterial, 2006*. Disponible en: http://www.sld.cu/servicios/hta/temas.php?idv=1765.

Ministerio de Salud Pública (2010). *Series del tiempo de mortalidad. Cuba 2007 2008*. Disponible en: http://files.sld.cu/dne/files/2010/10/series-tipificadas-de-mortalidad-2008.pdf.

Ministerio de Salud Pública (no date). *Metodología vigente para examen médico preventivo, periódico y a solicitud de las autoridades a conductores de vehículos a motor*. República de Cuba.

Ministerio del transporte (1999). Resolución 137 - 99 Revisión técnica de los vehículos a motor. *Gaceta Oficial de la República de Cuba Edición Ordinaria* No. 21, 13 de abril de 1999, ISSN 1682-7511.

National Highway Traffic Safety Administration (NHTSA) (2010). *Driving safety*. Available from: http://www.nhtsa.gov/Driving+Safety.

Organización Mundial de la Salud (2004). *Informe Mundial sobre prevención de los traumatismos causados por el transito: resumen*. Organización Mundial de la salud, ISBN 92 4 359131 2, Ginebra, Suiza,.

Oficina Nacional de Estadística (2010). *Accidentes de tránsito en cifras. Cuba 2009. Edición Julio 2010*. Oficina Nacional de Estadísticas de la República de Cuba. Disponible en: http://www.one.cu/aec2009/esp/23_tabla_cuadro.htm

Oficina Nacional de Estadística (2010). *Anuario Estadístico de Cuba. Transporte*. Oficina Nacional de Estadísticas de la República de Cuba. Disponible en: http://www.one.cu/aec2009/esp/13_tabla_cuadro.htm.

Paez Rodriguez D (2009). *Estudio de los accidentes de tráfico en Ciudad de la Habana 2006*. Disponible en: http://www.mappinginteractivo.com/plantilla-ante.asp?id_ articulo=1606.

Peden M, McGee K & Sharma G (2002). *The injury chart book: a graphical overview of the global burden of injuries,* World Health Organization; ISBN 92 4 156220 X, Geneva.

Salgado Martinez S (2010). *Reparan calles capitalinas*. Diario Granma, La Habana, lunes 19 de julio de 2010. Año 14 / Número 201, Avalilable from: http://www.granma.cubaweb.cu/2010/07/19/nacional/artic19.html.

Shults RA, Elder RW, Sleet DA, Nichols JL, Alao MO, Carande Kulis VG, et al, an the Task Force on Community Preventive Services (2001). Reviews of evidence regarding interventions to reduce alcohol-impaired driving. *American Journal Preventive Medicine,* Vol 21, No. 4S, pp. 66-84, ISSN 0749 3797.

Scielo Cuba (2011). *Published articles on traffic accidents in Cuba*. Available from http://scielo.sld.cu/cgi-bin/wxis.exe/iah/

World Health Organization (2009). *10 facts on global road safety*. Available from http://www.who.int/features/factfiles/roadsafety/en/

World Health Organization, (2009). *Global status report on road safety: time for action*. Geneva, World Health Organization. Available from. www.who.int/violence_injury_prevention/road_safety_status/2009

World Health Organization (2010). World Health Statistics, 2010. Available from http://www.who.int/whosis/whostat/ES_WHS10_Full.pdf, ISBN 978 92 4 156398 7.

World Health Organization (2011). Data and statistics. Available from http://www.who.int/research/en/.

Part 2

Disease Management

11

Health Infrastructure Inequality and Rural-Urban Utilization of Orthodox and Traditional Medicines in Farming Households: A Case Study of Ekiti State, Nigeria

Taiwo Ejiola Mafimisebi and Adegboyega Eyitayo Oguntade
The Federal University of Technology, Akure
Nigeria

1. Introduction

1.1 Background

Poverty is a pervasive problem in Africa and especially in Nigeria (World Bank, 2008). About 50.3% of the population of Sub-saharan Africa is reported to be living below the International Poverty Line of US$1.25 (UN, 2008). In Nigeria, about 55% of the population is living below the poverty line (World Bank, 2008). There is a geographical and sectoral dimension to the poverty situation in Nigeria. Poverty in Nigeria is more intense in the rural areas than the urban areas (Aigbokhan, 2000; Aigbokhan, 2008). Majority of Nigerians living in the rural areas are engaged either directly or indirectly in agriculture (NBS, 2006) and these are the people who are mostly trapped in poverty.

To develop appropriate policies to address poverty, there is a need for proper measurement of poverty. The use of money metric measures in indicating the level of poverty is gradually yielding place to other indicators of welfare which include deprivations in health, educational attainment, enjoyment of citizenship rights, social participation, life expectancy at birth and; maternal and child mortalities, among others (Okunmadewa, 1999; Srinivasan, 2001; Anderson, 2010). Among these indicators, health status and access to health facilities are keys to lifting people out of poverty or preventing them from falling into it (Republic of Sierra Leone, 2008). This is probably the reason while these health-related indicators are weighted heavily in the computation of the Human Development Index which is used for ranking countries in respect of welfare status (Herero *et al.* 2010).

Inadequate access to health services is one of the components of rural poverty which is prevalent in Nigeria (NBS, 2006). Inadequate access to health services determines, to a large extent, the decision of rural households to either patronize orthodox medicine (OM) or traditional medicine (TM) (Mafimisebi & Oguntade, 2010).

1.2 Justification for and focus of the study

Inadequate access to health services is a major issue confronting the poor in Nigeria. The Nigeria Core welfare Indicator study (NBS, 2006) revealed that 55.1% of Nigerians have access to OM health facilities while 7.5% consulted traditional healers in the four weeks preceding the survey. Obviously, Nigerians use both OM and TM for the maintenance of their health. In deciding which of these to use, access, in terms of availability and affordability, plays a significant role (Mafimisebi & Oguntade, 2010). Public policy affects both availability and affordability of OM services whereas for TM, availability and affordability are affected by the location of the prospective users (Mafimisebi & Oguntade, 2010). To this extent, the distribution of OM facilities requires public policy attention to ensure equitable access in terms of availability and affordability such that the decision to use either OM or TM will depend on users' preference. Given that affordability is a more critical factor in the rural and agriculture dependent areas because of higher level of poverty, public policy attention needs to be focused on access to OM services in the rural areas (Mafimisebi & Oguntade, 2010).

This study assesses the distribution of OM health infrastructure in Ekiti State, Nigeria, focusing on the rural-urban dichotomy that is prevalent in the establishment of OM health infrastructure in most states of Nigeria (NBS, 2007). It further looks at the use of OM and TM among farming households with special emphasis on the rural-urban dichotomy.

1.3 Approach to the study

This study was carried out in Ekiti State, Nigeria. It is one of the six states in South-west Nigeria and it has 16 Local Government Areas (LGAs). It is located between longitude 4° 45′ to 5° 45′ East of the Greenwich Meridian and latitudes 7° 15′ - 8° 5′ North of the Equator. Based on 2006 census, the state has a total population of 2,384,212 (National Bureau of Statistics (NBS), 2010). Ekiti State is largely agrarian (NBS, 2006) and hence it is typical of most states in Nigeria. The state was selected for this study because it is one of the states in the catchment area of the Federal University of Technology, Akure, the institutional base of the authors of this paper.

In this study, secondary data were used to assess the distribution of OM infrastructure. These data, which comprise the names and addresses, Local Government Area (LGA), ownership status and legal status of all orthodox health institutions in Ekiti State, were collected from the State Ministry of Health. The data were compared with similar data that were accessed from the NBS (NBS, 2007). In addition, the population figures by LGAs were also accessed from NBS (NBS, 2010) while the land areas of the LGAs were collected from the State Surveyor-General's office. For the assessment of rural-urban utilization of OM and TM, primary data were collected from farming households in two LGAs of Ekiti State, one of which is urban and the other rural. Two sets of primary data were collected; first, through the use of structured and pre-tested questionnaire administered on household heads and second, through focus group discussions (FGD) guided with a checklist of desired information. For the administration of the structured questionnaire, the multi-stage sampling method was used in selecting the respondents. In the first stage, Ado, an urban LGA , and Irepodun/Ifelodun, a rural LGA, were purposively selected. In the second stage, three communities in each LGA were randomly selected from the list of farming communities while in the third stage; twenty (20) households were systematically selected from the list of farming households in each community. This yielded a total of sixty (60) households each in the urban and rural LGAs. For the FGD, 206 other farmers participated. These FGD participants were not privileged to provide responses to the questionnaire and were not necessarily household heads.

The secondary data were analyzed through the use of Gini Coefficient and Index of Dissimilarity (ID) with a view to assessing the level of inequality in the distribution of health infrastructure in Ekiti State. To further assess the source of the inequality, both the number of persons and the land area per OM infrastructure, were analyzed focusing on the rural-urban dichotomy.

Gini Coefficient measures the degree of concentration (inequality) of a variable in a distribution of its elements. It compares the Lorenz Curve of a ranked empirical distribution with the line of perfect equality. The Gini Coefficient ranges from 0, where there is no concentration (perfect equality), to 1 where there is total concentration (perfect inequality). The ID is the summation of vertical deviations between the Lorenz Curve and the line of perfect equality. The closer the ID is to 1, the more dissimilar the distribution is to the line of perfect equality

The extent of inequality in the distribution of the health infrastructure was explored with the Gini Coefficient and the ID. The Gini Coefficient is calculated as:

$$G = 1 - \sum_{i=0}^{N} (\sigma Y_{i-1} + \sigma Y_i)(\sigma X_{i-1} - \sigma X_i)$$

Where

σX is cumulative proportions of the populations or land areas of the LGAs;

σY is the number of OM infrastructure in the LGAs; and

N is the number of LGAs.

The Index of Dissimilarity is calculated as:

$$ID = 0.5 \sum_{i=1}^{N} |X_i - Y_i|$$

Where,

X is the cumulative proportion of the populations or land areas of the LGAs,

Y is the cumulative proportion of the number of OM infrastructure in the LGAs; and,

N is the number of LGAs (Castillo-Salgado et.al., 2001; Dixon et.al., 1987; Rodrigue et.al., 2010).

For the primary data, qualitative description was used in presenting the result of the FGD. Descriptive statistics, which include frequencies and percentage, were used to describe the primary data on socio-economic and demographic characteristics of the respondents. The logistic regression was adopted in analyzing the influence of postulated independent variables on the probability of use of TM separately in the urban and in the rural locations. In using the logistic regression, we developed a dichotomous variable indicating whether the household uses TM more often than OM. This dichotomous variable is in this study called household's use of TM (HUTM). HUTM is 1 if a household uses TM more often and zero otherwise. The predictor variables are a set of socio-economic and demographic status indicators.

The estimating equation of the binary logit model is specified as follows:

$$Logit(p) = \ln(\frac{p}{1-p}) = \beta_0 + \beta_1 x_1 + \beta_2 x_2 + \cdots + \beta_7 x_7$$

p = probability that the household uses TM

x_1 = Age of household head (in years)

x_2 = Household size

x_3 = Sex of household head

x_4 = Household head's number of years of formal education

x_5 = Income from farm and non-farm sources (₦ per annum)

x_6 = Number of elderly people above 60 years in the household

x_7 = Religion (Christianity or Islam)

The equation is estimated by the maximum likelihood method because the procedure does not require the assumptions of normality or homoscedasticity of errors in predictor variable. The model was fitted separately for rural and urban households.

2. Health infrastructure inequality

2.1 Conceptual Issues on Health Infrastructure Inequality

According to WHO (1986), health is a state of complete physical, social and mental well-being, and not merely the absence of disease or infirmity. Health is considered a means to an end which can be expressed in functional terms as a resource which permits people to live an individually, socially and economically productive life. Health is also considered as a fundamental human right (WHO, 1986).

Health infrastructure (HI) has been seen from a number of perspectives. WHO (1998: 14) viewed HI as "those human and material resources, organizational and administrative structures, policies, regulations and incentives which facilitate an organized health promotion response to *public health* issues and challenges". Public Health Infrastructure (PHI), as defined by the Centers for Disease Control and Prevention (CDC) (2001), is the "underlying foundation that supports the planning, delivery and evaluation of all public health activities and practices". The three components of PHI identified by the CDC (2001) are workforce capacity and competency; information and data systems; and organizational capacity.

Turnock (2004) describes PHI as, "the systems, competencies, relationships and resources that enable performance of public health's core functions and essential services in every community." The conceptual framework for a public health system created by Handler *et al.* (2001) include structural capacity which is made up of information, organizational, physical, human and fiscal resources. In this paper, the focus is on the physical infrastructure component of HI. In Nigeria, physical infrastructure clearly indicates the presence of a HI. Most of the other components of HI are established around it.

According to WHO (1996), equity means fairness. Equity in health means that people's needs guide the distribution of opportunities for well-being. The WHO global strategy for achieving Health for All is fundamentally directed towards achieving greater equity in health between and within populations, and between countries. This implies that all people have an equal opportunity to develop and maintain their health, through fair and just access to resources for health. HI must therefore be equitably distributed in other to facilitate fair and just access to resources for health. HI is one of the socio-economic infrastructure that are considered critical for development in Nigeria. Others include education, water, electricity and transportation. The Nigeria Core Welfare Indicator study (NBS, 2006), measured Health access in terms of persons living in households with an OM health facility less than 30 minutes away. This clearly indicates the policy emphasis placed on the availability of physical HI in Nigeria.

The literature around health inequality is extensive. This literature touches on different aspects of health; HI distribution, status, access, outcomes, etc. HI distribution has been assessed from the perspective of inequality with the emphasis being on health inequality. Health inequalities can be defined as differences in health status or in the distribution of health determinants between different population groups (WHO, 2009). They are the result of 'a complex system operating at global, national and local levels which shapes the way society, at national and local level, organizes its affairs and embodies different forms of social position and hierarchy. The place people occupy on the social hierarchy affects their level of exposure to health-damaging factors, their vulnerability to ill health and the consequences of ill health (Marmot, 2009: 14). Health inequality refers to differences or variations in health-related quality of life and length of life profiles of different population groups in a nation (WHO, 2009).

The causes of urban health inequalities are associated primarily with socio-economic status, income, poverty, deprivation levels, unemployment, incapacity, worklessness, skills and educational level, housing conditions and social mobility as well as life chances (O'Brien *et.al.* 2010).

Inequality in health is not the same as inequity in health. Inequalities in health status between individuals and populations are inevitable consequences of genetic differences, of different social and economic conditions, or a result of personal lifestyles. Inequities occur as a consequence of differences in opportunity which result, for example in unequal access to health services, nutritious food, adequate housing and so on. In such cases, inequalities in health status arise as a consequence of inequities in opportunities in life (WHO, 1998). It should however be noted that public policy-induced inequality in HI and other socio-economic conditions will contribute to inequities in opportunities. According to Whitehead (1992), health inequities are 'differences in health which are not only unnecessary and avoidable but, in addition, are considered unfair and unjust'. This means that not all inequalities can be described as inequities. Whereas equality means sameness (equality of distributions), equity is *fairness* of distributions

Health status affects economic growth and sustainable development. There is evidence that investing in health brings substantial benefits to the economy (Anyanwu & Erhijakpor, 2007). According to WHO (2001), increasing life expectancy at birth by 10% will increase the economic growth rate by 0.35% a year. On the other hand, ill health is a heavy financial burden. About 50% of the growth differential between rich and poor countries is due to ill-health and life expectancy.

Harttgen & Misselhorn (2006) found that access to health infrastructure is important for child mortality which is one of the health outcomes covered by the MDGs. On the other hand, socio-economic factors, especially poverty, are often found to be strong determinants of health outcomes (Nolte & Mckee, 2004; Young, 2001; Leger, 2001). In most developing countries, health attainment indicators for the poor tend to be worse than the national average (Tandon, 2007). Also, the extent to which such health inequalities exist varies significantly across countries. Empirical evidence suggests that health inequalities have been persistent over time and, in many cases, have been growing (ADB, 2006). The rich can ignore government finance and health facilities; and access private sector health facilities on their own while the poor are more dependent on the public sector OM infrastructure and governments often do not have enough resources to expend on pro-poor health programmes and interventions (Tandon, 2007). Sachs (2004) has hence been calling for a scaling up of government health programmes in order to attain health-related MDGs.

2.2 Health Infrastructure Inequality and Health Policy in Nigeria

The MDGs had three out of eight goals directed at promoting health. These are reduction in child mortality, improvement in maternal health and combating HIV/AIDs, malaria and other diseases (UNDP, 2003). The first goal, which is the eradication of extreme poverty and hunger, is also indirectly related to health given the effect of poverty and hunger on the health status of individuals. This is an indication that the health sector requires significant public policy attention and commitment of resources. The governments of most states in South-west Nigeria, including Ekiti State, have laid emphasis over the years on free medical treatment, at least, for the vulnerable segment of the population (Ekiti State Planning Commission, 2004)) thus implying an alignment of public policy with the MGDs.

The National Health Accounts revealed that the bulk of health spending by Nigerians is on curative care, which utilizes 74% of the total healthcare. Preventive care is a distant second; this consumes only 1% of total healthcare in 2002. In some African countries, including Nigeria, government expenditure on health may have increased over the years but, it is still below the statutory recommendation (WHO 2001). WHO estimates that a minimum government expenditure of USD34 per person per year will be required to provide an essential package of public health interventions in order to achieve health related MDGs (WHO 2001). Nigeria is just striving to meet this target (NPC, 2004).

Nigeria's health policy which has identified primary healthcare as its fulcrum, defined a three tiered referral system for the management of patients. A network of primary healthcare centres in proximity to where people live, offering care of relatively low technology, is the first level of care from which patients gain entry into the healthcare system. Seriously ill patients beyond the management competence of primary healthcare workers are referred to secondary level general hospitals from where referrals are made to tertiary health facilities. The division of labour between the three complementary and easily recognizable levels seemed a rational, equitable and cost-effective way of dealing with the healthcare problems of the rural poor (Musa & Ejembi, 2004).

Health service management is decentralized at the three tier levels. In addition, some states have Health Management Board (HMB), which is responsible for direct service delivery while the Ministry of Health focuses on policy formulation, standard setting and; monitoring and evaluation. The private sector provides 65.7% of healthcare delivery in Nigeria. Efforts are on for increased public-private participation in healthcare delivery but there is yet to be a framework for collaboration (WHO, 2011). The underlying principles and values for the National Health Policy include: the principle of social justice and equity and the ideals of freedom and opportunity; health and access to quality and affordable healthcare is a human right; equity in healthcare and in health for all Nigerians is a goal to be pursued; and primary healthcare shall remain the basic philosophy and strategy for national health development (Federal Republic of Nigeria, 2004)

3. Results and discussion

3.1 OM health infrastructure inequality in Ekiti State

The Federal Republic of Nigeria placed health in the concurrent legislative list and thus all three tiers of government share the responsibility for the health sector. Ekiti State Government has the responsibility for Secondary Healthcare Services and the newly established University of Ado-Ekiti Teaching Hospital in Ado-Ekiti while the Local Governments have the responsibility of Primary Health Centres and the Health Posts in their wards.

The State Ministry of Health plans and develops health programmes. It also supervises the implementation procedures in line with the National Health Policy Guidelines. The Ministry, through the Hospital Management Board (HMB), provides Secondary Healthcare Services through seventeen (17) General and Three (3) Specialist Hospitals.

An overview of the available health infrastructure in Ekiti State is provided in Table 1. The table shows that there were 458 health facilities in the state. A total of 315 or 68.78% belongs to the public sector while private sector accounted for 31. 22%.

Healthcare Facilities	Number of Health Facilities	Percentage
Primary Healthcare	293	63.97
Secondary Healthcare	20	4.37
Tertiary Healthcare	2	0.44
Private Healthcare	143	31.22
Total	**458**	**100**

Source: Computed based on data obtained from Planning, Research and Statistics Department, Ekiti State Ministry of Health, Ado-Ekiti

Table 1. Distribution of Healthcare Facilities in Ekiti State (January 2011)

The distribution of the healthcare facilities by types across the LGAs is presented in Table 2. The table shows that Ado, an urban LGA, had the highest number of facilities with 75 while Irepodun/Ifelodun, a rural LGA, had 30.

LGA	Number of Primary Healthcare Facilities	Number of Secondary Healthcare Facilities	Number of Tertiary Healthcare Facilities	Number of Private Healthcare Facilities	Total
Ado	32	0	1	42	75
Efon	12	1	0	10	23
Ekiti East	14	1	0	11	26
Ekiti S/West	21	1	0	4	26
Ekiti West	25	2	0	3	30
Emure	12	1	0	15	28
Gboyin	17	2	0	6	25
Ido Osi	17	1	1	8	27
Ijero	29	1	0	5	35
Ikere	17	1	0	9	27
Ikole	22	2	0	4	28
Ilejemeje	10	1	0	2	13
Irepodun/ Ifelodun	18	1	0	11	30
Ise/Orun	14	1	0	4	19
Moba	15	1	0	4	20
Oye	18	3	0	5	26
Total	**293**	**20**	**2**	**143**	**458**

Source: Computed based on data obtained from Planning, Research and Statistics Department, Ekiti State Ministry of Health, Ado-Ekiti

Table 2. Distribution of Healthcare Facilities in Ekiti State by Types

Table 3 presents the results of the assessment of the distribution of health infrastructure in Ekiti State using the Index of Dissimilarity and Gini Coefficient. This is with a view to assessing the extent of inequality in the distribution across the LGAs. The distribution was assessed with respect to populations and the land areas of the LGAs with a view to determining if there was inequality in the distribution of the facilities. For the two indices used, the closer they are to 1, the more inequality exists in the distribution of the health facilities. The table indicates there was some inequality in the distribution of the health facilities whether considered from the point of view of the population or the land area since the values of the indices are all different from zero. The table reveals that all the indices for private hospitals were higher than the corresponding indices for public hospitals. This implies that inequality in the distribution of the private health facilities was higher than that of public facilities. The table also reveals that all the indices considered from the point of view of land areas were higher than the corresponding indices considered from the point of view of populations of the LGAs. This implies that inequality is higher when the distribution is assessed on the basis of land area than on the basis of population. Finally, the indices for both public and private hospitals combined were lower than the corresponding indices for private health facilities. This shows the moderating effect of the distribution of the public health facilities on inequality in the distribution of private health facilities.

Ownership Status	Population		Land Area	
	Dissimilarity Index	Gini Coefficient	Dissimilarity Index	Gini Coefficient
Public Hospitals Only	0.036	0.026	0.143	0.042
Private Hospitals Only	0.208	0.343	0.254	0.474
Both Public and Private Hospitals	0.064	0.017	0.164	0.099

Source: Authors' computation

Table 3. Concentration Indices for Health Facilities in Ekiti State

Table 4 presents information on the land area and healthcare facilities in Ado and Irepodun/Ifelodun LGAs and Ekiti State as a whole (All LGAs). Table 5 contains the estimated land area and number of persons per healthcare facility in Ado and Irepodun/Ifelodun LGAs and Ekiti State as a whole. The total land area of the state is 5,888.1 square kilometers out of which the land areas for Ado and Irepodun/Ifelodun LGAs are 297.9 square kilometers and 361.8 square kilometers, respectively. Ekiti State has a population of 2,384,212 while the populations of Ado and Irepodun/Ifelodun LGAs were 308,621 and 129,149, respectively. There were 458 healthcare facilities in Ekiti State out which 75 and 30 were in Ado and Irepodun/Ifelodun LGAs, respectively.

LGA	Land Area (Square Km)	Population	Private Healthcare Facilities	Public Healthcare Facilities	Public and Private Healthcare Facilities
Ado	297.9	308,621	42	33	75
Irepodun/ Ifelodun	361.8	129,149	11	19	30
All	5,888.1	2,384,212	143	315	458

Sources: Land Area- Surveyor-General's Office, Ekiti State, Population - National Bureau of Statistics, Abuja, Healthcare Facilities, Ekiti State Ministry of Health

Table 4. Land Area, Population and Healthcare Facilities in Ekiti State

Table 5 shows that the land area per private, public and; public and private (combined) healthcare facilities were larger for Irepodun/Ifelodun LGA compared to Ado LGA. This implies that, on the average, residents of Irepodun/Ifelodun LGA had to cover longer distances to access a healthcare facility than the residents of Ado LGA. There were more persons per private healthcare facility in Irepodun/Ifelodun LGA compared to Ado LGA in spite of the higher population of Ado LGA. This is because of the tendency of the private healthcare facility operators to concentrate their facilities in urban centres, where incomes are higher and the residents can afford to pay for services in line with the findings of Oguntade & Yusuf (2007).

There were more persons per public healthcare facility in Ado LGA compared to Irepodun/Ifelodun LGA in spite of the fact that government had established 33 healthcare facilities in Ado LGA compared to 19 healthcare facilities in Irepodun/Ifelodun LGA. This is because the population is much higher in Ado LGA than in Irepodun/Ifelodun LGA. When the number of both public and private healthcare facilities is taken into consideration, there were 4,305 persons per healthcare facility in Irepodun/Ifelodun LGA compared to 4,115 in Ado LGA. It thus appears that public healthcare facilities have moderated the effects of the concentration of private healthcare facilities in Ado LGA.

	Land Area per Private Hospital (Square Km)	Land Area per Public Hospital (Square Km)	Land Area per Public and Private Hospital (Square Km)	Persons per Private Hospital	Persons per Public Hospital	Persons per Public and Private Hospital
Ado LGA	7.09	9.03	3.97	7,348	9,352	4,115
Irepodun/ Ifelodun LGA	32.89	19.04	12.06	11,741	6,797	4,305
All LGAs	41.18	18.69	12.86	16,673	7,569	5,206

Source: Authors' computation

Table 5. Land Area and Persons per Healthcare Facility in Ekiti State

3.2 Implications of health infrastructure inequality in Ekiti State for access to OM services

Analysis of the distribution of healthcare facilities in Ekiti State revealed the presence of inequality. A further analysis of the distribution focusing at Ado, the most urbanized LGA, and Irepodun/Ifelodun LGA, a rural and largely agricultural LGA, gave an indication of the implication of the inequality in the distribution. While there was not much difference in the number of persons per healthcare facility in the urban and rural LGA studied, the land area per healthcare facility was three times larger in the rural LGA than in the urban LGA. This implies that residents of the rural LGA have to travel longer distances to access a healthcare facility compared with the residents of the urban LGA. The rural LGAs in Nigeria generally have poorer road networks and fewer commercial transportation facilities (Mafimisebi, 2010). Thus the residents of the rural LGAs are disadvantaged in terms of access to OM services. This may discourage the use of OM services in the rural LGAs and encourage the use of TM which is easily available and relatively cheaper (Mafimisebi & Oguntade, 2010).

The findings of this study corroborate the results of the Core Welfare Indicator Survey (NBS, 2006). The indicators of health access for Ekiti State obtained from the Core Welfare Indicator Survey (NBS, 2006) are presented in Table 6. The table shows that access to health facility in the State was 68.9%. Access to health facility in the urban areas was 72.8%, while in the rural areas, it was 64.6%. Access to prenatal care in Ekiti State was 99.9%. Delivery by health professionals was 92.1% while fully vaccinated children was 86.4%. In the urban areas, the percentage for fully vaccinated was 88.6, while the percentage for the rural areas was 84.3. The need for medical services was defined for those who were sick or injured in the four weeks preceding the survey. About 6.1% of households in the state indicated need for medical services. In the urban areas the percentage was 6.0, while in the rural areas it was 6.1. About 8.0% of households in Ekiti State used medical services within the four weeks preceding the survey. Lower number of households (7.5%) used medical services in the urban areas than in the rural areas (8.6%) within the four weeks preceding the survey. It appears there were more health challenges in the rural areas of the state. The results of this survey clearly indicate that access to health facility was higher in the urban areas than in the rural areas. However, the need for and the use of medical services were higher in the rural areas than in the urban areas.

Indicator	Urban (%)	Rural (%)	Whole State (%)
Access to health facility	72.8	64.6	68.9
Prenatal care	N.A.	N.A.	99.9
Delivery by health professional	N.A.	N.A.	92.1
Need medical services	6.0	6.1	6.1
Use medical services	7.5	8.6	8.0
Fully vaccinated children	88.6	84.3	86.4

N.A. - Not Available
Source: NBS (2006)

Table 6. Health Access Indicators for Ekiti State

4. Assessment of rural-urban utilization of TM and OM

This section discusses the results of the primary data analyzed on the use of TM and OM by farming households in Ekiti State. The focus of this section is the assessment of rural-urban utilization of TM and OM as against the assessment of access to OM facilities in the previous section.

4.1 Socio-economic characteristics of households

Table 4 presents the test of significance of difference of means of rural and urban socio-economic and demographic variables. The mean age of the farmers in Ado LGA was 51 years, while that of farmers in Irepodun/Ifelodun LGA was 59 years. Thus, farmers in Irepodun/Ifelodun LGA were older than those in Ado LGA. For both locations, however, it can be seen that most of the people engaging in farming activities were above 50 years old. Therefore, it could be concluded that farmers are aging in the study area and the need for sound health to remain productive will increasingly become important in the nearest future. Also, there is a need for young and more agile people, with interest in farming, to be encouraged to take over from these aging farmers.

The average household size in Ado LGA was 5.9, while that of Irepodun/Ifelodun LGA was 6.7 and there was no significant difference between these two values. The average farm size per household in Ado LGA was 1.49 hectares, while in Irepodun/Ifelodun LGA, it was 2.26 hectares. There was significant difference between the two average farm sizes at the 5% level. This may be as a result of the fact that land is more expensive per unit area in Ado LGA; a phenomenon which started about 15 years ago when Ado-Ekiti became the capital of Ekiti State. The influence of rapid urbanization of Ado-Ekiti has probably also spread to other towns in the LGA causing rising land prices. The phenomenon of rural urban migration has also contributed significantly to the rising population in Ado LGA leading to a relatively higher population density compared to other LGAs. Thus, farms are larger in Irepodun/Ifelodun LGA in spite of greater access by farmers in Ado LGA to extension services; due to the proximity of the Agricultural Development Programme Unit of the State Ministry of Agriculture with its headquarters in Ado-Ekiti.

Primary data analysis also revealed that average years of respondents' farming experience in Ado and Irepodun/Ifelodun LGAs were 28 years and 35 years, respectively. There was a significant difference in these mean values at the 1% level. This shows that farmers in Irepodun/Ifelodun LGA were more experienced in farming activities than their Ado LGA counterparts. This might be as a result of the fact that farmers in Irepodun/Ifelodun are exposed earlier in life to farming and allied activities being the major economic activities in most rural areas in Nigeria (NBS, 2006). In Ado LGA however, there are more opportunities to be engaged in the non-farm sector. This is because Ado LGA is host to the state capital.

Table 7 shows that the average years of formal education was 8.6 in Irepodun/Ifelodun and 11.3 in Ado LGA and there was a significant difference in these mean values at the 5% level. Thus, the tendency exists for a higher influence of the western education on Ado farmers compared with Irepodun/Ifelodun farmers.

4.2 Income from farming activities

The mean income from farming activities per household per annum was ₦76,748.56 for Irepodun/Ifelodun LGA and ₦124,822.94 for Ado LGA. There was statistically significant difference between the average incomes at the 1% level (Table 7). This is understandable because the rural areas are usually at a disadvantage compared with the urban areas in market prices (World Bank, 1993; Mafimisebi, 2010). Most rural dwellers are into farming as their main economic activity. The rural areas lack storage facilities and most farm products become perishable within few days of harvesting (Lancaster & Coursey, 1984). Thus, there is a glut of agricultural products in the rural markets where farmers witness low patronage and have to dispose of their products at lower prices. They can only sell at better and more remunerative prices obtainable in the urban markets if they own or can afford payment for transport facilities to convey their products to the urban centres. This easier, cheaper and timely access to urban markets in Ado and surrounding towns by farmers in Ado LGA may have been responsible for the significant difference in farm incomes between the two sets of farmers.

4.3 Expenditure on TM and OM by urban and rural farming households

The empirical results in Table 7 show that the average amounts of money expended per annum on OM for treatment of common ailments by farmers in urban and rural areas were ₦10,160 ($67.7) and ₦4,530 ($30.2), respectively. The corresponding amounts of money spent on TM were ₦2,118 ($14.1) and ₦730 ($4.9) per annum, respectively. There were significant difference in the expenditures on TM in Ado and Irepodun/Ifelodun LGAs at 5% level. The expenditures on OM in the two LGAs were also significantly different at 1% level. This means urban farmers spend more on both TM and OM than rural farmers.

The results show that expenditures on TM and OM in the urban LGA were higher than the corresponding expenditures in the rural LGA. This might be due to the higher level of income in the urban LGA. It also worth noting that expenditures on TM is expected to be lower than those on OM because TM resources are locally available compared with OM resources which are mostly imported. This might therefore account for the lower expenditures on TM in both LGAs. Similarly, TM resources are cheaper or almost free in the rural LGA (Mafimisebi & Oguntade, 2010) thus making TM expenditure in the rural LGA lower than in the urban LGA. The implication of this is that TM is more affordable and hence more accessible in the rural LGA (Mafimisebi & Oguntade, 2010).

The responses on the preferences of households in the use of OM and TM revealed that about 91.7% of the household heads in the rural LGA and 60.8% of the household heads in the urban LGA preferred the use of TM for common ailments that are not life-threatening and therefore would not require surgical interventions. For life-threatening ailments, 88.3% and 41.7.0% of the farming households in the rural and urban LGAs, respectively, preferred combining OM with treatment from TM.

Variables	Mean Value		Z-value	P-value
	Irepodun/ Ifelodun LGA (Rural)	Ado LGA (Urban)		
Age (yrs)	59	51	22.86	0.0342*
Household size	6.7	5.9	4.24	0.6643
Farm size hectares	2.26	1.49	16.112	0.0402*
Years of farming experience	35	28	12.108	0.0019**
Years of formal education	8.3	11.6	11.747	0.0474*
Household size (₦)	76,748.56	124,822.94	27.449	0.016**
Expenditure on OM	4,530	10,160	27.986	0.0023**
Expenditure on TM	730	2,118	11.625	0.0441*

*Significant at 5%, ** significant at 1%
Source: Data analysis

Table 7. Test of Significance of Difference of Mean Values of Rural and Urban of Socio-economic and Demographic Variables

Results from the FGDs showed that 100% and 50.0% of farmers groups in the rural LGA and urban LGA, respectively, indicated preference for TM when and if an ailment is capable of been treated by both methods. Also, 83.3% of farmer's groups in the rural LGA reported preferring to complement OM with TM in both cases of simple and complicated medical conditions. These findings tend to show that the rural dwellers have developed some preference for TM. This higher level of preference for TM in the rural LGA is in consonance with the findings of the Nigeria Core Welfare Indicator Study which revealed that 9.1% of the households the rural areas consulted traditional healer compared with 4.6% in the urban areas (NBS, 2006).

4.4 Factors determining use of TM

The estimates of the binary logistic regression for both rural and urban farmers are shown on Table 8. Generally, the binary logit model showed a commendably good fit to the data for both sets of farmers. The value of the Chi-square test was significant at 1% for rural and urban farmers. This indicates a rejection of the hypothesis that the model lacks explanatory power. The model correctly predicted 88.5% and 74.4% of the observations for rural and urban farmers, respectively. From Table 8, it could be seen that household size, education and income (significant at 1%) and the number of elderly people in a household (significant at 5%) had the greatest influence on use of TM by rural farmers. For farmers in the urban areas, age and education (significant at 5%) and household size (significant at 1%) exerted the greatest impact on use of TM.

Variable	Rural Households		Urban Households	
	Estimated Coefficient	Marginal Effects	Estimated Coefficient	Marginal Effects
Constant	-3.2992	----------	-4.0066	---------
Age of household head	0.3266	0.0254	1.4287*	0.0052
Size of household	1.2368**	0.0047	0.8896**	0.0122
Sex of household head	0.1084	0.0288	0.1175	0.0147
Education	-1.7347**	0.0193	-1.6264*	0.0246
Household income	-1.5489**	0.0176	0.0775	0.0064
Number of elderly people	0.9266*	0.0137	0.0636	0.0045
Religion of household head	0.0594	0.0094	0.0396	0.0066
Observation number		60		60
LR statistic (χ^2)		118.245**		136.844**
Degree of freedom		7.000		7.000
Log likelihood		-244.616		-219.927
McFadden R^2		0.522		0.473
% Predicted right		88.514%		74.447%

Note: The marginal effects are calculated at the mean of the predictor variables
*Significant at 5% level and ** significant at 1% level

Table 8. Logistic Model of Determinants of Use of TM

Additional insights can be obtained using the marginal effects calculated as the partial derivatives of the non-linear probability function, evaluated at each variable's sample mean. For instance, for the rural farmers, a unit increase in years of formal education and income, after the mean values, reduced the probability of use of TM by 0.0193 and 0.0176, respectively. This could be due to the fact that educated people have greater tendencies to accept western influence and regard TM as unhygienic, demonic, occultic and sinful

(Fasola, 2006, Chavunduka, 2009; Mafimisebi & Oguntade, 2010). In the same vein, higher incomes may tend to give a household access to the more expensive OM which is regarded as faster in action and status enhancing. On the contrary, an increase in household size and the number of elderly people in the household beyond the mean value will increase the probability of use of TM by 0.0047 and 0.0137, respectively. This is understandable because if household size increases in a scenario of constant or slowly rising income, per capital expenditure reduces making the household to prefer the cheaper TM to OM in the case of a health problem. In the same way, with increase in the number of elderly people that are usually repositories of TM knowledge, there is a higher probability of use of TM.

Surprisingly, age of household head that was statistically insignificant in the model for rural farmers was significant at 5% in the model for urban farmers. For urban farmers, a unit increase in the age of household head and household size will lead to 0.0054 and 0.0122 increases in the probability of using TM. This may be a result of the fact that higher age confers higher and better information on and knowledge of TM in Africa where such knowledge is most willingly shared among the elderly. On the other hand, a unit increase in income will translate to a 0.0064 fall in the probability of using TM.

5. Conclusions

Inadequate access to health services is one of the components of rural poverty which is prevalent in Nigeria. Inadequate access to health services determines, to a large extent, the decision of rural households to either patronize OM or TM. This study assessed the distribution of OM infrastructure in Ekiti State Nigeria, focusing attention on the rural-urban dichotomy. It further looked at the extent of patronage of TM and OM among farming households with special emphasis on the rural-urban dichotomy.

Result of the analyses indicates that inequality exists in the distribution of OM infrastructure in Ekiti State. There was a distinct rural-urban dichotomy in the provision of OM infrastructure in the state. This was caused largely by the concentration of private investment in OM infrastructure in the urban LGAs because of their profit motive. This emphasizes the need for the public sector to continue to moderate the distribution of OM infrastructure through its investment. In doing this, attention should be paid not only to the population of the LGAs but also to their land areas. In addition, the existence of private OM infrastructure in the respective LGAs should be considered in citing new public OM infrastructure.

The results from primary data analysis with respect to the urban LGA seem to establish an indirect nexus between poverty and utilization of TM. The fact that the use of TM increases with household size and age of household heads; two independent variables that are positively correlated with poverty in several studies, is an indication that as poverty increases in Nigeria, urban households have the tendency to revert to the use of TM. Similarly, for rural households, the use of TM increases with household size and the number of elderly people in the household. These two variables are also positively correlated with poverty, implying that increases in poverty among rural households will lead to increases in the use of TM. This is a justification for a welfare oriented health policy in Nigeria.

Given the tendency for the use of TM in Nigeria, steps that will improve the practice of TM, ensure sustainable use of TM resources and re-orientate farming households on how to properly and safely use TM, should be given important considerations in Nigeria's national health policy. Overall, the findings of the study clearly indicate the need for government in Nigeria to continue to play active role in the provision of health services in a sector that is increasingly being dominated by private entrepreneurs who are driven by the profit motive. In the current circumstances, farming households that are unable to access OM either because of the cost or distance to such facilities are being compelled to patronize TM; which is at the moment largely unregulated.

6. References

ADB (2006). Key Indicators 2006: Measuring Policy Effectiveness in Health and Education. Asian Development Bank, Manila.

Aigbokhan, B.E. (2000). Poverty, Growth and Inequality in Nigeria: A Case Study. *AERC Research Paper* 102. Nairobi. African Economic Research Consortium, 63 pp., Kenya

Aigbokhan, B.E. (2008). Growth, Income and Inequality in Nigeria. Economic Commission for Africa, ACGS/MPAMS Discussion Paper No.3, 33pp. http://www.uneca.org/acgd/mdgs/GrowthInequalityPoverty.pdf

Anderson, E. (2010). Growth Incidence Analysis for Non-Income Welfare Indicators: Evidence from Ghana and Uganda. Background Paper for the Chronic Poverty Report 2008- 09

Anyanwu, J.C., Erhijakpor, A.E.O. (2007). Health Expenditures and Health Outcomes in Africa, Economic Research Working Paper No 91, December

Castillo-Salgado C., Schneider C., Loyola E., Mujica O., Roca A. & Yerg T (2001). Measuring Health Inequalities: Gini Coefficient and Concentration Index. *Epidemiol Bull* 2001, 22:3–4

Centers for Disease Control and Prevention (CDC) (2001) *Public Health's Infrastructure: A Status Report,* (Atlanta, GA: CDC

Chavunduka, G (2009). Christianity, African Religion and African Medicine. World Council of Churches http://www.wcc-coe.org/wcc/what/interreligious/cd33-01.html.

Dixon, P. M., Weiner J., Mitchell-Olds T., & Woodley R (1987). Boot-Strapping the Gini Coefficient of Inequality. *Ecology*; 68: 1548-1551.

Ekiti State Planning Commission (2004). State Economic Empowerment and Development Strategy, Pp111.

Fasola, T.R.(2006). The Impact of Traditional Medicine on the People and Environment of Nigeria. In: *Sustainable Environmental Management in Nigeria* Ivbijaro M.F.A., Akintola F & Okechukwu R. U., 251-267

Federal Republic of Nigeria (2004). Revised National Health Policy, Federal Ministry of Health, Abuja, September

Handler, A., Issel, M. & Turnock, B. (2001). A Conceptual Framework to Measure Performance of the Public Health System. *American Journal of Public Health* 91, No. 8 http://www.ajph.org/cgi/reprint/91/8/1235

Harttgen, K. & Misselhorn, M. (2006). A Multilevel Approach to Explain Child Mortality and Under-nutrition in South Asia and Sub-Saharan Africa *Ibero America Institute for Economic Research (IAI), Discussion Papers*, September

Herrero, C., Martínez, R & Villar, A. (2010). Improving the Measurement of Human Development. Human Development Research Paper 2010/12 http://hdr.undp.org/en/reports/global/hdr2010/papers/HDRP_2010_12.pdf

http://www.who.int/countries/nga/areas/health_systems/en/index.html

Lancaster, P. A. & Coursey, D.G. (1984) *Traditional Post-Harvest Technology of Perishable Tropical Staples*. Food and Agriculture Organization of the United Nations, Rome. Available at http://www.fao.org/docrep/x5045e/x5045E00.htm#Contents (Accessed 15-04-2011)

Leger, S. (2001). The Anomaly that Finally Went Away *Journal of Epidemiology and Community Health*, 55: 79

Mafimisebi, T. E. (2010). Technology Adoption and Economic Development: Trajectories within the African Agricultural Industry. In: *Nanotechnology and Microelectronics: Global Diffusion, Economics and Policy*, Ekekwe, N. (Ed.) 298-313 , IGI Global Publishers, New York, USA

Mafimisebi, T.E. & Oguntade, A.E. (2010). Preparation and Use of Plant Medicines for Farmers' Health in Southwest Nigeria: Socio-Cultural, Magico-Religious and Economic Aspects, *Journal of Ethnobiology and Ethnomedicine*, 6:1doi:10.1186/1746-4269-6-1, http://www.ethnobiomed.com/content/6/1/1

Marmot, M. (2009). Marmot review: first phase report. Strategic review of health inequalities in England post-2010. Available at http://www.ucl.ac.uk/gheg/marmotreview/consultation/Marmot_Review_First_Phase_Report (Accessed 2/10/09)

Musa E. O. & Ejembi C. L. (2004). Reasons and outcome of paediatric referrals from first-level health facilities in Sabongari, Zaria, Northwestern Nigeria. *Journal of Community Medicine & Primary Health Care, Vol. 16(1): 10-15*

NBS (2006). Nigerian Core Welfare Indicators. National Bureau of Statistics. [http://www.nigerianstat.gov.ng/nbsapps/cwiq/2006/survey0/outputInformation/ cwiqreports.html] webcite Accessed on 14th October 2010

NBS (2007). Directory of Health Establishments in Nigeria, 2007. Available at www.nigerianstat.gov.ng (Accessed 14-04-2011)

NBS (2010). Federal Republic of Nigeria: 2006 Population Census. Available at www.nigerianstat.gov.ng (Accessed 14-04-2011)

Nolte, J. & Mckee, M. (2004). Does Health Care Save Lives? *The Nuffield Trust*, London, 58

NPC (2004). Nigeria: Draft National Economic Empowerment and Development Strategy-NEEDS, National Planning Commission, Abuja, 125 pp.

O'Brien, L., Williams, K. & Stewart, A. (2010). Urban health and health inequalities and the role of urban forestry in Britain: A review http://www.forestry.gov.uk/pdf/urban_health_and_forestry_review_2010.pdf/$FILE/urban_health_and_forestry_review_2010.pdf

Oguntade, A. E. & Yusuf N.A. (2007). Health Infrastructure inequality: A Case Study of Lagos State, Nigeria *The Social Sciences*. Vol. 2 (1): 51-55

Okunmadewa, F. (1999). International agencies response to poverty situation in Nigeria. *CBN Bullion* 23. 4: 66-70

Republic of Sierra Leone (2008). An Agenda for Change: Second Poverty Reduction Strategy (PRSP II) (2008 -2012) Available at http://www.imf.org/external/pubs/ft/scr/2008/cr08250.pdf.(Accessed 15-04-2011)

Rodrigue, J.P. (2009). *The Geography of Transport Systems*, Hofstra University, Department of Global Studies & Geography, 2009. Available at http://people.hofstra.edu/geotrans. Accessed on 14th October 2010

Sachs, J. D. (2004). Health in the Developing World: Achieving the Millennium Development Goals. *Bulletin of the World Health Organization*, 82 (12): 947–49

Srinivasan, T. N. (2001). Comment on Counting the World's Poor,' by Angus Deaton", *The World Bank Research Observer*, 16 (2) 157-168

Tandon, A. (2007) Measuring Government Inclusiveness: An Application to Health Policy *Asian Development Review*, Vol. 24, (1): 32-48 Available at www.adb.org/documents/ periodicals/adr/.../adr-vol24-1-tandon.pdf (Accessed 15-04-2011)

Turnock (2004). Public Health: What it is and What it Does, 3rd Ed., MA: Jones and Bartlett Publishers, Sudbury

UN (2008). End Poverty 2015: Millennium Development Goals Report. Available at http://www.un.org/millenniumgoals/pdf/Sub-Saharan%20Africa.pdf (Accessed 15-04-2011)

UNDP (2003). Millennium Development Goals, National Reports: A Look through a Gender Lens. Available at http://www.undp.org/women/docs/mdgs-genderlens.pdf (Accessed 15-04-2011)

Whitehead, M (1992). The Concepts and Principles of Equity in Health. *International Journal of Health Services*, 22: 429 - 445

WHO (1986). Ottawa Charter for Health Promotion. World Health Organization, Geneva

WHO (1996). Equity in health and health care. World Health Organization, Geneva

WHO (2011) Health systems policies and service delivery WHO African Region: Nigeria

WHO, (1998). Health Promotion Glossary. WHO/HPR/HEP/98.1 Available at http://www.who.int/hpr/NPH/docs/hp_glossary_en.pdf (Accessed 15-04-2011)

WHO, (2001) WHO Country Cooperation Strategy: Nigeria, World Health Organization Regional Office for Africa, Brazzaville Available at http://www.who.int/countries/nga /about/ccs_strategy02_07.pdf (Accessed 15-04-2011)

World Bank (2008). Country Assistance Evaluation. Nigeria: Independent Evaluation Group Approach Paper. Available at *lnweb90.worldbank.org/oed/oeddoclib.../nigeria_cae_approach_paper.pdf* (Accessed 15-04-2011)

World Bank, (1993). A strategy to Develop Agriculture in Sub-Saharan Africa and a Focus for the World Bank. Africa Technical Department Series, 2003, 83-900

World Health Organization (2001) Macroeconomics and Health: Investing in Health for Economic Development, Available at http://www3.who.int/whosis/cmh (Accessed 15-04-2011)

Young, F. W. (2001). An Explanation of the Persistent Doctor-Mortality Association. *Journal of Epidemiology and Community Health*, 55: 80-84.

12

A New Economic and Social Paradigm for Funding Recovery in Mental Health in the Twenty First Century

Robert Parker
*Northern Territory Clinical School,
Darwin, Northern Territory,
Australia*

1. Introduction

Mental illness is a significant factor in disease related disability throughout the world. About 16% of the global burden of disease not attributable to communicable disease has been attributed to mental disorders (Prince et al 2007) with substance abuse disorders contributing to a further 4% of this burden (ibid). In Australia, "Mental Disorders" were considered to be the third major cause of health loss (behind cancer and cardiovascular disease) in 2003 but were estimated to increase at a significant rate to move ahead of cancer and become the second major cause of "health loss" by 2013 (Begg et al 2008). This burden of mental illness is particularly pronounced in the youth of Australia with disability-adjusted life years (DALY's) for mental illness calculated to be above 90,000 (compared to the next highest of 48,000 DALY's due to injury) for the 15 to 24 year old age group in 2003 (Eckersley 2011). Along with the current burden of disease attributed to mental illness, there is a number of challenges facing societies in the developed and developing world that are likely to lead to an increase in mental illness. Sartorius (pers comm) has recently outlined some of these challenges. They include: weakening of community resilience mechanisms, increasing awareness of gaps and unreachable opportunities, migration of people, talents and capital with the subsequent loss of social capital in some societies, the challenges of increased urbanisation on community supports and family structures, the changing nature of privileged families in developed society with less children, longer life spans and more fragile family structures, the decrease of middle class "norms" in developed countries and the additional increase of the middle class in developing countries with potential economic and social alienation from less privileged groups, the changing role of women and the implications that this has for child care and care of the elderly and the changing paradigms of medicine itself with increasing use of technology in addition to evolving ethical issues such as euthanasia.

The severity of personal disability from mental illness is pervasive.

The poetry of Anne Sexton in the poem "Sickness unto Death" (1977) helps describe some of this inner experience for severe mood disorder:

"God went out of me
As if the sea dried up like sandpaper,
As if the sun became a latrine
God went out of my fingers,
They became stone
My body became a side of mutton
And despair roamed the slaughter house..."(Porter 1991)

The recent poem by Sandy Jeffs (2009) describes her life affected by schizophrenia.

"I am many things, in many places
Fool that I may be, mad that I may be.
I am, in all my precarious guises
The creation of a cruel mind"

People suffering from severe mental illness currently face significant levels of poor health (Symonds & Parker 2007), high levels of unemployment (Dunne E et al 2008), homelessness (Browne & Hemsley 2010), alienation from family members (Druss et al 2009) and services (Luhrmann 2008). The economic cost of these issues to society generally is significant with people affected by schizophrenia estimated to have provided a direct cost to the United States economy of $62.7 billion in 2002 (Wu et al 2005)

2. Primary health care

The above issues have gained increasing importance against a background of increasing international recognition about what should constitute the ideal of health for individuals and communities. The Declaration of Alma-Ata (1978) defined health as "a state of complete physical, mental and social wellbeing and not merely as the absence of disease and infirmity" as a fundamental human right. The Declaration further called on all governments to formulate national policies, strategies and plans of action to launch and sustain primary health care as part of a comprehensive national health system and in co-ordination with other sectors". The Ottawa Charter for Health Promotion (1986) built on the initial foundations of the Declaration of Alma-Ata. The Charter reported that health "is therefore seen as a resource for everyday life, not the objective for living" and "as a positive concept emphasizing social and personal resources as well as physical capacities". The Charter goes on to define the prerequisites for health as: "peace, shelter, education, food, income, a stable eco-system, sustainable resources, social justice and equity".

The Declaration of Alma-Ata was produced in the context of a new "global approach" to health developed initially through the creation of the World Health Organisation (WHO) as a key agency of the United Nations and then the broad visionary strategy of the drive to "Health for All by the year 2000" by the then WHO director, Hafldan Mahler. This coincided with the increasing involvement of the World Bank as the major external funder for health sector development in developing countries and it has been noted that the Bank has "positioned itself operationally and intellectually at the fulcrum of international health development" (Walt 2006).

In the context of the above initiatives mental health is currently defined by the World Health Organisation as "a state of well being in which the individual recognises his or her own abilities, can cope with the normal stresses of life, can work productively and fruitfully and is able to make a contribution to his or her community" (Herrman et al 2005)

3. Amartya Sen and the concept of human agency

Apart from health, there has also been an appreciation of economic opportunities associated with the empowerment of human agency, ideas further developed by Amartya Sen, who was awarded the Nobel Prize for Economic Science in 1998. Sen (1999) defines "agency" as "someone who acts and brings about change and whose achievements can be judged in terms of their own values and objectives, whether or not we assess them in terms of some external criteria as well". Sen then goes on to discuss the way that *instrumental effectiveness* of freedom may enhance this potential for agency. "This instrumental role of freedom concerns the way different kinds of rights, opportunities and entitlements contribute to the expansion of human freedom in general and thus to promoting development". Sen then defines his instrumental freedoms as (1) political freedoms (civil rights), (2) economic freedoms (the opportunities to utilize economic resources for the purposes of consumption, production and exchange), (3) social opportunities (arrangements for education, health care etc), (4) transparency guarantees (transparency and trust in personal interaction) and (5) protective security (unemployment benefits, famine relief etc). These instrumental issues then underpin *substantive freedoms* for humanity such as political and civil liberty, social inclusion, literacy and economic security. The work of Sen is having as significant impact on individuals concerned with enhancing the agency of deprived groups such as those people affected by severe mental illness and this will be further discussed later in the chapter. Henry (2007) further defines the issues that Sen promotes "Sen also notes that a second subset of other relevant capabilities of considerable interest to the classical economists – such as the capability to live without shame, the capability to participate in the activities of the community, and the capability of enjoying self-respect – provides a basis for relative poverty comparisons....policy makers should be concerned with opportunities. Specifically, they should be concerned to ensure that individuals are endowed with capabilities that allow them the *freedom* to choose to live their lives in ways that have real meaning and real value....".

The concepts that Sen defines have been usefully applied to Indigenous disadvantage in Canada and Australia (as described below). They may have also particular importance in supporting strategic policy initiatives to develop a mental health Recovery framework.

4. Effective funding models for primary health care: The indigenous paradigm in Canada and Australia

The broad spectrum of disadvantage experienced by those afflicted by severe mental illness is to a degree, similar to the current predicament of the Indigenous populations of Australia and Canada. Recent innovative government policies to redress this disadvantage have been based on the definitions of Primary Care previously described in addition to policies based on the desire to enhance substantive freedoms as promoted

In Canada in 2002, First Nations tribes constituted 976,305 people or about 3 percent of the population (Indian and Northern Affairs Canada Communications Branch 2004) Kirmayer et al (2000) note that First Nations Tribes have had contact with European culture since the sixteenth century. They comment " the history of European colonisation of North America is a harrowing tale of the indigenous peoples' decimation by infectious disease, warfare and active suppression of culture and identity that was tantamount to genocide (ibid). Kirmayer et al note that it is likely that 90% of an original population of 7 million Canadian First Nations people died as a direct and indirect result of European contact (ibid). The authors comment that First Nations people were removed to settlements that were chosen by government or mercantile interests rather than by the Indigenous Canadians themselves. This often resulted in major social dislocation for the community structures. In addition, from 1879 to 1973, there was a Government policy of removing First Nation children from their homes to church run boarding schools where their heritage was denigrated and suppressed. In addition, these children were subject to physical, emotional and sexual abuse (ibid).

Indigenous First Nations Canadians have high unemployment rates (25%) compared to the general Canadian population (10%) with particularly high rates on reservations (31%) (MacMillan et al 1996). First Nations people generally live in poor housing and only a limited number of communities have adequate water and waste disposal (ibid). They have high infant mortality rates of 13.8 per 1000 live births for all Canadian Indian infants compared to 7.3 for all Canadian infants. Age standardised mortality ratios for Canadian First Nation women is almost double that for Canadian women generally whilst the aged standardised mortality rates for First Nation men is about 50% above that for Canadian men generally with higher death rates for men on reserves. The leading cause of death for Canadian First Nation people between 1986 and 1988 was injury and poisoning that accounted for 31% of all deaths in this population compared to 7.5% of all Canadians (ibid).

Suicide rates for Indigenous Canadians are two to three times higher than Canadians generally. There is a particularly high suicide rate for the Inuit people with the suicide rate in Inuit youth being up to 5 times the rate of Canadian youth generally (ibid). Canadian First Nation communities also report high rates of alcohol abuse, other substance abuse and family violence (ibid) that are probably relevant is respect to the high suicide rates. Solvent abuse, including petrol, glue and cleaning products in isolated First Nation communities (ibid, p1576). Kirmayer et al (2000) also report that there are generally high rates of mental illness in many Indigenous Canadian communities. They note "the high rates of suicide, alcoholism and violence and the pervasive demoralisation seen in Aboriginal communities can be readily understood as the direct consequences of a history of dislocations and the disruption of traditional subsistence patterns and connection to the land". However, conversely, the First Nation communities with more "cultural control" factors such as employment of First Nations people in key positions in the community (such as the police) and with increased community governance appear to have less suicide (Chandler & Lalonde 1998).

A response to the significant disadvantage of Canada's First Nations Peoples, very much developed in the spirit of primary health as outlined in the Ottawa Declaration was the Canadian Aboriginal Horizontal Framework (Canada's Performance 2005). This government policy was co-ordinated between the Canadian Federal government and Provincial governments to address the disadvantage in Canadian First Nation social determinants across a "wide front". Leadership from the top was a key initial factor in the development of the Framework with the then Canadian prime minister Paul Martin committing to a round table discussion with all levels of Canadian government and First Nation leaders. A policy retreat with members of the Canadian Committee on Aboriginal Affairs and First Nations leaders followed. There was also a commitment to the development of an Aboriginal report card to track progress with the Canadian health strategy.

The Canadian Aboriginal Horizontal Framework was then developed as a strategic guide to funding priorities and co-operation between the various levels of government as well as allowing the establishment of performance indicators. The Framework appears to place the "pillars" of health at equal value. The "pillars" were: Health, Lifelong Learning, Safe and Sustainable Communities, Housing, Economic Opportunity, Lands and resources and Governance and Relationships. Each of the "pillars" of the Framework was then be divided into "sub pillars". As an example, Safe and Sustainable communities were divided into: Community Infrastructure, Social Support and Community Well-being and Community Safety and Justice. Unfortunately, the policy appears to have been wound back following the election of the Conservative Government in Canada in 2006. However, the policy remains an important example of the way that a government can enact policy to remedy the broad range of disadvantage with financial "strategic pillars" attached to the relevant issues of "Primary Health" as outlined in the Ottawa Charter.

In Australia, Archaeological evidence suggests that Aboriginal people have been present for the last 45000-50,000 years. The ethnographic evidence from early contact suggests that Aboriginal people who survived infancy were relatively fit and disease free (Flood 2006). Further, Australia's native foods supported a nutritious, balanced diet of protein and vegetables with adequate vitamins and minerals with little salt sugar and fat. Life on the move kept people physically fit (ibid).

In terms of "mental health", traditional Aboriginal culture had a number of strong reinforcing factors that have been well defined by Professor(s) Helen and Jill Milroy (Milroy et al 2003). Aboriginal sense of self was seen in a collective sense, intimately connected to all aspects of life, community, spirituality, culture and country. The culture also provided for everyone through sharing rules and relationships and kinship were of prime importance, defining social roles. Aboriginal people were also given a sense of meaning and understanding of life experience through their connection to country and their Dreaming. Spiritual beliefs offered guidance and comfort and offered a sense of connectivity and belonging despite distress, death and loss. Lore, the body of knowledge that defined the culture and the tribal elders who contained and interpreted the Lore were highly valued. Customary law defined rules and consequences. Over 200 traditional languages and other methods of communication allowed a rich expression of interaction in the above social context and formal ceremony allowed a method of dealing with life's transitions thought birth, initiation and death. Men and women had defined economic and cultural roles within the tribe. Children were well protected within the group with a range of "aunties" and older siblings able to take over the child care role if the mother was stressed.

Franklin and White (1991) describe the elements of destruction of this optimum physical and mental good health of the Aboriginal people following the British colonization of Australia in 1788. These elements were the introduction of new diseases, the removal of ancestral land which led to psychological distress and spiritual despair and the herding of Aboriginal people into reserves and settlements, destroying lifestyle and leading to marginalisation and poverty. Other specific policies such as the Stolen Generations from the 1930s to the 1960s where Aboriginal children were forcibly removed from their parents and raised in Mission settlements reinforced government social Darwinist ideology and led to the destruction of family life with resulting emotional desolation for many individual Aboriginal people.

The current significant disadvantage of Aboriginal health and social determinants is well recognized. Hospitalization rates for cardiovascular disease in Aboriginal and Torres Strait Islander was 80% higher than for other Australians in the North West of Australia in 2002 to 2004. (AHMAC 2006) Rheumatic heart disease was nine times more common for Aboriginal and Torres Strait Islanders than other Australians (ibid). Diabetes and renal failure also figure prominently in Aboriginal health issues. In 2004-2005, three times as many Aboriginal and Torres Strait Islanders were reported to have diabetes compared to other Australians (ibid). Hospitalization rates for Aboriginal and Torres Strait Islander people with diabetes are six times higher than for other Australians (ibid). End Stage Renal Disease, often the consequence of poorly controlled diabetes was eight times higher for Aboriginal and Torres Strait Islander peoples than other Australians (ibid). Given these alarming health statistics, it is not surprising that life expectancy for Aboriginal and Torres Strait Islander people is 17 years less than for other Australians (ibid), an issue now well recognized in the "CLOSETHEGAP" (HREOC 2008) agenda.

Aboriginal and Torres Strait Islander disadvantage is also apparent in other social indices. The 2002 National Aboriginal and Torres Strait Islander Social Survey estimated that 26% of the Aboriginal and Torres Strait Islander population over 15 were living in overcrowded housing. The overcrowding becomes more apparent in remote areas where it is estimated that 62% of Aboriginal and Torres Strait Islanders live in overcrowded housing (AHMAC 2006). In respect to education, the National Schools Statistics Collection reported that the retention rate of Aboriginal and Torres Strait Islander students in Year 7/8 to Year 10 was 88.3% compared to 98.6% for other students. Unfortunately, the retention rate for Aboriginal and Torres Strait Islander students from Year7/8 to year 12 of high school was only 39.5% compared to 76.6% for other students (ibid). Given this trend in education, the accompanying statistics of significant Aboriginal and Torres Strait Islander disadvantage in employment and income to the rest of Australia are no surprise along with data from the prisons that shows that Aboriginal and Torres Strait Islander people are twelve times more likely to be in prison compared to the remainder of the Australian population (ibid).

Poverty and racism also provide a framework for the above statistics. Walter & Saggers (2007) point to the significant association between poverty and adverse health outcomes. They note that a significant proportion of Australia's Indigenous population live in a situation of "absolute poverty" as defined by the United Nations where they have severe deprivation of basic human needs including food, safe drinking water, sanitation facilities, health, shelter education and information. Some diseases such as scabies and diarrhea are directly related to inadequate sanitation and living conditions (ibid). The issues of Indigenous poverty appear particularly marked in rural areas. In addition, the failure of a recent plethora of policies to advance Aboriginal health has been attributed to a pervasive culture of "welfare colonialism", an aspect of continuing poverty. "Welfare Colonialism" (Anderson 1997) affects Aboriginal communities where most Aboriginal populations rely heavily on the provision of public sector resources. Over time, the mechanisms to deliver these overlie the traditional methods of Aboriginal governance, reducing the capacity of the communities to develop leadership in the solutions to their problems. In addition, the continuing experience of widespread racism against Aboriginal people generally within the Australian community appears to have a continuing negative effect, particularly on the mental health of Aboriginal people (Paradis 2007).

The Australian government policy environment has also recently produced a number of innovative solutions in respect of government approaches to the above Aboriginal and Torres Strait Islander disadvantage leading to the formal Council of Australian Governments financial funding strategy, the National Indigenous Reform Agreement. The Agreement in 2008 was prefaced by a paper written by Ken Henry, Secretary of the Australian Treasury. Henry (2007) suggested a broad based approach across Australian Government Departments to address Aboriginal and Torres Strait Islander health disadvantage, similar in some ways to the Canadian Framework. Henry described three key interdependent foundations to current Aboriginal and Torres Strait Islander disadvantage in Australia. Poor economic and social incentives, the underdevelopment of human capital and an absence of the effective engagement of Aboriginal and Torres Strait Islander Australians in the design of policy frameworks that might improve these incentives and capabilities. Henry commented that he and other Secretaries in the Australian Government Secretaries Group on Aboriginal and Torres Strait Islander Affairs had identified seven platforms that need to be prioritized within a framework of Aboriginal and Torres Strait Islander capability development. These included: basic protective security for women and children, early childhood development, a safe and healthy home environment, an accessible primary care health service, ensuring that incentives in the welfare system do not work against promotion of investment in human capital, real job prospects as a result of education and governance systems that support political freedom and social opportunities of local Indigenous people to be engaged in policy development.

The proposal by Henry resulted in the formation of the Council of Australian Governments National Indigenous Reform Agreement in 2008. The building blocks of the strategic financial agreement between the Australian Federal and State Governments were based on the primary care principles outlined in the Ottawa Charter. The Building Blocks outlined by the Agreement are: Early Childhood (early learning, development and socialization opportunities), Schooling (infrastructure, workforce, curriculum, student literacy and numeracy achievement. and opportunities for parental engagement and school/community partnerships), Health (access to effective, comprehensive primary and preventative health care), Economic Participation (real jobs, business opportunities, economic independence and wealth creation), Healthy Homes (adequate water and sewerage systems, waste collection electricity and housing infrastructure), Safe Communities (improved, accessible law and justice responses, effective policing. "safe houses", child protection and alcohol policy) and Governance and Leadership (capacity building so that Indigenous Australians can play a greater role in exercising their rights and responsibilities as citizens) (COAG 2008). The Agreement also has specific funding of $ 4.6 Billion overall for the "Building Blocks" to allow their progression by the Australian Commonwealth and State governments. COAG continues to monitor the progress and outcomes of the funding strategy.

The above discussion of government programs for the Indigenous peoples of Canada and Australia shows that government is able to construct realistic funded policy initiatives based on the accepted international principles defining primary health.

5. The Recovery Movement in mental health

The Recovery Movement in mental health has gained increasing momentum in recent years. Leff & Warner (2006) note that " the model refers both to the subjective experiences of hope, healing, empowerment and interpersonal support experienced by people with mental illness, their carers and service providers and to the creation of recovery-oriented services that engender a positive culture of healing and a support for human rights". The authors add that, as a result of the Recovery Movement, there is renewed interest in fighting the stigma that leads people with mental illness to lose their sense of self, to provide access to the services and education that give consumers the knowledge and skills to manage their illness, empowering consumers to share responsibility with providers in the healing process and providing access to peer support that validates the possibility of recovery (ibid). Recent discussion about the Recovery Movement has also focused on the "capabilities" approach of

Amartya Sen. Davidson et al (2010) note "the capabilities approach diverts our attention away from the possession of resources to the exercise of freedoms. This shift is not meant to deny the crucial role that resources play in social and political life but rather places emphasis on the fact that the usefulness of wealth lies in the things that it allows us to do-the substantive freedoms it helps us to achieve". The authors go on to argue that Sen's concepts of active agency and freedoms should apply to the "here and now" in respect to people's choices on a daily basis rather than some theoretical ideal future. In addition, the pursuit of agency generates diversity as each individual will pursue such agency according to individual need and a supporting system needs to accommodate such diversity (ibid). The end result should be to "increase the access of people with serious mental illness to opportunities and supports that allow them to live a decent and self determined quality of life" (ibid). Sen's economic concepts are also closely aligned to emerging discussions of social capital that are discussed later in the chapter.

Piat et al (2010) review a range of government initiatives to develop the recovery model. The US President's New Freedom Commission identified a fragmented health system and gaps in care as obstacles to recovery and this led to all 50 US States adopting recovery mission statements and implementing at least one evidence-based service. In New Zealand, discrimination and stigma were identified as most problematic and this led to a significantly enhanced role for psychiatric patients (consumers) within the system with good consumer-provider being identified as a key indicator for recovery orientated services (ibid).

Unfortunately, the economic basis of supporting effective recovery does not appear to have matched the theoretical process of empowerment and particularly so in the developed world. The observation that people suffering from schizophrenia often have a better outcome from disease in the third world (Warner 1986) may be related to the situation where economic opportunity (such as having meaningful work on a family farm or in a family kitchen) along with a place to sleep and adequate diet may be much easier to provide within the economic restraints and social supports of third world countries. Warner (ibid) has also commented on the nature of work in less developed countries that may be protective for someone suffering from severe mental illness. He notes that the person's family is less likely to emotionally smother the individual and the tasks allocated to the individual are likely to be geared to the level of performance that the person can actually achieve. In comparison, the costs of providing adequate housing and meaningful employment to individuals in developed countries are often significantly higher. In addition, it often has been difficult for governments to provide coordinated sustained funding for such programs across a range of different government departments that have responsibility for each program. The difficult task of addressing the above issues in the developed world is exemplified in a recent evaluation of the cost of mental illness in Canada in 2003. The review found that the cost of undiagnosed mental illness was about 28% of a total cost of $50,847 million dollars with direct medical costs of treating mental illness contributing only about 10% of this amount with the remainder being attributed to lost productivity (Lim et al 2008).

6. The Australian mental health plans and the Canadian Mental Health Commission

Federal Governments in both Australia and Canada have attempted to develop strategies to enhance services for those people affected by severe mental illness in a variety of ways.

Since the early 1990's, the Federal, in co-ordination with the State and Territory Governments of Australia have developed four successive mental health plans through the Australian Council of Health Ministers. The most recent plan of 2009-2014 has the following five priority areas for government action in mental health:

1. Social inclusion and recovery
2. Prevention and early intervention
3. Service access, coordination and continuity of care
4. Quality improvement and innovation and
5. Accountability - measuring and reporting progress. (DOHA 2009)

The authors of the plan note that "the plan is ambitious in its approach and for the first time includes a robust accountability framework. Each year, governments will report progress on implementation of the plan to the Council of Australian Governments. The plan includes indicators for monitoring change in the way the mental health system is working for people living with mental illness as well as their families and carers. Health ministers have agreed to develop targets and data sources for each of the indicators in the first twelve months of the plan." (ibid). Although the plan stresses "A Whole of Government Approach", it is unlikely that it will develop the appropriate sustained funding strategy to support outcomes similar to that initiated by the Council of Australian Governments National Action Plan on Mental Health 2006-2011 (COAG 2006), a government response to substantial deficiencies in public mental health provision outlined in the "Not For Service" Report (MHCA 2005). This contrasts with the normal rather disorganised system of mental health funding in Australia where one recent review (AHHA et al 2008) commented "there is still no single agency, organization or level of government with the remit and responsibility for the setting of strategic mental health policy or for the oversight, monitoring or operationalisation of mental health care. Funding methodologies and funding amounts vary between jurisdictions and have traditionally not been based on population need. This and the range of agencies and providers involved in the provision of mental health care has lead to inequities in access, service provision and health outcomes".

The Canadian Government established the Mental Health Commission for Canada in 2007. After extensive consultation with a range of stakeholders in Canada, the Commission published it's strategy document in 2009 (MHCC 2009). The strategy has seven goals: the engagement of people suffering from mental illness in the process of recovery, mental health promotion and mental illness prevention, a responsive mental health system, recognition of the role of families, equitable and timely access to effective treatments and support, actions informed by best evidence with measurable outcomes and support for research and social inclusiveness (ibid). The Commission was allocated $130 million by the Canadian Federal Government for 10 years in 2008 with the money being targeted towards the three key initiatives of the Commission which were to conduct a 10-year anti-stigma campaign, build a pan-Canadian Knowledge Exchange Centre, and elaborate a national mental health strategy for Canada (Government of Canada 2008). However, there does not appear to be any overall funding strategy for mental health in Canada apart from this with services being provided through it's Medicare system and mental health services bundled in with other general health services through the Regional Funding Authorities within each Province (Block et al 2008) It has been estimated that funding of mental health for Canada in 2003-2004 was 5% of total health spending which was lower than most developed countries (Jacobs et al 2008). Other authors have argued that the funding models of Medicare in Canada have led to the restriction of community services and other professional services such as psychologists for people suffering from mental illness (Mulvale et al 2007, Moulding et al 2009)

7. A new paradigm for mental health funding

Given the complexities of developing sustainable funding models for mental health, one solution would be to develop policy and funding strategies around a series of "pillars or "building blocks", similar to the Canadian Aboriginal Horizontal Framework and Council of Australian Governments National Indigenous Reform Agreement. This would align government policy to internationally accepted principles of health care and may allow a broader government overview and responsibility for the various components necessary to develop mental health. Funding could be allocated to each "pillar" and benchmarks attached to each pillar to assess progress. The "pillars" suggested are: Physical Health, Social Inclusion, Education, Effective Treatments, Substance Abuse, Mental Health Response to Disaster, Housing and Governance. Each one of these will be discussed in turn with a view to relevance and with mention of previous and current programs that could provide a basis of funding.

8. The physical health of people suffering from severe mental illness

There is a significant amount of information that people who suffer from serious mental illness also are at increased risk of increased morbidity and premature mortality from co-morbid medical illness. Viron & Stern (2010) talk of patients suffering from severe mental illness losing over 25 years of potential life with 87% of years of potential life lost being attributable to medical illness. They further comment that the mortality gap, based on data from 1997 to 2000 is 10 to 15 years wider than it was in the early 1990's. Observations at the beginning of the twentieth century noted that physical morbidity and mortality were greater amongst psychiatric patients than in the general population. Other commentators have noted the lack of thorough medical evaluation and inadequate treatment of medical disorders amongst psychiatric patients (Felker B et al 1996) . The issue of co-morbid medical conditions is particularly prominent in patients suffering from schizophrenia. This is not surprising given the social isolation, problems with adequate housing and the lack of organisation of proper meals and poor diet reported for this group of patients (Jablensky et al 2006, Brown et al 1999). High rates of tobacco and other substance use in this group also add to the disease burden (Jeste et al 1996).

Apart from the obvious issues of significant disability related to the illness process itself, there also appear to be a number of medical and health system barriers to recognition and management of medical illness in people with schizophrenia. Such barriers include a reluctance of non-psychiatrists to treat people with serious mental illness, frequent changes of treating doctor, lack of adequate follow up due to patients' itinerancy and lack of motivation and the available time and resources for an appropriate review of medical issues of people who may be uncooperative or have trouble communicating their physical needs (Lambert et al 2003). Higher rates of poverty in those experiencing severe mental illness (d'Amore et al 2001) along with stigma related to the experience of mental illness (Barney et al 2006) may also be further barriers patients with mental illness developing an effective relationship with a General Practitioner. The atypical antipsychotic medications may also lead to an increased prevalence of endocrine disorders such as Type 2 Diabetes (Lambert & Chapman 2004), thus necessitating increased medical vigilance in this regard.

As a way of attempting to improve the co-ordination of the care of medical illness in those patients with serious mental illness, there has been a significant stimulus to develop shared care models between psychiatric specialists and general practitioners. Such models include a Consultation-Liaison model (Gask et al 1997), collaborative case discussions between specialist psychiatrists and groups of General Practitioners (Davies et al 1997) and shared care projects with extensive education for involved General Practitioners (Meadows 1998). There have also been substantive improvements in remuneration for shared care in Australia with the Medicare Plus program encouraging a collaborative care mode.

The General Practice Clinic operated within a mental health service (Symonds & Parker 2007) compensates for a number of the barriers to health engagement discussed above and allows for a high quality of health care with extended clinical review times and health screening significantly above the Australian national average. Other recommendations for improved health care for people suffering from severe mental illness are: improved health screening and health promotion along with systemic models of medical and mental health care integration such as the VHA system in the USA (Viron & Stern 2010). Increased awareness by psychiatrists of the metabolic effects of psychotropic medication along with improved information to carers of people affected by severe mental illness in respect to appropriate medical care (De Hert et al 2010). Better co-ordination of a range of specialist services such as occupational therapists, pharmacists and dieticians in respect to the medical health care of people affected by severe mental illness may also be useful (Heald et al 2010).

9. Social Inclusion

A socially inclusive society is defined as one where all people feel valued, their differences are respected, and their basic needs are met so they can live in dignity. Social exclusion is the process of being shut out from the social, economic, political and cultural systems which contribute to the integration of a person into the community (Cappo 2002). Leff & Warner (2006) have outlined factors that lead to social exclusion for people affected by severe mental illness. These include the disabilities produced by the illness itself (such as the negative features of schizophrenia which include apathy and reluctance to engage with others), disabilities produced by professional care (including institutionalization and side effects of medication), stigmatizing attitudes of the public and self stigma of individuals (which may affect recognition of illness and ability to obtain appropriate treatment), media influences, poverty and discrimination in housing and employment.

Some of these factors are going to be considered in other sections of this chapter. The key focus on this area of social inclusion in the current context is addressing stigma and the maintenance of people suffering from severe mental illness within their social group. Sartorius (2010) discusses a range of barriers to effective campaigns to reduce stigma. He notes that anti-stigma campaigns have to be longer than a year to be effective. Sartorius comments that other factors that have been proven to reduce stigma such as legislation to effect employment and housing, ongoing promotion of useful strategies (such as education of health care professionals, public education forums for members of the public by people who have suffered from mental illness and avoidance of pejorative comments in the media) and permanent networks of interested business people, professionals, patients and their families that respond to local issues within cultures and communities.

To an extent, the *headspace* Model of Care for young people suffering from severe mental illness in Australia attempts to fulfill some of the above requirements in an organizational sense. A principal aim of *headspace* is "to establish a highly accessible, more specialized multidisciplinary model of care to target the core health needs of young people"(McGorry et al 2007). To enable these objectives, *headspace* has developed a number of funded centers within Australian local communities with the aim of building greater awareness of youth mental health within these communities and building capacity within these communities to ensure early detection and early intervention of emerging mental illness and substance use disorders, create a youth and family friendly environment, benefit from significant improvements in access, service integration and quality through co-location, secondment of clinical staff and outreach and access evidence-based interventions for the treatment of mental and substance use disorders (ibid).

The engagement of family members of people suffering from severe mental illness in the treatment process is crucial. This is because of the therapeutic value that family members may bring to the care of the person through their knowledge of expert and longitudinally developed information about the person which is helpful for appreciation of psychosocial deficits and current mental state in addition to their involvement in any case planning for the person's further management (Furlong & Leggatt 1996) Further evidence that therapeutic family interventions, particularly behavioural education, in reducing relapse for people suffering from schizophrenia and thus improving the cost-effectiveness of treatment (Mihalopoulos et al 2004) add emphasis to the value of family intervention in the illness.

The psychological effects of any chronic illness in relation to the family members of the person so affected are well recognised (Bloch et al 1994) Such factors include the issues surrounding the illness itself (acute onset, chronicity, acute exacerbation), the life-cycle stage of the family and the meaning of the illness to the family. Such "meaning" will be influenced by the family's previous experience of illness and belief systems about illness (ibid). Whilst these issues are relevant in the case of family members of someone suffering from schizophrenia, there is additional evidence of the devastating additional effect of the illness on family, leading to comments such as that recently made in a textbook of mental health law that "like other service providers but perhaps more than other service providers, the family and friends of the individual will have an emotional and practical interest in the fate of that individual" (Bartlett & Sandland 2003)

The family burden of living with a person suffering from a major mental illness such as schizophrenia is well described. It has been noted that stigma associated with the illness spreads to the whole family and may cause them to avoid talking about how they are feeling or deem themselves as social outcasts, leading to barriers between them and mental health professionals (Teschinsky 2000)

Recent reviews of the pressures faced by carers of people suffering from severe mental illness describe the "Objective Burden" that involves disruption to the household routines, finances and relationships and a "Subjective Burden" which involves the psychological consequences of the individual's illness for the family (Martens & Addington 2001, Wong et al 2008). The "Subjective Burden" of the illness appears to be higher for relatives of people experiencing first onset illness associated with schizophrenia (Martens & Addington 2001) and promotes the beneficial therapeutic value of psycho-education for the family in respect to information about the illness, illness management skills, communication skills and problem solving skills (Motlova 2007) therefore being an effective way of reducing this distress through empowerment of family members. Culture and differing family belief systems may be particularly important in this regard (Lesser 2004) The legal issues of confidentiality allowing such engagement with families are complex but can be negotiated in legislation, such as recent Mental Health Acts in Victoria and the Northern Territory of Australia (Parker et al 2010)

Participation in the workforce is an important factor in social inclusion. Warner (1983) comments that a key factor for any work for people affected by severe mental illness is that there should be stable expectations geared to the level of performance that the individual can actually achieve and this is more difficult to achieve in industrial society where there are high productivity requirements and competitive performance ratings. Further issues that may interfere with effective workforce participation in developed countries are co-morbid substance abuse and physical illness (Cornwell et al 2009). Employment programs for people affected with severe mental illness that are integrated into public mental health services appear to be one way to improve outcomes. One example of this is the Individual Placement and Support Approach in the United States that has been found to have almost a three fold increase in employment participation (60% versus 22%) (Waghorn et al 2007). A recent collaboration between Mental Health Services and the Vocational Education Sector in New South Wales that integrates supported education along with supported employment for mental health consumers is hoping to have similar results, maximising chances for consumer choice in employment and enhanced long term employment outcomes (VETE 2011, J McMahon pers comm). Apart from the economic benefits of the participation of people affected by severe mental illness in paid employment, there are also other personal benefits for those such engaged such as increased pride, self esteem, empowerment and facilitation with coping (Dunn et al 2008).

A range of issues may assist with social inclusion of individuals affected by severe mental illness in the third world. It has been noticed that cultural mechanisms may be more accepting of mental illness in these countries (Kermode et al 2009, Postert 2010). However, Rahman & Prince (2008) note that there is a significant amount of stigma experienced by families of people affected by severe mental illness in third world countries. They go on to suggest the incorporation of mental health treatment into primary care services as a way of reducing this stigma along with the training of primary care workers in the use of psychotropic medication. It has also been noted that regular use of such medication (with a subsequent reduction of difficult behaviours) may lead to greater social function and acceptance of the person within their community (de Jong & Komproe 2006).

10. Education

It has been recognised for a considerable period of time now that education in itself leads to empowerment in health. The review by DeWalt et al (2004) displayed that patients with poor literacy had poorer health outcomes including knowledge, intermediate disease markers, measures of morbidity, general health status and use of health resources. Cutler and Lleras-Muney (2006) suggest a range of mechanisms for education to enable health behaviours. They note that the effect of education increases with increasing years of education. Education in relation to income and occupational choice has some relationship to health empowerment but that different thinking and decision making patterns as a result of increased education may also have significant effects on health behaviours.

Henry (2007) comments on required "development platforms" which need to be in place for education to be effective. These include: security from violence, promotion of early childhood development, a home environment that is conducive to regular patterns of sleep and study, free from overcrowding and distraction and ready access to suitable primary health service infrastructure. A good example of the essential nature of such platforms to improved educational outcomes has been the success of the Clontarf Foundation education programs with Indigenous male adolescents in Australia. The Clontarf Foundation, a not for profit, organisation, was established in Western Australia in 2000. It was established to improve the discipline, life skills and self esteem of young Aboriginal men so that they can participate meaningfully in society. The Foundation currently has contact with 2000 young Aboriginal men in Western Australia and the Northern Territory. The Foundation's programmes to young Aboriginal men are delivered through a network of 25 Academies, each of which operates in partnership with (but independently of) a school or college. Australian Rules Football (AFL) is used to attract the young men to school and then keep them there. In order to remain in the program, participants must continue to work at school and embrace the objectives of the Foundation, Each Academy has an individual staff member who, in addition to delivering the football program, acts as a mentor and trainer addressing many of the negatives impacting on the young men's lives. Many of the Academy staff are ex AFL players. Participation by young Aboriginal men in the Clontarf Foundation has resulted in significantly increased retention rates for the participants through to the completion of secondary education and then on to participation in the workforce. By the end of 2008, 41 (76%) graduates of the 2007 program were employed. In April 2009, 51 of the 76 graduates of the 2008 program were in full time employment (Clontarf Foundation 2010)

Examples of successful education programs in mental health are: initiatives to improve mental health literacy, education programs to empower carers of people affected by severe mental illness and mental health training for police.

Health literacy appears to be a key component of improved education and health outcomes. Health literacy has been defined as "the ability to gain access to, understand and use information in ways which promote and maintain good health (Jorm et al 1997) Jorm and his colleagues found that health literacy in respect to mental health was not well developed amongst a sample of the Australian population and that this lead to unwillingness to accept help from mental health professionals or to a lack of adherence to advice given (ibid).

A potential solution to poor health literacy are the "mental health first aid training programs" developed for the Aboriginal and Torres Strait Islander Population of Australia (Kanowski et al 2009) in addition to the wider Australian population (Kitchener & Jorm 2006) The programs aim to provide help to a person developing a mental health problem or in a mental health crisis (Kanowsky et al 2009) and are aimed at Instructors who develop the skills for staff working in Aboriginal and Torres Strait Islander primary health organisations. The programs are based on education about a range of symptoms of mental illness as well as a response to a range of potential mental health scenarios such as helping a suicidal person, a person experiencing a panic attack, a person who has experienced a traumatic event and a psychotic person who is perceived to be threatening (Kitchener & Jorm 2006). It was estimated that in 2005, 350 people who worked area health services, non government organisations, government departments or as private practitioners had completed the Instructor training in Australia (ibid).

A further, school based initiative in mental health literacy is the "Mind Matters" Curriculum that was developed for Australian Secondary Schools (Wyn et al 2000) The project is based on a model of school change developed by the World Health Organisation and involves curriculum materials about emotional and mental health issues in addition to creating a school environment that is safe, responsive to student needs and that assists students in their ability to cope with challenges and stress (ibid).

Psycho-education for the family involving information about the illness, illness management skills, communication skills and problem solving skills (Motlova 2007) has been demonstrated to be an effective way of reducing this distress. It has been shown that, as a result of the training, families become empowered to better manage their relative's mental illness and their reactions to it. A recent evaluation of formal group training provided to carers of people affected by early psychosis resulted in the carers reporting less isolation, improved confidence, greater understanding of psychosis, reduction in guilt and increased confidence in their caring role (Riley et al 2011).

Education of other professional groups who have involvement with people affected by severe mental illness is also an important aspect to the strategy to improve knowledge and skills and effect better management of these individuals. A good example of this is the Mental Health Intervention Team Course offered by the New South Wales Police Force (Donohue D et al 2009). It is recognised that police often are at the fore front of interactions with people who are severely affected by mental illness and may significantly aroused as a result. Kesic et al (2010) in a review of fatalities as a result of interaction with police in Victoria found that 54.2% (26/48) of the victims had a history of DSM IV Axis I disorder, 39.6% of the 48 events had a history of substance abuse/dependence, 10.4% had formal diagnosis of Axis II personality disorder and that 87.5% were known in some capacity to mental health services or police. It was also estimated that in any given year, Currently New South Wales Police Officers can expect to attend approximately 22,000 mental health related incidents (about 30% of total call outs per year) with some of the incidents posing the biggest risk to their safety (Donohue et al 2009).

The New South Wales Police Mental Health Intervention Team course runs over four days and includes formal education sessions in respect to mental illness, substance abuse, legal issues and available services in addition to "real situation" education scenarios such as role plays. The formal aims of the course are: to reduce the rate of injury to police and mental health consumers on interaction, improve awareness amongst front line police of the risks involved in mental health incidents, improve collaboration with other government and non government agencies in the response to, and management of mental health crisis incidents and reducing the time taken by police in the handover of mental health consumers to the health care system. An important aspect to the education is the participation of mental health consumers and carers in educating police about the way that they are affected by symptoms and the way that they would like to be approached during acute exacerbations of their illness. The effect of severe mental illness on the carers was also well appreciated by the police participants of the course that I attended and police commented that they found the sessions with mental health consumers and carers some of the most valuable learning that they took from the course. Police (ranging from Area Commanders to constables) who attend the course are awarded a course badge as a formal "police appointment" to be worn on their uniform at the conclusion of the course. To an extent, this also allows people who are severely affected by mental illness and who are in crisis to recognise that attending police, wearing the badge, have training to assist them.

11. Effective treatments

Effective treatments (underpinned by rigorous and continuing research) are an essential component of any broad strategy for quality mental health service delivery. The treatments have specific costs that obviously inform public policy in respect to what particular economies and cultures are prepared to fund. As an example, the Tolkien II team have estimated that the average cost of treating a case of depression in Australia in 2005 was $175,566 with psychological therapies and medication. Tolkien II Team (2006). Effective therapeutic interventions are also a major area of concern for key stakeholders of mental health services with this area being considered most important in a recent European survey of Mental Health Recovery initiatives (Turton et al 2010).

A crucial issue that informs the above economic models is the use of Evidence Based Practice as a gold standard for funding decisions. There are complexities with this issue, however. Tanenbaum (2005) defines three potential controversies and a caveat in respect to evidence base practice in mental health policy. The first controversy is how restrictive should the definition of the evidence be and whether dominant definitions privilege some forms of treatment over others. The second controversy raised by Tanenbaum is that there is a significant difficulty translating research findings into clinical practice and this relates to a larger controversy in mental health about whether practice is in fact applied science. It also focuses on a significant paradox where the 'significantly filtered" study populations of pharmaceutical trials often have little in common with the complex patients treated by clinicians (Westen 2005). Tanenbaum's third controversy is "the definition of *effective* health care and who decides the benchmarks for *effectiveness*".

Notwithstanding the above controversies, there has been increasing emphasis in recent times on evidence based guidelines for the treatment of mental illness with initiatives such as the American Psychiatric Association Practice Guidelines (APA 2011) and the Clinical Practice Guidelines introduced by the Royal Australian and New Zealand College of Psychiatrists (RANZCP 2011)

However, research has consistently shown that education efforts alone do not appear to strongly influence healthcare provider practitioner behaviours in comparison to a range of factors that have been demonstrated to influence such behaviours such as consumer demand for services, financial incentives and penalties, administrative rules and regulations and feedback on practice patterns (Mueser et al 2003). The authors go on to suggest six Evidence-Based Packages that may be useful in the management of people affected by severe mental illness. These are collaborative psychopharmacology, assertive community treatment, family psycho education, supported employment, illness management and recovery skills and integrated dual diagnosis treatment. Mueser et al also propose an implementation strategy for the packages that will enhance their success. These involve standardized complementary training and consultation packages for mental health centres in addition to discussion with health authorities in respect to financing, regulatory and contracting mechanisms to support the introduction of the Evidence-Based Packages (ibid). Specific attitudes of mental health providers that may need to be addressed in the adoption of Evidence-Based Packages are the intuitive appeal of the package, the strength of the requirement to adopt the package on the individual, the openness to new practice and the divergence of usual practice with research based/ academically developed interventions (Aarons 2004)

Further issues that considerably affect the implementation of evidence based practice are the pressure on policy makers to justify the allocation of resources and demonstrate add on value, the need for practitioners to have confidence in the likely success of implementing the interventions and that the people who are likely to benefit see that the program and it's process of implementation are participatory and relevant to their needs. A further challenge is the application of existing evidence to good practice on the ground, particularly in disadvantaged and low income countries (Barry & McQueen 2005)

Given the above difficulties, an effective best practice model will probably be optimally provided by a knowledge of basic science, best evidence via knowledge of epidemiology and randomised controlled studies along with interpretation and individualisation related to clinical experience and available resources (Belmaker R pers comm.). However, effective treatments will continue to be a constant objective of appropriate funding priority in mental health and require a governance mechanism to review their ongoing usefulness and economic priority.

12. Substance abuse and mental illness

In the current era, no effective mental health policy can be expected to succeed without some measures to control substance abuse that precipitates and sustains mental illness. Although this area is complex and may appear somewhat overwhelming, a brief overview of a major area of practice and public health appears to show a number of factors worthy of policy intervention in a broad sense.

There is substantial evidence that children exposed to trauma in their domestic environment are at later risk of severe mental illness such as schizophrenia (Harley et al 2010) and substance abuse (ibid). There are a number of explanatory models for this with stress exacerbating genetic vulnerability to mental illness (Xie et al 2009) and people using substances to self medicate PTSD resulting from childhood trauma as well as increased substance abuse in the context of dysfunctional personalities (Jonson-Reid et al 2009))and aberrant emotional attachment (Rees 2005).

Alcohol abuse continues to be a major contributor to childhood trauma (Nelson et al 2010) with the children of alcoholic parents exhibiting higher rates of anxiety and depression (Eiden et al 2009). In addition, alcohol has further effects such as the higher rates of anxiety and depression in children affected by foetal alcohol syndrome (Hellemans et al 2009)

There is also a growing body of evidence in respect to the close association of substance abuse and mental illness, particularly in respect to cannabis and amphetamine abuse. Paparelli et al (2011) in their review article point to emerging consistent evidence between cannabis abuse and an increased risk of psychiatric symptoms and chronic illness. The authors also discuss the increased risk of psychosis as a result of repeated amphetamine and methamphetamine abuse and point to evidence of probable neuronal damage due to repeated methamphetamine abuse. The issue of brain damage related to amphetamine use was also demonstrated in a recent pilot study that appeared to show that 1:5 of young people who presented to a hospital ED in the context of amphetamine abuse had an occult brain lesion, as a result of their amphetamine abuse, on MRI scans (Fatovich et al 2010).

A range of strategies have been suggested for successful intervention with mental illness and substance abuse. Legislative measures such as increased excise on alcohol, improved policing of drink driving and reducing availability of alcohol to young people through a minimum legal purchase age have been shown to be highly effective in reducing alcohol related harm in Germany (Walter et al 2010). Recent information from Australia indicates that improved policing in respect to amphetamine abuse may have been a factor in reducing inpatient admissions from psychosis secondary to psycho-stimulants (Sara et al 2011). Innovative primary care approaches to managing cannabis abuse (Lubman & Baker 2010) and stimulant abuse (Frei 2010) have also found to be useful. Such management approaches involve improved screening for substance abuse and mental health problems, education and self monitoring for affected individuals, developing harm reduction strategies and patient empowerment through exploring options for change and negotiating a change plan.

13. Mental health response to disaster and trauma informed care

Some of the earliest written records in human history from Sumeria in 2000BC record the anguish and suffering of the population following the destruction of Nippur (Kinzie & Goetz 1996). In more modern times, there has been increasing recognition in a more rigorous scientific manner on the significant psychological and psychiatric sequelae resulting from people affected by disasters (Norris et al 2002)

This increased recognition has also occurred in the co-incident context of political recognition of high public expectation in respect to the quality of services that government in the developed world provides to it's citizens involved in a disaster. As an example of this the British Foreign Secretary, Jack Straw, on the anniversary of the 2004 tsunami, apologised to British families caught up in the disaster who had not received adequate support, commenting that British citizens have "very high expectations of what the British government can deliver and fair enough" (Eyre 2008). This co-incident context is of significant concern given projected estimations that in Australia, 65% of men and 50% of women may be exposed to a traumatic event during their lifetime (Forbes et al 2007) and with the current prevalence for PTSD being 1.3%, or 20,000 cases per year (ibid).

In recent years, there also has been increased identification of the effect of historical trauma as a subjective experiencing and remembering of events in the mind of an individual or the life of a community, passed from adults to children in cyclic processes and how this intergenerational trauma can lead to the breakdown of a functional society (Atkinson et al 2010). In this context, Professor Helen Milroy (pers comm) also describes the phenomenon of "Malignant Grief" as an end result of persistent intergenerational trauma and stress experienced in Australian Indigenous communities. Professor Milroy defines Malignant Grief as a process of irresolvable, collective and cumulative grief that affects Australian Indigenous individuals and communities. The grief causes individuals and communities to lose function, become progressively worse and ultimately leads to death. Professor Milroy further comments that the grief has invasive properties, spreading throughout the body and that many of Australia's Indigenous people die of this grief.

Enhanced clinician skills for clinicians to assist people affected by disaster and trauma as the need arises can be incorporated into organisational development within mental health services (Guscott et al 2007). On occasion, specific programs may need to be developed to address mass population trauma such as the one organised by the Peking Institute of Mental Health to assist clinicians and volunteers working with the Chinese population effected by the Sichuan earthquake in 2008 (Parker et al 2009). In addition, enhanced education resources devoted to the appropriate response of mental health clinicians to those affected by disaster (Ursano et al 2007) can guide appropriate economic and managerial responses by governments and health organizations.

14. Housing

Homelessness amongst people affected by severe mental illness is a continuing concern. In a recent series of nationwide meetings to discuss mental health policy and service provision in Australia, the lack of appropriate housing for the mentally ill was a consistent and significant theme in the discussions amongst a wide group of stakeholders (R Irving pers comm.). It has been estimated that 46% of homeless people in the United States may have a mental illness (O'Hara 2007) with another review estimating prevalence rates of psychosis at around 10 to

13% and a prevalence of affective disorders at around 20 to 40 % in homeless people (Schanzer et al 2007) Homelessness is also associated with higher rates of readmission to inpatient units along with longer inpatient stays (ibid). Additionally, homelessness is linked with excess mortality and particularly so with homeless people who abuse substances (Morrison 2009). Poverty, disabling health, behavioural issues co morbid substance abuse, competition for available public housing stock along with complex processes in applying for such stock all limit the opportunity for the mentally ill to access appropriate housing (O'Hara 2007). In addition, conventional categorical funding streams, bureaucratic program requirements, narrow administrative approaches to resource allocation and management and staff skills not geared to supporting the mentally ill in normal housing have been thought to have limited successful involvement by mental health services in this area (ibid).

It has also been noted that housing is a significant aspect of the recovery for people affected by severe mental illness with the concept of a "home" providing "roots, identity, security, belonging and a place of emotional wellbeing" (The PLoS Medicine Editors 2008). The "home" concepts that appear to be valued by the mentally ill are considered to be markers of ontological security: namely constancy, daily routines, privacy and a secure base for identity construction (Padgett 2007). It appears that different levels of housing support may be appropriate in this regard with supervised housing being more appropriate for people with severe disability from mental illness with a graduation to independent housing in the context of recovery (Tsai et al 2010).

Apart from the humanitarian aspects of the provision of a "home" to enhance recovery for people affected by severe mental illness, there also appear to be economic benefits generally with potential savings from repeated and lengthy hospital admissions that should encourage further strategies in this area.

15. Governance

The development of effective governance processes to enable the mental health of a population should be the major concern of any government and health authority. Effective governance processes should have a continuing "flow on" effect over many years with demonstrated benefit for people affected by severe mental illness, their families and communities. Mulvale et al (2007) point to the way that historical factors can mitigate against good governance in developing a modern mental health system that reflects recovery principles. Alternatively, O'Connor and Paton (2008) elaborate key aspects of a modern clinical governance framework (safety of patients and staff, consumer and family focus and participation, a skilled and valued workforce, incidents as learning opportunities, continuous improvement of clinical care, structures of accountability) and the ways that such aspects can be supported at various levels of a health system in the developed world. Governance systems should also be underpinned by strong ethical principles in respect to the appropriate treatment for people affected by mental illness. A good example of such ethical principles is the Code of Ethics produced by the Royal Australian and New Zealand College of Psychiatrists (RANZCP 2010).

In an economic sense, it appears that the key objective of any governance system for mental health would be to maximise the potential of people affected by mental illness in respect to their human value and their contribution to their community and society in general. Porter (2010a) argues that any value in an individual's health status is measured by outputs rather than inputs and depends on actual patient outcomes, not the volume of services delivered.

Porter further notes that such outcomes should involve survival, functional status, sustainability of outcome and "others". Eriksson (2011) comments on a number of preconditions to enhance individual social capital, a significant component of human value, which then results in enhanced health. These are a Macro Structure (Social and Political conditions, Income distribution) and Social Network Characteristics (Internalised Norms, Group Solidarity and Reciprocity) that lead to enhanced social support, social influence, social control, social participation and material resources) which lead to health benefits such as access to support, health enhancing behaviours, increased status and rewards, enhanced cognitive skills, belongingness and meaning of predicament along with improved access to health services and job opportunities. Eriksson (ibid) reports that trust and reciprocity are essential cognitive features of such collective and individual social capital and that these appear to be core elements for creating a health supporting environment, one of the five action areas for health promotion defined by the Ottawa charter. It could, therefore be argued that elements of the above should underpin any governance to enhance mental health.

Other key aspects of governance as outlined by O'Connor and Paton above is the development of appropriate mental health legislation and mental health service policies to protect patients, their carers and the community and comparative surveillance of such developments. The Mental Health Atlas (World Health Organisation 2005) reports and compares the presence in and population coverage of mental health legislation and mental health service policies in a range of world regions. The Atlas similarly reports on workforce for mental health. However, statistics do not necessarily supply the full picture of emerging trends. An example is the significant potential decline in numbers of mental health nursing workforce in Australia. Changes to nurse education in the 1980's along with the changing nature of work in psychiatric nursing appear to have significantly reduced the entry of young people into the profession. As a result, there may be major problems replacing the current workforce as they retire, leading to a severe workforce shortage in about a decade.

Mental health consumer employment within mental health services is an emerging and welcome development with consumer assisted services enhancing consumer outcomes with improved social functioning and reduced symptom severity and hospitalization (Nestor & Galletly 2008). However, it is essential that such consumer consultants be supported with training in addition to appropriate pay and conditions (ibid). The value of the role of family and carers in the management of people affected by severe mental illness is also being increasing recognised (Parker et al 2010).

The increasing use of outcome measures to assess disability and recovery as well as benchmarking where mental health services are gauged against each other and a number of key performance indicators (Coombs et al 2011) is another emerging mechanism in governance that needs to be considered. Porter (2010b) goes on to suggest a revised tier of hierarchies that is appropriate to assessing health outcomes. Tier One is whether the patient's health status is achieved or retained. Tier Two is the process of recovery of the patient and involves the time taken to achieve recovery and best attainable function in addition to the "disutility" of the care process (complications of treatment such as missed diagnoses and the ability to work whilst undergoing treatment). Tier Three involves the sustainability of the treatment process itself as well as any new health problems related to treatment. Such work encourages different ways of viewing different aspects of recovery in mental health and may allow a more accurate estimation of the economic basis of mental health management.

16. Conclusion

The previous chapter has briefly outlined eight potential "mental health pillars of wisdom" that should be a strategic focus in any mental health funding formula to emphasise Recovery. The formula can obviously be adjusted to local economic social and cultural needs but provides a more comprehensive vision of a future for the provision of mental health. The "pillars" are also useful entities to attach specific funding priorities as well as benchmarks to assess achievement in each area.

17. References

Aarons G (2004) Mental Health Provider Attitudes Toward Adoption of Evidence-Based Practice: The Evidence-Based Practice Attitude Scale; *Ment Health Serv Res;* 6 (2): 61-74.

AHHA et al (2008) Australian Healthcare and Hospitals Association, The Mental Health Services Conference of Australia and New Zealand & PricewaterhouseCoopers; *Mental Health Funding Methodologies: Roundtable Discussion Paper*

AHMAC (Australian Health Ministers Advisory Council), (2006). *Aboriginal and Torres Strait Islander Health performance Framework Report,* AHMAC Canberra

Anderson I (1997) "The National Aboriginal Health Strategy" in Gardner H (ed) *Health Policy in Australia* Oxford University Press

APA (2011) American Psychiatric Association Practice Guidelines (http://www.psych.org/mainmenu/psychiatricpractice/practiceguidelines_1.aspx (Accessed January 2011)

Atkinson J, Nelson J & Atkinson C (2010) Trauma, Transgenerational Transfer and Effects on Community Wellbeing in Purdie N, Dudgeon P & Walker R (eds) *Working Together: Aboriginal and Torres Strait Islander Mental Health and Wellbeing Principles and Practice.* Australian Government. Canberra

Barney L, Griffiths K, Jorm A & Christensen H (2006) Stigma about depression and it's impact on help-seeking intentions. *Australian and New Zealand Journal of Psychiatry ;* 40: 51-54

Barry M & McQueen D (2005) The Nature of Evidence and It's use in Mental Health Promotion in Herrman H, Shekar S & Moodie R (Eds) *Promoting Mental Health: concepts, emerging evidence, practice*: Report of the World Health Organisation, Department of Mental Health and Substance Abuse in collaboration with the Victorian Health Promotion Foundation and the University of Melbourne

Bartlett P & Sandland R (2003) *Mental Health Law: Policy and Practice.* Second edition. Oxford University Press, Oxford.

Begg S, Vos T, Barker B, Stanley L & Lopez A (2008) Burden of disease and injury in Australia in the new millennium: measuring health loss from disease, injuries and risk factors. *Medical Journal of Australia*: 188 (1): 36-40

Bloch S, Hafner J, Harari E & Szmukler G (1994) *The Family in Clinical Psychiatry.* Oxford University Press, Melbourne.

Block R, Slomp M, Patterson S, Jacobs P, Ohinmaa AE, Yim R & Dewa C (2008) The Impact of Integrating Mental and General Health Services on Mental Health's Share of Total Health Care Spending in Alberta *Psychiatric Services* 59 (8): 860-863

Brown S, Birtwistle J, Roe L & Thompson C. (1999) The unhealthy lifestyle of people with schizophrenia. *Psychological Medicine.,* 29: 696-701

Browne G & Hemsley M (2010) Consumer participation in housing: reflecting on consumer preferences. *Australasian Psychiatry* 18(6): 579-583

Canada's Performance 2005: The Government of Canada's Contribution. Part 4: Aboriginal Peoples http://www.tbs-sct.gc.ca/report/govrev/05/cp-rc09_e.asp (accessed March 2008)

Cappo (2002) *Social inclusion initiative. Social inclusion,participation and empowerment.* Address to Australian Council of Social Services National Congress, Hobart,28–29 November.

Chandler M & Lalonde C (1998) Cultural Continuity as a hedge against suicide in Canada's First Nations. *Transcultural Psychiatry* 35(2): 191-219

Clontarf Foundation 2010 http://www.clontarffootball.com/ (accessed April 2010)

COAG (2006) Council of Australian Governments *National Action Plan on Mental Health 2006-2011* http://www.coag.gov.au/coag_meeting_outcomes/2006-07-14/docs/nap_mental_health.pdf (accessed March 2011)

COAG (2008) Council of Australian Governments *National Partnership Agreement on Indigenous Economic Participation* http://www.coag.gov.au/intergov_agreements/federal_financial_relations/docs/national_partnership/national_partnership_on_indigenous_economic_participation.pdf (accessed March 2011)

Coombs T, Walter G & Bronn P (2011) Overview of the National Mental health Benchmarking Project. *Australasian Psychiatry* 19 (1): 37-44

Cornwell K, Forbes C, Inder B & Meadows G (2009) Mental Illness and its effect on Labour Market Outcomes. *The Journal of Mental Health Policy and Economics*; 12; 107-118.

Cutler D & Lleras-Muney A (2006) Education and Health: Evaluating Theories and Evidence: *National Bureau of Economic Research Working Paper 12352*: National Bureau of Economic Research, Cambridge MA

D'Amore J, Hung O, Chiang W & Goldfrank L (2001) The epidemiology of the homeless population and it's impact on an urban emergency department. *Academic Emergency Medicine*, 8: 1051-1055

Davidson L, Rakfeldt J & Strauss J (2010) *The Roots of the Recovery Movement in Psychiatry.* Wiley-Blackwell Oxford

Davies JW, Ward WK, Groom GL, Wild AJ & Wild S. (1997) The case conferencing project: a first step towards shared care between general practitioners and a mental health service. *Australian and New Zealand Journal of Psychiatry*; 31(5):751-755

Declaration of Alma-Ata (1978) http://www.who.int/hpr/NPH/docs/declaration_almaata.pdf (Accessed March 2011)

De Hert M, van Winkel R, Van Eyck & Peuskens J (2010) Physical Health management in psychiatric settings: *European Psychiatry* 25 S22-S28

de Jong JT & Komproe IH (2006) A 15 year open study on a cohort of West African out patients with chronic psychosis *Soc Psychiatry Psychiatr Epidemiol* 41 (11); 897-903

De Walt D, Berkman N, Sheridan S, Lohr K & Pignone M (2004) Literacy and Health Outcomes: *J Gen Intern Med* 19: 1228-239

DOHA (Australian Department of Health and Ageing) (2009) *Fourth National Mental Health Plan – An agenda for collaborative government action in mental health* 2009–2014 Canberra: http://www.health.gov.au/internet/main/publishing.nsf/content/mental-pubs-f-plan09

Donohue D, Murphy S & Cowan D (2009) *Mental Health Intervention Team Course: Participant Guide*: NSW Police College, Goulburn

Druss BG, Hwang I, Petuhova M, Sampson NA, Wang PS & Kessler RC (2009) Impairment in role functioning in mental and chronic medical disorders in the United States: results from the National Comorbidity Survey Replication. *Molecular Psychiatry*; 14; 728-737

Dunn E, Wewiorski N & Rogers ES (2008) The Meaning and Importance of Employment to people in Recovery from Serious Mental illness: Results of a Qualitative Study; *Psychiatry Rehabilitation Journal* 32(1); 59-62

Eckersley R (2011) Troubled Youth, an island of misery in an ocean of happiness, or the tip of an iceberg of suffering? *Early Intervention in Psychiatry*; 5 (Suppl 1); 6-11

Eiden R, Molnar D, Colder C, Edwards E & Leonard K (2009) A Conceptual Model Predicting Internalizing Problems In Middle Childhood Among Children of Alcoholic and Non-alcoholic Fathers: The Role of Marital Aggression *J Stud Alcohol Drugs* 70; 741-750

Eriksson M (2011) Social capital and health-implications for health promotion. *Global Health Action*. 4; 5611 -DOI:10:3400/GHA.V4i0:5611

Eyre A (2008) Meeting the needs of people in emergencies; a review of UK experiences and capability. *Emerging Health Threats Journal* 1:e9. doi: 10.3134/ehtj;08.009

Fatovich D, McCoubrie D, Song S, Rosen D, Lawn N & Daly F (2010) Brain abnormalities detected on magnetic resonance imaging of amphetamine users presenting to an emergency department: a pilot study. *Medical Journal of Australia*: 193 (5) 266-268

Felker B, Yazel J & Short D (1996). Mortality and medical co-morbidity among psychiatric patients: a review. *Psychiatric Services*; 47: 1356-1363

Flood J (2006) *The Original Australians: Story of the Aboriginal People*. Allen and Unwin Sydney

Forbes D, Creamer M, Phelps A, Couineau, Bryant R, McFarlane A, Devilly G, Mathews L. Raphael B, Doran C, Merlin T & Newton S (2007) Australian guidelines for the treatment of adults with acute stress disorder and post traumatic stress disorder *Australian and New Zealand Journal of Psychiatry*; 41: 637-646

Franklin M-A & White I (1991) The history and politics of Aboriginal health in Reid and Trompf (eds) *The Health of Aboriginal Australia* Harcourt Brace Janovich; Sydney

Frei M (2010) Party drugs: Use and harm reduction. *Australian Family Physician* 39 (8) 558-561

Furlong M & Leggatt M (1996) Reconciling the patient's right to confidentiality and the family's need to know. *Australian and New Zealand Journal of Psychiatry*. 30; 614-622

Gask L, Sibbald B & Creed F(1997) Evaluating models of working at the interface between mental health services and primary care. *British Journal of Psychiatry* 1997;170:6-11

Government of Canada (2008) http://www.hc-sc.gc.ca/ahc-asc/media/nr-cp/_2008/2008_134-eng.php (Accessed December 2010)

Guscott W, Guscott T, Malingambi G & Parker R (2007) The Bali Bombings and the Evolving Mental Health Response to Disaster in Australia: Lessons from Darwin. *Journal of Psychiatric and Mental Health Nursing*, 14 :239-242

Harley M, Kelleher I, Clarke M, Lynch F, Arsenault L, Connor D, Fitzpatrick C & Cannon M (2010) Cannabis use and childhood trauma interact additively to increase the risk of psychotic symptoms in adolescence *Psychological Medicine* 40; 1627-1634

Heald A, Montejo A, Millar H, De Hart M, McCrae J & Correll C (2010) Management of Physical Health in patients with schizophrenia: practical recommendations *European Psychiatry* 25: S41-S45

Hellemans K, Sliwowska J, Verma P & Weinberg J (2009) Prenatal alcohol exposure: Fetal programming and later life vulnerability to stress, depression and anxiety disorders; *Neuroscience and Behaviour Reviews*: 34; 791-807.

Henry K (2007). *Addressing Extreme Disadvantage through Investment in Capability Development.* Closing Keynote Address to the Australian Institute of Health and Welfare Conference "Australia's Welfare 2007" www.treasury.gov.au/documents/1327/PDF/Health_and_Welfare_Conference.pdf - (accessed March 2008)

Herrman H, Shekar S & Moodie R (Eds) (2005) *Promoting Mental Health: concepts, emerging evidence, practice*: Report of the World Health Organisation, Department of Mental Health and Substance Abuse in collaboration with the Victorian Health Promotion Foundation and the University of Melbourne

HREOC (Human Rights and Equal Opportunity Commission). (2008) *CLOSETHEGAP: National Indigenous Health Equality Targets* , HREOC, Sydney.

Indian and Northern Affairs Canada Communications Branch (2004) *The Landscape: Public Opinion on Aboriginal and Northern Issues.* Minister of Public Works and Government Services. Canada

Jablensky A, McGrath J, Herrman H, Castle D, Gureje O, Evans M, Carr V, Morgan V, Korten A & Harvey C. 2000Psychotic disorders in urban areas: an overview of the Study on Low Prevalence Disorders. *Australian and New Zealand Journal of Psychiatry*; 34: 221-236

Jacobs P, Yim R, Ohinmaa AE, Eng , Dewa CS, Bland R, Block R & Slomp M (2008) Expenditures on mental health and addictions for Canadian provinces in 2003 and 2004 *Canadian Journal of Psychiatry* 53(5): 306-313

Jeffs S (2009) *Flying with paper wings: reflections on living with madness.* Vulgar Press Melbourne

Jeste D, Gladsjo J, Lindamer L & Lacro J. (1996) Medical Co-Morbidity in Schizophrenia. *Schizophrenia Bulletin*.: 22(3); 413-430

Jonson-Reid M, Presnall N, Drake B, Fox L, Bierut L, Reich W, Kane P, Todd R & Constantino J (2010) The Effects of Child Maltreatment and Inherited Liability on Antisocial Development: An Official Records Study: *J Am Acad Child Adoles Psychiatry*; 49 (4); 321-343

Jorm A, Korten A, Jacomb P, Christensen H, Rodgers B & Pollitt P (1997) "Mental health literacy" : a survey of the public's ability to recognise mental disorders and their beliefs about the effectiveness of treatment; *Medical Journal of Australia*: 166: 182-185

Kanowski L, Jorm A & Hart L (2009) A mental health first aid training program for Australian Aboriginal and Torres Strait Islander peoples: description and initial evaluation: *International Journal of Mental Health Systems* 3: 10 Published online 2009 June 3. doi: 10.1186/1752-4458-3-10.

Kermode M, Bowen K, Arole S, Pathare A & Jorm A (2009) Attitudes to people with mental disorders: a mental health literacy survey in the rural area of Maharashtra, India *Soc Psychiatry Psychiatr Epidemiology*; 44 (12): 1087-96

Kesic D, Thomas S & Ogloff J (2010) Mental illness among police fatalities in Victoria 1982-2007: case linkage study: *Australian and New Zealand Journal of Psychiatry*; 44: 463-468

Kinzie JD & Goetz RR (1996) A Century of Controversy Surrounding Post Traumatic Stress-Spectrum Syndromes: The Impact on DSM III and DSM IV, *Journal of Traumatic Stress*; 9(2): 159-179

Kirmayer L, Brass G & Tait C (2000). The Mental Health of Aboriginal Peoples: Transformations of Identity and Community. *Canadian Journal of Psychiatry*, 45: 607-616

Kitchener B & Jorm A (2006) Mental health first aid training: a review of evaluation studies: *Australian and New Zealand Journal of Psychiatry*; 40: 6-8.

Lambert T, Velakoulis D & Pantelis C. (2003) Medical co-morbidity in schizophrenia. *Medical Journal of Australia* 2003; 178: S67-70

Lambert T & Chapman L. (2004) Diabetes, psychotic disorders and antipsychotic therapy: a consensus statement. *Medical Journal of Australia*, 181 (10), 544-548

Leff J & Warner R (2006) *Social Inclusion of People with Mental illness*. Cambridge University Press. Cambridge UK

Lesser J (2004) All Care and Whose Responsibility. *Psychiatry, Psychology and Law* 11 (2); 236-243

Lim K-L, Jacobs P, Ohinmaa A, Schopflacher D & Dewa CS (2008): A new population-based measure of the economic burden of mental illness in Canada; *Chronic Diseases in Canada*; 28 (3) 92-98

Lubman D & Baker A (2010) Cannabis and mental health: Management in Primary care. *Australian Family Physician* 39 (8) 554-557

Luhrmann T (2008) "The Street Will Drive You Crazy"; Why Homeless Psychotic Women in the Institutional Circuit in the United States Often Say No to Offers of Help. *American Journal of Psychiatry*; 165; 15-20

MacMillan H, MacMillan A, Offord D & Dingle J (1996). Aboriginal health. *Canadian Medical Association Journal*. 155(11), 1569-1578

Martens L & Addington J (2001) The psychological well being of family members of individuals with schizophrenia. *Soc Psychiatry, Psychiatr Epidemiology*. 36: 128-135

McGorry P, Tanti C, Stokes R, Hickie I, Carnell K, Littlefield L & Moran J (2007) *headspace*: Australia's National Youth Mental Health Foundation-where young minds come first; *Medical Journal of Australia*; 187(7) S68-S70

Meadows G. (1998) Establishing a collaborative model for primary mental health care. *Medical Journal of Australia* 1998; 168(4): 162-165

MHCA (2005) Mental Health Council of Australia. *Not For Service: Experiences of Injustice and Despair in Mental Health Care in Australia*, Canberra. http://www.hreoc.gov.au/disability_rights/notforservice/documents/NFS_Final doc.pdf (Accessed March 2011).

MHCC (2009) Mental Health Commission of Canada: *Toward Recovery and Well-Being: A Framework for a Mental Health Strategy in Canada*: Ottawa

Mihalopoulos C, Magnus A, Carter R & Vos T (2004) Assessing cost-effectiveness in mental health: family interventions for schizophrenia and related conditions. *Australian and new Zealand Journal of Psychiatry*: 38: 511-519

Milroy H, Milroy J, Parker R & Phillips N (2003) *Aboriginal and Torres Strait Islander Mental Health* Education Unit for the PCP Course offered by the NSW Institute of Psychiatry. Sydney

Motlova L (2007) Schizophrenia and the Family. *Neuroendocrinology Letters* 28 (Suppl 1), : 147-159

Morrison D (2009) Homelessness as an independent risk factor for mortality: results from a retrospective cohort study. *International Journal of Epidemiology*; 38; 877-883

Moulding R, Grenier J, Blashki G, Ritchie P, Pirkis J & Chomienne M-H (2009) Integrating Psychologists into the Canadian Health Care System: The Example of Australia; *Canadian Journal of Public Health* 100(2) 145-147

Mueser K, Torrey W, Lynde D, Singer P & Drake R (2003) Implementing Evidence-Based Practices for people with Severe Mental Illness; *Behaviour Modification* 27 (3) 387-411

Mulvale G, Abelson J & Goering P (2007) Mental health service delivery in Ontario, Canada: how do policy legacies shape prospects for reform? *Health Economics, Policy and Law* 2; 363-389

Nelson E, Lynskey M, Heath A, Madden P & Martin N (2010) A Family Study of Adult Twins with and without a History of Childhood Abuse: Stability of Retrospective Reports of Maltreatment and Associated Family Measures *Twin Res Hum Genet* 13 (2) 121-130

Nestor P & Galletly S C (2008) The employment of consumers in mental health services; politically correct tokenism or genuinely useful? *Australasian Psychiatry* 16(5); 344-347

Norris F, Friedman M, Watson P, Byrne C, Diaz E, & Kaniasty K (2002). 60,000 Disaster Victims Speak :Part 1, An Empirical Review of the Empirical Literature, 1981-2001, *Psychiatry*; 65(3) 207-260.

O'Connor N & Paton M (2008) "Governance of" and "Governance by": implementing a clinical governance framework in an area mental health service; *Australasian Psychiatry* 16(2): 69-73

O'Hara A (2007) Housing for People with Mental Illness: Update of a Report to the President's New Freedom Commission. *Psychiatric Services*. 58 (7) 907-913

Ottawa Charter for Health Promotion (1986) http://www.who.int/hpr/NPH/docs/ottawa_charter_hp.pdf (Accessed march 2011)

Padgett D (2007) There's No Place Like (a) Home: Ontological Security Among People with Serious Mental Illness in the United States. *Soc Sci Med*; 64 (9): 1925-1936

Paparelli A, Di Forti M, Morrison P& Murray R (2011) Drug-induced psychosis; how to avoid star gazing in schizophrenia research by looking at more obvious sources of light. *Frontiers in Behavioural Neuroscience*: Volume 5, Article 1, 1-9

Paradis Y (2007) Racism in Carson B, Dunbar T, Chenhall R & Bailie R (eds) *Social Determinants of Indigenous Health* Allen and Unwin Sydney.

Parker R, Chee N, Coglan A, Fraser J & Raphael B (2009) The China-Australia Training on Psychological Crisis Intervention for Medical and Volunteers following the Sichuan Earthquake. *Medical Journal of Australia* 190 (9) 508-509

Parker R, Leggatt M & Crowe J (2010) Public Interest and Private Concern: The Role of Carers for People suffering from severe mental illness in the Twenty First Century *Australasian Psychiatry* 18 (2) 163-166.

Piat M , Sabetti J & Bloom D (2010) The Transformation of Mental Health Services to a Recovery Orientated System of Care: Canadian Decision Maker Perspectives: *International Journal of Social Psychiatry* 56(2): 168-177

Porter M (2010a) Value in Health Care: Supplementary Appendix 1 to What is Value in health care ? *N Engl J Med*; 363; 2477-81

Porter M (2010b) Value in Health Care: Supplementary Appendix 2 to What is Value in health care ? *N Engl J Med*; 363; 2477-81

Porter R (ed) (1991) *The Faber Book of Madness* Faber and Faber London

Postert C (2010) Moral agency, identity crisis and mental health; an anthropologist's plight and his Hmong ritual healing. *Cult Med Psychiatry*; 34 (1): 169-185)

Prince M, Patel V, Shekhar S, Maselka J, Phillips MR & Rahman A (2007) No health without mental health *Lancet*; 370; 859-877

Rahman A & Prince M (2008) Mental health in the Tropics: *Annals of Tropical Medicine and Parasitology* 102 (2) 89-110)

RANZCP (2010) Royal Australian and New Zealand College of Psychiatrists Code of Ethics (Accessed March 2011) http://www.ranzcp.org/images/stories/ranzcp-attachments/Resources/College_Statements/code_ethics_2010.pdf

RANZCP (2011) Royal Australian and New Zealand College of Psychiatrists (http://www.ranzcp.org/resources/clinical-practice-guidelines.html Accessed January 2011)

Rees C (2005) Thinking about children's attachment. *Arch Dis Child*; 90; 1058-1065

Riley G, Gregory N, Bellinger J, Davies N, Mabbott G & Sabourin R (2011) Carer's education groups for relatives with a first episode of psychosis: an evaluation of an eight week education group; *Early Intervention in Psychiatry*; 5; 57-63

Sara G, Burgess P, Malhi G & Whiteford H (2011) Amphetamine availability and admissions for psychosis in New South Wales, 2001-2009. *Australian and New Zealand Journal of Psychiatry*; 45: 317-324

Sartorius N (2010) Short-lived campaigns are not enough *Nature* 468; 164-166

Schanzer B, Dominguez B, Shrout P & Caton C (2007) Homelessness, Health Status and Health Care Use. *American Journal of Public Health*. 97 (3) 464-469)

Sen A (1999) *Development as Freedom*. Oxford University Press. Oxford

Symonds D & Parker R (2007) The Top End Mental Health Services General Practice Clinic: an initiative for patients with serious mental illness. *Australasian Psychiatry* 15 (1): 58-61

Tanenbaum S (2005) Evidence-Based Practice As Mental health Policy: Three Controversies and A Caveat; *Health Affairs* 24 (1); 163-173

Teschinsky U (2000) Living with Schizophrenia, the Family Experience. *Issues in Mental Health Nursing*. 21: 387-396.

Tolkien II Team (2006) *Tolkien II A Needs Based costed stepped care model for Mental Health Services*; Sydney: World Health Organization Collaborating Centre for Classification in Mental Health

The PLoS Medicine Editors (2008) Homelessness is just not a housing problem. *PLoS Med* 5(12): e1000003.doi:10 :1371/journal.pmed:1000003

Tsai J, Bond G, Salyers M, Godfrey J & Davis K (2010) Housing Preferences and choices among adults with mental illness and substance use disorders: A qualitative study. *Community Mental Health*; 46 (4); 381-388

Turton P, Wright C, White S, Killaspy H & DEMoBinc Group (2010). Promoting Recovery in Long-Term Institutional Mental Health Care: An International Delphi Study. *Psychiatric Services* 61 (3) 293-299

Ursano R, Fullerton C, Weisath L& Raphael B (2007) *Textbook of Disaster Psychiatry*. Cambridge University Press. Cambridge

VETE (2011) Vocational Education, Training and Employment Service, FACT SHEET ONE: Introduction to the Vocational Education, Training and Employment (VETE) Service http://www.sswahs.nsw.gov.au/mhealth/content/pdf/vete_factsheet_1.pdf (Accessed April 2011)

Viron M & Stern T (2010 The Impact of Serious Mental Illness on Health and Healthcare ; *Psychosomatics* 51(5) : 458-465)

Waghorn G, Collister L, Killackey E & Sherring J (2007) Challenges to implementing evidence-based supported employment in Australia: *Journal of Vocational Rehabilitation*; 27; 29-37

Walt G (2006) *Health Policy: An Introduction to Process and Power*. Eighth Impression. Zed Books. London

Walter M & Saggers S (2007) Poverty and Social Class in Carson B, Dunbar T, Chenhall R & Bailie R (eds) *Social Determinants of Indigenous Health* Allen and Unwin Sydney.

Walter U, Suhrcke M, Gerlich M & Boluarte T (2010) The opportunities for and obstacles against prevention; the example of Germany in the areas of tobacco and alcohol. *BMC Public Health* 10: 500 doi:10.1186/1471-2458-10-500

Warner R (1983) Recovery from schizophrenia in the Third World. *Psychiatry*; 46; 197-212

Westen D (2005) Are Research Patients and Clinical Trials Representative of Clinical Practice in Norcross J, Beutler L & Levant R (eds) *Evidence-Based Practices in Mental Health: Debate and Dialogue on Fundamental Questions* American Psychological Association. Washington DC.

Wong C, Davidson L, McGlashan T, Gerson R, Malaspina D & Corcoran C (2008) Comparable family burden in families of clinical high risk and recent onset psychosis. *Early Intervention in Psychiatry*. 2: 256-261

World Health Organisation (2005) *Mental Health Atlas*. World Health Organisation. Geneva

Wu EQ, Birnbaum HG, Shi L, Ball DE, Kessler RC, Moulis M & Aggarwal J (2005) The Economic Burden of Schizophrenia in the United states in 2002. *Journal of Clinical Psychiatry*; 66; 1122-1129

Wyn J, Cahill H, Holdsworth R, Rowling L & Carson S (2000) Mind Matters, a whole-school approach promoting mental health and wellbeing. *Australian and New Zealand Journal of Psychiatry*; 34; 594-601.

Xie P, Kranzler H, Polling J, Stein M, Anton R, Brady K, Weiss R, Farrer L & Gelernter J (2009) Interactive Effect of Stressful Life Events and the Serotonin Transporter 5-HTTLPR Genotype on Post Traumatic Stress Disorder Diagnosis in 2 Independent Populations; *Arch Gen Psychiatry* 66(11): 1201-1209

13

Three Decades of the Integrated Child Development Services Program in India: Progress and Problems

Niyi Awofeso[1,2] and Anu Rammohan[3]
[1]*School of Population Health, University of Western Australia,*
[2]*School of Public Health and Community Medicine, University of New South Wales*
[3]*Discipline of Economics, School of Business, University of Western Australia*
Australia

1. Introduction

It is understood that life success, health and emotional wellbeing have their roots in early childhood. Investing resources to support children in their early years of life brings long-term benefits to them and to the whole community. Early childhood development outcomes are therefore important markers of the welfare of children, and can predict future health and human capital. Well conducted research studies show that Early Child Development programs benefit children, families, and communities, and are associated with; higher and timelier school enrolment, higher school completion rates, improved nutrition and health status, child morbidity and mortality, improved social and emotional behaviour, and increased earning potential and economic self-sufficiency as an adult (Reynolds et al., 2001; Young, 1996).

Over the past three decades, India has experienced high prevalence of malnutrition despite increasing agricultural production and enviable economic growth. Some analysts have attributed this to poverty, spending patterns which favour festivals and non-essential foodstuffs over staple food, and high rates of infectious and chronic diseases (Banerjee & Duflo, 2006; Radhakrishna & Ravi, 2004). India's governments have sought to address chronic malnutrition through an extensive network of food-based social safety net, price controls for staple foods, income support, food-for-work programmes and direct provision of nutritious food to children. By far the biggest nutrition supplementation programme in India is the Integrated Child Development Services (ICDS).

Early childhood care and education services were prioritised in India's 1986 National Policy on Education as a crucial input into primary education and a significant support for women wishing to work in the formal sector. An inter-ministerial survey in 1972 revealed that child care programmes in India were not having the desired impact owing to resource constraints, inadequate coverage, and a fragmented approach. Consequently, India's ICDS was established in 1975 with the following objectives; (1) lay the foundation for the physical, psychological and social development of children; (2) improve the nutritional and health status of children in the age group 0-6 years and reduce the incidence of mortality, sickness, malnutrition and school dropout; (3) enhance, through improved health care and education, the ability of mothers to look after the normal needs of their children, and; (4) achieve effective co-ordination of policy and implementation among various departments responsible for child development (Kaul, 1993). The ICDS is estimated to be the world's largest integrated early childhood program, with over 40,000 centres established nationwide. The program covers over 4.8 million expectant and nursing mothers and over 23 million children under the age of six. Of these children, more than half participate in early learning activities. The network consists of 3907 projects, covering nearly 70 per cent of the country's community development blocks and 260 urban slum pockets.

ICDS programs are delivered through a network of projects in slum, rural or tribal areas. Rural or urban projects cater for populations of about 100,000 people divided into 100 centres or *Anganwadis* (literally courtyards), while tribal projects cater for populations of about 35,000 people divided into 50 centres. Each centre has a trained paraprofessional or Anganwadi worker - generally a local woman proposed by the community and trained for three months in health and nutrition education, community support and participation, pre-school education and record maintenance. Each project has four or five supervisors and one Child Development Officer who is responsible for the management and implementation of the entire programme in her/his jurisdiction (Lokshin et al, 2005). For children aged below 6 years, the core services offered for children are supplementary nutrition, immunisation, basic health care such as anti-helminth treatment, referral services to hospitals and health centres, non-formal pre-school education. For mothers, the core services offered are tetanus immunisation for expectant mothers, supplementary nutrition and health education (Muralialharari & Kaul, 1993). The ICDS services are delivered almost exclusively at the Anganwadi, or childcare centre. Each centre is run by an Anganwadi worker and one helper, who undergo three months of institutional training and four months of community-based training. The cost of the ICDS program averages $10-$22 per child a year (Dasgupta *et al*, 2005).

As at March 2008, the ICDS comprised 6120 operational projects and 1053006 *Anganwadi* centres, which reached about 58.1 million children (and 10.23 million pregnant or lactating women) , compared with 27.5 million children enrolled in 2000 (Kapil, 2002).

Despite increasing funding of the ICDS program over the past three decades, the ICDS has so far fallen short of its stated objectives. India's sub-optimal maternal and child health and education programs are exemplified by the following trends: India slipped from Millennium Development Goals (MDG) rank 128 in 2008 to 134 in 2009; India accounts for 50% of the world's hungry; At least 46% of Indian children are undernourished; in 2006, on average 254 women died giving birth to a child for every 100,000 live births relatively modest reduction from 327 in 1990. The states of Assam, Bihar, Chhattisgarh, Jharkhand, Madhya Pradesh, Orissa, Rajasthan, Uttar Pradesh and Uttaranchal had the highest numbers ranging from 480 to 312. Kerala at 95, Tamil Nadu at 111 and West Bengal at 141 fared less badly; Across India 74 children died before they reached the age of five for every 1,000 live births in 2005-06 as compared to 125 in 1990. At this rate India is likely to miss the target of reducing under-five mortality rate to 42 for 1,000 live births by 2015; About 400,000 infants die in the first 24 hours of their life and 90 per cent of deaths are due to preventable diseases like pneumonia and diarrhoea; India ranks 171 out of 175 countries in the world in public health spending; Despite 10.7% of the national budget devoted to education, only 61.9% of adult Indians aged over 15 years in 2008 (73.2% males and 56.9% females) were literate; India's measles vaccination coverage in India increased from 54% in 2000 to 70% in 2008, but this coverage is much lower than the 2008 global coverage of 83%. India achieved 23% measles mortality reduction between 2000 and 2008, but still accounts for two- thirds of the remaining global mortality from measles in 2008.; the proportion of underweight (severe and moderate) children below three years of age declined only marginally during 1998-99 to 2005-06, from about 47 to 46% and at this rate of decline is expected to come down to about 40% only by 2015 (UN, 2010; UNESCO, 2010; WHO, 2009).

The lack-lustre trends in children's nutrition in India occurred despite increased funding for the ICDS program, from $US35m in 1990 to $US170m in 2000, and a 2005 decision by the Indian government to accord high priority to the expansion of the ICDS program. Although major reforms in public health, and particularly in maternal and child health, are urgently required in India, it is debatable whether the management of the ICDS program is appropriate for the formidable maternal and child health challenges it was established to address. It is noteworthy that India's youth literacy rate increased from 61.9% in 1991 to 79.3% in 2008. India's 2009 MDG report (GI, 2010) projects a youth literacy rate of at least 98% by 2015. Thus, this chapter will be focussed on health-related components of the ICDS program.

A 2006 World Bank study of the ICDS (Lokshin et al, 2005) determined that the programme had little overall effect on nutritional outcomes, and that the only significant effect of the programme was a positive effect on boys' stunting in the data from the 1992 survey, but not in 1998. For girls, the effect was not significant. At regional levels, the only significant finding was a *negative* impact in the poor Northern states, and in the Northeastern states. There, children living in an ICDS village had a higher probability of being underweight in the 1998 survey. This chapter examines health management aspects of the operations of the ICDS program, with a focus on under-nutrition of children aged 0 - 3 years. Our central thesis is that sub-optimal health management is a major encumbrance to the realisation of the objectives of the ICDS program, especially in relation to improving children's nutrition levels.

Since malnutrition in India is mainly caused by inadequate nutrition, infectious diseases and poor sanitation, we also review public policies on food security. Public health services remain an important and cost-effective means of lowering the population's susceptibility to disease. According to Jalan and Ravallion (2003), the number of child deaths due to unsafe water is higher in India than any other country. Furthermore, World Bank estimates show that nearly a fifth of the rural Indian population does not have access to safe drinking water. It is therefore important that India's public and child health programs be complemented with community-based programmes that are specifically aimed at preventing under-nutrition and the spread of infectious diseases. India's public health and family health programs should include (at least on paper) infrastructure (water, sanitation, food storage, buildings), income generation, and provision of welfare and health safety nets. Community involvement and ownership are crucial, in contrast to the top-down delivery of health care in India (parts of which, like supplies, equipment, and trained personnel, remain necessary). Community-based, nutrition programmes have an important role in ensuring wide and timely coverage of key health services, such as immunization. Women's visits to health services, whether for curative or preventive child health care, are excellent opportunities for health workers to provide health and nutrition preventive services to women (e.g., education, counselling, and micronutrient supplements). This chapter utilises data on India's Family health surveys as well as government reports and scholarly articles to review health management facets of the ICDS, and proposes integrated strategies for revitalising India's child health services.

2. Review of health management aspects of ICDS

ICDS services are provided through a vast network of ICDS centres, better known as "Anganwadi". The term Anganwadi developed from the idea that a good early child care and development centre could be run with low cost local materials even when located in an 'Angan' or courtyard. The Anganwadi centre is operated by a modestly paid Anganwadi worker, assisted by an Anganwadi helper or *Sahayika*. The local Anganwadi is the cornerstone of the ICDS programme. The basic responsibility for implementing the programme rests with the State Government. The nodal department responsible for implementing ICDS at the state level is typically the Women and Child Development Department, or sometimes a related department (e.g. the Social Welfare Department). One Anganwadi worker is allotted to a population of 1000. However, this differs by state, with relatively affluent states having a better staff to child ratios. In order to provide supplementary nutrition, cooked food is provided to the children in the age group of 2-6 years, expectant and lactating mothers and adolescent girls. The Supplementary Nutrition Programme aims to provide up to 300 calories and 8-10 grams of protein to the children and 500 calories and 20-25 grams of protein to the lactating mothers, pregnant ladies and adolescent girls. Severely malnourished children are given double diet as compared to a normal child. Immunization services are provided to all children below six years of age, who are immunized against tuberculosis, diphtheria, whooping cough, tetanus, polio and measles.

Of all childhood nutrition programmes in India, the ICDS is the only one with federal legislative backing. For example, in 2006, On 13 December 2006, India's Supreme Court stipulated that the Government of India shall sanction and operationalize a minimum of 14 lakh AWCs in a phased and even manner starting forthwith and ending December 2008. The ruling stated that, while maintaining the upper limit of one AWC per 1000 population, the minimum limit for opening of a new AWC is a population of 300 may be kept in view. All the State Governments and Union Territories were directed to fully implement the ICDS scheme by, inter-alia, allocating and spending at least Rs.2 per child per day for supplementary nutrition out of which the Central Government shall contribute Rs.1 per child per day; allocating and spending at least Rs.2.70 for every severely malnourished child per day for supplementary nutrition out of which the Central Government shall contribute Rs.1.35 per child per day; allocating and spending at least Rs.2.30 for every pregnant women, nursing mother/adolescent girl per day for supplementary nutrition out of which the Central Government shall contribute Rs.1.15. (Right to Food campaign, 2007) .

Tarozzi and Mahajan (2007) documented an increase in gender inequality in nutritional status in India over the 1990s, with the nutritional status of boys improving substantially more than that of girls. Gragnolati et. al (2005) attribute much of the child malnutrition in India to the high levels of exposure to infection and inappropriate infant and young child feeding and caring practices in the first two to three years of a child's life. A persistent decline in per capita calorie consumption in India over the last twenty years has been documented (Deaton and Dreze, 2008; Ray, 2007) The declining trend occurred across all income levels, and at a point when the nutritional measures for children are worsening.

Program placement: Coverage of ICDS is modest relative to need. In 2009, it benefitted 34 million children aged 0-6 years and 7 million pregnant and lactating mothers. Programme coverage is especially high in the southern region, the north-eastern region, and the non-poor states of the northern region. Of the villages sampled by the NFHS, a third had an ICDS programme in place in 1992, and the figure had risen to more than half in 1998. The need for the ICDS program appears to be particularly high in the poor northern states of Bihar, Madhya Pradesh, Orissa, Rajasthan and Uttar Pradesh, where the proportion of stunted and underweight children exceeded 50% in the 1992 and 1998 surveys. The proportion of villages covered by ICDS activities in these region increased, on average from 28% to 43% between 1992 and 1998, compared with increases from 58% to 82% between 1992 and 1998 in the rich northern states of Gujarat, Haryana, Maharashtra and Punjab. The programme coverage is regressive relative to need, expenditure per child, and economic performance of the states. The states with the highest prevalence of stunted and underweight children, such as Bihar and Uttar Pradesh tend to have the lowest programme coverage. In 2001/2002, government expenditure per undernourished child in the 'rich' north states averaged 235 rupees, compared with 97 rupees in the 'poor' north states. Bihar (the poorest state) receives only Rs 25 per malnourished child, while Punjab (the richest state) receives Rs 334. Ironically, due to poor governance, Bihar spent only 76% of its ICDS allocation in 2003, compared with 98% of allocated ICDS funds spent by Punjab in the same year (Lokshin et al, 2005). The average resident in Bihar is at least four times poorer than the average person in Punjab. Bihar's government health expenditure per person in 2005 was 84 rupees, compared with 251 rupees in Punjab. Bihar's 2007 per capita income was 13663 rupees, compared with Punjab's 27,873 rupees (Berham & Ahuja, 2008). Based on wealth rankings, richer villages have a higher probability of being covered by the programme than poorer ones. For example, only half of the villages from the lowest two income deciles had the ICDS programme in place in 1998, while about 80 per cent of the richest villages in India were covered (Radhakrishna & Ravi. 2004).

Equity issues: Program placement closely reflect equity issues, but extend to include analysis of persistent inequalities in maternal and child health outcomes based on income level., caste, gender or rural residence. A recent analysis of trends in infant undernutrition in India between 1992 and 2005 using the nationally representative family health survey (Subramanyam et al, 2010) revealed that the overall prevalence (%) of underweight was 49.14, 43.82 and 40.26 in 1992, 1998 and 2005 respectively. The corresponding prevalence (%) of stunting was 52.43, 50.65, and 44.73. Social disparities in undernutrition over these 14 years either widened or stayed the same. The absolute rates of undernutrition decreased for everyone regardless of their social status. The disparities by household wealth were greater than the disparities by maternal education. There were no disparities in undernutrition by caste, gender or rural residence. Maternal education is improving, with the female literacy parity index of youths increasing from 0.64 in 1991 to 0.81 in 2001, and projected to reach parity by 2015. The bulk of the increase was in the poor states. For example, in Bihar, the female literacy rate in 2001 was 34%, compared with male literacy rate of 60%. By providing bicycles for year 9 and 10 students, and providing school uniforms free of charge to women, Bihar increased its year 9 enrolment of girls in year 9 by 170,000 in 2007, compared with 2006 prior to the commencement of the scheme However, addressing income inequity, the most influential determinant of infant undernutrition in India, remains a major challenge. The proportion of people below the national poverty line estimated for 1990 was 37%. By the year 2004-05, the poverty headcount ratio declined to 28%. The poorer and relatively populous states such as Bihar, Jharkhand, Chhattisgarh, Madhya Pradesh had about 193.5 million of people below poverty line in 2004-05 (64% of total people below poverty line) and are expected to have nearly 198 million people below poverty line in 2015 (71% of total people below poverty line (GI, 2010). Despite claims of rapid economic growth by Bihar and several other poor states, outmigration, poverty and inefficient health administration have not translated economic gains into significant improvements in maternal and child health.

Public health facilities are typically allocated on the basis of population (Koenig *et al.*, 2000). However, the quality of services is likely to depend on the level of economic development in the region; owing to the difficulties of relocating skilled medical personnel in remote areas.

In India, the Panchayati Raj Act has placed emphasis on building local government, and devolving health activities to them.

However, a rapid rise in private providers of healthcare, with a subsequent increase in its utilisation can in turn influence the quality of care in public facilities (Peters *et al.*, 2002). According to Bhargava *et al.* (2005) the healthcare infrastructure in India has evolved gradually over time and comprises of public facilities, private providers and NGO's. Initially, healthcare was available mainly in urban areas via government facilities and from private practitioners offering services to those who can afford them. Urban settings are considered to be more attractive to medical personnel, thereby restricting the pool of medical practitioners prepared to work in rural areas. This increase in supply of urban doctors has improved the quality of medical services in urban areas.

Government health expenditure in India is relatively low compared to other countries in the region and has actually declined over the last two decades. According to Bhalotra (2007), while government health expenditure constituted 1.3% of the GDP in 1990, this had declined to 0.9% in 1999. Relative to other countries in the region, India devotes a smaller share of its income to health spending than, for example, Bangladesh (1.4%) or Sri Lanka (1.8%) (Deolalikar 2005), and it spends a disproportionate part of its health budget on (curative) hospital services which are less pro-poor than (preventive) public health expenditures (Peters *et al.* 2002).

Jalan and Ravallion (2003) found a significantly lower prevalence and duration of diarrhoea among children living in households with piped water. Health gains from piped-water tend to be lower for children with less well-educated women in the household. It is possible that education is acting as a proxy for knowledge about how to assure that water is safe to drink and how best to treat illness. The income effect on the child-health benefits from piped water is also found at given levels of education, though it is not as pronounced. This is consistent with a previous study by Rajna et al (1998) which used data from the 1992-1993 National Family and Health Survey in India to show that improvements in health services, maternal education and provision of safe drinking water have had a desirable impact on child survival in Uttar Pradesh.

Health workforce: The World Health Report 2008 and the 62nd World Health Assembly resolution strongly reaffirmed the principles of primary health care. These principles include equity, solidarity, social justice, universal access to services, multi-sectoral action, decentralization and community participation as the basis for strengthening health systems and optimising the quality of health services (WHO, 2008). Member states were urged to train and retain adequate numbers and mix of health workers able to work in a multidisciplinary context (GO, 2006). The ICDS was conceptualised as a primary health care initiative, but not enough has been done so far to develop and retain adequate health workforce in terms of quantity, quality and distribution. There are around 1.5 million women workers engaged in the Anganwadi projects across India. Although each ICDS is staffed by several Anganwadi and community health officers (most of whom are Anganwadi with several years' experience), and headed by a maternal and Child Development Officer, the front-line staff is the Anganwadi, local women proposed by an ICDS village and trained in health and nutrition for at least three months. The Anganwadi workers are not normally gazetted as government workers, but are rather paid as casual staff. Anganwadi workers are expected to have completed high school. Those with less than high school education are employed as Anganwadi helpers. In announcing the 2008-2009 Budget, Indian Finance Minister Chidambaram stated that minimum salaries would be increased for Anganwadi workers to Rs 1500 ($US36) per month and helpers to Rs 750 ($US18) per month. In the public sector, the national minimum wage since 2009 is Rs 100 per day. On 4 May 2010, hundreds of Anganwadi workers from various parts of India staged a protest march in New Delhi demanding higher wages, job security and status of government servants with privileges of pension and allied retirement benefits. The wide inequity in remuneration between Anganwadi workers and the least paid Indian government employees is a major demotivating factor for the core human resource sector of the ICDS programme. There are also wide regional differences in salaries paid to Anganwadi, and this is a major source of perceived unfairness and demotivation for relatively lower paid staff. For example, in Puducherry, Anganwadi workers are paid Rs 12,000 per month workers and Anganwadi helpers paid Rs 6,000 monthly, compared with Rs 2000 monthly for Anganwadi workers and Rs 1200 monthly for helpers in Kamataka. Such perceived unfairness, coupled with other workforce-related encumbrances affecting Anganwadis, contribute to sub-optimal performance of this cadre of workers (Figure 1).

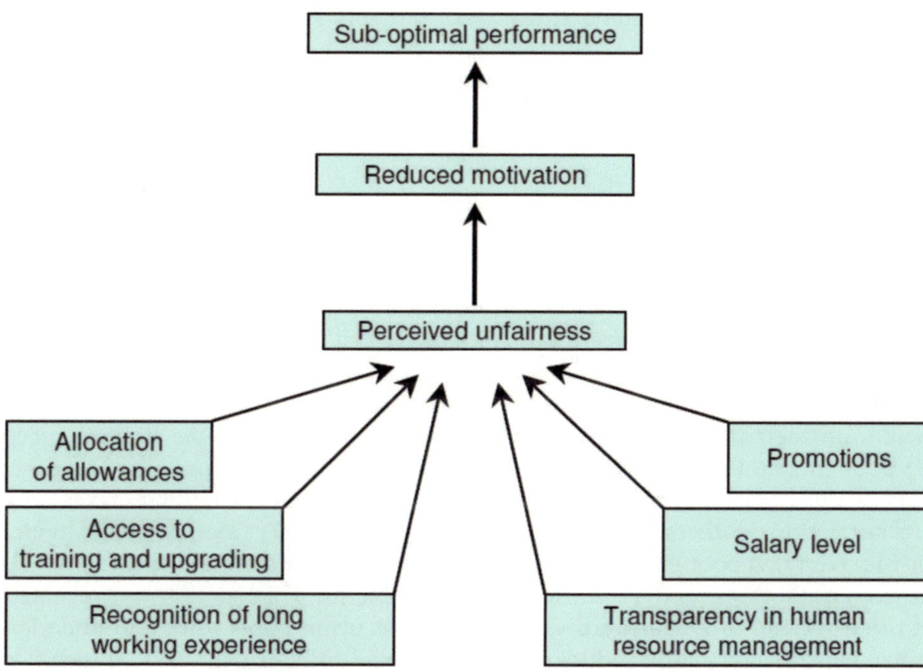

Fig. 1. Factors influencing health workers performance (Source; http://www.biomedcentral.com/content/pdf/1472-6963-11-34.pdf)

There are wide variations in the competence of Anganwadi workers, with some workers, particularly in the wealthier states having tertiary educational qualifications. It is in the most vulnerable states such as Bihar that qualified Anganwadi workers are in short supply. The distribution of Anganwadi workers is not fluid - being almost exclusively women, Anganwadi staff generally work in their areas of residence. Cultural encumbrances as well as lack of formal recognition of this cadre of workers are additional disincentives for mobility to underserved areas. Thus, areas with low female literacy are unlikely to have qualified Anganwadi workers. Such health workforce shortages explain why the ICDS program may paradoxically result in negative maternal and child health outcomes in poorer and remote regions of India where female education is low. Consequently, many centres, particularly in the poorer states such as Orissa are staffed by Anganwadi helpers, and these staff lack the necessary qualifications for the level of in-service training they are regularly invited to attend (GO, 2006; Udani et al, 1990). It is unrealistic to expect a high school graduate with three months training to adequately perform some of the tasks entrusted to Anganwadi workers, such as pre-school and health education, maintenance of records of births and deaths, administration of pulse-polio drops, and provision of supplementary nutrition to pregnant and lactating mothers and children up to the age of six. Access to Anganwadi training is inequitable. As at January 2008, Andhra Pradesh, whose maternal and child health indicators are higher than the national average, had 66 accredited Anganwadi training centres, while Bihar had none and Sikkim had only one, despite these two states having high levels of infant malnutrition and inferior maternal health outcomes compared with national average. In relation to food provision, for example, many states provide pre-packaged food which the Anganwadi workers describe as unpalatable to enrolled children. As a result, some Anganwadi workers have had buy food for severely malnourished children from their paltry salaries - a source of significant job dissatisfaction. Since 2009, Anganwadi workers and helpers have been advocating that the food preparation and supply must be localised and the responsibility for food procurement and preparation must be given to women's organisation instead of contractors, as is the case in Kerala and Tamil Nadu (Radhakrishna & Ravi, 2004).

Strategic approach to addressing undernutrition: A 2008 study of reasons for poor performance of health workers entailed interviews of Anganwadi and mothers in rural Wardha, Sewagram. Mothers of children enrolled in ICDS programs in this region lamented the poor quality of supplementary food. They reported that *Khichari*, a preparation of rice and dal (pulses), a common supplementary food, contained very little oil and dal component. So children refused to eat it every day. Although, there was variety in the supplementary food available, such as use of sprouted grains and green peas, they were less frequently prepared. Anganwadi, on their part listed the 12 most common reasons for the limited success of ICDS: 1) poor cooperation from villagers; 2) poor understanding of parents; 3) mothers do not follow medical advice; 4) mothers are busy with farm work; 5) Irregular and poor health check-up service; 6) mothers do not follow dietary advices; 7) poor personal hygiene of families; 8) poverty; 9) poor environmental sanitation; 10) poor child care practices; 11) poor support from authorities, and 12) various social problems. This survey also revealed that most of the workload of Anganwadi workers is taken up in paperwork and attendance at workshops, which significantly reduce the time devoted to their core ICDS duties (Dongre et al, 2008). Although the ICDS is the most well-known of India's national dedicated maternal and child health nutrition and education program, there are at least two other national and 10 regional nutrition and education programs in India, including National Mid-day Meal Scheme, the National Rural Health Mission, Comprehensive Rural Health Project, Integrated Nutrition and Health Program and the Public Distribution System. These programs appear to compete rather than collaborate with one another in the achievement of optimal maternal and child health outcomes (Tarozzi, 2002; Mann et al, 2010). India's public health system, on which all maternal and child health programs rely is poorly funded and poorly functioning. From an expenditure perspective, government spending on health per capita increased from Rs 202 to Rs 257 between 2000 and 2005. Adjusting for inflation, this increase is modest - Rs 215 in 2005. However, as percentage of GDP, India's government health spending actually fell from 1.12% in 1999 to 0.97% in 2005 (Berman & Ahuja, 2008). In terms of fulfilment of public health functions, a 2004 World bank evaluation found that although India's public health system has the capacity to carry out its public health functions, the system has major weaknesses in relation to persistently overlooking fundamental public health functions such as public health regulations and their enforcement; "deep management flaws", which hinder effective use of resources, including inadequate focus on evaluation; on assessing quality of services; on dissemination and use of information; and on openness to learning and innovation; "the central government functions too much in isolation and needs to work much more closely with other key actors, especially with sub-national governments, as well as with the private sector and with communities." (Das Gupta et al, 2004). Given inadequate funding and flawed management of the public health system, the platform on which the ICDS relies is weak. India's weak public health system partly explains the insignificant impact of the program on maternal and child health outcomes. Child malnutrition is mostly the result of high levels of exposure to infection and inappropriate infant and young child feeding and caring practices, and has its origins almost entirely during the first two to three years of life. The ICDS program, while successful in many ways, has not made a significant dent in child malnutrition. This is mostly due to the priority that the program has placed on food supplementation, targeting mostly children after the age of three when malnutrition has already set in. Compared to 1990, 10,000 fewer children in India died daily before reaching their fifth birthday in 2009. However, India still accounted for 21% of global under-five mortality in 2009. The infant mortality rate declined 40%, from 83.8% in 1990 to 50.3% in 2009, while the under-five mortality rate declined 45%, from 118 in 1990 to 65.6 in 2009 (UN, 2010). The slower decline in infant mortality rate reflects, in part the inappropriate strategy of the ICDS in focussing food supplementation on children aged 37 to 59 months, with less attention paid to encouraging breast feeding and providing adequate supplementary feeding to infants.

Maternal feeding and caring behaviour: Maternal feeding and caring behaviour is mediated by sociocultural environments of households, including the impact of religion and parental education and wealth status. A 2005 study of 408 children aged 1 - 3 years enrolled in an ICDS program in north India found that 199 (48.7%) children were underweight and 79.2% of children had dietary calories intake below 80% of recommended dietary intake. Advice regarding breast feeding and/or complementary feeding was given by Anganwadi workers to only 179 (43.8%) women (Prinja et al, 2008). The ICDS program has not achieved any major success in improving behavioural outcomes such as timely initiation of breast feeding (16.7%) and complementary feeding (39.9%). Prevalence of exclusive breast feeding has remained low at 28.2%. Although other factors including socio-economic conditions, socio-cultural beliefs and literacy status determine child feeding practices, the low proportion of women who reported to have been advised by the Anganwadi worker regarding breast feeding and complementary feeding reflects the deficiency of the program (Prinja et al, 2008). The percentage of pregnant women who had at least three antenatal care visits in 2008 was 51%, and only 47% of deliveries were attended by skilled birth attendants. Antenatal care attendance is a strong predictor of maternal caring behaviour (Halim et al, 2010). An important gap in maternal feeding practices is exclusive breastfeeding for the first four months of infancy. A 2003 study in urban and rural areas of Latur and Osmanabad districts of Maharashtra State revealed that exclusive breastfeeding for the first four months was undertaken by 40% of mothers. Such inadequacies predispose infants to malnutrition and infection (Kameswararao, 2004).

Micronutrient deficiencies – Iron and vitamin A: According to the World Health Organization's 2009 Global health risks' report (WHO, 2009), iron deficiency anaemia accounted for 400,000 deaths and 1.5% of the global Disability Adjusted Life Years in 2004. This cost is disproportional borne by developing nations as 60% of the morbidity and 95% of the mortality related to iron deficiency are derived from the poorest nations of the world. Despite increased national and international awareness and recent governmental intervention programs, the prevalence of anaemia among Indian women has remained higher than 45% since 1990, and anaemia trends remain strongly correlated with iron deficiency. A 2007 Indian government "12 by 12 initiative", aimed at ensuring that all Indian adolescents have 12g/dL haemoglobin by 2012, listed the main causes of anaemia in India as low dietary intake, poor availability of iron, chronic blood loss due to hookworm infestation, and malaria (MOHFW, 2006). Although serum iron monitoring is not a major duty of Anganwadi workers, they can contribute to screening for iron deficiency indirectly through growth monitoring, which is a core duty. Unfortunately, it has been been reduced to routine of weight recording, with less than 3% of mothers in one ICDS-related study having knowledge of nutritional status of their child in terms of the growth chart (Prinja et al, 2008). Despite mothers stating that lack of nutritious food is the prime reason for their infants' undernutrition, the food provided by many Anganwadi centres is not palatable and most enrolled pupils do not eat adequately. In India as at 2008, 60.8 million children are chronically undernourished, representing 48% of all undernourished children aged less than 5 years globally. Almost all these undernourished children suffer from iron deficiency anaemia (Pada, 2010). In India, anaemia is the second most common cause of maternal death, accounting for 20% of total maternal deaths. Multiple studies show that at least 45% of all Indian women are anaemic, based on WHO criteria. Most anaemic mothers are malnourished, and are more likely to deliver malnourished babies (WHO, 2008). The main underlying cause of vitamin A deficiency as a public health problem is a diet that is chronically insufficient in vitamin A that can lead to lower body stores and fail to meet physiologic needs (e.g. support tissue growth, normal metabolism, resistance to infection). Deficiency of sufficient duration or severity can lead to disorders such as xerophthalmia (xeros = dryness; -ophthalmia = pertaining to the eye), the leading cause of preventable childhood blindness, anaemia, and weakened host resistance to infection, which can increase the severity of infectious diseases such as measles and risk of death. Good plant sources of vitamin A include spinach, carrots and oranges. Based on biochemical measurement, vitamin A deficiency is a public health problem in India, with over 5% of children affected [Figure 2] (WHO, 2009b). Although biochemical retinol measurements are not part of Anganwadi workers duties, they could be easily trained in detecting vitamin A deficiency using characteristic eye signs of vitamin A deficiency, such as bitot spots - superficial, irregularly-shaped, foamy grey or white patches that appear on the conjunctiva, the membrane that covers most of the eyeball. More importantly, the foodstuffs supplied at ICDS centres need to be prepared such that they are nutritious, balanced and palatable. Given the high incidence of nutritional blindness in India, provision vitamin A supplements may be included in the duties of Anganwadi staff. In a longitudinal study designed to assess the impact of a massive-dose vitamin A programme on the incidence of keratomalacia, 50 000 preschool children in 450 slum areas in India's Hyderabad city were given 200 000 IU of vitamin A once every 6 months. During the study period, the incidence of keratomalacia in areas covered by the programme decreased by about 80%, while in control areas the reduction was of the order of 20%. To test whether large doses of vitamin A supplements prevented keratomalacia, a case-control analysis was done, with patients with severe protein-energy malnutrition being used as controls. The high odds ratio clearly indicated that keratomalacia was more likely to occur in children not receiving supplements (Vijayaraghavan et al, 1984)

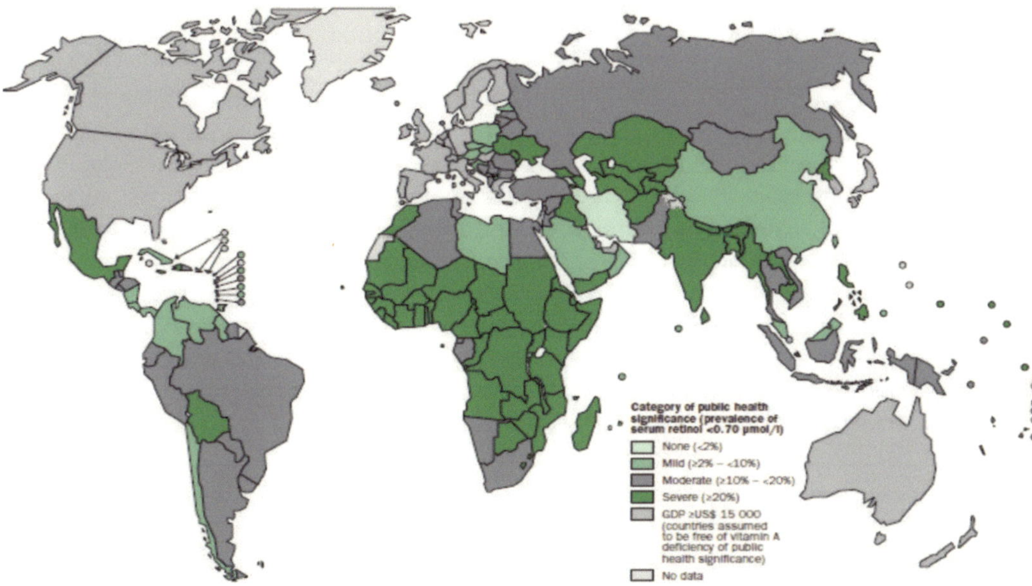

Fig. 2. Global Vitamin A deficiency prevalence (Source: WHO, 2009b).

ICDS infrastructure: The infrastructure for ICDS clinics is sub-optimal to facilitate achievement of its objectives. Although total budgetary allocation for the ICDS scheme increased from Rs. 529300.00 Lakh in 2007/2008 to Rs. 670500.00 Lakh in 2009/2010, this budget translates to less than 2 rupees per enrolled child and mother per day, and there is very little to show for such funding increases in the area of infrastructure. For example, a report of unannounced visits by the Karnataka State Commission for Protection of Child Rights to ICDS centres in 13 districts between July 2009 and July 2010 revealed cramped Anganwadi centres with no toilets for children, stale bread passed on as 'hot meals', drab walls without any charts as characteristic findings. Commission chairperson Nina Naik stated that there is an urgent need for "revisiting and redesigning the current ICDS programme in the interest of children". Low attendance was also found to be rampant, with just 20-25% of the enrolled children in the 3-6 year bracket going to ICDS centres. "Community seemed to have no confidence in the service and retain children at home or admit the 5-6 year olds into private pre-school services," observed the report. Similarly, a 2009 study of 65 ICDS centres in 10 districts of Madhya Pradesh found that, of the 65 centres studied only 24 (37%) have suitable buildings. Only 72% of the studied centres had their own Salter children weighing machine, only 66% of the centres had adult weighing machines, and only 58% had growth registers (Samvad, 2009). A major contributor to poor ICDS infrastructure is corruption. For example, a recent Times of India report stated that, in the state of Assam, although the government allots Rs 175000 for each ICDS building, the state spends only Rs 30,000 in each of the buildings in reality (Times of India, 2011).

Inadequate systems capacity building input into ICDS

Capacity building is any action that improves the effectiveness of individuals, organizations, networks, or systems—including organizational and financial stability, program service delivery, program quality, and growth. Capacity building is a long-term process that improves the ability of an individual, group, organization, or ecosystem to create positive change and perform better to improve public health results (MSH, 2010). A number of activities which have taken place under the banner of organisational capacity building in relation to the ICDS program have focussed on erecting buildings and providing training programs to Anganwadi workers.

A systems capacity building approach to improving the ICDS looks beyond training, and even the ICDS itself, into structural factors which may impact on child health and development. The starting point for improving child health and development is the Indian nubile female. Poorly nourished women are more likely to give birth to underweight infants, a major risk factor for both child as well as maternal morbidity and mortality (Kelly et al, 1996).A recent maternal nutrition study in Pune found that 33% of Indian women have a BMI less than 17, implying significant underweight, compared with 14% of men (Chorghade et al, 2006). Improving maternal nutrition in India would entail addressing cultural, socio-economic and, knowledge-based and attitudinal impediments, a task beyond the scope of ICDS, but within the scope of India's public health system. Effective systems capacity building comprises optimal interaction of nine components [Box 1 and Figure 3] (Potter & Brough, 2004):

- *Performance capacity*: Are the tools, money, equipment, consumables, etc. available to do the job? A doctor, however well trained, without diagnostic instruments, drugs or therapeutic consumables is of very limited use.
- *Personal capacity*: Are the staff sufficiently knowledgeable, skilled and confident to perform properly? Do they need training, experience, or motivation? Are they deficient in technical skills, managerial skills, interpersonal skills, gender-sensitivity skills, or specific role-related skills?
- *Workload capacity*: Are there enough staff with broad enough skills to cope with the workload? Are job descriptions practicable? Is skill mix appropriate?
- *Supervisory capacity*: Are there reporting and monitoring systems in place? Are there clear lines of accountability? Can supervisors physically monitor the staff under them? Are there effective incentives and sanctions available?
- *Facility capacity*: Are training centres big enough, with the right staff in sufficient numbers? Are clinics and hospitals of a size to cope with the patient workload? Are staff residences sufficiently large? Are there enough offices, workshops and warehouses to support the workload?
- *Support service capacity*: Are there laboratories, training institutions, bio-medical engineering services, supply organizations, building services, administrative staff, laundries, research facilities, quality control services? They may be provided by the private sector, but they are required.
- *Systems capacity*: Do the flows of information, money and managerial decisions function in a timely and effective manner? Can purchases be made without lengthy delays for authorization? Are proper filing and information systems in use? Are staff transferred without reference to local managers' wishes? Can private sector services be contracted as required? Is there good communication with the community? Are there sufficient links with NGOs?
- *Structural capacity*: Are there decision-making forums where inter-sectoral discussion may occur and corporate decisions made, records kept and individuals called to account for non-performance?
- *Role capacity*: This applies to individuals, to teams and to structure such as committees. Have they been given the authority and responsibility to make the decisions essential to effective performance, whether regarding schedules, money, staff appointments, etc?

Box 1. Nine component elements of systems capacity building applicable to improving the effectiveness of ICDS programme

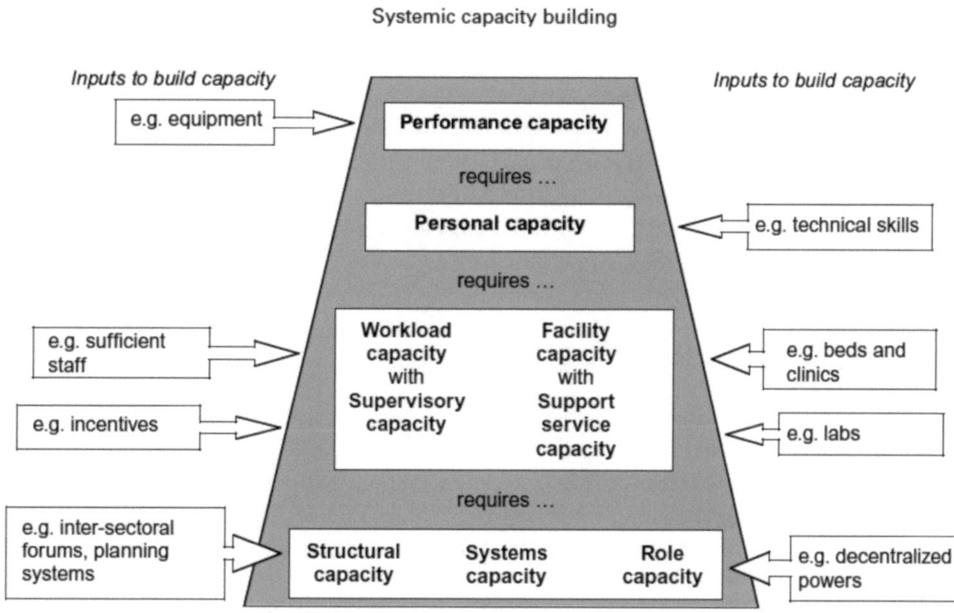

Fig. 3. Pyramid of effective capacity building

3. Conclusion

The ICDS has not met its objectives, three decades on, due in part to poor health management. A systems capacity building approach is proposed to improve the health and development of mothers and children in India. This approach entails a revitalised India's public health, rather than the ICDS, as a major facilitator of maternal and child health improvements. Issues that need to be addressed include; (1) Revitalising India's public health system, and providing adequate funding to make it more responsive to the needs of the whole population, instead of the over-reliance of vertical programmes such as ICDS; (2) Introducing sustainable poverty reduction programmes, particularly in areas with high maternal and child malnutrition. Improvement in maternal education is also very important in reducing maternal and child health. Remarkably, such improvements are already underway; (3) Expanding the depth and breadth of the training curriculum of Anganwadi workers and professionalising the cadre within India's public service. These workers require adequate remuneration commensurate with their job description, over and above the minimum wage in India's public sector; (4) Devolving the supply of ICDS food from pilfering contractors to local women groups. Employment of dieticians to facilitate adequate quantity (at least 500 calories per meal) and quality (i.e. rich in all food classes) of the meals served at Anganwadi centres. Home visits should be introduced, particularly for malnourished children, to work with the mothers of such children in the provision of nutritious meals at their respective homes; (5) Streamlining the wide array of existing maternal and child health programs, most of which have not demonstrated evidence of effectiveness, to assure quality implementation; (6) Targeting children from 1-3 years, as most of the malnutrition in children develop from this period, and most long term consequences of malnutrition may be minimised if this cohort of children are properly monitored nutritionally; Training and employment of health administrators to adequately manage the ICDS program; Focusing more on program outcomes, linked to child nutrition measures, rather than ICDS processes such as numbers of centres established; (7) Fortifying the food handed out by the PDS and those prepared at ICDS centres with micronutrients and vitamins, as this would be an economical and effective way to lower rates of anaemia and vitamins, and increase maternal and child nutrition; (8) Standardised building and equipment plans for ICDS centres should be established nationally, and only ICDS centres that meet minimum standards for building and equipment within a specified budget range should be allowed to operate. Such an approach will enhance the functioning of ICDS centres, and reduce fraudulent practices related to the construction of these sites.

4. References

Allen, Lindsay H. and Stuart R. Gillespie. (2001). 'What Works? A review of the efficacy and effectiveness of nutrition interventions', Manila: UN Administrative Committee on Coordination Subcommittee on Nutrition, in collaboration with the Asian Development Bank.

Berman, P, Ahuja R (2008). Government health spending in India. *Economic and Political Weekly*, June 28, pp 209-216.

Banerjee, AV & Duflo, E. (2006). The economic lives of the poor. *Journal of Economic Perspectives* 21 (1), pp 141-168.

Bhalotra, Sonia (2007), 'Spending to Save? State Health Expenditure and Infant Mortality in India', IZA Discussion Paper No. 2914.

Bhargava, A., Chowdhury, S, and Singh, K.K.(2005), Healthcare infrastructure, contraceptive use and infant mortality in Uttar Pradesh, India, Economics and Human Biology, 3, 388-403.

Das Gupta, M, Michael Lokshin, M & Ivaschenko, O (2005), Improving Child Nutrition Outcomes in India Can the Integrated Child Development Services Program Be More Effective?, *World Bank Policy Research Working Paper 3647*, June 2005.

Das Gupta M, Rani M. India's Public Health System: How Well Does It Function at the National Level? World Bank Policy Research Working Paper 3447, November 2004.

Deaton, A. and J. Dreze (2009). Food and Nutrition in India: Facts and Interpretations. *Economic and Political Weekly*, XLIV(7), 42 - 65.

Deolalikar, A. (2005), *Attaining the Millennium Development Goals in India: How Likely and What Will It Take To Reduce Infant Mortality, Child Malnutrition, Gender Disparities and Hunger-Poverty and to Increase School Enrollment and Completion?* Oxford University Press, New Delhi, 2005.

Dongre, AR, Deshmukh, PR & Garg, BS (2008). Eliminating childhood malnutrition: discussions with mothers and Anganwadi workers. *Journal of Health Studies*, 1 (2-3), pp 48-52.

Government of India [GI] (2010). *Millennium Development Goals: India Country report 2009.* New Delhi: Ministry of Statistics and Programme Implementation, India.

Government of Orissa [GO] (2006). Training of trainers' manual for Anganwadi workers - Kishori Shakti Yojana and Balika Mandal as strategies for empowering adolescent girls. Orissa, 2006. URL: http://www.wcdorissa.gov.in/download/KSYTrainingoftrainerManualforAWWs.pdf Accessed 30-January 2011.

Gragnolati, Michele, Shekar, M , Das Gupta, M, Bredenkamp, C and Lee, Yi-Kyoung (2005), 'India's undernourished children: A Call for reform and Action', Health, Nutrition and Population (HNP) Discussion Paper, The World Bank.

Greiner, Theodore, and David F. Pyle.2000. "Nutrition Assessment – India", paper presented at the World Bank-UNICEF Joint Nutrition Assessment Workshop, Oct 11-12, 2000.

Halim, N, Bohara, AK, Xiaomin, R. Healthy mothers, healthy children: does maternal demand for antenatal care matter for child health in Nepal? *Health Policy and Planning*, 2010, doi: 10.1093/heapol/czq040.

Jalan, Jyotsna and Martin Ravallion (2003) 'Does Piped Water Reduce Diarrhea for Children in Rural India?' *Journal of Econometrics* Vol. 12(1): 153-73.

Kameswararao, AA (2004). Breast Feeding Behaviour of Indian Women. *Indian Journal of Community Medicine*, 19 (2), pp62-64

Kapil, U (2002). Integrated Child Development Services (ICDS) scheme: a program for holistic development of children in India. *Indian Journal of Paediatrics*; 69 (7), pp 597-601.

Kaul V. (1993). Integrated child development services in India. *Childhood*, 1 (4), pp 243-245.

Kelly A, Kevany J, de Onis M, Shah PM. (1996). WHO collaborative study of maternal anthropometry and pregnancy outcomes. International Journal of Gynecology & Obstetrics, 53 (3), pp 219-223.

Koenig, M., Foo, G., Joshi, K., (2000), 'Quality of care within the Indian family welfare programme: a review of recent evidence', *Studies in Family Planning*, 31, 1–18.

Lokshin, M, Das Gupta, M, Gragnolati, M & Ivaschenko O (2005). Improving Child Nutrition? The Integrated Child Development Services in India. *Development and Change* 36 (4), pp 613–640.

Management Sciences for Health (2010). Challenges Encountered in Capacity Building: Review of Literature and Selected Tools. Position Paper No. 10, 2010, p 2.

Mann, V, Eble, A, Frost, C, Premkumar, R, Booneb, P (2010). Retrospective comparative evaluation of the lasting impact of a community-based primary health care programme on under-5 mortality in villages around Jamkhed, India. *Bulletin of WHO*, 88 (10), pp 727-736.

Ministry of Health and Family Welfare [MOHFW], Government of India. *Micronutrient National Investment Plan (IMNIP) for 2007-2011.* Delhi; MOHFW, URL: http://www.micronutrient.org/CMFiles/MI%20Around%20the%20World/Asia/India-MN-Investment-Plan.pdf Accessed 23 January 2011.

Muralialharari R, Kaul V (1993). *Responding to children's needs: Integrated Child Development Services in India.* In: Elderling L, Leseman P. Early intervention and culture: preparation for literacy; the interface between theory and practice. UNESCO, ISBN 92-3-102937-1, Paris.

Pada, G (2010). Child malnutrition in India - putting the smallest first. The Economist, 23 September, URL:
http://www.economist.com/node/17090948 accessed 27 January 2011

Peters, D., Yazbeck, A., Sharma, R., Ramana, G., Pritchett, L.,Wagstaff, A.(2002) Better Health Systems for India's Poor. World Bank, Washington, DC.

Prinja, S, Verma, R, Lal, S. (2008). Role of ICDS program in delivery of nutritional services and functional integration between Anganwadi and health worker in north India. *The Internet Journal of Nutrition and Wellness.* 2008 Volume 5 Number 2.

Radhakrishna , R & Ravi, C. (2004). Malnutrition in India - trends and determinants. *Economic and Political Weekly*, 39 (7), pp 671-676.

Ray, R. (2007). Changes in Food Consumption and the Implications for Food Security and Undernourishment: India in the 1990s. *Development and Change* 38(2), 321 - 343.

Reynolds, AJ, Temple, JA, Robertson DL & Mann EA (2001). Long-Term Effects of an Early Childhood Intervention on Educational Achievement and Juvenile Arrest: A 15-Year Follow-Up of Low-Income Children in Public Schools. *Journal of the American Medical Association*, 285 (18), pp. 2330-2346.

Right to Food Campaign (2007). Anganwadis for all: a primer. New Delhi (restricted circulation. URL: http://www.righttofoodindia.org/data/icds06primer.pdf Accessed 29 January 2011), Delhi.

Samvad V. Moribund ICDS: a study on the ICDS and Child Survival issues in Madhya Pradesh. Right to Food Campaign Madhya Pradesh Support Group, Vikas Samvad and Sanket-Centre for Budget Studies, Bhopal. URL: http://southasia.oneworld.net/Files/ICDS.pdf Accessed 29 January 2011.

Subramanyam, MA, Kawachi, I, Berkman, LF & Subramanian SV (2010). Socioeconomic inequalities in childhood undernutrition in India: analyzing trends between 1992 and 2005. *PLoS One*. 5(6): e11392.

Tarozzi, A (2002). *The Indian Public Distribution System as provider of food security: evidence from child anthropometry in Andhra Pradesh*. Princeton University, Economics Paper 185, 208 Fisher Hall, Princeton, NJ 08544.

Tarozzi, A. and A. Mahajan (2007). Child Nutrition in India in the Nineties. *Economic Development and Cultural Change*, 55(3), 441 - 486.

Times of India. Anganwadi workers' agitation on Thursday. January 31, 2011. URL: http://timesofindia.indiatimes.com/city/guwahati/Anganwadi-workers-agitation-on-Thursday/articleshow/7393484.cms Accessed 31 January 2011.

Udani RH, Chothani S, Arora S, Kulkarni CS. (1990). Evaluation of knowledge and efficiency of Anganwadi workers. *Indian Journal of Paediatrics*, 47 (4), pp 289-292.

UNESCO (2010). *Global Education Digest 2010*. UNESCO Institute of Statistics, ISBN: 978-92-9189-088-0, Quebec.

United Nations (2010). *Millennium Development Goals 2010*. New York: United Nations, ISBN 978-92-1-101218-7, New York.

Vijayaraghavan, KN, Rao, NP, Sarma R, Reddy V. (1984) impact of massive doses of Vitamin A on incidence of nutritional blindness. *The Lancet* 324, Issue 8395, pp 149-151.

World Health Organisation South East Asia Regional Office (2009). *Report of the regional consultation on measles*. WHO, SEA-Immun-57, New Delhi.

World Health Organization (2009). Global Health Risks: mortality and burden of disease attributable to selected major risks. WHO, ISBN 978 92 4 156387 1, Geneva.

World Health Organization (2009b). Global prevalence of vitamin A deficiency in populations at risk 1995–2005. WHO, ISBN 978 92 4 159801 9, Geneva.

World Health Organization (2008). The World Health Report 2008: primary health care - now more than ever. Geneva: World Health Organization, 2008.

World Health Organisation (2008). Worldwide prevalence of anaemia 1993-2005. WHO, ISBN 978 92 4 159665 7, Geneva.

Young, M. (1996). *Early Child Development: Investing in the Future*. The World Bank, ISBN 0-8213-3547-2, Washington, DC.

14

Disease Management of Avian Influenza H5N1 in Bangladesh - A Focus on Maintaining Healthy Live Birds

Muhiuddin Haider and Bethany Applebaum[1]
University of Maryland, USA

1. Introduction

Since March 22, 2007 when the Bangladesh Government declared highly pathogenic Avian Influenza H5N1 present, the disease has become a major public health concern throughout Bangladesh. Avian Influenza (AI) affects all poultry, wild and domestic, including poultry at commercial farms, live bird markets, and in backyard farms, putting many people at risk of contracting the disease. Avian Influenza affects both poultry and humans; therefore efforts in managing the disease necessitate a multi-sector approach.

This chapter provides an overview of selected[2] aspects of H5N1 disease management efforts in Bangladesh, focusing specifically on prevention efforts that decrease the risk involved with live birds transmitting the virus. An analytic model to examine field-level data is used to explore how using behavioral change communication, social mobilization, and the coordination between human and animal health to maintain healthy live-bird facilities can be used to manage H5N1 in Bangladesh. Specifically, this chapter will provide suggestions for continual disease management with a focus on how multi-sector activities, behavioral change communication, logistics management, interventions impacting live birds, and linking research to practice can contribute to successful disease management programs. Current efforts to reduce the prevalence of AI are addressed, as well as gaps in the effort and future steps to reduce the prevalence of H5N1.

2. An overview of AI in Bangladesh

Highly Pathogenic Avian Influenza (HPAI) is an emerging zoonotic infectious disease, which is caused by the H5N1 subtype of the type A strain of the influenza virus (World Health Organization [WHO], 2006a). The virus is found in, and transmitted through, the feces, saliva, and eye and nasal discharge of infected birds (Centers for Disease Control [CDC], 2008). It is transmitted to healthy birds through contact with infected birds or

---

[1] The authors would like to acknowledge the contributions and assistance provided by Nicole I. Wanty, M.A.A. and Mohammed Zakaria that helped in the completion of this chapter.

[2] It is important to note that this chapter does not consider an exhaustive list of all possible aspects of disease management for H5N1. For example, this chapter does not explore the clinical management of H5N1 in Bangladesh. As this chapter will demonstrate, the need for clinical management of AI can be decreased, if not completely eliminated, by managing H5N1 in the live birds.

contaminated droppings. Humans contract HPAI through direct contact with infected birds. Symptoms of human infection include conjunctivitis, sore throat, sore muscles, and severe respiratory diseases such as pneumonia. The mortality rate for humans is high, capable of reaching 100 percent mortality in as few as two days (CDC, 2007).

Some of the factors that contribute to spread of HPAI from birds to humans include slaughtering poultry and preparing the meat in the home, direct contact with sick or infected birds, and the consumption of infected poultry. Poultry farmers sell infected birds in an attempt to mitigate their losses from culling (Otte et al.) and backyard farmers may choose to eat a sick bird, rather than waste limited resources. Human infection may also occur through direct contact with the feces of contaminated birds. For example, when children ingest soil contaminated with the feces of infected birds (WHO, 2006a) or poultry droppings and waste are used as fertilizers. Disposal of infected carcasses in bodies of water that are used by domestic purposes, including drinking, laundry, swimming, and bathing places people at risk as well. Infected carcasses are also fed to other animals, such as pigs, which may also increase the risk of human infection (Otte et al.).

While human-to-human transmission of HPAI infection is rare, scientists believe that under the right conditions, the H5N1 virus may mutate into a form transmissible from person-to person. The World Health Organization believes the H5N1 virus has already met all of the prerequisites for a pandemic, except the ability to spread from human-to-human. Therefore, the WHO has labeled the H5N1 virus as the most likely virus to start the next pandemic and many people believe that it is only a matter of time until an HPAI pandemic occurs (WHO, 2006a). In light of these forecasts and the unique ability of the influenza virus to spread, it is estimated that human-to-human contagious virus could affect all continents within three months (WHO, 2006a).

Since 2007, AI has become a major public health concern throughout Bangladesh, because it affects poultry at commercial farms, live bird markets, and backyard poultry farms throughout the country, which puts many people at risk of exposure to the disease. Avian Influenza affects the health of both poultry and humans, which necessitates a multi-sector approach to manage the health, social, and economic factors of the disease. Stakeholders from all levels of government as well as the private sector need to work together in the areas of animal health, human health, public awareness, public communication, and capacity building.

Animal health issues require the involvement of veterinarians, commercial poultry farmers and stakeholders, and backyard poultry farmers. These individuals are necessary for disease management because they can directly help minimize threat of H5N1 in humans by controlling infections in poultry, strengthening disease prevention and preparedness capability, strengthening surveillance measures and capacity, strengthening disease surveillance and diagnostic capacity, and improving bio-security in poultry production and trade.

In terms of human health, the involvement of the Department of Health is crucial for coordinating and improving the overall response capacity for disease outbreaks. The Departments of Health workers are necessary to implement and support monitoring for disease and progress evaluation of disease management. In addition, it is important to involve private sector physicians and health professionals to monitor disease outbreaks in the human population.

Multi-sector activities should focus on building capacity and infrastructure to support disease management. This includes training individuals associated with poultry production and poultry marketing about Avian Influenza-related issues and relevant prevention techniques, providing supplies necessary for improving hygiene-related practices, training relevant individuals on communicating with media personnel and other stakeholders, providing adequate compensation following culling operations, and developing programs for monitoring, evaluating, and implementing technical support for projects.

Raising public awareness and increasing communication to the public about Avian Influenza disease management and outbreaks is crucial. Efforts in this vein should focus on improving communication services and methods for information dissemination. This includes developing materials for communication such as websites, printed materials, and audio/video materials. Additionally, it is important to continue developing new communication technologies, such as a web-based SMS gateway, and creating new strategies to disseminate information to target audiences.

Some of the coordination and planning efforts that have been put in place for Avian Influenza disease management include but are not limited to the following:

- the creation, implementation, and revision of the National Avian Influenza and Human Pandemic Influenza Preparedness and Response Plan
- creating and training response teams
- performing bio-security audits at commercial farms
- improving bio-security measures of live bird markets through cleaning, spraying, training personnel, improving sanitation, and constructing separate slaughter places
- developing and distributing Commercial Farm Bio-security Guidelines
- obtaining funding from international stakeholders for disease management coordination, prevention, and containment, including strengthening disease management capacity and rehabilitation programs for farmers with infected flocks
- obtaining the cooperation and collaboration of relevant organizations and NGOs
- developing communication materials and methods for the distribution of information for preparedness, protection, reporting, response, and policy compliance

These efforts have primarily focused on the importance of maintaining the health and safety of live birds. Thus far, the efforts from the Bangladesh government and development partners have been effective in enabling the country to prevent the Avian Influenza H5N1 from reaching an epidemic proportion in poultry populations and preventing human infection.

3. Animal health approaches

In order to prevent the spread of HPAI (High Pathogenic Avian Influenza) between birds and to human, biosecurity measures need to be maintained at commercial and backyard poultry farms and at live bird markets. In Bangladesh, poultry production occurs in commercial and backyard farms, and distribution occurs at live bird markets, all of which have been greatly impacted by Avian Influenza.

This is the appropriate time to save the poultry industry. The general population is familiar with Avian Influenza, but they are not properly aware of what they should do to protect human and poultry health from infectious diseases. Biosecurity may be one of the most important elements for prevention and control of Avian Influenza.

3.1 Commercial farms

Commercial poultry farms, both layer and broiler, are situated in risky locations and operated under unhygienic conditions. Commercial farms are not maintaining minimum biosecurity level with many farms lacking a gate, footbath, and delineated farm boundaries. In addition, many farm workers do not know how to maintain biosecurity to protect the poultry and themselves from disease.

Commercial poultry businessmen are concerned about Avian Influenza and facing many challenges. The government decided to destroy infected farms as well as other adjacent farms that were situated within five kilometers of the affected farm. During this time, many quality farms were destroyed and the owners did not receive adequate compensation. The government compensation was 90 taka for each chicken, although one the market price of one chicken is approximately 150 taka. Finally the government revised their decision to only destroy farms situated within one kilometer of an affected farm. For this reason, many small and medium poultry businessmen left the poultry business and they are engaged in different business opportunities, such as garments factory, or no business at all. This means that many former small and medium poultry businessmen are unable to support their families. In addition, many of them obtained a loan from the bank to cover start-up costs and are now unable to pay the loan (USAID/Bangladesh 2010).

Unfortunately, most of the commercial farms are not maintaining minimum biosecurity. The Department of Livestock Services (DLS) provides technical support to the farms, but the support is inadequate. The situation requires a combined effort from multiple stakeholders to improve biosecurity level for commercial farms. Private and public sectors should work together to achieve sustainable health for both human and poultry populations. In this regard, human health workers and animal health workers should work together to combat Avian Influenza or other infectious diseases.

3.2 Backyard farms

In rural areas, 80 to 90 percent of households raise backyard poultry. Poultry meat is a major source of nutrition, and it is an income source for the majority of impoverished women. Generally, the practices used to rear backyard poultry are unhygienic. Many households keep the birds inside the home or bedroom. Chickens and ducks are kept together in one shed, constructed from bamboo or muddy soil. This makes it difficult to clean the shed properly. Many communities are still unaware of Avian Influenza and how the disease can be spread between poultry or from poultry to humans. Large portions of the population lack knowledge regarding biosecurity, poultry, and human health (USAID/Bangladesh 2010).

In addition, backyard poultry farming methods and scavenging (free-ranging) poultry may put commercial poultry at risk, especially given the lack of biosecurity at commercial farms. The backyard and commercial farmers should be aware of this addition risk. Backyard poultry, which have a greater likelihood of coming into contact with wild, infected foul, should not enter into the commercial farm premises. If backyard poultry enter a commercial farm property, the disease can enter the commercial poultry population and the virus can spread from chicken to chicken.

The national assessment of backyard poultry rearing practices in Bangladesh aimed to describe poultry raising practices over time, specifically as it relates to human-poultry interaction and hygiene practices. It has sought to describe the contribution of poultry production to income and nutrition and describe the epidemiology of poultry illness in terms of incidence, seasonality, clinical signs, outcomes, and pathogens responsible for poultry illness.

Since March 22, 2007, there have been a series of outbreaks of Avian Influenza in Bangladesh, which have resulted in the deaths of a large number of poultry. This has had both a social and economic impact on the population of Bangladesh. Many backyard poultry and mini-farm holders (100-1,000 birds) are particularly vulnerable. As of October 2010, the government had culled almost 2 million chickens and destroyed almost 26 million eggs.

Although there is a policy to provide compensation for all species of poultry culled and the eggs destroyed, the compensation is not equivalent to what the farmers could have received from healthy birds. Even though compensation rates have increased, the compensation provided to these farmers is not enough money to be able to re-establish themselves in the poultry practice. The main objective of a rehabilitation program for the farmer at the community level is to help restock and repopulate their flocks, bringing them back into the poultry practice. These programs raise awareness about Avian Influenza and biosecurity practices, as well as leads to the mobilization of resources between the public and private sectors.

To implement the rehabilitation program, the Ministry of Fisheries and Livestock (MoFL) developed and approved rehabilitation policy guidelines. District committees and six selected NGOs implemented the program as per the rehabilitation policy guidelines to assist a total of 14,000 backyard poultry holders and 2,240 mini farmers. The NGOs were involved in the assessment of the situation as the policy affected farmers and their families, the submission of a field assessment report to the district committee, assistance in training, procurement, distribution as well as utilization of inputs (new birds, feed, funds for renovations, medical services) as well as supervision, monitoring, follow-up and reporting of the rehabilitation program. The backyard poultry holders received ten fowl of improved variety at the age of 4-5 months, twenty five kilograms of poultry feed, money for renovations or the replacement of a poultry house, medical services like vaccinations and de-worming for one year, and a two-day long awareness and skills development training. Mini farmers received two hundred one-day-old broiler chicks and fifty kilograms of poultry feed (USAID/Bangladesh 2010).

This rehabilitation program has helped restore confidence among the affected community and has helped small entrepreneurs re-enter the poultry trade. The rehabilitation policy is a unique approach to public-partnerships to re-engage community members in poultry rearing, while decreasing the threat of Avian Influenza. The policy is also complimentary to the Avian Influenza containment program, restocking and repopulating with healthy poultry. To make the policy a success in terms of sustainability, improved biosecurity and preventative measures are need, as well as increased awareness and social commitment of the community.

Additionally, backyard poultry holders have been working on identifying risk factors for characterizing the dispersion of Avian Influenza in backyard flocks. This work has included identifying risk factors for the susceptibility of backyard poultry flocks to Avian Influenza H5 virus as well as assessing the dispersion of the virus within 10km of affected farms.

3.3 Live bird markets

Live bird markets are an important consideration in disease management for Avian Influenza because infectious diseases are easily spread from one market to another, exposing many animals and humans to the disease. The live bird markets of Bangladesh are very dirty and unhygienic. Vendors, transporter, slaughterers, processors and even consumers are not aware about spreading of disease and contamination. It might be one of the sources of infectious diseases like avian influenza.

Once a virus develops in one market, it can easily be transported to other markets and farms by way of contaminated equipment, birds, people, and vehicles. In addition to animal infections, many human infections around the world have been traced to live bird markets, including the single human case of Avian Influenza, which was identified in Bangladesh on May 22, 2008. Consequently, there is great need for biosecurity in the live bird markets.

Live bird market surveillance for Avian Influenza in Bangladesh has involved identifying Avian Influenza subtypes and strains that are circulating in domestic waterfowl in live bird markets in Bangladesh, exploring every day practices of poultry rearing, particularly human interactions with poultry, exploring poultry raisers' perceptions and practices regarding sick poultry, and exploring human and poultry interactions in the local poultry markets.

Currently, the biosecurity in live bird markets is low. Slaughterers and poultry processors do not use protective gear such as masks and gloves. Birds are processed and slaughtered in the same place, rather than using the more hygienic process of completing these two processes in separate locations. After processing the birds, the waste (offal, blood, and feathers) are not properly stored and disposed of. Vendors throw the waste from their stalls elsewhere on the market premises. Cleaning crews are not aware of the need to use proper protective gear or the need for spraying and disinfection methods. Additionally, consumers come to the markets without wearing masks or gloves, and are, therefore, exposed to the hazards that result from the unhygienic practices (USAID/Bangladesh 2010).

The United States Agency for International Development's (USAID) Stamping Out Pandemic and Avian Influenza (STOP AI) helps countries prepare for, respond to, and recover from HPAI outbreaks. The project delivers technical assistance and training, and promotes collaboration between animal and human health professionals. STOP AI aims to mobilize public and private sector partners as well as NGOs to implement systematic and sustained behavioral changes that will result in measureable improvements in biosecurity. Stop AI has put forth a framework in which the public animal health system, private sector poultry industry, public health system, civil society, as well as donors and NGOS work together to provide and implement a systematic, commercially-viable Avian Influenza surveillance, biosecurity, and outbreak response program/plan. This framework includes developing public-private partnerships and providing on-demand national level assistance. In developing this framework, STOP AI conducted a baseline market survey in Bangladesh, held stakeholder workshops to share survey data and an action plan, and adopted training materials for ground-level stakeholders such as farmers, veterinarians, and cleaners. Recommendations include renovating, upgrading, cleaning, and disinfecting live bird markets. In order to carry out these activities, capacity building is required to train stakeholders and acquire supplies such as sprayers, pressure washers, detergents, masks, and gloves (USAID/Bangladesh 2010).

Implementing effective biosecurity is not without challenges and requires the combined efforts of stakeholders in both the public and private sectors. One challenge is that differing political views can delay development work. People in the private sector engaged in biosecurity endeavors tend to do so for personal interests, and may not be motivated or willing to make concessions not within their personal interest. Similarly, the poultry industry-related stakeholders want and need to see direct benefits in order to become engaged in practicing biosecurity. The industry stakeholders also need training on how to apply the biosecurity measures.

Another difficulty lies in the cost-sharing of funds; direct spending of cost-share funds without a sub-contract is difficult to manage within municipality regulations. As such, it is easier to work in a private live bird market than in a public market. In a private market, there are fewer hoops to jump through than in the public sector because it only requires dealing with the owner for making decisions regarding cost-sharing. However, the public sector is needed for developing the necessary infrastructure to sustain effective biosecurity at the live bird markets. Additionally, collecting cost-share money from stakeholders can be difficult because they rely on donors to pay all funds. For the sustainability of the program, it is necessary to have a plan regarding who will pay for live bird market cleaners and disinfection operations. It is also important that enough time be given for training cleaners after the renovations of live bird markets are complete(USAID/Bangladesh 2010).

3.4 Waterfowl

Thus far, the affected domestic poultry seems to be limited to chickens. However, there has been an investigation by the Department of Forestry to determine whether H5N1 is infecting wild waterfowl in Bangladesh. This work has focused on investigating if contact between wild and domestic waterfowl is associated with H5N1 in wild migratory birds as well as determining whether infection with influenza A impairs flight or migration using satellite. This study plans to examine 600 wild waterfowl and shorebirds to be tested by Rapid Test, PCR, and ELISA. Thus far, 34 birds of 11 species have been sampled, and there have not been any reported outbreaks in waterfowl (USAID/Bangladesh 2010).

Prevention efforts examining wild migratory birds is vital to preventing the spread of infection among domestic poultry populations. Migratory birds may transport the disease along migration paths and infect poultry along those routes.

4. Human health approaches

Integrating human health as part of Avian Influenza disease management requires coordination between stakeholders at all levels and involves multiple components. Although the clinical aspects of human health management of Avian Influenza are beyond the scope of this chapter, it is important to note that is an imperative part of disease management. We will address the following 6 components related to human health in this section: planning, surveillance, laboratory work, research, capacity building, and communications.

Planning for both preparedness and response to an outbreak in Bangladesh has involved developing and implementing the National Avian Influenza and Pandemic Influenza Preparedness Plans and Pandemic Contingency Plan by a national multi-sectoral planning team. The goal of the plan is a comprehensive and coordinated response to address H5N1 in domestic poultry and minimize transmission to humans. The plan addresses multiple sectors and works to strengthen capacity among many other aspects of H5N1 prevention.

Surveillance efforts on Avian Influenza have focused on high-risk group surveillance, hospital-based surveillance, population-based surveillance, drug trials, and the previously discussed surveillance at live bird markets. For example, the Avian Influenza Contact Follow-Up Monitoring Committee regularly follows up in affected districts with people exposed to poultry. People involved in culling infected poultry or in close contact (less than 1 meter) with infected poultry were given a single dose of anti-viral tablets for 7 days and followed up for 14 days. People with household contacts (more than 1 meter) and health care worker contact (unprotected) or other contact were followed up for 14 days without any anti-viral tablets. Follow up was done daily by health care workers to detect influenza-like illness, which was defined as fever, cough and respiratory distress. Suspected cases were reported to the Institute of Epidemiology, Disease Control & Research (IEDCR) and necessary follow-up steps were taken (USAID/Bangladesh 2010).

Other human-health related approaches to managing Avian Influenza include laboratory-based research, such as pharmaceutical development and testing. For example, a drug trail based in Kamalapur has been evaluating the effectiveness of treatment with Oseltamavir on interrupting the transmission of influenza (May 2008- December 2010). Oseltamavir is the generic version of Tamiflu, an anti-viral that slows the spread of the influenza virus between cells.

Hospital-based influenza surveillance has been increasing. In 2007, twelve hospitals participated in surveillance efforts. Six of the 12 hospitals were run by the government, and six were privately-run hospitals. The hospitals were distributed among six divisions in Bangladesh. By 2010, fourteen hospitals distributed in all seven divisions of Bangladesh participated in the influenza surveillance program (USAID/Bangladesh 2010).

Population-based surveillance has involved collecting both epidemiological and biological data. Samples were collected from cullers and poultry workers to examine the sero-prevalence of antibodies for H5N1. Additionally, there has been a longitudinal assessment of the effect of influenza on the cognitive development of urban poor children in Bangladesh. For this surveillance, a certain amount of laboratory capacity is necessary to analyze the samples and data. IEDCR has been a WHO-accredited lab since 2007, and IEDCR regularly participates in activities involving H5N1.

It is important to note that Avian Influenza is not easily transmitted to humans. If we were able to prevent and/or manage the disease among the live birds, many of the human-health related aspects of disease management would not be needed. As such, efforts should focus on capacity building, logistics management, and communication for behavior change that will help prevent, manage, or even eradicate Avian Influenza in live birds.

5. Capacity building

Capacity building is crucial for disease management strategies at all levels. If the necessary human resources, infrastructure, and commodity supplies are not in place, behavioral change for Avian Influenza disease management and prevention will not be sustainable, or in some cases even be able to occur.

Community-level capacity building includes training and education for community members and local disease surveillance. Capacity building at live bird markets is one of the most crucial aspects of disease prevention. For capacity building at the live bird market, it is crucial that the management and ground-level workers be trained in and implement bio-security measures. In order for that to happen, there needs to be a supply of hygiene and cleaning commodities, such as soap, clean towels and sprayers, as well as a supply of clean water, which requires government assistance. Thus, the infrastructure and capacity for logistics management, which is discussed later in this chapter, must be built-up.

Similarly, manpower and logistics management of the Veterinary Service need to be further developed to carry out surveillance and respond to outbreaks of Avian Influenza. Additionally, illness surveillance centers and active surveillance measures among high risk groups need to be developed. This will involve training workers and volunteers, as well as increasing community awareness of Avian Influenza.

Another important aspect of disease management is building the capacity for appropriate laboratory and epidemiological work, which includes developing the physical laboratories and training personnel, as well as stocking the laboratories with necessary supplies.

6. Logistics management

In addition to building capacity and infrastructure support for disease management, it is important to take into the account the logistics of implementing the various aspects of disease management. Logistics management considers issues pertinent to implementing disease management strategies such as space and equipment availability, staffing and human resource skills, supplies of relevant commodities, recordkeeping and reporting, and transportation.

In the case of Avian Influezna in Bangladesh, USAID's DELIVER Project has aimed to coordinate plans to "meet the challenges presented by existing and emerging pandemic threats by establishing and operating a secure, reliable global mechanism to store, transport, rapidly deliver, and track in-country distribution of current and future USAID Avian Influenza International Stockpile (AIIS) and outbreak response assets." To achieve these objectives, it has been necessary to work in close partnership with stakeholders from the planning process to implementation, develop a sustainable project design, emphasize the ownership of the stakeholders, gradually phase in the project and stakeholder involvement, and prepare stakeholders to take over by building capacity in private sector to sustain the project (USAID/Bangladesh 2010).

In conjunction with various stakeholders, DELIVER has been able to create a dedicated storage floor in the Department of Livestock Services (DLS), introduce warehousing best practices as well as a uniform logistics recording and reporting system, and design, develop and introduce a digital livestock management system. Additionally, DELIVER has trained personnel on logistics management, computer inventory management, and online reporting. As a result, they have been able ensure proper warehousing, distribution and in-country stock of Avian Influenza commodities (detergent, sprayers, decontamination kits, flu detection kits). Similarly, they have cooperated with Directorate General of Health Services (DGHS) and WHO to ensure proper storage and supply of H1N1 vaccines. Sufficient inventory is kept at a central warehouse and commodities are positioned in proximity to potential outbreak areas. DLS has the ability to respond quickly within a few hours to a reported outbreak in any upazila (district). Additionally, DLS can see the current report and inventory online at any time and use it to make supply decisions (USAID/Bangladesh 2010).

DELIVER was able to establish a regular field logistics monitoring system for problem solving, capacity building, and troubleshooting. Sustaining the inventory management and web-based reporting system within DLS is challenging though because DLS is an environment of frequent staff turnover. Another challenge is using the available data in forecasting, procurement, and supply decisions. The goals for the future are all focused on sustaining and continuing to build the capacity to sustain and strengthen these efforts (USAID/Bangladesh 2010).

7. Communication

Communication is a crucial aspect of disease management. It includes all forms of communication from daily media surveillance to the distribution of printed materials aimed at raising awareness of Avian Influenza control measures (e.g. hygiene, cleaning/washing, and waste disposal).

The majority of the communication messages have focused on five target audiences: slaughter at home, restaurants, consumers, truckers, and vendors at live bird markets. Additionally, there have been regular press briefings issued, as well training and orientation sessions for the media personal reporting on Avian Influenza issues. As a result of improved communication, people have better access to accurate information on prevention and treatment of H5N1. People are also better informed on basic bio-security and hygienic preventive measures, where to receive services in the case of an outbreak, and the government policy on H5N1 as it relates to the compensation, bio-security, and rehabilitation plans (USAID/Bangladesh 2010).

In an attempt to improve communication and information access for the public, current communications efforts are looking to establish and implement web-based SMS communications plans. This technology has the potential to be used to update the relevant stakeholders at all levels with information regarding Avian Influenza. This includes everything from the current market price of birds to outbreak alerts to best practices (USAID/Bangladesh 2010).

One example of disease management from a communication-based approach is illustrated through the piloting of an intervention to reduce the risk of transmission of Avian Influenza to humans in rural Bangladesh. This intervention involved developing, modifying and disseminating a set of culturally appropriate messages on slaughtering and handling practices for sick and dead poultry. Once the original communications materials were developed, their acceptability and feasibility in the community was explored and the message was disseminated at five courtyard meetings. Using observation, informal conversation, in-depth interviews, and group discussions to collect data, researchers found that villagers verbally expressed willingness to follow the messages if their poultry have "bird flu." However, in practice, they were unwilling to avoid slaughtering or selling sick poultry as they would lose household income(USAID/Bangladesh 2010).

Research has shown that barriers to practicing AI preventative measures fall into two categories. The largest barrier that prevents the practice of AI preventive measures is the attitudes of the population. While people may express a willingness to follow the practices, in practice, the perceived risk of AI infection in humans is too low to outweigh the immediate cost of losing income from the poultry. In addition, there is little value given to the prevention of AI. In general, the cost of prevention for any poultry farmer in greater in the short term and the benefits are reaped over the long term. This leads to negligence and carelessness towards the practice of AI preventive measures. The second barrier that prevents the practice of AI preventive measures is a lack of awareness. The lack of awareness begins with a failure to initially identify the disease in backyard and semi-commercial farms. Populations also lack awareness about high-risk behaviors that can lead to the contraction of the disease in humans and the prevention measures for the points of contraction. Finally, there is a lack of awareness about AI vaccination for poultry (USAID/Bangladesh 2010).

8. Conclusion

The lessons learned from current and past AI initiatives are invaluable. Stop AI found that backyard farmers and women were the most likely to follow bio-security practices than other groups and men. Other initiatives found that containing the disease is much more challenging than assumed and bio-security of farms should be given the highest priority.

Coordination among donors and agencies is critical and an area that needs to be further strengthened. In addition, prudent communications has the potential to reduce the risk of market collapse due to infection of AI and prevent more cases in both humans and animals.
While many lessons have been learned, there are still many gaps that need to be addressed to the problem of AI in Bangladesh. There needs to be a clear understanding of the epidemiology of the H5N1 virus. Research on the development of cheap and easily available quick diagnostic techniques needs to be expanded. In addition, more manpower is needed to improve the logistics of the Veterinary Service to carry out surveillance and respond to outbreaks of AI. Finally, improved coordination between stakeholders and donors is required to adequately address the problem of AI.
The need for clinical management of AI H5N1 may be decreased and possibly eliminated by managing H5N1 in live birds.
To achieve this goal, there are further steps that need to be taken. First a coordination, information, and cooperation model should be developed focused on increasing common understanding to prevent the threat of emerging and re-emerging zoonotic diseases of economic importance in the region. In addition, more emphasis should be placed on "risk" oriented communication rather than "fear" oriented communication. A cost-effective method for diagnosis and response should be developed, as well as increased capacity building. In spite of the challenges, with hard work, transparence, strong coordination, and willingness, focusing efforts on improving and sustaining animal health is a feasible approach for managing AI.
The current public health approach to avian influenza focuses on control and management after an outbreak has already occurred. However it would be possible to utilize resources more strategically by adopting a prevention-centered approach. By preventing an outbreak before it occurs, resources can be directed toward broader improvements in sanitation and hygiene practices that will positively affect not only avian influenza control efforts, but those of many other communicable diseases. In addition, focusing resources on prevention can avert significant morbidity and mortality.
Efforts to support a prevention-centered approach to pandemic avian influenza can be used to strengthen the nation's public health infrastructure, more broadly, which will ultimately result in greater public health and security gains than any reactionary response could possibly hope to. While the necessity has previously been to control and mitigate outbreaks once they have occurred, we are in a strategic position to move towards a more sustainable focus on prevention. It is time to seize the opportunity to get ahead of the threat and to focus resources on stopping outbreaks before they occur.

9. References

Centers for Disease Control and Prevention. (2007. May 07) Avian Influenza (flu): Key facts about avian influenza. Retrieved from http://www.cdc.gov/flu/avian/gen-info/facts.htm

Centers for Disease Control and Prevention. (2008. May 28) Avian Influenza (flu): Key facts about avian influenza. Retrieved from http://www.cdc.gov/flu/avian/gen-info/facts.htm

World Health Organization. (2006a, February). Avian Influenza ("bird flu"). Retrieved from http://www.who.int/mediacentre/factsheets/avian_influenza/en/

World Organization for Animal Health [OIE]. 2010. October 5): Avian influenza facts and figures: H5N1 timeline. Retrieved from http://www.oie.int/Eng/info_ev/en_AI_factoids_H5N1_Timeline.htm

Otte, J., Hinrichs, J., Rushton1, J., Roland-Holst, D., & Zilberman, D. (2008) Impacts of avian influenza virus on animal production in developing countries. *Perspectives in Agriculture, Veterinary Science, Nutrition and Natural Resources 2008.*

USAID/Bangladesh. 2010. Unpublished paper; presented at the API Dissemination Workshop,MOFLS, Dhaka Bangladesh 2010.

World Organization for Animal Health [OIE]. 2010. October 5): Avian influenza facts and figures: H5N1 timeline. Retrieved from http://www.oie.int/Eng/info_ev/en_AI_factoids_H5N1_Timeline.htm

World Health Organization. (2010c). WHO Egypt. Retrieved from [1]http://www.who.int/countries/egy/en/

15

Affectation Situation of HIV/AIDS in Colombian Children

Ana María Trejos Herrera, Jorge Palacio Sañudo
Mario Mosquera Vásquez and Rafael Tuesca Molina
Fundación Universidad del Norte, Barranquilla
Colombia

1. Introduction

Acquired immunodeficiency syndrome (AIDS) is a global emergency and one of the most formidable challenges to human life and human dignity. The Declaration of Commitment on HIV/AIDS, adopted unanimously by the member states of the United Nations at the Special Session of the General Assembly (UNGASS) in New York and the Millennium Declaration, adopted by 189 nations and signed by 147 heads of state and government called for global action to build a global response to HIV/AIDS. (United Nations General Assembly Special Session on HIV/AIDS [UNGASS], 2001).

Globally, the number of children under 15 living with HIV has increased from 1.6 million [1.4 million - 2,1 million] in 2001 to 2.0 million [1.9 million-2, 3 million] in 2007, while young people between 15 and 24 represent an estimated 45% of new HIV infections worldwide. (Joint United Nations Programme on HIV/AIDS [UNAIDS] & World Health Organization [WHO], 2007).

With an adjustment in early 2006, the National Institute of Health (NIH) reported 54,805 cases of Colombian HIV infection and AIDS. The general behavior of the notification has been toward increased, with the rate for the period 1983-2005 to 5.36 cases per 100,000 population and for the last decade 1995-2004 to 7.85 cases per 100,000 population. The reported annual incidence should be used with caution in response to underdiagnosis, the underreporting and delayed reporting that characterized the passive surveillance of HIV/AIDS in the country. (Programa Conjunto de las Naciones Unidas sobre el VIH/SIDA [ONUSIDA] Grupo Temático para Colombia & Ministerio de la Protección Social de Colombia Dirección General de Salud Pública, 2006).

This chapter aims to analyze the situation of involvement for HIV/AIDS in Colombian children based on a study conducted in five cities - Colombian regions: (1) Barranquilla, Santa Marta and Cartagena, (2) Cali and Buenaventura (Instituto Colombiano de Bienestar Familiar [ICBF], Save the Children, Unicef & Universidad del Norte, 2006). The study shows that the delivery of HIV/AIDS diagnosis in children affected is not an established practice in the Colombian context. The low rate of disclosure indicates that within the integrated health management is a priority to develop strategies or clinical models of revelation that support processes of professionals who provide health services to affected families.

This project arose from the need to understand the situation of involvement and quality of life of children and adolescents seropositive for HIV in five Colombian cities, to articulate and assess the scope of the public policies at the time. Our study included children under 18 years of age with three situations of HIV/AIDS affectation: (1) children seropositive or seronegative for HIV, orphans HIV/AIDS (father, mother or both who had died from the disease), (2) children seropositive for HIV and, (3) children seropositive or seronegative for HIV, having lived with HIV positive people.

In 2006, only (3.8%) for 11 children in five Colombian cities were aware of their diagnosis of HIV/AIDS seropositivity compared with [96.2% (n=275)] who were unaware of the situation of HIV/AIDS affectation. The reasons for delaying the delivery of diagnosis that were reported by health professionals and caregivers of affected children, are related to prevent psychological harm or emotional stress to the child; situations cause fear of stigmatization and discrimination against the inadvertent disclosure of the child to others, and lack training regarding the procedure and age to provide this information by professionals providing health services to these children.

Furthermore, due to the importance of quality of life related to health (HRQOL) of children and their caregivers affected in the diagnosis, care and treatment of HIV/AIDS, the chapter will also address the evaluation of the following dimensions of quality of life: (1) Mobility, (2) Personal Care, (3) Activities of Daily Living, (4) Pain/Discomfort and (5) Anxiety/Depression using EuroQol (EQ-5D) instrument, as necessary to make decisions regarding front the care of these children.

Although current antiretroviral treatments managed to increase survival and quality of life of people affected by HIV/AIDS, it is also true that as a chronic disease requiring ongoing treatment, not exempt of adverse effects, to which should be add an important psychosocial impact. Based on this, relevant psychosocial variables have been also analyzed, such as family function instrument employing the Family Apgar and the perception of social support both children and their caregivers using the instrument Social Support (MOS) and scan variables Clinic children were seropositive for HIV/AIDS, which are also explored throughout this chapter.

Similarly results are displayed on the levels of information about the disease who have children who are aware of their diagnosis of HIV/AIDS seropositivity, as well as the caregivers of children who are still unaware of their situation involvement, which will allow to assess the degree of knowledge or misinformation that has this affected population and how can this affect or not confronting the diagnosis. In the same way, will address findings related to usage patterns and access to health services and education which will show that the health and education services in the Colombian context must overcome some obstacles in ensuring not only access to care but also increase the availability, fairness, integrity and quality from the perspective of rights and in order to benefit the child population under 18 years affected with HIV/AIDS.

This will be discussed by combining data from both quantitative and qualitative methodology, provided by the research tools employed and by the focus groups conducted with: (1) children who are aware of their diagnosis of HIV/AIDS, (2) caregivers of children who know their status of involvement for HIV/AIDS and (3) Professionals who provide health services to children affected population, which contain relevant evidence that allow further appreciation of the difficulties felt by the affected children in our country.

2. Illness status disclosure to children with HIV/AIDS

One of the factors that most worries the caregivers of children with HIV and professionals who provide health services is the issue of who, when and how they will reveal to the child that he/she has a chronic and stigmatizing disease that requires demanding treatment and involves the issue of death. (Nagler et al., 1995) explain that the HIV/AIDS carries stigma, which has profound psychological, social and emotional implications for the sufferer. For this reason, too many families make the decision to hide the child's HIV diagnosis, including members of the same family.

FACTORS THAT INHIBIT ILLNESS STATUS DISCLOSURE

1. *Cause damage or psychological harm to the child.* (Abadía-Barrero & Larusso, 2006; Bikaako-Kajura et al., 2006; Boon-Yasidhi et al., 2005; Davis & Shah, 1997; Instituto Colombiano de Bienestar Familiar [ICBF], Save the Children, Unicef & Universidad del Norte, 2006; Instone, 2000; Lester et al., 2002; Lipson, 1993; Myer et al., 2006; Oberdorfer et al., 2006; Tasker, 1992; Wiener et al., 1996; Wiener & Figueroa, 1998; Wiener et al., 1998).
2. *Concern about child discloses his/her HIV illness status to others.* (Bikaako-Kajura et al., 2006; Boon-Yasidhi et al., 2005; Davis & Shah, 1997; Instituto Colombiano de Bienestar Familiar [ICBF], Save the Children, Unicef y Universidad del Norte, 2006; Instone, 2000; Kouyoumdjian et al., 2005; Meyers & Weitzman, 1991; Oberdorfer et al., 2006; Tasker, 1992; Ledlie, 1999; Lester et al., 2002; Lewis et al., 1994; Waugh, 2003; Weiner & Figueroa, 1998; Weiner et al., 1998).
3. *Caregiver's difficulty accepting that the child is old enough to understand HIV diagnosis.* (Abadía-Barrero & Larusso, 2006; Bikaako-Kajura et al., 2006; Boon-Yasidhi et al., 2005; Flanagan-Klygis et al., 2002; Kouyoumdjian et al., 2005; Oberdorfer et al., 2006) .
4. *Parental guilt.* (Lee & Johann-Liang, 1999; Lipson, 1993; Ledlie, 1999; Tasker, 1992; Waugh, 2003).
   Fear about having to answers painful and difficult questions. (Cohen, 1994; Davis & Shah, 1997; Lee & Johann-Liang, 1999; Lipson, 1993; Tasker, 1992; Waugh, 2003; Weiner & Figueroa, 1998; Wiener et al., 1998)
5. *Fears that disclosure will negatively affect their child's health or cause hastening disease progression.* (Lipson, 1993).
6. *Fear that the child associate to caregiver with socially disapproved behaviors such as homosexuality and promiscuity.* (Kouyoumdjian et al., 2005)
7. *Belief that child will feel the same emotional reaction that caregiver felt when knew the bad news..* (Lipson, 1993).

Fig. 1. Factors that inhibit illness status disclosure to children with HIV/AIDS.

Colombian caregivers were afraid that the child would get depressed, be isolated, anxious or worried about having this chronic disease. Caregivers also fear that once the illness status is disclosed, the child will tell others, which will lead him and his family to situations of stigma and discrimination with potentially serious consequences such as expulsion from residence, school, and refusal to play with the child, among others. Similarly, professionals who provide health services to these children showed a lack of consensus on the procedure and age for disclosing illness status.

Researchers found that children were aware of their illness and impending death, despite their parent´s stance of protective communication. (Hardy et al., 1994). Given the number of visits they make to the hospital or clinic and the acquaintances they meet, complete unawareness by a certain age is doubtful. Although kept in secrecy, children often showed curiosity or knowledge about their treatments (Lee & Johann-Liang, 1999). They may listen in on a conversation about AZT treatment between the doctor and their parent or ask other patients about their condition (Lipson, 1993). The stigma of HIV/AIDS leads families to keep the diagnosis secret from the child, other family members and schools.

The American Academy of Pediatrics guidelines for the illness status disclosure to children and adolescents with HIV infection says it is imperative that all adolescents have knowledge of their illness status and that disclosure should be considered for children under school age according to their level of cognitive development, age, family dynamics, psychosocial maturity and other clinical variables (Committee on Pediatric AIDS [COPA], 1999).

Disclosure of HIV diagnosis to children is becoming increasingly important because antiretroviral therapy becomes more widely available, however internationally rates of disclosure seem to be low. Some factors can inhibit and facilitate the decision making of caregivers to disclose illness status to their children with HIV/AIDS (See Figure 1).

Disclosure of HIV diagnosis should be viewed as a process, rather than an event, it is related to the child's cognitive development and aims to provide him/her with age appropriate information.

3. Health-Related Quality of Life (HRQOL) in children affected with HIV/AIDS

Advances in HIV treatment have allowed that quality of life of people affected with HIV/AIDS increased. Quality of Life related to Health subscales provides an overall vision of health and allows make important decisions about patient care. To have a benchmark of the health status of the pediatric patient should be a priority for institutions that provide health services.

For this reason we use EuroQol (EQ-5D) to estimate how Colombian caregivers perceive the Health-Related Quality of Life of their children. EQ-5D is a standardized instrument for use as a measure of health outcome. Applicable to a wide range of health conditions and treatments, it provides information about mobility, self-care, usual activities, pain/discomfort and anxiety/depression.

Results shows in Mobility subscale that 94.4% (N=269) of children with HIV/AIDS do not have trouble walking, 5.6% (N=17) have some problems or confined to bed. In Self-Care subscale, 96.1% (N=275) do not have problems bathing or dressing; 3.9% (N=11) of children have some problems or are unable to bathing or dressing. In Usual Activities subscale results shows that 96.1% (N=275) do not have problems to perform their usual activities, 3.9% (N=11) of children have some problems or are unable to perform their usual activities. In Pain/Discomfort subscale caregivers perceive that 84.6% (N=242) of their children do not have pain or discomfort, however 15.4% (N= 44) of children have some problems or may be experiencing pain and discomfort. Finally, caregivers perceive that 90.2% (N=258) of their HIV-positive children do not have anxiety or depression while 9.8% (N=28) may be experiencing anxiety or depression according to caregiver's report (See Table 1.)

Health-Related Quality of Life N=(286)	No Problems		Some Problems		Confined to bed/Unable to Perform	
	F	%	F	%	F	%
Mobility	269	94.4%	16	5.2%	1	0.4%
Self-Care	275	96.1%	7	2.5%	4	1.4%
Usual Activities	275	96.1%	8	2.9%	3	1%
Pain/ Discomfort	242	84.6%	40	14%	4	1.4%
Anxiety/ Depression	258	90.2%	25	8.7%	3	1.1%

Table 1. Health-Related Quality of Life (HRQOL) in Colombian children affected with HIV/AIDS measured by their caregivers.

The above results indicate that Colombian children affected with HIV/AIDS have a good level of health. Worth noting that all these children are affiliated to the social security health and are receiving Highly Active Antiretroviral Treatment (HAART). However, the highest percentage of problems found in Pain/Discomfort subscale with 15.4% of children who have some problems or may be experiencing pain and discomfort according to caregiver's report.

(The World Health Organization [WHO], 2003) defines health as a state of complete physical, mental, and social well-being and not merely the absence of disease or infirmity. It follows that measurement of health must not only include estimates of the frequency and severity of diseases, but also well-being and quality of life. This is particularly true for patients with HIV/AIDS because of the chronic and debilitating nature of the illness, stigma, and a high rise of premature death (Nojomi et al., 2008).

4. Family Functioning and social support in families affected with HIV/AIDS

Family Functioning play a very important role in coping with HIV illness. Understanding aspects of this interaction between children's health and their family is important to keep and increase quality of life, coping and adherence to treatment, well-being and psychological adjustment for a HIV-positive child. A family with good parental relationships would mean the family members are willing to solve problems together, showing concern for each other, and there will be fewer quarrels. In this sense, it is necessary for a child with a chronic illness such as HIV could find in his/her family some solid foundations that allow him/her to deal with this diagnosis.

For estimated this variable, we used Family Apgar to assess a family member's perception of family functioning by examining his/her satisfaction with family relationships. 73.8% (N=211) of Colombian children are in a norm functionality family. This mean, responder's perception about his/her family has the basic features to be functional and harmonic in the domains: adaptation, partnership, growth, affection and resolve. 18.2% (N=52) of families affected with HIV/AIDS report moderate dysfunction while 8% (N=23) families report severe dysfunction (See Table 2).

In every family has a complex dynamic patterns governing their living and functioning. Of this dynamic is appropriate and flexible, in other words, functional, contribute to family harmony and provide its members the ability to develop strong feelings of identity, safety and welfare (Sherboune & Stewart, 2003; Cohen et al., 1985).

Family Functioning N=(286)	F	%
Norm Functionality	211	73.8%
Moderate dysfunction	52	18.2%
Severe dysfunction	23	8%

Table 2. Family Functioning in families affected with HIV/AIDS.

Interest in the concept of social support has increased dramatically over the last few years, due to the belief that the availability of support may impact favorably on a person's health and emotional well-being (Sherbourne, 1988). Consider the psychological impact of HIV/AIDS social support may play a small but potentially important role in helping HIV-positive people to cope with illness.

(Leserman et al., 1992) found that subjects primarily coped with the threat of AIDS by adopting a fighting spirit, reframing stress to maximize personal growth, planning a course of action, and seeking social support; satisfaction with one's social support networks and participation in the AIDS community were related to more healthy coping strategies (e.g., fighting spirit, personal growth). These results suggest that health professionals should encourage more adaptive coping strategies, help the patients to use existing sources of positive social support, and assist patients in finding community support networks.

The availability of someone to provide help or emotional support may protect individuals from some of the negative consequences of major illness or stressful situations (Barrera, 1981).

Investigators (Brandt & Weinert, 1981; Brown & Brady, 1987; Broadhead et al, 1988; Cohen & Syme, 1985; Cohen & Wills, 1985; Duncan-Jones, 1981; House & Kahn, 1985; Norbeck et al., 1981; Reis, 1988; Sarason et al., 1983) have attempted to measure the functional components of social support under the belief that the most essential aspect of social support is the perceived availability of functional support. (Cohen & Hoberman, 1983; House & Work, 1981; Wills, 1985). Functional support refers to the degree to which interpersonal relationships serve particular functions.

The functions most often cited are (1) emotional support which involves caring, love and empathy, (2) instrumental support (referred to by many as tangible support), (3) information, guidance or feedback that can provide a solution to a problem, (4) appraisal support which involves information relevant to self-evaluation and, (5) social companionship, which involves spending time with others in leisure and recreational activities. (Ahumada et al., 2005; Fleming et al., 2004; Gill et al., 2002; Sherbourne, 1988).

A 20-item MOS questionnaire was administered to all participants. This questionnaire limits the evaluation scale of the entire network of the interview subjects; participants performed their social support excluding people that do not have a good relationship. Four degrees of functional social support (Call et al., 2000): An emotional/informational, tangible, affectionate, and positive social interaction were administered and shows a Global Index of families affected with HIV/AIDS. 74.1% of families have a maximum social support, 22.7% have a medium social support and 3.1% have a minimum social support (See Table 3).

Social Support N=(286)	F	%
Maximum	212	74.1%
Medium	65	22.7%
Minimum	9	3.1%

Table 3. Social Support in families affected with HIV/AIDS.

5. Clinical status of children with HIV/AIDS

Health-related quality of life (HRQOL) is increasingly recognized as an important measure for assessing the burden of chronic diseases (Hays et al., 2000). HIV-specific parameters, such as low CD4 cell count and high virus load, have previously been shown to adversely affect HRQOL in some studies of HIV-infected patients (Casado et al., 2011; Niuwerk et al., 2001).
Other studies show weak HRQOL associations with disease stage and CD4 cell count (Niuwerk et al., 2001). Similarly, the effect of HAART on HRQOL has been assessed with some studies (Call et al., 2000).
According to international definitions on the concept of childhood affected by HIV/AIDS, participating minors must comply with the following affectation categories as criteria of population inclusion, nonexcluding amongst themselves: 1. HIV/AIDS seropositive and/or seronegative children, and adolescents, orphaned by HIV/AIDS (father, mother, or both deceased because of the disease). 2. HIV seropositive children and adolescents. 3. HIV seropositive and/or seronegative children and adolescents, cohabitating with HIV seropositive individuals.
80 children were HIV-positive in five Colombia cities. 80% (N=64) were receiving antiretroviral therapy and most 34.9% (N=30) had HIV load undetectable or low 20% (N=15) (See Table 4). As we mentioned earlier, Colombian children affected with HIV/AIDS have a good level of health because all these children are affiliated to the social security health and are receiving Highly Active Antiretroviral Treatment (HAART); 80% (N=64) children are receiving HAART (See Table 4).

Viral Load N=(80)	F	%
High	10	13.8%
Medium	8	10%
Low	15	20%
Undetectable	30	34.9%
Unclassified	17	21.3%
Antirretroviral Therapy (N=80)	**F**	**%**
YES	64	80%
NO	14	17.5%
Unknown	2	2.5%

Table 4. Viral Load and Antiretroviral Therapy in HIV-positive children.

6. Health service utilization and barriers to health services in children with HIV/AIDS

The results of this investigation shows the dynamics of the demand of services by children affected with HIV/AIDS, and the information will be useful in planning and organizing care for families with HIV. We found in Colombian families affected with HIV/AIDS a pattern of frequent use (50.8% N=145) of the health service (See Table 5).

Health Services Utilization (N=286)	F	%
Frequent	145	50.8 %
Regular	74	25.9 %
Occasional	37	12.9 %
Sporadic	30	10.4 %

Table 5. Health Services Utilization in Colombian families affected with HIV/AIDS.

Families affected with HIV have to face some barriers in health service provision such as: Arrival Time to heath service (half hour to an hour or more than an hour) 60.4% (N=138); Waiting Time exceeding 30 minutes in 53.8% (N=154) and 85.7% (N=245) of the children affected are not receiving Home Care even though they needed it; Health professional argue against this latter finding that caregivers do not provide personal information for fear of discrimination (See Table 6).
No significant results were found for other barriers explored: Respectful and Friendly Service; Discretion and Confidentiality Service; Subsidizes Antiretroviral Therapy; Acquisition of Antiretroviral Therapy with own money and Transportation, however many of the families reported in the focus groups did not have resources for transportation to health service (See Table 6).

Barriers to Health Services	Category	N	%
Arrival Time (N=286)	Less than half an hour	148	51.7%
	Half hour to an Hour	102	35.7%
	More than an Hour	36	12.6%
Transportation (N=286)	One Bus	127	43.6%
	More than one Bus	25	9.1%
	Mototaxi	35	12.5%
	Particular Transport	29	10.5 %
	Other: (walking; bike)	70	24.3%
Waiting Time in Service (N=286)	Immediately (15′)	39	13.6%
	Family should wait (15′ A 30′)	93	32.6%
	More than 30′	154	53.8%
Respectful and Friendly Service (N=286)	Yes	259	70.6%
	No	26	29.1%
	Sometimes	1	0.3%

Barriers to Health Services	Category	N	%
Discretion and Confidentiality Service (N=286)	Yes	265	92.7%
	No	20	7%
	Sometimes	1	0.3%
Home Care (N=286)	Monthly	4	1.4%
	2 to 3 months	14	4.9%
	Every 6 months	7	2.4%
	1 time per year	16	5.6%
	Never	245	85.7%
Entity that subsidizes Antiretroviral Therapy (N=64)	Subsidized by the foundation	4	6.5%
	Subsidized by the health lender (EPS)	6	10.4%
	Subsidized insurance scheme (ARS)	33	50.6%
	Subsidized by distrital or departamental health secretary	21	32.5%
Acquisition of Antiretroviral Therapy with own money (N=64)	Yes	4	6.7%
	No	60	93.3%

Table 6. Barriers of Health Services in Colombian families affected with HIV/AIDS.

87.4% of Families affected with HIV reports that health attention has not been denied (See Table 7).

Denial of Health Services (N=286)	F	%
YES	36	12.6 %
NO	250	87.4 %

Table 7. Denial of Health Services in Colombian families affected with HIV/AIDS.

7. Conclusion

The low rate of disclosure of HIV status to children found in the study indicates that it is a priority to develop disclosure clinical model in the Colombian context. For this reason since 2008 our institution is conducting the investigation: "Evaluation of the effects of a disclosure clinical model in HIV-positive children 7 - 18 years old in adherence to treatment and psychological adjustment". Research Project awarded with the Fellowship for Research from the Department of Research and Projects. Awarded in the 2008 Call for Proposals for Doctorate Programs at Universidad del Norte

This research aims to provide a clinical model to help affected families overcome fears that lead them to delay the delivery of HIV diagnosis. Mainly, caregivers want to avoid psychological or emotional harm to child and they fear that child tell the diagnosis to others and be discriminated against.

According to the above, health professionals do not know for sure at what age a child should know their HIV diagnosis. Some believe that at 10 years a child is old enough to manage this information. Some believe that children should learn about biosecurity practices and adherence to treatment without knowing the diagnosis in a playful way, through stories, comics and other fun techniques. Health professionals recognize that children perceive that something happens with his/her bodies by going through periods of illness and drugs.

Caregivers and health professionals explain to children that drugs are for flu, pneumonia, heart problems, fever and other low-impact diseases, but do not tell the child that he/she has HIV/AIDS.

Colombian families interviewed showed a positive degree of satisfaction with Family Functioning and Social Support. Children have good quality of life, low virus load and have access to Antiretroviral Treatment. Some barriers were identified in health services utilization.

On the other hand, we consider important to offer some recommendations to access to Colombian children affected with HIV/AIDS. Not all health services in the Colombia cities have pediatrics patients with HIV. Once identified health services, health teams evaluate the research protocol, this assessment could take 2 or 3 months. Also, it is important to know that caregivers take children to health services once a month and informed consent must be obtained through a detailed explanation of the research and get his/her signature as the child's legal representative.

Health services should provide to researches a private place for interviews. Many health services were not including in this study for lack of such space.

This type of researches must have a budget to be allocated to pay transportation costs of caregivers and HIV-positive children. These families have economic limitations to move to health services.

Another recommendation is to consider extending the running time for such studies because of the difficulties identified in the location and recruitment of subjects.

8. Acknowledgment

The authors acknowledge the support of the financial organizations and especially the willingness of those who made this study possible: children and adolescents affected by HIV/AIDS and caregivers of the five cities: Cali, Buenaventura, Barranquilla, Santa Marta y Cartagena.

Moreover, we extent our heartfelt thanks to all institution that offer services to families affected with HIV/AIDS, especially those who were agreed to cooperate with aims of this research:

In Cali city: Emsanar, Lila Mujer, Fundamor and Casa Gami.

In Buenaventura city: Fundación Si Buenaventura.

In Barranquilla city: Fundación François Xavier Bagnoud, Fundación Esperanza por la Vida, Susalud EPS, Fundación Grupo Estudio Barranquilla and Unidad Especial de Salud y Ambiente (UESA).

In Santa Marta city: Heres Salud E.U., Fundación Luz de Esperanza and Sistemas Integrales de Salud de Colombia (SISCO).

In Cartagena city: Unidad Médico Quirúrgica, Fundación Amigos Positivos, Sistemas Integrales de Salud de Colombia (SISCO) and Vivir Bien.

9. References

Abadía-Barrero C & Larusso M. The Disclosure Model versus a Developmental Illness Experience Model for Children and Adolescents Living with HIV/AIDS in São Paulo, Brazil. *AIDS Patient Care and STDs* 2006. Volume 20, Number 1.

Ahumada R, Castillo L, Muñoz B y Moruno M. Validación del Cuestionario MOS de Apoyo Social en Atención Primaria. *Medicina de Familia (And)* Vol. 6, N.° 1, abril 2005

Barrera M. *Social support in the adjustment of pregnant adolescents: assessment issues.* In Social Nerworks and Social Support (Edited by Gottlieb B.). Sage, Beverly Hills, CA 198 1.

Bikaako-Kajura W, Luyirika E, Purcell DW, Downing J, Kaharuza F, Mermin J., et al. Disclosure of HIV status and adherence to daily drug regimens among HIV-infected children in Uganda. *AIDS Behaviour* 2006, 10(Suppl. 4), S85-S93.

Boon-Yasidhi V, Kottapat U, Durier Y, Plipat N, Phongsamart W, Chokephaibulkit K & Vanprapar N. Diagnosis Disclosure in HIV-Infected Thai Children. *J Med Assoc Thai* 2005.

Brandt P. A. & Weinert C. The PRQ-A social support measure. *Nurs. Res.* 30, 277-280, 1981.

Broadhead W. E., Gehlbach S. H., DeGruy F. V. and Kaplan B. H. The Duke-UNC Functional Social Support Questionnaire: Measurement of social support in family medicine patients. *Med. Care* 26, 709-721, 1988.

Brown S P., Brady T., Lent R. W., Wolfert J. and Hall S. Perceived social support among college students: Three studies of the psychometric characteristics and counseling uses of the social support inventory. *J. Counseling Psycho/*34, 337-354, 1987.

Casado A, Consiglio E, Podzamaczer D, Badia X. Highly active antirretroviral treatment (HAART) and health-related quality of life in naïve and pretreated HIV-infected patients. *HIV Clin Trials* 2001; 2:477–82.23.

Cohen S & Hoberman H. Positive events and social supports as buffers of life change stress. *J. appl. Sot. Psycho/*13, 99-125, 1983.

Cohen S., Mermelstein R., Kamarck T. & Hoberman H. *Measuring the functional components of social support.* In Social Support: Theory, Research and Applications (Edited by Sarason I.). Martines Nijhoff. Holland, 1985.

Cohen FL. Research on families and pediatric human immunodeficiency virus disease: A review and needed directions. *Developmental and Behavioral Pediatrics* 1994, 15(3), S34-S42.

Cohen S. & Syme S L. *Issues in the study and application of social support.* In Social Support and Health (Edited by Cohen S. and Syme S. L.). Academic, Orlando, 1985

Cohen S. & Wills T. A. *Stress, social support, and the buffering hypothesis.* Psychol. Bull. 98, 310-357. 1985.

Committee on Pediatric Aids. Disclosure of illness status to children and adolescents with HIV infection. *Pediatrics* 1999.103:164-166.

Call SA, Klapow JC, Stewart KE, et al. Health-related quality of life and virologic outcomes in an HIV clinic. *Qual Life Res* 2000; 9:977–85.

Davis J K & Shah K. Bioethical aspect of HIV infection in children. *Clinical Pediatrics* 1997, 36, 573-579.

Duncan-Jones P. The structure of social relationships: Analysis of a survey instrument-Part 1. Sot. *Psychiaf.* 16, 55-61, 1981.

Flanagan-Klygis E, Ross LF, Lantos J, Frader J & Yogev R. Disclosing the diagnosis of HIV in pediatrics. *AIDS and Public Policy Journal* 2002, 17(1), 3-12.

Fleming C, Christiansen D, Nunes D, Heeren T, Thornton D, Horsburgh R, James M , Graham C and Craven D. Health-Related Quality of Life of Patients with HIV Disease: Impact of Hepatitis C Coinfection. *Clinical Infectious Diseases* 2004; 38:572–8

Gill CJ, Griffith JL, Jacobsen D, Skinner S, Gorbach SL, Wilson IB. Relationship of HIV viral load, CD4 counts, and HAART use to healthrelated quality of life. *J Acquir Immune Defic Syndr* 2002; 30:485–92.

Hardy MS, Armstrong FD, Routh DK, Albrecht J & Davis J. Coping and communication among parents and children with human immunodeficiency virus and cancer. *Developmental and Behavioral Pediatrics* 1994, 15(3), S49-S53.

Hays RD, Cunningham WE, Sherbourne CD, et al. Health-related quality of life in patients with human immunodeficiency virus infection in the United States: results from the HIV Cost and Services Utilization Study. *Am J Med* 2000; 108:714–22.

House J. S. & Kahn R. *Measures and concepts of social support.* In Social Support and Health (Edited by Cohen S. and Syme S. L.). Academic Press, San Francisco, 1985.

House J. S. *Work, Stress and Social Support.* Addison- Wesley, Reading, MA, 1981.

Instituto Colombiano de Bienestar Familiar [ICBF], Save the Children, Unicef y Universidad del Norte. *Calidad de Vida, Apoyo Social y Utilización de Servicios de Salud y Educación en niños, niñas, adolescentes y acudientes afectados con VIH/SIDA en cinco ciudades-región colombianas: (1) Cali y Buenaventura y, (2) Barranquilla, Santa Marta y Cartagena.* Informe Final de Investigación 2006. Departamento de Investigaciones Universidad del Norte (DIP): Barranquilla.

Instone SL. Perceptions of children with HIV infection when not told for so long: implications for diagnosis disclosure. *J Pediatr Health Care* 2000. Sep-Oct; 14(5):235-43.

Joint United Nations Programme on HIV/AIDS [UNAIDS] & World Health Organization [WHO], 2007). Aids Epidemic Update. 27/08/2010. Available from: http://data.unaids.org/pub/epislides/2007/2007_epiupdate_en.pdf

Kouyoumdjian F, Meyers T & Mtshizana S. Barriers to disclosure to children with HIV. *Journal of Tropical Pediatrics* 2005. Vol. 51. No 5.

Lee CL & Johann-Liang R. Disclosure of the Diagnosis of HIV/AIDS to children born of HIV-infected mothers. *AIDS Patient Care and STDs* 1999, 13(1), 41-45.

Ledlie S. Diagnosis Disclosure by Family Caregivers to Children who have Perinatally Acquired HIV Disease: When the Time Comes. *Nursing Research* 1999. 48(3):141-149.

Lester P, Chesney M, Cooke M, Weiss R, Whalley P, Perez B, Glidden D, Petru A, Dorenbaum A & Wara D. When the Time Comes To Talk About HIV: Factors Associated With Diagnostic Disclosure and Emotional Distress in HIV-Infected Children. *JAIDS Journal of Acquired Immune Deficiency Syndromes* 2002. 31:309-317.

Leserman, J, Perkins, DO, Evans, DL. Coping with the threat of AIDS: the role of social support. *Am J Psychiatry* 1992 149: 1514-1520.

Lewis SY, Haiken HJ & Hoyt LG. Living beyond the odds: A psychosocial perspective on long-term survivors of pediatric human immunodeficiency virus infection. *Developmental and Behavioral Pediatrics* 1994, 15(3), S12-S17.

Lipson M. *What do you say a child with AIDS*. The Hastings Center Report 1993. 23; 2: research library core. Pag. 6.

Meyers A & Weitzman M. Pediatric HIV disease: The newest chronic illness of childhood. *Pediatric Clinics of North America* 1991, 38(1), 169-194.

Myer L, Moodley K, Hendricks F & Cotton M. Healthcare provider's perspectives on discussing HIV status with infected children. *Journal of Tropical Pedia*trics 2006, 52(4), 293-295.

Nagler S, Adnopoz J & Forsyth B. *Uncertainly, stigma and secrecy: psychological aspects of AIDS for children and adolescents*. In: Andiman W, Geballe S, Guende, eds. Forgotten Children of the AIDS Epidemic 1995. New Haven, CT: Yale University Press; 1-10.

Niuwerk PT, Gisolf EH, Reijers MH, Lange JM, Danner SA, Sprangers MA. Long-term quality of life outcomes in three antiretroviral treatment strategies for HIV-1 infection. *AIDS* 2001; 15:1985–91.

Nojomi M, Anbary K & Ranjbar; M. Health-Related Quality of Life in Patients with HIV/AIDS. *Arch Iranian Med 2008;* 11 (6): 608 - 612.

Norbeck J. S., Lindsey A. M. & Carrieri V. L. The development of an instrument to measure social support. *Nurs. Res.* 30, 264-269, 1981.

Oberdorfer P, Puthanakit T, Louthrenoo O, Charnsil C, Sirisanthana V & Sirisanthana T. Disclosure of HIV/AIDS diagnosis to HIV-infected children in Thailand. *Journal of Pediatrics and Child Health* 2006. 42:283-288.

Programa Conjunto de las Naciones Unidas sobre el VIH/SIDA (ONUSIDA)., Ministerio de la Protección Social de Colombia y Dirección General de Salud Pública (2006). Infección por VIH y Sida en Colombia. Estado del Arte 2000-2005. *Pro-Offset Editorial Ltda: Bogotá D.C.*

Reis J. A factorial analysis of a compound measure of social support. *J. clin. Psychol.* 44, 876890, 1988.

Sarason I G., Levine H. M., Basham R. B. and Sarason B. R. Assessing social support: The social support questionnaire. *J. Person. Sot. Psvchol.* 44, 127-139, 1983.

Sherboune C & Stewart A. The MOS social support survey. *Sot. Sci. Med.* Vol. 32, No. 6, pp. 705-714, 1991.

Sherbourne C D. The roll of social supports and life stress events in use of mental health services. *Med. Care* 27, 1393-1400, 1988.

Tasker M. How can I tell you. Secrecy *and disclosure with children when a family member has AIDS*. Bethesda, MD 1992: Association for the care of children Health.

The World Health Organization [WHO], 2003. WHO Definition of Health. 23/02/2011. Available from: http://www.who.int/about/definition/en/print.html

United Nations General Assembly Special Session on HIV/AIDS. Declaration of Commitment on HIV/AIDS. Resolution A/Res/S-26/2, 27 June 2001 (www.unaids.org/UNGASS/docs/AIDSDeclaration_en.pdf), hereinafter cited as Declaration of Commitment.

Waugh S. Parental Views on Disclosure of Diagnosis to their HIV-positive Children. *AIDS Care* 2003. Vol. 15 No 2, pp. 169-176.

Wiener L, Battles H, Heilman N, Sigelman C & Pizzo P. Factors associated with disclosure of diagnosis to children with HIV/AIDS. *Pediatr AIDS HIV Infect* 1996. 7(5):310-324.

Wiener LS & Figueroa V. Children speaking with children and families about HIV infection. In P. A. Pizzo & C. M. Wilfert (Eds.), *Pediatric AIDS* 1998: The challenge of HIV infection in infants, children and adolescents (pp. 729-758). Baltimore: Williams and Wilkins.

Wiener LS, Septimus A & Grady C. Psychosocial support and ethical issues for the child and family. In P. A. Pizzo & C. M. Wilfert (Eds.), *Pediatric AIDS* 1998: The challenge of HIV infection in infants, children and adolescents (pp. 703-727). Baltimore: Williams and Wilkins.

Wills T. A. *Supportive functions of relationships*. In Social Support and Health (Edited by Cohen S. and Syme S. L.). Academic, Florida, 1985.

16

Strengthening Health Systems in Yemen: Review of Evidence and Implications for Effective Actions for the Poor

Abdulwahed Al Serouri[1], John Øvretveit[2],
Ali A. Al-Mudhwahi[3] and Majed Yahia Al-Gonaid[3]
[1]*Faculty of Medicine and Health Sciences, University of Sana'a,*
[2]*MMC Karolinska Institute MMC, Stockholm,*
[3]*Primary Health Care Sector, MoPHP,*
[1,3]*Republic of Yemen*
[2]*Sweden*

1. Introduction

Decisions about how best to use resources are always political decisions, but can be more effective if they are also informed by research. International reports and donor policies emphasise how research can help make health strategies more effective and the need for evidence based policies (WHO, 2004; Green & Bennet, 2007, Moynihan et al., 2008, WB, 2005).

The aim is to review international and Yemeni experiences in order to find evidence of proven effective strategies which would make the best use of the resources available for improving health.

2. Health system strengthening (HSS)

A "successful strengthening strategy" is defined as changes which are implemented, which improve the quantity or quality of health services, especially for the poor, and which are sustained. This includes financing strategies to help poor people to access health services.

Concepts of "the health system" recognise that the lowest level "system" is not just a set of health services but also includes the patient or citizen, their family and community, which may do more than health services to protect and care for a person's health.

3. Evidence basis for future strategy

3.1 Why does Yemen need to strengthen its health system and health services?

Health research and health sector reviews in Yemen report evidence of:

3.1.1 Health needs

- There are significant levels of unmet health needs, especially for poor people in rural districts where 71% of the population lives, and great variations in needs between areas (MoPHP, 2010).
- Maternal, infant and child mortality rates are amongst the highest in the world (366/100,000 and 69/1000, 102/1000 respectively), and there are high rates of many preventable diseases (MoPHP, 2010).
- There are significant levels of dissatisfaction among patients and providers with health services and systems, relating to access and quality (HESAS, 2003, Al Serouri, 2004). Poor health services have been proposed as one factor contributing to civil unrest, and secessionist movements (Sidhom, 2010).

3.1.2 Poor matching of resources to needs

- Health service coverage about 67% of the population but only 35% for the rural population (MoPHP, 2010)
- Mal-distribution of human resources, with distribution favouring urban areas, and 42% of physicians working in four governorates, and a shortage of employed female staff (MoPHP, 2010)
- Poor Health Information System (HIS) data, and poor planning of services in relation to needs (MoPHP, 2010)
- A large private sector, primarily in urban areas, with limited government regulation and supervision (MoPHP, 2010)

3.1.3 Inefficient use of resources

- Poorly equipped facilities (HESAS, 2003)
- Shortages of drug and supplies (HESAS, 2003)
- Limited budget for the operational costs, staffing, and incentives for health services of government facilities (HESAS, 2003)
- Deficiencies in health management skills and systems (HESAS, 2003)
- Most public health programs, including child health, infectious diseases, nutrition and other programs provided as vertical programmes, available in less than 40% of health facilities (MoPHP, 2000).

3.2 Which strengthening strategies are effective in low income countries?

WB 2005 classified HSS strategies as three types:

3.2.1 Provider based strategies

Performance improvement; Human resource management; Financial management; Information management; Pharmaceuticals and supplies management; Equipment management; Facilities/capital works management; Auxiliary support services; Marketing services and products; Reorganizing providers; Public sector provider reorganization

3.2.2 Government and financing strategies

Policy & strategy development; Information on the health of the public; Financing: Securing public resources for health, Allocating health resources, Pooling resources, Payment mechanisms.

3.2.3 Households and community empowerment strategies

Building individual/household capacity; Building community capacity; Transferring authority, responsibility, and resources

Evidence from research outside of Yemen shows four strategies are effective for strengthening health services in a number of low income settings:

- Removal of financial barriers to health care access
- Increasing the number of health workers
- Changing physician behaviour (e.g. more rational drug prescribing)
- Changes to drug procurement systems.

However the evidence is not strong because many specific interventions are grouped within these categories, and some of the specific interventions have had more success than others.

Case studies reported in a WB 2005 HSS study found that different strategies used to reduce financial barriers for access all had positive results. These were: the Ghana strategy which used a "National Health Insurance Scheme"; Uganda and Zambia abolished user fees; and Vietnam introduced user fees with exemptions; and used social health insurance for the poor.

The research shows different strategies have been used to increase the number of health workers, including using paid or unpaid community health workers (CHWs), all of which had positive results, the latter especially for the poor. Where numbers have been increased, this has clearly strengthened health services (WB, 2005).

Strategies that involve strengthening accountability and which link financing to measures of performance and accountability (e.g. through contracting), have been found to be effective over the short-term, and over a number of settings. Evidence from the WB 2005 case studies show positive results when the Afghan government contracted not-for-profit providers and also related finance to performance. Ghana's decentralization of finance and performance-based contracts also produced positive results. However, the payment schemes and measurement had limitations, and there were also negative results, such as loss of income for large hospitals with high demand and utilisation by low- or no-income population. These cases show evidence that the payment and measurement needs careful design and piloting to reduce negative consequences.

As regards the payment of incentives to health workers to increase the quantity and quality of services, there is moderate evidence that strategies of this type are successful.

3.3 Is there evidence of strategies which have been effective in Yemen to strengthen health services?

There is evidence that some centrally-managed "vertical" disease programmes e.g. the National Malaria Control Programme have successfully reduced disease burden e.g. malaria had dropped in the Tihama region from 46 to 11 %, and in Socotra, an island in the Indian Ocean, the prevalence rate had fallen from 36 to 1% (NMCP, 2003). However, the National Health Strategy (2010-2025) noted that some vertical disease control programs does not have the capacity effectively to detect, control, prioritize, and plan the public health management of these diseases. Furthermore, the cost-effectiveness and long term sustainability of such vertical programs still questionable (MoPHP, 2010).

On the other side, there is evidence of a successful programme for strengthening primary care units to provide immunization on an outreach basis with financial incentives, increasing the coverage of Penta3 by 29%. More recently, there is some evidence that vertical programmes (Malaria, TB, IMCI, nutrition, and bilharzia) can be integrated into PHC and district services using the same approach, and can improve preventative and curative services (MoPHP, 2009). The results of such integrated outreach activities showed remarkable improvements according to the following:

- Coverage of EPI: increase in Penta 3 coverage by 35 %, 34% in Measles and 72% for Tetanus Toxoid 2.
- Coverage of other services: IMCI, RH, & Nutrition services were provided for a new target population including under 5 children and child bearing age women.
- Costs: The cost per child during the EPI outreach was 1.3$ whereas the cost for the integrated outreach was 1$.

Many donors are currently building upon the service delivery model developed under the GAVI-funded Health Sector Strengthening project. The proposed future World Bank Yemen Health and Population Project (2010-2015) intends to draw on the experience of the EPI and GAVI programmes in order to develop strengthening strategies to reach the MDG goals 4 and 5. UNICEF will be supporting community-based services in the governorates of Sana'a and Ibb to complement the routine outreach services supported by GAVI project in these two governorates. JICA is supporting community-based services in six districts in Yemen in three governorates based on the experience that was implemented by GAVI funded HSS Project.

However the evidence suggests that some PHC facilities and districts are less able to integrate these vertical programmes, and require additional actions to strengthen management and systems so as to be able effectively to provide a wider range of services (MoPHP, 2010).

3.4 Are disease-specific programs an effective way to strengthen health services?

There are some studies of disease-specific programmes in other lower income countries (e.g. strategies to improve reproductive health services), as well as some unsystematic literature reviews of these strategies. Some of this research considers the scale-up of successful pilot programs (Øvretveit, 2008, Øvretveit, 2011).

However, the research does not provide a clear answer to this question. There is some weak evidence that disease-specific programmes do divert resources from other programmes and do distort overall health services away from local needs. There is evidence from Zambia where there is a chronic shortage of health workers that "vertical" programmes for providing HIV/AIDS anti-retroviral therapy (ART) diverted scarce personnel from providing other needed services (Øvretveit, 2008).

There is also some evidence that these programmes can strengthen health systems beyond their specific area of interest. But the evidence is inconclusive and appears to depend on how the strategy is implemented - careful implementation of certain types of HIV/AIDS programmes can also strengthen other services, but again the research is limited and cannot be generalised (Øvretveit, 2008).

One overview of research into health systems constraints for the MDGs (Travis, 2004) categorised the disadvantages of vertical delivery systems described in the literature as follows:

3.4.1 Duplications

Running parallel systems for delivering drugs to health facilities will increase transport costs, and increase the number of forms that health workers need to complete to secure their drug supply.

3.4.2 Distortions

Creating a separate cadre of better paid health workers for the specific tasks of a programme may deplete staff from other key functions and/or de-motivate staff who do not benefit from higher pay or better conditions.

3.4.3 Disruptions

Programmes often train health workers by taking them away from their jobs for several days or weeks, leaving their posts vacant. This training tends to be uncoordinated across programmes, and may result in the same worker receiving several training courses in a year, with a substantial loss of services being delivered.

3.4.4 Distractions

Similarly, the specific and uncoordinated reporting requirements of vertical programs/donors can lead to several forms being filled by a sole health worker for the same problem, distracting them from more productive uses of their time.

Although the Travis 2004 overview provided limited evidence, it concluded that:

> *"Disease or service-specific strategies to strengthen health systems on their own are unlikely to bring about the improvements in health systems needed to achieve the MDGs. ...Such an approach must be complemented by a substantial additional body of knowledge and action that takes the functioning of the health system as its core concern".*

3.5 Can actions to strengthen disease-specific programs that are effective in one area be successfully spread within a country?

There is some moderate evidence from research that such programmes can be successfully "scaled up". This means that more studies have found successful scale up than those which have found less successful scale up. However, there is a publication bias towards reporting the "scale ups" that were successful, and not reporting the unsuccessful ones.

One example is the strengthening strategy used to scale up NGO-CHW projects across one set of districts in Zambia. The original model was refined, and then a pilot scale up programme was made, which was then itself developed to allow spread in other regions. The HIV/AIDS CHW model was extended to provide programmes including malaria control, and immunization (Øvretveit, 2008) .

There is evidence that success appears to depend on how the implementation is carried out, and on certain enabling factors in the environment, as well as on the type of disease specific programmes: more complex multiple-component programmes appear to be less successful in scale up, but this may be because the capacity was not there to ensure continual coordination in some cases. Research based guidance for scale-up is given in Øvretveit , 2006.

3.6 Are many strengthening strategies together more successful?

The evidence (WB, 2005) is that they can be, but often are not because of a lack of resources and management capacity at different levels to coordinate and implement the different strategies. There is some evidence that multiple compatible strategies, where different changes reinforce each other, are likely to have a more significant, long-term effect than single-action strategies alone (e.g. integrated delivery of health service, multiple component healthcare reforms). But the risks of failed implementation are higher because:

3.6.1 Consensus and support

It is more difficult to obtain consensus and support for each component of a multiple-action strategy than for a single approach.

3.6.2 Management and oversight

More complex multiple-action strategies demand greater management capacity if the actions are to be mutually-reinforcing. Persistent oversight is needed for effective consensus building, planning, coordination, review, and readjustment. Management capacity may not be able to provide these.

3.6.3 Timing

Because of limited resources and capacity, the specific actions for multiple-action strategies will need to be phased-in at different times so that these resources and capacity are not overwhelmed by the demands of many actions at one time.

3.6.4 Implementation of non-mutually reinforcing actions

There is a possibility that specific actions will not be implemented, or may be implemented in ways that undermine other components of the strategy. For example, incentives to provide specific services (e.g. special payments for immunization), can reduce incentives to provide other services for which there is greater need (Øvretveit, 2006).

Overall, the evidence shows that, the more complex the strengthening strategy (e.g. many changes, phased changes, with a large overall change), the more support is required (expert facilitators, external training and supervision). Multiple component and sophisticated strengthening strategies can be more effective only if properly implemented - it is costly to provide this support nationally and some level of ongoing support or supervision is often required (Øvretveit, 2006).

3.7 Is how the strategy implemented more important than the type of strategy?

One conclusion from this review of research is that that almost any strategy might be possible to implement, if certain conditions and implementation methods are present. There is positive evidence for this from successful implementation, as well as negative evidence from the failed implementations which did not have supportive conditions or were not well-managed.

A systematic review of 150 studies using high quality experimental designs (Øvretveit et al., 2008) noted that many of the strategies studied had significant amounts and types of resources to ensure full implementation: similar results could only be expected if the resources or conditions were repeated. One common element in the few studies with many positive outcomes was efforts to assess needs and constraints. In these studies 'constraint reduction plans' were found in 66% of the randomized interventions. However, many interventions that did not use this approach also had positive outcomes. Also, the research often did not describe to what extent these constraint reduction plans were implemented.

Overall there is evidence, that, of all the fully implemented strategies, some were effective in strengthening service delivery for poor people. What appears to be important is targeting poor people, ensuring regular measurement of impact, and oversight to ensure the poor benefit.

There is also research into strategies used for scale-up which have proven successful. There are useful frameworks for scale up of successful pilot strengthening approaches in Yemen including one by Cooley & Kohl 2005. Their tested framework gives a three-step process to carry out ten key tasks which their study suggests were needed for effective scaling up. Key choices to be made in deciding how to apply a strengthening intervention more widely (e.g. in scale-up) are: the sequencing of elements of the strengthening programme; and the pace of spread (e.g. rapid or phased); the areas to spread to and the sequence of areas.

A Community-based Health Planning and Services (CHPS) initiative in Ghana (Nyonator et al., 2006) gives some possible lessons for how to carry out a strengthening strategy in Yemen. The model aimed to reorient primary health care from clinics to communities, by relocated nurses to live and work in community-constructed clinics and using volunteers to mobilizing traditional social institutions to get community support. The scale up strategy used decentralized planning to adapt the operational details to local circumstances.

The study notes actions which helped to overcome constraints to scale-up by comparing slow and faster implementing districts. One was to use "peer exchange" to discuss the details of practical changes which would be needed and to use the original pilot as a demonstration model for visits. This is combined with training for upgrading clinical skills, new referral arrangements, quality assurance, and community-based health management.

The study notes that once the initiative gets started in one or two zones there is spread of the new approach within districts, but spread is slow across district boundaries because of staff exchanges. So within- and across- district involvement of leaders from neighbouring communities was necessary. It also notes a resource constraints problem to scale up where often fewer resources are available than were used in the pilot. The "faster" districts had found additional funds, usually not from government, for example "private practitioners" -paramedics who are community financed rather than salaried employees.

The action taken to address some of the problems of nurses working in areas they were not from, was a "community engaged" approach to decentralized training. Communities select nurse trainees, who are sent to a local training centre where fees are paid by the districts and communities to be served by the trainees. On graduation, nurses return home, rather than to a post in a distant location.

The study provides an analysis of issues and principles some of which may apply in other settings and for other strengthening-strategies. The first highlighted was the role of research: not just evidence from a district which replicated the pilot, both of which convinced policy-makers and others that the pilot would work elsewhere, but to identify problems and guide the scale-up. The second was the need for specific guidelines about parts of the programme that needed to be changed, the steps needed to get the operational change, and for monitoring whether change was taking place. The third observation was that the pilot was useful as a demonstration of the model and as a training centre. There was a need to resource the pilot founding implementation team to pass on their experience and motivation. A fourth item was the value of many ways of communicating the evidence and progress as well as sustaining the effort: newsletters documented community and worker experience with the programme and conferences, demonstration exchanges, and staff meetings. The report notes that "CHPS is thus a complex story. Its core strategy is based on a complex experiment, multiple replication efforts, and diverse sources of evidence. But, its core agenda is quite simple for stakeholders to understand and embrace".

Fig. 1. Example of lessons from research from a health service strengthening strategy

3.8 How important is it to adapt the strategy to fit the situation, and to continue to adapt it?

There was some evidence from the review that adaption - taking a strategy and adapting it to the country and local conditions - was associated with fuller strategy implementation. In addition, that continuous strategy adaption in scale up led to fuller implementation and that adaptation was easier in small-scale interventions. In Ghana, a scale-up of a child and maternal health service strengthening pilot was made using an approach adapted for the situation using peer demonstration, diffusion, and teamwork (Phillips et al, 2006).

There are different examples of intervention approaches which decisions makers can use. A two-phased approach involves a pilot, then feedback, and then further modification of the intervention, followed by regional or national dissemination. A three-phased approach may prove to be even more effective. If time and resources allow, the initial pilot may be followed by additional pilots at the same time within different country contexts, allowing for more detailed guidance for decision-makers. There is evidence that implementation effectiveness is increased by providing continuous feedback to the strategy team and leaders about health service needs, constraints, implementation progress, and health service impact. This can be done by independent researchers.

Data from the WB, 2005 HSS case studies show that the planning of all the strategies in each country included some type of assessment of constraints and adaptation of ideas to the country situation. There was great variation after initial national planning in, continual adaptation (e.g. whether annual reviews and re-planning were carried out to adjust the strategy to changing circumstances), and also in adaptation by lower levels to the situation and needs of local areas.

There is evidence that strategies with not only initial, but also continual and local adaptation were more successful from the examples of decentralization in Ethiopia, Ghana Uganda, and Zambia (Øvretveit et al., 2008).

3.9 Is stakeholder involvement and consultation necessary to effective implementation?

Overall there is some limited evidence from the research that consulting or involving those who make the change, or who can stop it, is necessary for implementation. But there are also counter examples from authoritarian governance situations such as China where success was due to strong implementation structures without consultation (Kaufman, et al 2006). The research can help decision makers be more aware of the different approaches to consultation and involvement of different parties and levels of the health system, and of examples where this has been done. Research does not show if involvement and consultation is always necessary or which type is most effective in which situations.

The research reports adaptation by decision makers or implementers alone, after consultation. It also reports consultation and stakeholder involvement with little adaptation, and as pre-implementation preparation or as a form of education (Fajans, 2006)

The evidence suggests that some pre-implementation consultation can increase the speed and depth to which a strategy is implemented, but much depends on the country's history and culture. Many studies refer to lack of stakeholder consultation, or of lack of involvement and commitment as one explanation for less successful implementation. Where there has been successful implementation, widespread involvement in a process for agreeing the strategy is often reported as building commitment and as a key factor explaining successful implementation.

3.10 Are there strategies which are less dependent on the environment, which work in most countries?

There was no strong evidence from the review of research that some strategies were more "robust" than others, and less influenced by some of the conditions which appeared to affect implementation of all the strategies. A number of studies reported success where implementation had included constraints assessment and actions to reduce constraints (table 1 at end of this review). The implications are that, if decision makers take action to ensure that as many of these conditions as possible are met, this would increase the likelihood of implementation of the strategy (Travis, 2004).

3.11 Should we implement a strategy if we are uncertain if we have the right resources?

The research reviewed shows that one condition profoundly influencing all strengthening strategies are whether there are adequate resources for the change, for example as indicated by average per-capita income of the country, health care expenditure, and availability of health workers and capable managers (WB, 2005).

Findings from the WB, 2005 HSS case studies show that some strategies were not implemented because of lack of resources initially, or a reduction in available resources later, typically when donor or project finance ceased. There was evidence from the cases that availability of finance was a necessary but not sufficient condition for health service strengthening: some human resource strategies had financial resources, but a shortage of health workers prevented full implementation (e.g. in Ethiopia, Afghanistan).

4. Conclusions from the review of research into health service strengthening strategies

There is evidence of high levels of unmet health needs in Yemen, and of the potential for health services to prevent and alleviate suffering, especially of poor people. There is evidence of a number of deficiencies in the allocation of services, their performance and accessibility. This evidence suggests that changing the allocation of resources and increasing efficiency could do much to meet existing needs. However, the changes will not be easy to make, will take time, and will need capable management and incentives for change at all levels. Central and local government will need support to build the capacity, commitment and persistence to make the changes needed.

Research in Yemen has found vertical programmes have been effective, but possibly at the expense of generic primary health care and district services. Research found that PHC could provide EPI successfully on an outreach basis, and this "integration" model has recently been used for Malaria, TB, IMCI, nutrition, and bilharzias in a GAVI programme. Evidence shows that some PHC and districts can successfully provide prevention and care for these diseases and clients, but others need additional strengthening so as to be able to do so.

Research from other lower income countries shows the strength of service delivery (amount, accessibility for those most in need and quality) is most strongly influenced by the resources available for the service. This, in turn, depends on the amount of finance from government and private (individual and other), the number and skills of health workers, the facilities and supplies (especially drugs), and participation of the community in different ways including volunteer services.

Other specific factors have a greater or lesser influence on the strength of service delivery in different situations (e.g. pay and conditions of government workers can be critical for motivation and retention in most situations).

5. Practical implications for Yemen from the research

A future strengthening strategy will be more effective if it implements changes which have already proven successful for increasing the quantity and quality of health services in Yemen and elsewhere.

5.1 General principles for design and implementation of strengthening strategies

Use research and evidence from elsewhere, but combine it with local knowledge and adapt a change or strategy to the local situation:

1. Research suggests that the consequences of a strengthening strategy are difficult to predict, and that a strategy successful in one region could be unsuccessful in another. Adapting the strategy so that it can be implemented may require local research and/or community consultation.
2. Carry out a "barrier analysis" to assess constraints and hindrances to implementation.
3. Consultation can improve the design and planning of a strategy and can speed implementation, but much depends on the local situation.
4. Involve all levels: each levels of the health and local government system has a role in strengthening health services which needs to be specified, ideally through consultation, and then developed through training and other actions.
5. Pilot test any strategy first, and revise it using feedback from the pilot.
6. Scale up successful pilots using a tested method for scale up (e.g. the Cooley & Kohl, 2005 three-step approach describe above).
7. Include feedback to strategy implementers from continual monitoring of progress, of constraints and of new opportunities arising from the changing situation.
8. Flexibility and adaptation: have regular formal and informal review points where the strategy is modified for the changing situation.

5.2 Strengthening health services

Research suggests the following actions could effectively strengthen health services in Yemen:

1. Careful and phased implementation of the "GAVI vertical integration" model in PHC beyond the pilot districts. This can be informed from lessons from scale up strategies elsewhere, including strengthening governorate, district and PHC management which may not currently have the capacity to carry out the integration, adapting the model locally, and using information about implementation to make these adaptations.
2. Removal of financial barriers to health care access, using one or a mixture of the strategies reported to be effective, such as payment exemptions for the poor or social health insurance schemes.
3. Increase income for health services with effective systems to use and account for the finance, and by a combination of extra government allocations and income generating methods.
4. Increasing the number and skills of health workers, especially in rural areas, by rapidly expanding paramedic training, and possibly by more use of community health workers.
5. Improving pharmaceutical management

   There is less strong evidence to suggest the following strengthening strategies would be effective, but enough to suggest they should be seriously considered for Yemen:
6. Appropriate licensing of practitioners and health service accreditation, and enforcement of penalties.

5.3 Strengthening management and systems

For these health service strengthening actions to be carried out, actions to strengthen the health system will be needed. These are actions which increase the capability of managers at all levels and how they work together, and improve the management systems such as for management information and human resource management.

For most strategies, managers at all levels need to be developed and given time to plan and implement strengthening interventions (rather than solely manage routine operations), with some managers dedicated full-time to implementing the strengthening intervention. Aspects of leadership associated with successful strengthening changes include: a clearly communicated mandate from top management that gives authority, resources, and accountability to leaders and teams throughout the organization, as well as respected "change champions," and implementation teams.

The evidence suggests that some strategies which require stronger management capacity should not be pursued on more than a pilot basis until the capacity has been developed. Strategies which might be considered later, and which have proven to have some success with adequate management systems are:

1. Performance based contracting or other ways of linking financing to measures of performance and accountability
2. Payment of incentives to health workers to increase the quantity and quality of services.

5.4 Reduce constraints to health service strengthening

In planning and implementing a strategy, decision makers would be advised to assess and address the following factors which have been reported in research to enable/hinder implementation of most types of strategies:

Enabling/Hindering Factor	Description
Resources for the strengthening strategy	Funding for the strengthening strategy
	Number of personnel engaged in carrying out the strengthening intervention
	Competence of managerial and front-line personnel (e.g. professionalism, skills, expertise in change processes), particularly their ability to adapt the intervention to local circumstances (i.e. through an assessment of constraints, opportunities, resources)
Management and governance capacity	Ability/power of each management level to prompt the level below to take action
	Ability of each management level to hold others accountable (i.e. impose rewards, sanctions)
	Degree of corruption
	Degree of local community participation and assistance in the implementation process
Political stability and support	Frequency of changes in government, or leadership implementing the strategy
	Degree and consistency of support by powerful interest groups
	Degree of consensus among powerful interest groups
	Degree and consistency of popular support

Source: Øvretveit, 2006

Table 1. Enabling/Hindering Factor

5.5 Practical steps for developing a strategy

The following draws on the research reviewed to describe a series of steps which is likely to result in an effective strengthening strategy which is implementable:

1. Create a structure which includes key stakeholders to formulate a service-strengthening strategy for the country and each region
2. Combine actions to strengthen delivery of disease specific programmes with actions to strengthen health services and the health system overall.
3. Use the constraints-based list below to guide national and local information gathering on the nature, severity and possible solutions for national and local constraints to:
   - Finance for health services
   - Human resources and management and planning
   - Employee and provider motivation and payment systems
   - Quality and performance improvement programmes and methods
   - Necessary changes to organisation
   - Drug supply and better prescribing
   - Management development and management system development especially for management information and use
   - Good governance including community participation in health services
   - Cross-sector interventions which strengthen health services
4. Consider from this report and others which evidence about constraint-reduction actions is most applicable to your country, and the strength of the evidence.
5. Combine this information with the national information described above to formulate sub-strategies to reduce each of the constraints. Consider which actions would produce significant short term results and which are longer term actions.
6. Consider which actions in each sub-strategy are the same or similar and then prioritise these in the overall strengthening strategy.
7. Sequence the strategy in relation to priorities, funding availability and your assessment of the absorptive- and change-coping capacity of the system.
8. Create a structure for implementation involving stakeholders, and with systems to allocate the resources to each sub strategy, and to monitor and to regularly review the strategy.

6. Acknowledgment

This report was commissioned by the MoPHP, Primary Health Care Sector to help inform future strategy to strengthen health services and health systems in Yemen. The grant is from GAVI for Health System Strengthening (HSS).

7. References

Al Serouri, A.W. (2004). Towards Quality Health Care In Yemen Republic: I- Quality from Clients' perspective. The Yemeni Journal of Medical and health Research, 2004, 3: 1-6.

Cooley, L., Kohl, R. (2005). *Scaling-up – a conceptual and operational framework.* Washington D.C., In: *Management Services International,* accessed 30 March 2010, Available from: <http://www.vibrantcommunities.ca/downloads/SSI_downloads/kohl_scaleup.pdf>

Fajans P, Nguyen Thi Thom, Whittaker M, Satia J, Tran Thi Phuong Mai, Can, Do Thi Thanh Nhan, Newton N (2006). Strategic choices in scaling-up: introducing injectable contraception and improving quality of care in Viet Nam. In: Simmons Fajans P, Ghiron L, eds. Scaling-up health service delivery: from pilot innovations policies and programmes. Geneva, World Health Organization, 2006.

Green, A., Bennet, S. (Eds) (2007). *Sound choices: enhancing capacity for evidence-informed health policy*. WHO Geneva

HESAS (2003). Improvement Programme For Clinical Services (SIP). Situation Assessment in 10 Health Centers and 9 Health Units of 10 Governorates. March 2003.

Kaufman J, Zhang E, Xie Z (2006). Quality of care in China: from pilot project to national programme. In: Simmons R, Fajans P, Ghiron L, eds. Scaling-up health service delivery: from pilot innovations to policies and programmes. Geneva, World Health Organization.

MoPHP (2000). Health Sector Reform in the Republic of Yemen Strategy for Reform

MoPHP (2009). Annual Progress Report for GAVI supported activities in 2008. Sana'a Yemen

MoPHP (2010). National Health Strategy 2010-2025. Ministry of Public Health and Population, Sana'a, Yemen.

Moynihan, R., Oxman, A.D., Lavis, J.N., Paulsen, E. (2008). Evidence-Informed Health Policy: Using Research to Make Health Systems Healthier – Report from the Kunnskapssenteret (Norwegian Knowledge Centre for the Health Services), No. 1-2008. Oslo: Norwegian Knowledge Centre for the Health Services; 2008.

NMCP (2003). The National Malaria Control Programme In Yemen. Progress Report

Nyonator, F.K., Akosa, A.B., Awoonor-Williams, J.K., Phillips, J.F., Jones, T.C. (2006). Scaling-up experimental project success with the community-based health planning and services initiative in Ghana. In: *Scaling-up health service delivery: from pilot innovations to policies and programmes.* Simmons R., Fajans P., Ghiron L. Geneva, World Health Organisation.

Phillips JF, Jones TC, Nyonator FK, Ravikumar SR (2006). Evidence-based scaling-up of health and family service innovations in Bangladesh and Ghana. In: Simmons R, Fajans P, Ghiron L eds. Scaling-up health service delivery: from pilot innovations to policies and programmes. Geneva, World Health Organization, 2006.

Sidhom, Y (2010). Responsive Governance for a More Stable Yemen. http://www.rti.org/newsletters/witw/2010aug-sep/index.cfm?starting_up=2.

Øvretveit, J. (2006). Strengthening Health Services in Low Income Countries: Guidance for decision makers implementing strategies. Washington: World Bank, HDNHE, and MMC, Karolinska Institute, Stockholm.

Øvretveit, J. (2008). Strengthening health services in Zambia: case study, World Bank and Karolinska Institute MMC, Stockholm.

Øvretveit, J 2011. Widespread focused improvement: lessons from developing countries for scaling up specific improvements to health services International Journal for Quality in Health Care 2011; Volume 23, Number 3: pp. 239–24610.1093/intqhc/mzr018

Øvretveit, J., Peters, D., Siadat, B., Thota, A. (2008) Summary of Review of Research into Strengthening Health Services in Low Income Countries, Washington: World Bank, Parent, F, Coppieters, Y. 2001. A process of change in first-line health services in Chad. Health Policy and Planning 16(1): 122–123.

Travis, P., Bennett, S., Haines, A., Pang, T., Bhutta, Z., Hyder, A.A., Pielemeier, N.R., Mills, A., Evans T. (2004). Overcoming health-systems constraints to achieve the Millennium Development Goals. *Lancet*; 364: 900-06.

WB (2005). Health Services Delivery - Lessons from Low and Middle-Income Countries Concept Note," David Peters, The World Bank, Washington.

WHO (2004). World report on knowledge for better health: strengthening health systems, WHO Geneva.

17

Performance Measurement Features of the Italian Regional Healthcare Systems: Differences and Similarities

Milena Vainieri and Sabina Nuti
Istituto di Management - Laboratorio Management & Sanità, Scuola Superiore Sant'Anna, Pisa Italy

1. Introduction

A growing number of factors among which rising costs, technological advancements, aging population, health market failure and medical errors, led many industrialized countries to manage their health services and goals through performance measurement (Arah et al, 2003; Kelley & Hurst., 2006; Smith, 2002). In this context it became a commonplace for countries to formally assess the performance of their healthcare system (Mc Loughlin et al., 2001).
Since the 1980s the introduction of "New Public Management" (NPM) principles has promoted a number of reforms in order to drive a more efficient, effective and accountable public sector (Hood, 1995a; Lapsley, 1999; Saltman et al. 2007). OECD countries have applied these principles in different ways with different emphasis (Hood 1995b).
Among the NPM principles, the one asking the public sector to adopt more explicit and measurable standards of performance measurement, has motivated countries to create different performance measurement systems (PMS).
In the Italian health sector, the development of PMS can be traced back to the 90s reforms that introduced managerial tools and devolved the organization and assessment of healthcare services to Regions. This devolution, enforced by the recent federalist reform of 2009, has led Regions to shape their own organizational structures and relationships among health system actors (Censis, 2008; Formez, 2007). As a consequence of these reforms, Italy has now 21 Regional Health Systems with significant differences from each other.
On the basis of these considerations the Italian health sector provides with an interesting scenario in order to detect and analyze the differences and similarities in PMS adopted by the Regional governments.
This chapter attempts to provide a cross sectional analysis of the Italian Regional PMS characteristics using evidences of an empirical study carried out in 2008-2009.

2. Theoretical frameworks

As a consequence of NPM reforms, especially those concerning PMS, academics and international organizations such as the World Health Organization (WHO) and the Organization for Economic Cooperation and Development (OECD) developed conceptual frameworks and models in order to help countries in building effective tools (Arah et al., 2006; Kelley et al., 2006; Murray & Evans, 2003; Smith, 2002; Veillard et al., 2005).

Both WHO and OECD based their frameworks on three main goals of health systems: (a) health improvement and outcomes; (b) responsiveness and access; and (c) assuring fairness of financial contribution. (Arah et al 2003).
These organizations declined these goals into four dimensions of performance: (a) health improvement/outcomes (b) responsiveness (c) equity, (d) efficiency.
Using these four dimensions, Hurst & Jee Hughes (2001) compared PMS adopted by a group of countries. The study highlights that countries do not covered all dimensions moreover often common dimensions are drill down differently.
On the basis of this evidence a first aim of this paper is to map the differences and similarities of IRHSs regarding the dimensions of performance monitored by Regional top managers and/or policy makers.
Another burning topic related to PMS in healthcare is the use of pay for performance mechanism as a governance tool (Van Herck et al 2010, Mannion & Davies 2008).
It is recognized that management tools should be managed in a coordinated way, especially the linkages between rewarding system (one of the two perspective of the pay for performance) and budgeting (Flamholtz et al., 1985; Ouchi, 1979). The connection between them is a crucial factor that can determine the effectiveness of PMS at the organizational level. To this extent it appears worthy to analyze the differences in the connection between PMSs and the rewarding system.
Finally another important topic related to PMS is benchmarking. Arah et al (2003) pointed out that a group of countries, that adopted a national PMS in health care, uses benchmarking as a mechanism to drive change in terms of improvement. In this perspective benchmarking is applied in order to gather information which can help the organization to improve its performance (Watson, 1993).
Although benchmarking gained growing relevance in health PMS at several levels, from international to organizational level (Johnston, 2004; NHS executive, 1999; Pink et al,2001; Nuti et al. 2009), in the Italian health sector it was not widespread yet at national or regional level (Banchieri, 2005).
In such circumstances a last issue that the empirical study aims to analyze regards differences and similarities in the attitude of Italian Regional Health System (IHRS) towards the use of benchmarking.

3. Research methods

The study, reported in this chapter, is based on semi-structured interviews carried out in the Italian Regional Health Systems (IRHSs); Regional documents (Regional law or Regional publications) and secondary data (i.e. Italian studies and reports).
Concerning interviews, all Regional health councillors and Regional heads of health departments were invited to participate in the study.
The collection of field data mainly took place between 2008 and 2009.
The interviews focused mainly on three topics:

- the description of tools used for measuring the performance of health services;
- the linkage between PMS and rewarding system;
- regional attitude towards benchmarking.

Nevertheless there was a questionnaire, interviews were conducted following an open approach so that interviewees could highlight their meanings and perception about the PMS and the field situation (Patton, 1990). Due to the open approach Regional interviewees were not forced to answer to all the items included in the questionnaire; as a consequence some items remained uncovered.

A total of 15 Regions (over 21) participated in the study. Some Regions did not participate in the study because of institutional reasons such as the election or judgmental inquiries. Taking into account these issues the answer rate was high and the responses were quite balanced across Italian Regions (see table 1).

Regions	Regions participating on the study	Area	Population	N° of Public Health Authorities	Financial deficit
Piedmont	Yes	North	4,352,828	21	Recovery Plan (2010)
Lombardy	Yes	North	9,545,441	45	
Bolzano	Yes	North	487,673	1	
Trento	Yes	North	507,030	1	
Veneto	Yes	North	4,773,554	23	
Friuli Venezia Giulia	Yes	North	1,212,602	9	
Liguria	Yes	North	1,607,878	8	Recovery Plan (deficit covered by other regional resources)
Tuscany	Yes	Centre	3,638,211	16	
Umbria	Yes	Centre	872,967	6	
Marche	Yes	Centre	1,536,098	5	
Campania	Yes	South	5,790,187	19	Recovery Plan
Apulia	Yes	South	4,069,869	10	Recovery Plan (2010)
Basilicata	Yes	South	591,338	4	
Sicily	Yes	South	5,016,861	18	Recovery Plan
Sardinia	Yes	South	1,659,443	12	Recovery Plan (deficit covered by other regional resources)
Lazio	No	Centre	5,493,308	21	Recovery Plan
Abruzzo	No	South	1,309,797	4	Recovery Plan
Molise	No	South	320,074	1	Recovery Plan
Calabria	No	South	1,998,052	11	Recovery Plan (2009)
Emilia Romagna	No	North	4,223,264	17	
Valle d'Aosta	No	North	124,812	1	

Sources: Minister of Health, 2010 data and National Institute for Statistics.

Table 1. A snapshot of the main statistics and comments of the IHRSs

Conducted interviews generally lasted between 1 and 2 hours. They were recorded and sent to the interviewees for their validation. In addiction preliminary results of the cross-regional analysis were presented to those who participated in the study in a feedback seminar held in 2009. The discussions evolved on this occasion represented an effective means of the cross-validation of the preliminary interpretations on the IHRSs responses on the characteristics of PMSs which were collected in a research report (Nuti & Vainieri, 2009) .

Findings coming from interviews are also supported and integrated by the documental analysis and the secondary data collected during the research.

4. Results

This paragraph reports the results of the three research topics analyzed regarding differences and similarities in: the PMS dimensions; the IRHSs' integration tools and in the regional attitude towards the use of benchmarking. Quotation are reported in italics.

4.1 Differences and similarities in the PMS dimensions

A first description given by regional policy makers and regional managers on the adopted tools (reported in the table 2) outlines that often Regions adopt more than one tools in order to cover all dimensions identified by the OECD. Sometimes Regions complain to be overwhelmed by a plethora of indicators (see Piedmont and Apulia quotation).

Many Regions that developed multidimensional PMS declared to have applied the following conceptual frameworks: Basilicata and Bolzano based their PMS on balanced scorecard approach (Basilicata regional law 329/2008 and Bolzano county law 1809/2009); Trento PMS is based on EFQM (European Foundation for Quality Management) framework (Panizza, 2010); Marche PMS is based on the value chain; Lombardy based its PMS on JCHA (Joint Commission on Hospital Accreditation) while Tuscany developed its own framework with the help of the Scuola Superiore Sant'Anna of Pisa (Nuti et al, forthcoming a).

Regions	**Information about PMS framework**
BASILICATA	Region uses more than one tools. They are then systematized in an annual BSC. BSC is the theoretical framework declared by the interviewees. Standards are set by the regional law 329/2008. There are both common and specific targets across Health Authorities.
CAMPANIA	The recovery plan's dimensions are monitored
FRIULI VENEZIA GIULIA	There are more tools that monitor the dimensions declared. Measurements are carried out by the Regional Agency for healthcare. Most of indicators are based on hospital data. *The 90% of primary care services measures is an indirect indicator of primary care performance because it comes out from hospital information systems such as the hospitalization rate for the heart failure…*
LIGURIA	Mainly the recovery plan's dimensions are monitored. *Liguria is one of the regions that have to follow a recovery plan from the financial deficit so that many actions, objectives and tools are determined by this particular situation*
LOMBARDY	The theoretical framework declared by interviewee is the JCHA: Joint Commission Hospital Accreditation.
MARCHE	Supply chain model is the theoretical framework declared by interviewee.
PIEDMONT	There is a plethora of tools with lots of information. *Our capacity to produce reports is higher than our capacity to read it.* There is an observatory on equity and epidemiologic aspects that supports analysis for health policy.
BOLZANO	BSC is the theoretical framework declared by interviewees. As regards as the customer and citizens satisfaction, it was carried out by the regional statistician department using panel. *Primary care measures are weak, we are not able to gather reliable information. So our systems are biased by the hospital side.*

Regions	Information about PMS framework
TRENTO	EFQM model is the theoretical framework declared by interviewees but is not the only tool adopted.
APULIA	Many tools are adopted in order to monitor performance. *There are too much indicators that are not systematized yet.*
SARDINIA	Indicators are derived by the Regional Health Plan. A top down approach was used in this stage.
SICILY	Many control systems have been introduced with the recovery plan. *There is a general lack of control systems.*
TUSCANY	Theoretical framework on Performance Evaluation System (PES) had been developed in 2004 in collaboration with the Mes lab, study centre of Scuola Superiore Sant'Anna of Pisa that is still in charge of the measurements and surveys. PES provides Region with a striking visual picture of the overall performance of health authorities.
UMBRIA	The epidemiological observatory makes periodical studies on equity and outcome. There is more than one tool.
VENETO	There is more than one tool. Regional Agency for healthcare helps Regional health department in the measurement and the process of evaluation.

Table 2. Information about regional PMS framework

The dimensions covered by all principal tools quoted by Regions are reported in table 3.

Regions	(a) health improvement /outcomes	(b) responsiveness	(c) equity (of health outcomes, access and finance respectively);	(d) effciency (both macroeconomic and microeconomic).
Basilicata	X	X		X
Campania	X			X
Friuli Venezia Giulia	X	X	X?	X
Liguria	X			X
Lombardy	X	X		X
Marche	X	X		X
Piedmont	X		X	X
Bolzano	X	X		X
Trento	X	X	X?	X
Apulia	X	X		X
Sardinia	X		X?	X
Sicily	X			X
Tuscany	X	X	X	X
Umbria	X		X?	X
Veneto	X	X	X?	X

Table 3. OECD dimensions covered by regional PMS.

Efficiency is the dimension with the highest level of commonalities across Regions. It can be addressed to the fact that Regions developed PMSs first focusing on standards and targets concerning managerial efficiency and cost containment, and then they extended their attention to other issues (Ancona , 2008). The predominance of the efficiency dimension emerges when there are consistent problems on keeping financial equilibrium and the Italian central government asks Regions for a recovery plan. Table 1 summarizes the Regions with a recovery plan in the period of interviews. Thus Regions under central government pressure for reducing financial deficit are mainly focused on costs containment. As a consequence the other dimensions (ie. Responsiveness) are considered less urgent and, as a matter of facts, they are not strictly monitored (this is well highlighted by the quotation of Liguria Region reported in table 2).

Regions	**PMS' Dimensions**
BASILICATA	1. Acute care 2. Territorial services 3. Primary care and prevention 4. Continuty of care 5. Integration between social and sanitarian care 6. Customer satisfaction (normative fulfilment) 7. Financial perspective 8. Human resources
CAMPANIA	Efficiency and financial aspects
FRIULI VENEZIA GIULIA	1. Efficiency 2. Equity 3. Promoting the good clinician practices 4. Improvements on population's health status The customer satisfaction is carried out by civic audits.
LIGURIA	There are indicators of efficiency, appropriateness and health production.
LOMBARDY	1. Financial and efficiency perspective 2. Outcome 3. Customer satisfaction (periodical surveys)
MARCHE	1. Population's characteristics; 2. Need 3. Demand 4. Supply 5. Access 6. Outcome/output 7. Financial perspective
PIEDMONT	1. Efficiency 2. Financial perspective 3. Ad hoc analysis (equity) Customer satisfaction is carried out by civic audits.

Regions	PMS' Dimensions
BOLZANO	1.Efficiency and economic sustainability 2. Appropriateness 3. Quality and outcome 4. Customer and citizens satisfaction (periodical survey on a panel)
TRENTO	1. Regional strategies 2. Financial perspective 3. Efficiency 4. Quality 5. Appropriateness 6. Equity
APULIA	1. Efficiency 2. Financial dimension 3.Clinical performance 4.Appropriateness 5.Regional strategies 6.Customer satisfaction
SARDINIA	1. Activation of some pathway projects 2. Activation of projects mainly based on developing health information services 3. Financial perspective 4. Specific indicators for each Health Authorities
SICILY	1. Appropriateness 2. Quality 3. Clinical risk management
TUSCANY	1. Population health, 2. Regional policy targets, 3. Quality of care, 4. Patient satisfaction, (periodical surveys) 5. Staff satisfaction, 6. Efficiency and financial performance
UMBRIA	1. Quality 2. Efficiency 3. Appropriateness
VENETO	1. Efficiency 2. Quality (for specific areas) 3. Appropriateness 4. Regional strategies

Table 4. Details of regional PMS dimensions

The health improvement and outcome is the other dimension declared by all Regions. That is due to the fact that some indicators included in the recovery plan are those related to an appropriate use of resources such as the number of medical DRGs discharged by surgical wards. Apart these indicators there are a lot of differences concerning the type of indicators included: only few Regions declare to include quality indicators or clinical risk (safety) indicators (see table 4) in addiction other differences concern the technique applied in order to

calculate some indicators for instance the large (or null) use of dichotomous (yes/no) indicators or the use of specific indicators related to the treatment of particular chronic conditions.
Responsiveness and equity are the dimensions less monitored and also those that register a high number of differences.
Regarding responsiveness, common indicators are those related to waiting times. Besides this type of indicators, other monitored topics concern patient satisfaction. Nevertheless lots of Regions declare to monitor patient satisfaction, methods are quite different from each others for instance some Regions, such as Lombardy and Bolzano, run sample surveys; others use the civic audit and finally others, such as Basilicata, control that surveys have been executed by Health Authorities without having information about the results (see table 4).
Concerning Equity, the Commission on Social Determinants of Health (CSDH) of WHO asserted that the systematic and continuous measuring of equity indicators is a fundamental step in order to close the gap of inequities (CSDH, 2008).
Only some Regions declare to have monitored equity. Most indicators related to equity require surveys so that many Regions seldom measured these type of indicators. The only two Regions that are able to measure systematically equity in access for some services (ie. Hospital discharges) are Piedmont and Tuscany (see table 5).

Regions	**Equity dimension**
Basilicata	*None at the moment.*
Bolzano	*We are still studying systematic indicators on equità. Nowadays we focus on immigrants.*
Liguria	*We are planning to control this aspect.*
Lombardy	Equity is pursued using indicators focused on frailty people.
Piedmont	Many ad hoc survey have been run on various topics. Inequalities are studied by the epidemiologic observatory, they have developed very high competences on these issues. In years Piedmont Region records the education degree in the hospitalization data so that we could control whether there are differences among social classes for inpatients.
Apulia	*We pay attention on frailty classes. We reorganized the exemptions on the basis of those classes.*
Sardinia	*We don't have equity indicators. At the moment we look at frailty classes such as mental health, elderly or drug addicted.*
Tuscany	*We have indicators coming from survey related to the educational degree and systematic indicators related to the access of educational classes for inpatient services.*
Trento	There is an ad hoc survey conducted by the specialized centre of Trento regarding all services. This study looked at indicators concerning the access per gender, age, education and so on.
Umbria	*We don't have systematic indicators on equity. Administrative data don't have reliable information on education or income. Many surveys have been conducted by the university centre on this topic. Some of them are really important.*
Veneto	*Although equity is one of the key issue of our regional strategic plan, we don't have indicators that control this aspect in a systematic way.*

Table 5. Regional responses on equity dimension

Information gathered by interviews and documental analysis highlight that Regions with comprehensive tool covering almost all OECD dimensions are those that are supported by internal (such as regional agency or epidemiologic observatory) or external (such as university centres) institutions. In this perspective it seems that innovative management tools are associated to a fertile cultural environment (ie. specialized university centre or observatory).

4.2 Differences and similarities in IRHS integration tools

Responses about integration between PMS and rewarding system can be classified into three groups (as reported in figure 1).
In the first group there are Regions that have coped with central pressure on the deficit control, they suspended the CEOs rewarding system or linked it to normative fulfilments (Case A).
In the second group (Case B) there are Regions (Basilicata and Sardinia) which show full integration between rewarding system and performance measurement system. These regions have recently implemented performance measurement systems and in order to enforce them, they decided to strictly link the rewarding system. To this extent the rewarding system introduces an innovative way of measuring performance.
The last group of Regions (Case C) is characterized by a partial integration of rewarding and performance measurement systems. These Regions decided to make a selection of measures to be rewarded adding to the PMS' measures also other type of decisions.

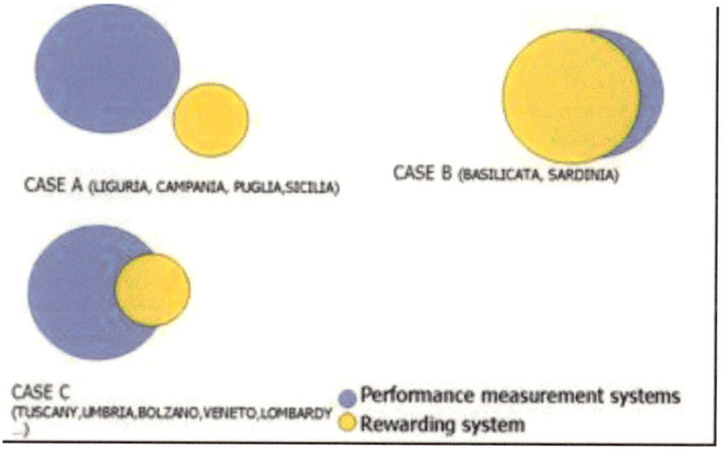

Fig. 1. Integration between performance measurement systems and rewarding system.

In general PMS covers much more topics than the rewarding system as it is represented in case A and C. These two groups collect the majority part of the Regions that participated in the study. The only case where the rewarding system is almost overlapping with the PMS adopted is the case B. It seems that when Regions seek to implement new reliable control system they use the rewarding system as a driver of change.

4.3 Differences and similarities in the regional attitude towards the use of benchmarking

Benchmarking is seen by all Regions, with the exception of Apulia, as an interesting opportunity to improve their performance.

These responses seem to be particularly influenced by contextual factors (described in table 1) such as the size of the Region and the environmental pressure. Indeed small regions such as Umbria feel, more than others, the necessity to look outside regional boundaries in order to gain the advantages of benchmarking (see table 6 Umbria, Trento and Bolzano quotations).

Regions	Responses on the openness to benchmarking
BASILICATA	*We are in favour of a general evaluation of health services. A minimum set of shared performance indicators can activate useful benchmarking processes.*
CAMPANIA	--
FRIULI VENEZIA GIULIA	*It is a must to enhance regional accountability. It is possible to identify a National set of indicators to be monitored at a Regional level. Sharing indicators and criteria is essential in order to guarantee a real comparison among Regions overcoming the risk of self referral assessment.*
LIGURIA	*We start participating in a regional network that could enable learning processes thanks to benchmarking outside our regional boundaries.*
LOMBARDY	*No wind is good for whom that does not know the rhumb line. It's a strategic problem, benchmarking can be a crucial help in defining the rhumb line. Above all in the European context*
MARCHE	--
PIEDMONT	*We are in favour of a benchmarking within the Regions because we believe that we would be at a good level of performance and we would have the same problems of other Regions but we ask for a regional network that smoothly runs the comparison*
BOLZANO	*We are the first ones who want to start benchmarking mechanism as a learning tool*
TRENTO	*It could be defined National guidelines in order both to compare regional health system and to support Regions develop effective tool using the same methodological issues.* *A performance evaluation system at a National level may activate useful benchmarking processes across regional health services and may help improving local performance evaluation systems.*
APULIA	*[...] Although we get data benchmarking, at this stage we prefer adopting a soft approach: in our opinion the measurement process has to be a supportive management tool. The assessment linked to performance benchmarking across health authorities could lead to disadvantages above all in terms of relationships.*
SARDINIA	--
SICILY	*We are definitely open to benchmarking.* *Benchmarking enabled us to identify and face the unacceptable gaps between Sicily and other Regions.*
TUSCANY	*Data benchmarking across health authorities can enable Regions to overcome self referral attitude and it can enhance learning and assessment processes in order to highlight best practices*
UMBRIA	*It is important to be able to compare measures at National level. It is more useful doing benchmarking with similar units outside its own Region than going on regional averages as in the case of Perugia teaching hospital that is the sole regional teaching hospital*
VENETO	*We are in favour of benchmarking at the National level. Results should be read by everyone. Indicators should be shared. Regions should create a linkage between National and Regional performance evaluation systems.*

Table 6. Regional responses on the openness benchmarking

Moreover uncertainty about the future due to the economic crisis, the Italian fiscal federalism reform and the European parliament spectrum imposes health sector and policy makers to share information about performance and successful strategies as affirmed by Lombardy (see table 6).
Although there is enthusiasm about benchmarking across Regions, this technique is not commonly applied within regional boundaries as governance tool.
Particularly interesting are the cases of Tuscany and Lombardy that both use benchmarking as learning tool among health authorities. Indeed while the former applies benchmarking to all indicators in a full transparent way (Nuti et al., forthcoming a), the second uses it especially for outcome indicators keeping clear the label of health authorities.
Even though most of Regions declare to be willing to compare their performance with others (see table 6) they show some reserve on how benchmarking should be done.
Some Regions declared that benchmarking should be done by National Government after having shared the selection of indicators, some says that the comparison should be run by an external benchmarking agency, others prefer having a regional supervision on how to run comparison finally someone asks only for a comparison on methodology.
Figure 2 summarize the regional positions, pointing out the different visions that go from a regional system (where there is maximum autonomy on measuring performance, no benchmarking across Regions) to a national system (where everything is decided and done by National Government).

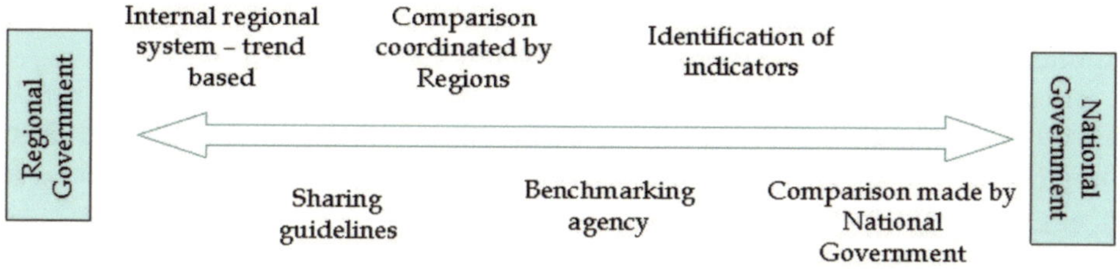

Fig. 2. Different visions on benchmarking.

Regions that are less willing to compare their performance are those that traditionally have had more autonomy (such as Trento) or those that have gone through a period of drastic cuts (such as Apulia). Regions more willing to enable benchmarking process and to go beyond regional boundaries are those that already measure their health service.

5. Discussions and conclusions

Italian regional devolution on health care has led each Region to develop its own PMS.
Although national reforms have pushed the adoption of managerial tools, the study points out that still few Regions have developed PMS capable to measure all the topical dimensions of the OECD framework (Efficiency, Responsiveness, Equity and Health improvement/outcome). In particular dimensions less controlled are: responsiveness and equity. Besides another weakness of the Italian regional PMSs is that often policy makers and regional managers use a plethora of tools in order to control the performance of health service and health system organizations. This highlights that in most cases regional policy level lacks of strategic tools capable of summing up the overall performance in an easy, integrated and systematic way.

Similarities concerning the dimensions covered by all PMSs seem to be dictated by path dependency or national pressure on financial deficit. Indeed past choices, such as the DRG financing system, have had an enduring influence on narrowing the range of viable alternatives in fact health informative systems are mainly oriented to hospital services (as Friuli Venezia Giulia and Bolzano complained in table 2). Moreover national pressure on financial deficit have shaped lots of regional PMSs so that these PMSs are focused on the efficiency and financial performance dimension paying less attention to the other ones.
Pioneer Regions in the development of PMS or area indicators are those that declared to have adopted a specific framework or those that have specialized regional study centres (often linked to University) that have spurred Regions to look beyond traditional measures (ie. Piedmont with the equity research group or Tuscany with the MeS lab).
Another interesting result pointed out by the study is the role played by the rewarding systems. The rewarding system is often integrated with PMS even if they do not completely overlap. A different situation regards Regions that are not used to measure performance in a systematic and coordinated way. Here, the rewarding system is the means by which Regions, such as Basilicata, introduce comprehensive PMSs. To this extent rewarding system can be seen as the driver of innovation.
Scholars suggest benchmarking as another driver of change. Although most Regions acknowledge that benchmarking processes may help spreading innovation and improvements there are still few Regions that adopt benchmarking within regional boundaries (Lombardy and Tuscany), sometimes because they are small Region (like Bolzano or Umbria), sometimes because they don't want to enable negative competition (like Apulia). Most Regions declare to be open to compare their performance across regional health authorities or teaching hospitals but there are quite different visions on how this comparison should be done. From one side there is the vision related to the fear of loosing autonomy (like Regions that want to share only the criteria on how to assess performance), on the opposite side there is the vision that consider performance benchmarking as a powerful tool in order to support regional decisions and strategies (like Regions that ask for public evidence in order to overcome unacceptable differences).
This paper has provided with a first picture of the similarities and differences of the Regional PMSs seeking to identify the factors that may have influenced the PMS design.
These hypotheses on factors that affect PMSs design, should be tested throughout other studies above all with the new scenario that has been emerging on the performance control: from one hand a group of Regions decided to start a network in which they compare and evaluate the performance of health services throughout the help of a benchmarking agency; from the other hand on April 2010 the Ministry of Health published on the website its national performance evaluation system (Nuti et al forthcoming b).

6. References

Ancona A. (2008) I sistemi di valutazione dei servizi sanitari. *I quaderni di monitor;* I supplemento al n.20

Arah O.A., Klazinga N.S., Delnoij M.J., Ten Asbroek A.H.A., Custers T. (2003) Conceptual frameworks for health systems performance: a quest for effectiveness, quality, and improvement. *International Journal for Quality in Health Care;* 15(5): 377-398

Arah OA, Westert GP, Hurst J, Klazinga N.S.(2006) A conceptual framework for the OECD Health Care Quality Indicators Project. *International Journal for Quality in Health Care*; September:5-13

Banchieri G. (2005) *Confronti. Pratiche di benchmark nella sanità pubblica italiana*, Italpromo Esis Publishing Editore.

Censis.(2008) *I modelli decisionali nella sanità locale*. Censis.Roma.

Flamholtz E.G., Das T.K., Tsui A.S. (1985) Toward an integrative framework of organizational culture. *Accounting, Organizations and Society*; 10(1):35-50

Formez. (2007) I sistemi di governance dei servizi sanitari regionali. *Formez*; 57

Hood, C. (1995b). The new public management in the 1980s: variations on a theme. *Accounting Organizations and Society*, Vol 20 n2/3 pp 93-109

Hood, C. (1995a). Contemporary Public Management: A New Global Paradigm? *Public Policy and Administration*. 10(2): 104-117.

Hurst J., Jee-Hughes M.Performance (2001) Measurement and Performance Management in OECD Health Systems. *OECD Labour Market and Social Policy Occasional Papers*; 47

Johnston D.J. (2004) Increasing value for money in health systems. *European Journal of Health Economics*; 5:91-94

Kelley E, Hurst J. (2006) Health Care Quality Indicators Project: Conceptual Framework. *OECD Health Working Papers*; 23 doi:10.1787/440134737301

Lapsley, I.(1999) Accounting and the New Public Management: Instruments of Substantive Efficiency or a Rationalising Modernity?, *Financial Accountability and Management* 15(3/4): 201-207

Mannion R & Davies H TO (2008) Payment for performance in health care. *BMJ*; 336: 306-308

McLoughlin V., Leatherman S., Fletcher M., Wyn Owen J. (2001) Improving performance using indicators. Recent experiences in the United States, the United Kingdom, and Australia. *International Journal for Quality in Health Care*; 13(6): 455-462

Modell S, Jacobs K, Wiesel F.(2007)A process (re)turn? Path dependencies, institutions and performance management in Swedish central government. *Management Accounting Research*;18: 453–475

Murray C.L.J., Evans D.B. (2003) *Health Systems Performance Assessment Debates, Methods and Empiricism*. World Health Organization. Geneva.

NHS Executive. (1999) *The NHS Performance Assessment Framework*.The Stationery Office.London.

Nuti S, Vainieri M. (2009) *Fiducia dei cittadini e valutazione della performance nella sanità italiana*. Edizioni ETS. Pisa.

Nuti, S., Bonini, A, Murante, A.M. & Vainieri, (2009) M.Performance assessment in the maternity pathway in Tuscany region. *Health Services Management Research*; 22, 115-121.

Nuti, S., Seghieri, C., Vainieri, M (forthcoming a) Assessing the effectiveness of a performance evaluation system in the public healthcare sector: some novel evidence from the Tuscany Region experience. *Journal of Management and Governance*.

Nuti, S., Seghieri, C., Zett S., Vainieri, M (forthcoming b) Assessment and improvement of the Italian Healthcare system: first evidences from a pilot national performance evaluation system". *Journal of Healthcare Management*.

Ouchi W.G. (1979) A conceptual framework for the design of Organizational Control Mechanism. *Science*; 25

Panizza G. (2010) Relazione sullo stato del Servizio Sanitario Provinciale Anno 2009 (dati 2008) *infosalute n.8* Giunta della Provincia Autonoma di Trento

Patton M.Q. (1990) *Qualitative evaluation and research methods*. SAGE Publication..

Pink G.H. McKillop I. Schraa E.G. Preyra C. Montgomery C. Baker R. (2001) Creating a Balanced Scorecard for Hospital System. *Health Care Finance*;2(3):1-20

Saltman R.B., Bankauskaite V.,Vrangbaek K. (2007) *Decentralization in health care*. Mc Graw Hill Open Univesity Press.

Smith P.C. (2002) *Measuring Up. Improving Health Systems Performance in OECD Countries*. OECD.Ottawa.

Van Herck P, De Smedt D, Annemans L, Remmen R, Rosenthal M B and Sermeus W. (2010) Systematic review: Effects, design choices, and context of pay-for-performance in health care. *BMC Health Serv Res.*; 10: 247.

Veillard J, Champagne F, Klazinga N., Kazandjian V, Arah O.A.,Guisset A.L. (2005) A performance assessment framework for hospitals: the WHO regional office for Europe PATH project. *International Journal for Quality in Health Care*; 17:487-496

Watson G. (1993) *Strategic Benchmarking: How to Rate Your Company's Performance Against the World's Best*. Wiley & Sons.

CSDH (2008) *Closing the gap in a generation: health equity through action on the social determinants of health*. Final Report of the Commission on Social Determinants of Health. Geneva, World Health Organization.

Part 3

General Issues

18

Causal Inference in Randomized Trials with Noncompliance

Yasutaka Chiba
Division of Biostatistics, Clinical Research Center,
Kinki University School of Medicine,
Japan

1. Introduction

In human clinical trials, ethical considerations for study subjects override the scientific requirements of trial design. Noncompliance with an intervention or study procedure for ethical reasons is thus inevitable in practice (Piantadosi, 1997).
The Coronary Drug Project (CDP) trial (CDP Research Group, 1980) was a typical example of trials with noncompliance. The CDP trial was a large, double-blinded, randomized trial testing the effect of the cholesterol-lowering drug, clofibrate, on mortality. Patients were randomly assigned to the clofibrate or placebo groups and were followed for at least 5 years, documenting clinic visits and examinations. During each 4-month follow-up visit, the physician assessed compliance by counting or estimating the number of capsules returned by the patients. In the protocol, good compliers were defined as patients taking more than 80% of the prescribed treatment. Table 1 summarizes the incidence of death during the 5-year follow-up period, based on the treatment assigned and compliance status. Patients who left the trial before the end of the 5-year follow-up period were excluded.

Group	No. of patients	Deaths	Compliance status	No. of patients	Deaths
Clofibrate	1065	194	More than 80%	708	106
			Less than 80%	357	88
Placebo	2695	523	More than 80%	1813	274
			Less than 80%	882	249
Totals	3760	717			

Table 1. The compliance status and incidence of death during a 5-year follow-up period in the CDP trial.

In the clofibrate group, 708 patients were considered good compliers; 106 died during the follow-up period. There were 357 patients considered poor compliers; 88 died. Comparing the compliance status of the proportion of patients that died yields 106/708 – 88/357 = –9.68%. From this result, clofibrate seems to have been beneficial. However, when we make the same comparison for the placebo group, it yields 274/1813 – 249/882 = –13.12%. Surprisingly, we obtain the result that the placebo was more beneficial than clofibrate. However, nobody would interpret the result as being that the placebo had the effect of decreasing death.

Which subgroups to compare to estimate the treatment effect correctly is an important problem. From the viewpoint of treatment compliance, it is considered best to compare the proportion of deaths for the compliers in each group: 106/708 – 274/1813 = –0.14%. This comparison is called the per-protocol (PP) analysis. The PP analysis generally yields biased estimates of treatment effects, because whether patients comply with the assigned treatment is not randomized and several factors may affect it. This problem can be avoided by intention-to-treat (ITT) analysis, in which patients are analyzed according to the assigned treatment regardless of the treatment actually received (Fisher et al., 1990; Lee et al., 1991): 194/1065 – 523/2695 = –1.19%. The ITT estimate may represent the effect of the treatment intended, but generally does not represent the treatment effect itself (Schwartz & Lellouch, 1967; Sheiner & Rubin, 1995).

Noncompliance data may be obtained from actual clinical trials, as in the CDP trial. To estimate the treatment effect correctly from such data, we should consider the expected outcomes if all patients had received the test treatment and the control, and compare them. The effect yielded from such a comparison is called the average causal effect (ACE) (Robins & Tsiatis, 1991; Robins & Greenland, 1994). Several researchers have discussed methodology to estimate ACE (Pearl, 2000; Manski, 2003; Sato, 2006), but as yet, no standard methodology has been developed. Nevertheless, we can derive bounds on ACE using the deterministic causal model (e.g., Pearl, 1995; Cai et al., 2007; Chiba, 2009b). In this chapter, we discuss how estimates from major analyses, such as ITT and PP, are biased and present bounds on ACE under certain assumptions.

To achieve these objectives, this chapter is organized as follows. In Section 2, notation and definitions are provided. Sections 3 and 4 discuss noncompliance by switching the treatment, which, in contrast to the CDP trial, means that non-compliers in a sub-population assigned to treatment A receive treatment B and those assigned to treatment B receive treatment A. We discuss biases from major analyses such as ITT and PP in Section 3, and discuss the bounds on ACE in Section 4. Section 5 discusses noncompliance by receiving no treatment, as in the CDP trial. As in many publications, the instrumental variable (IV) assumption is used in these sections, but this assumption is relaxed in Section 6. Finally, Section 7 offers some concluding remarks. The derivations of equations and inequalities presented in this chapter are outlined in Section 8.

2. Notation and definitions

In the following sections, R is the randomization indicator, where $R = 2$ for subjects randomized to the test treatment and $R = 1$ for subjects randomized to the control. Similarly, X indicates actual (received) treatment that may not be randomized under protocol violations such as noncompliance, where $X = 2$ for subjects who received the test treatment, $X = 1$ for subjects who received the control, and $X = 0$ for subjects who received no treatment. The observed outcome is Y and $Y_{X=x}$ is the counterfactual value (or equally potential outcome) of Y if treatment X was set to x (Rubin, 1974, 1978, 1990). ACE is defined as $\text{ACE} \equiv \text{E}(Y_{X=2}) - \text{E}(Y_{X=1})$. Note that ITT and PP estimators are represented by $\text{ITT} \equiv \text{E}(Y \mid R = 2) - \text{E}(Y \mid R = 1)$ and $\text{PP} \equiv \text{E}(Y \mid X = 2, R = 2) - \text{E}(Y \mid X = 1, R = 1)$, respectively. Furthermore, we use the notation $E_{xr} = \text{E}(Y \mid X = x, R = r)$ and $p_{x\mid r} = \Pr(X = x \mid R = r)$; then, $\text{PP} \equiv E_{22} - E_{11}$.

We require the consistency assumption that $Y_{X=x} = Y$ for all subjects, so that the value of Y that would have been observed if X had been set to what it in fact was is equal to the value of Y that was in fact observed. Thus, this assumption indicates that $\text{E}(Y_{X=x} \mid X = x) = \text{E}(Y \mid X = x)$ and furthermore $\text{E}(Y_{X=x} \mid X = x, R = r) = \text{E}(Y \mid X = x, R = r)$ $(= E_{xr})$. We assume that $Y_{X=x}$ is independent from X given R and Z, where Z is a confounder or a set of confounders between X and Y. In Sections 3-5, we also require the instrumental variable (IV) assumption, which states that the potential outcome $Y_{X=x}$ is not affected directly by the treatment assignment R; rather, $Y_{X=x}$ is influenced only by the treatment actually received (Holland, 1986; Angrist et al., 1996). Thus, subjects' potential outcomes are independent of treatment assignment and are constant across the sub-populations of subjects assigned to different treatment arms. The IV assumption is formalized as follows:

ASSUMPTION 1: Instrumental variable (IV)

$$\mathrm{E}(Y_{X=x} \mid R = 2) = \mathrm{E}(Y_{X=x} \mid R = 1).$$

This assumption may hold in successfully blinded randomized trials, because subjects are not aware of their assigned treatments and so the assigned treatments do not affect the potential outcomes. However, this often may not hold in unblinded trials, in which subjects are aware of the assigned treatment and this knowledge may affect the potential outcomes, and needs to be critically evaluated. Assumption 1 is used in Sections 3-5, but is relaxed in Section 6.

3. Biases of estimates

In this section and the next section, we discuss noncompliance by switching the treatment, which means that non-compliers in a sub-population assigned to treatment A receive treatment B and those assigned to treatment B receive treatment A. In this type of noncompliance, all subjects have the value $X = 1$ or 2 (and not $X = 0$) for both $R = 1$ and 2. Thus, $p_{0|r} = 0$ and $p_{1|r} + p_{2|r} = 1$. The derivations of equations in this section are given in Section 8.1.

In this section, we discuss how estimates from major analyses, such as ITT and PP, are biased. To do so, we introduce the following R-specific bias factors due to confounding between X and Y (Brumback et al, 2004; Chiba et al., 2007):

$$\alpha_r \equiv \mathrm{E}(Y_{X=2} \mid X = 2, R = r) - \mathrm{E}(Y_{X=2} \mid X = 1, R = r),$$

$$\beta_r \equiv \mathrm{E}(Y_{X=1} \mid X = 2, R = r) - \mathrm{E}(Y_{X=1} \mid X = 1, R = r),$$

where $r = 1, 2$. α_r and β_r are confounding effects that would arise from R-stratified comparisons of those with $X = 2$ versus those with $X = 1$. When $\alpha_r > 0$ and $\beta_r > 0$, $\mathrm{E}(Y_{X=x} \mid X = 2, R = r) > \mathrm{E}(Y_{X=x} \mid X = 1, R = r)$, which means that the subjects who received the test treatment tend to have larger outcome values than those who received the control, leading to positive confounding. Conversely, when $\alpha_r < 0$ and $\beta_r < 0$, $\mathrm{E}(Y_{X=x} \mid X = 2, R = r) < \mathrm{E}(Y_{X=x} \mid X = 1, R = r)$, which means that the subjects who received the test treatment tend to have smaller outcome values than those who received the control, leading to negative confounding. No confounding occurs between X and Y when $\alpha_r = \beta_r = 0$.

Under Assumption 1, using α_r and β_r, $\mathrm{E}(Y_{X=2})$ and $\mathrm{E}(Y_{X=1})$ are expressed as:

$$\mathrm{E}(Y_{X=2}) = E_{2r} - \alpha_r p_{1|r}, \tag{3.1}$$

$$\mathrm{E}(Y_{X=1}) = E_{1r} + \beta_r p_{2|r}. \tag{3.2}$$

Using these equations, ITT $\equiv \mathrm{E}(Y \mid R = 2) - \mathrm{E}(Y \mid R = 1)$ can be expressed by a function of ACE $\equiv \mathrm{E}(Y_{X=2}) - \mathrm{E}(Y_{X=1})$ and bias factors:

$$\text{ITT} = \text{ACE} + \{\alpha_2 - (E_{22} - E_{12})\}p_{1|2} + \{\beta_1 - (E_{21} - E_{11})\}p_{2|1}. \quad (3.3)$$

Thus, the ITT estimator is generally a biased estimator of ACE, and can be unbiased when $\alpha_2 = E_{22} - E_{12}$ and $\beta_1 = E_{21} - E_{11}$, i.e., $\text{E}(Y_{X=2} | X = x, R = r) = \text{E}(Y_{X=1} | X = x, R = r)$ for $x \neq r$. This equation implies that the ITT estimate can be unbiased when no treatment effect exists for all subjects (under the sharp null hypothesis: $Y_{X=2} = Y_{X=1}$ for all subjects). Furthermore, equation (3.3) shows that, if we know whether the treatment effect is positive or negative, we can know the sign of bias of the ITT estimate.

Likewise, it can be demonstrated that the PP estimator is generally a biased estimator of ACE, because the difference between equation (3.1) with $r = 2$ and equation (3.2) with $r = 1$ derives:

$$\text{PP} = \text{ACE} + \alpha_2 p_{1|2} + \beta_1 p_{2|1}. \quad (3.4)$$

This equation shows that the PP estimate can be unbiased when $\alpha_2 = 0$ and $\beta_1 = 0$, which imply that whether subjects receive the test treatment or control treatment is randomly determined (no confounder exists between X and Y). Furthermore, if we know the common sign of confounding effects (the common signs of α_r and β_r), we can know the sign of the bias of the PP estimate.

In addition to the ITT and PP estimators, the IV estimator has been developed (Cuzick et al., 1997; Greenland, 2000; Hernán & Robins, 2006). The estimate is calculated by the following formula:

$$\text{IV} \equiv \{\text{E}(Y | R = 2) - \text{E}(Y | R = 1)\} / (p_{2|2} - p_{2|1})$$

for $p_{2|2} \neq p_{2|1}$. Although the IV estimator may yield a less biased estimate of ACE, it is also generally biased. This is because the IV estimator is expressed using bias factors as follows (Chiba, 2010a):

$$\text{IV} = \text{ACE} - w_1(\alpha_1 - \beta_1) + w_2(\alpha_2 - \beta_2), \quad (3.5)$$

where $w_r = p_{1|r}p_{2|r} / (p_{2|2} - p_{2|1})$ and $p_{2|2} \neq p_{2|1}$. Thus, the IV estimate can be unbiased when $\alpha_r = \beta_r$, i.e., $\text{E}(Y_{X=2} - Y_{X=1} | X = 2, R = r) = \text{E}(Y_{X=2} - Y_{X=1} | X = 1, R = r)$. Similar to the ITT estimate, the IV estimate can also be unbiased when no treatment effect exists for all subjects (under the sharp null hypothesis: $Y_{X=2} = Y_{X=1}$ for all subjects). Additionally, the IV estimate can be unbiased even when $\text{E}(Y_{X=2} - Y_{X=1} | X = x, R = 2) = \text{E}(Y_{X=2} - Y_{X=1} | X = x, R = 1)$ (Robins, 1989).

Furthermore, as an alternative to the IV estimator, Chiba (2010b) proposed the following estimator of ACE:

$$\text{IV}' \equiv (E_{22}p_{1|1} + E_{12}p_{2|1} - E_{21}p_{1|2} - E_{11}p_{2|2}) / (p_{2|2} - p_{2|1}).$$

This estimator is also generally a biased estimator of ACE, and the estimate can be unbiased under $\alpha_1 = \alpha_2$ and $\beta_1 = \beta_2$, which may be reasonable when the influence of confounding between X and Y is equal in both assigned groups.

4. Bounds on average causal effect

In randomized trials with noncompliance by switching the treatment, we cannot generally estimate ACE in an unbiased manner (Section 3). Thus, in this section, we discuss bounds on ACE. We introduce the bounds under some assumptions in Section 4.1, and illustrate them by using data from a classic randomized trial in Section 4.2. The derivations of inequalities in this section are outlined in Section 8.2.

4.1 Assumptions and bounds

In Section 4.1.1, we introduce bounds on ACE under Assumption 1 only. Because the bounds generally have a broad width, we present the bounds with narrower widths by adding some plausible assumptions in Sections 4.1.2 and 4.1.3.

4.1.1 The instrumental variable

When the outcome Y has a finite range $[K_0, K_1]$, the bounds on ACE under Assumption 1 are as follows (Robins, 1989; Manski, 1990):

$$\max\left\{\begin{matrix} K_0 p_{1|1} + E_{21} p_{2|1} \\ K_0 p_{1|2} + E_{22} p_{2|2} \end{matrix}\right\} - \min\left\{\begin{matrix} E_{11} p_{1|1} + K_1 p_{2|1} \\ E_{12} p_{1|2} + K_1 p_{2|2} \end{matrix}\right\}$$
$$\leq \mathrm{ACE} \leq \min\left\{\begin{matrix} K_1 p_{1|1} + E_{21} p_{2|1} \\ K_1 p_{1|2} + E_{22} p_{2|2} \end{matrix}\right\} - \max\left\{\begin{matrix} E_{11} p_{1|1} + K_0 p_{2|1} \\ E_{12} p_{1|2} + K_0 p_{2|2} \end{matrix}\right\}. \quad (4.1)$$

Note that $K_0 = 0$ and $K_1 = 1$ in the case of a binary outcome. Furthermore, using a method of linear programming in the case of a binary outcome, Balke and Pearl (1997) presented the following bounds under Assumption 1 only:

$$\max\left\{\begin{matrix} P_{12|2} + P_{01|1} - 1 \\ P_{12|1} + P_{01|2} - 1 \\ P_{12|1} - P_{12|2} - P_{11|2} - P_{02|1} - P_{11|1} \\ P_{12|2} - P_{12|1} - P_{11|1} - P_{02|2} - P_{11|2} \\ -P_{02|2} - P_{11|2} \\ -P_{02|1} - P_{11|1} \\ P_{01|2} - P_{02|2} - P_{11|2} - P_{02|1} - P_{21|1} \\ P_{01|1} - P_{02|1} - P_{11|1} - P_{02|2} - P_{01|2} \end{matrix}\right\} \leq \mathrm{ACE} \leq \min\left\{\begin{matrix} 1 - P_{02|2} + P_{11|1} \\ 1 - P_{02|1} + P_{11|2} \\ P_{02|2} + P_{01|2} + P_{12|1} + P_{01|1} - P_{02|1} \\ P_{12|2} + P_{01|2} + P_{02|1} + P_{01|1} - P_{02|2} \\ P_{12|2} + P_{01|2} \\ P_{12|1} + P_{01|1} \\ P_{12|2} + P_{01|2} + P_{02|1} + P_{12|1} - P_{11|1} \\ P_{12|1} + P_{01|1} + P_{12|2} + P_{11|2} - P_{11|1} \end{matrix}\right\}, \quad (4.2)$$

where $P_{yx|r} = \Pr(Y = y, X = x \mid R = r)$ $(y = 0, 1)$. Inequality (4.2), which is the bounds on ACE having the narrowest width without adding any other assumptions, gives bounds with a narrower width than inequality (4.1) in some situations. However, these bounds generally have broad widths. Thus, in Sections 4.1.2 and 4.1.3, we derive bounds with narrower widths by adding some plausible assumptions.

4.1.2 The monotone treatment response

To derive narrower bounds, Manski (1997) presented the following monotone treatment response (MTR) assumption:

ASSUMPTION 2.1: Monotone treatment response (MTR)
$Y_{X=s} \geq Y_{X=t}$ *for all subjects, where* $s \geq t$.

For $(s, t) = (2, 1)$, the MTR means that a subject takes a larger outcome value if he/she received the test treatment than if he/she received the control. This holds when it is apparent that the test treatment has a positive effect.

Under Assumptions 1 and 2.1, the lower bound on ACE is improved as follows:

$$\mathrm{ACE} \geq \max\{\mathrm{ITT}, -\mathrm{ITT}\}. \quad (4.3)$$

Thus, we can say that ACE is not less than the ITT estimate when the MTR holds. Note that the second and third terms in equation (3.3) are not less than 0 under the MTR, because $E(Y_{X=2} \mid X = x, R = r) \geq E(Y_{X=1} \mid X = x, R = r)$, i.e., $a_2 \geq E_{22} - E_{12}$ and $\beta_1 \geq E_{21} - E_{11}$, hold under the MTR.
Using the reverse sign of the inequality in Assumption 2.1, the following reverse MTR (RMTR) assumption can be applied:

ASSUMPTION 2.2: Reverse monotone treatment response (RMTR)
$Y_{X=s} \leq Y_{X=t}$ *for all subjects, where* $s \geq t$.

In contrast to the MTR, for $(s, t) = (2, 1)$, the RMTR means that a subject takes a smaller outcome value if he/she received the test treatment than if he/she received the control. This holds when it is apparent that the test treatment has a negative effect. Under Assumptions 1 and 2.2, the upper bound on ACE is improved as ACE ≤ min{ITT, –ITT}, implying that ACE is not more than the ITT estimate when the RMTR holds.
Assumptions 2.1 and 2.2 are very strict assumptions, because the inequalities must hold for all subjects. In the case of a binary outcome variable, we can use an alternative assumption that is weaker than Assumptions 2.1 and 2.2, but can derive the same bound as those under these assumptions. This is introduced below after the concept of principal stratification (Frangakis & Rubin, 2002).
Based on principal stratification, four types of potential outcomes are defined as follows: doomed $\{Y_{X=2} = 1, Y_{X=1} = 1\}$, which consists of subjects who always experience the event, regardless of the treatment received; preventive $\{Y_{X=2} = 0, Y_{X=1} = 1\}$, which consists of subjects who do not experience the event when they receive the test treatment but do when they receive the control; causative $\{Y_{X=2} = 1, Y_{X=1} = 0\}$, which consists of subjects who experience the event when they receive the test treatment, but not when they receive the control; and immune $\{Y_{X=2} = 0, Y_{X=1} = 0\}$, which consists of subjects who never experience the event, regardless of the treatment received (Greenland & Robins, 1986). Because X and Y are binary, the potential outcomes could be any of these four types. Note that Assumption 2.1 implies that no preventive subject exists: $\Pr(Y_{X=2} = 0, Y_{A=1} = 1) = 0$, because $Y_{X=2} = 0$ and $Y_{X=1} = 1$ cannot hold simultaneously under $Y_{X=2} \geq Y_{X=1}$. Likewise, Assumption 2.2 implies that no causative subject exists.
We can obtain inequality (4.3) even under the following assumption (Chiba, 2011):

ASSUMPTION 3.1
$$\Pr(Y_{X=2} = 1, Y_{X=1} = 0 \mid X = x, R = r) \geq \Pr(Y_{X=2} = 0, Y_{X=1} = 1 \mid X = x, R = r).$$

This assumption indicates that the number of causative subjects is not less than the number of preventive subjects within all strata with $X = x$ and $R = r$. Thus, Assumption 3.1 is weaker than Assumption 2.1, because Assumption 2.1 requires that no preventive subject exists but this is not the case for Assumption 3.1.
Likewise, the following assumption, 3.2, can derive the same upper bound as that under Assumption 2.2:

ASSUMPTION 3.2
$$\Pr(Y_{X=2} = 1, Y_{X=1} = 0 \mid X = x, R = r) \leq \Pr(Y_{X=2} = 0, Y_{X=1} = 1 \mid X = x, R = r).$$

In contrast to Assumption 3.1, this assumption implies that the number of causative subjects is not more than the number of preventive subjects within all strata with $X = x$ and $R = r$. Again, note that Assumption 2.2 implies that no causative subject exists and thus Assumption 3.2 is a weaker assumption than Assumption 2.2.

4.1.3 The monotone treatment selection

The other assumption to derive narrower bounds is the following monotone treatment selection assumption (Manski & Pepper, 2000; Chiba, 2010c):

ASSUMPTION 4.1: Monotone treatment selection (MTS)
$$E(Y_{X=x} \mid X = s, R = r) \geq E(Y_{X=x} \mid X = t, R = r) \text{ for } s \geq t.$$

For $(s, t) = (2, 1)$, the MTS means that subjects who received the test treatment tend to have larger outcome values than those who received the control within each study treatment-arm subpopulation. For example, when patients with a worse condition prefer to receive the new treatment ($X = 2$), it should be anticipated that the incidence proportion of a bad event ($Y = 1$) such as death will be higher, compared with those who receive the standard treatment ($X = 1$); this indicates that the MTS holds.

Under Assumptions 1 and 4.1, the upper bound on ACE is improved as follows:

$$\text{ACE} \leq \min\{E_{21}, E_{22}\} - \max\{E_{11}, E_{12}\}. \tag{4.4}$$

Specifically, when $\min\{E_{21}, E_{22}\} = E_{22}$ and $\max\{E_{11}, E_{12}\} = E_{11}$, the upper bound is equal to the PP estimator. Thus, ACE is no more than the PP estimate when the MTS holds. Note that this is also verified from equation (3.4) because Assumption 4.1 implies that $\alpha_r \geq 0$ and $\beta_r \geq 0$.

Similar to the RMTR, the following reverse MTS (RMTS) assumption can be applied:

ASSUMPTION 4.2: Reverse monotone treatment selection (RMTS)
$$E(Y_{X=x} \mid X = s, R = r) \leq E(Y_{X=x} \mid X = t, R = r) \text{ for } s \geq t.$$

In contrast to the MTS, for $(s, t) = (2, 1)$, the RMTS means that subjects who received the test treatment tend to have smaller outcome values than those who received the control within each study treatment-arm subpopulation. The lower bound on ACE under the RMTS is ACE $\geq \max\{E_{21}, E_{22}\} - \min\{E_{11}, E_{12}\}$, implying that ACE is not less than the PP estimate when the RMTS holds.

It is obvious that the combination of Assumptions 2.1 and 4.1 improves both the lower and upper bounds:

$$\max\{\text{ITT}, -\text{ITT}\} \leq \text{ACE} \leq \min\{E_{21}, E_{22}\} - \max\{E_{11}, E_{12}\}.$$

Likewise, under the combination of Assumptions 2.2 and 4.2, bounds on ACE are

$$\max\{E_{21}, E_{22}\} - \min\{E_{11}, E_{12}\} \leq \text{ACE} \leq \min\{\text{ITT}, -\text{ITT}\}. \tag{4.5}$$

These inequalities show that ACE exists between ITT and PP estimates under these combinations of assumptions.

By extending a theory developed in the context of observational studies (VanderWeele, 2008a; Chiba, 2009a), Chiba (2009b) presented another assumption that derives the same upper bound as that under the MTS (Assumption 4.1):

ASSUMPTION 5.1: Monotone confounding (MC)
Both $E(Y \mid X = 2, R = r, Z = z)$ *and* $\Pr(X = 2 \mid R = r, Z = z)$ *are non-decreasing or non-increasing in z for all r, and the components of Z are independent of each other.*

For an assumption corresponding to the RMTS (Assumption 4.2), Assumption 5.1 is changed as follows:

ASSUMPTION 5.2: Reverse monotone confounding (RMC)
One of $E(Y \mid X = 2, R = r, Z = z)$ *and* $Pr(X = 2 \mid R = r, Z = z)$ *is non-decreasing and the other is non-increasing in z for all r, and the components of Z are independent of each other.*

Although the MTS and MC (RMTS and RMC) give the same upper (lower) bound on ACE, the relationship between them has not been clear. In Section 8.2, we demonstrate that the MC implies the MTS, but it is unclear whether the converse holds.

4.2 Application

For illustration, the assumptions and bounds presented in this section are applied to data from the Multiple Risk Factor Intervention Trial (MRFIT) (MRFIT Research Group, 1982). The MRFIT was a large field trial to test the effect of a multifactorial intervention program on mortality from coronary heart disease (CHD) in middle-aged men with sufficiently high risk levels attributed to cigarette smoking, high serum cholesterol, and high blood pressure. Intervention consisted of dietary advice on ways to reduce blood cholesterol, smoking cessation counseling, and hypertension medication. All subjects were randomly assigned to the intervention program or the control group.

For this illustration, attention is restricted to the effects of cessation of cigarette smoking. This restriction follows other studies (Mark & Robins, 1993; Matsui, 2005; Chiba, 2010a) and was applied due to the paucity of differences achieved for the other risk factors. Table 2 summarizes the incidence of subject mortality due to CHD during the 7-year follow-up period based on the assigned treatment and the actual subject smoking status 1 year after study entry. R represents the assigned group ($R = 2$ for the test group and $R = 1$ for the control group), X is the actual smoking status 1 year after entry ($X = 2$ for smoking cessation and $X = 1$ for continued smoking), and Y is the incidence of CHD deaths ($Y = 1$ for dead and $Y = 0$ for alive). ITT and PP analyses yielded ITT = 69/3833 – 74/3830 = −0.13% and PP = 11/991 – 70/3456 = −0.92%, respectively. IV and IV′ estimates were −0.82% and −0.72%, respectively.

Group	No. of subjects	CHD deaths	Smoking status at 1 year	No. of subjects	CHD deaths
Test	3833	69	Quit	991	11
			Not quit	2842	58
Control	3830	74	Quit	374	4
			Not quit	3456	70
Totals	7663	143			

Table 2. The status of cigarette smoking and the incidence of mortality due to CHD in the MRFIT during a 7-year follow-up period.

To derive the ACE bounds, it is necessary to discuss whether the assumptions in this section hold. It is clear that cessation of cigarette smoking prevents death from CHD. Thus, Assumption 2.2 (RMTR: $Y_{X=2} \leq Y_{X=1}$ for all subjects) holds (i.e., no causative subject, who died when they quit smoking but lived when they continued smoking, exists). However, it is possible that such subjects do exist, because the stress of quitting smoking might lead to CHD and this stress would have been lower if the subject had continued smoking (i.e., a causative subject existed). Under this observation, Assumption 2.2 does not hold. However, Assumption 3.2 would still hold, because even if a few causative subjects exist, the number would be the smallest in the four principal strata.

In general, health-conscious individuals may tend not to die from CHD and quit smoking compared with individuals who are not health-conscious. Trial subjects would likely have had similar tendencies, and subjects who quit smoking would logically tend not to have died from CHD. Therefore, it is considered that Assumption 4.2 (RMTS: $E(Y_{X=x} \mid X = 2, R = r) \leq E(Y_{X=x} \mid X = 1, R = r)$ for $x = 1, 2$ and $r = 1, 2$) is valid. Although Assumption 1 may not hold because this trial was an unblinded trial (the details are discussed in Section 6), we here use this assumption for illustrative purposes.

The arguments presented above demonstrate that Assumptions 3.2 and 4.2 can be assumed. Thus, from inequality (4.5), the bounds on ACE become $-0.92\% \leq \text{ACE} \leq -0.13\%$. This result indicates that quitting smoking would prevent death from CHD. Note that the bounds under Assumption 1 only become $-11.31\% \leq \text{ACE} \leq 72.60\%$, where inequalities (4.1) and (4.2) yield the same bounds. While the bounds under Assumption 1 only do not give enough information about ACE, adding Assumptions 3.2 and 4.2 greatly improves the bounds.

5. Noncompliance by receiving no treatment

While noncompliance by switching the treatment was discussed in Sections 3 and 4, this section discusses noncompliance by receiving no treatment, which means that non-compliers receive no treatment. In this type of noncompliance, subjects who are allocated to $R = 2$ take the value of $X = 0$ or 2 (and not $X = 1$) and those who are allocated to $R = 1$ take the value of $X = 0$ or 1 (and not $X = 2$). Thus, $p_{0|2} + p_{2|2} = 1$ and $p_{0|1} + p_{1|1} = 1$. The derivations of equations and inequalities in this section are similar to those in Sections 3 and 4, and can be achieved straightforwardly by replacing $x = 1, 2$ in Sections 3 and 4 to $x = 0, 1$ and $x = 0, 2$. Thus, they are omitted.

5.1 Biases of estimates

By following a similar discussion to Section 3, we show that the ITT and PP estimators generally yield biased estimates of ACE. Unfortunately, the IV estimator cannot be defined in this type of noncompliance.

To express the biases of ITT and PP estimators, we introduce the following bias factors instead of α_r and β_r in Section 3:

$$\gamma \equiv E(Y_{X=2} \mid X = 2, R = 2) - E(Y_{X=2} \mid X = 0, R = 2),$$

$$\delta \equiv E(Y_{X=1} \mid X = 1, R = 1) - E(Y_{X=1} \mid X = 0, R = 1).$$

Similar to α_r and β_r, γ and δ are also confounding effects. γ is interpreted as a confounding effect that would arise from comparisons of those with $X = 2$ versus those with $X = 0$ for the test treatment group. When $\gamma > 0$, $E(Y_{X=2} \mid X = 2, R = 2) > E(Y_{X=2} \mid X = 0, R = 2)$, which means that the subjects who received the test treatment tend to take larger outcome values than those who received no treatment. Conversely, when $\gamma < 0$, $E(Y_{X=2} \mid X = 2, R = 2) < E(Y_{X=2} \mid X = 0, R = 2)$, which means that the subjects who received the test treatment tend to take smaller outcome values than those who received no treatment. Whether subjects in the test treatment group actually receive the treatment is randomly determined when $\gamma = 0$. δ is interpreted using a similar process in the control group.

Biases of ITT and PP estimators can be explained in a similar manner to Section 3, using γ and δ. Because $E(Y_{X=2})$ and $E(Y_{X=1})$ are expressed as $E(Y_{X=2}) = E_{22} - \gamma p_{0|2}$ and $E(Y_{X=1}) = E_{11} - \delta p_{0|1}$, the ITT estimator is given by:

$$\text{ITT} = \text{ACE} + \{\gamma - (E_{22} - E_{02})\}p_{0|2} - \{\delta - (E_{11} - E_{01})\}p_{0|1}.$$

Therefore, the ITT estimator is generally a biased estimator of ACE, and can be unbiased when $\gamma = E_{22} - E_{02}$ and $\delta = E_{11} - E_{01}$, i.e., $E(Y_{X=r} | X = 0, R = r) = E(Y_{X=0} | X = 0, R = r)$ for $r = 1, 2$. This equation indicates that the ITT estimate can be unbiased when no effect of the treatments exists against no treatment for all subjects (under the sharp null hypothesis: $Y_{X=x} = Y_{X=0}$ for all subjects, where $x = 1, 2$).
The PP estimator is given by:

$$\text{PP} = \text{ACE} + \gamma p_{0|2} - \delta p_{0|1}.$$

Thus, the PP estimate can be unbiased when $\gamma = 0$ and $\delta = 0$, implying that whether subjects receive the assigned treatment is randomly determined (no confounder exists between X and Y).
In contrast to the case of noncompliance by switching the treatment, it may be difficult to know the signs of biases of ITT and PP estimates.

5.2 Bounds on average causal effect

We extend the bounds concept introduced in Section 4.1 to the case of noncompliance by receiving no treatment.
The bounds under Assumption 1 only are as follows:

$$(E_{22}p_{2|2} + K_0p_{0|2}) - (E_{11}p_{1|1} + K_1p_{0|1}) \leq \text{ACE} \leq (E_{22}p_{2|2} + K_1p_{0|2}) - (E_{11}p_{1|1} + K_0p_{0|1}), \quad (5.1)$$

where $[K_0, K_1]$ is a finite range of outcome Y. In the case of a binary outcome, this inequality is simplified to:

$$P_{12|2} + P_{01|1} - 1 \leq \text{ACE} \leq 1 - P_{02|2} - P_{11|1}.$$

As in Section 4.1, the MTR and MTS assumptions and these reverse assumptions can be applied to obtain bounds on ACE with narrower widths. For example, for $(s, t) = (2, 0)$, Assumption 2.1 is $Y_{X=2} \geq Y_{X=0}$, which means that a subject takes a larger outcome value if he/she received the test treatment than if he/she received no treatment. This holds when it is apparent that the test treatment has a positive effect compared with no treatment. The similar interpretation is given for $(s, t) = (1, 0)$ $(Y_{X=1} \geq Y_{X=0})$ in place of the test treatment to the control.
Under Assumptions 1 and 2.1, the lower bound of $E(Y_{X=x})$ becomes $E(Y_{X=x}) \geq E(Y | R = x)$ for $x = 1, 2$, which is derived using $t = 0$ in Assumption 2.1. Likewise, $E(Y_{X=x}) \leq E(Y | R = x)$ under Assumptions 1 and 2.2. Although these bounds of $E(Y_{X=x})$ do not give a bound on ACE in contrast to that in Section 4.1.2, Assumption 2.1 can derive the following bounds by combination with inequality (5.1)[1]:

$$E(Y | R = 2) - (E_{11}p_{1|1} + K_1p_{0|1}) \leq \text{ACE} \leq (E_{22}p_{2|2} + K_1p_{0|2}) - E(Y | R = 1).$$

Similar to Assumptions 3.1 and 3.2, in the case of a binary outcome variable, we can make weaker assumptions that derive the same bounds as those under Assumptions 2.1 and 2.2, using the principal stratification approach. In the case of noncompliance by receiving no treatment, four types of potential outcomes, based on principal stratification, are re-

[1] If $(s, t) = (2, 1)$ in Assumption 2.1 is used as in Section 4.1, the lower bound on ACE is improved to 0.

defined as follows: doomed $\{Y_{X=x} = 1, Y_{X=0} = 1\}$, which consists of subjects who always experience the event, regardless of whether they receive the assigned treatment; preventive $\{Y_{X=x} = 0, Y_{X=0} = 1\}$, which consists of subjects who do not experience the event when they receive the assigned treatment but do when they receive no treatment; causative $\{Y_{X=x} = 1, Y_{X=0} = 0\}$, which consists of subjects who experience the event when they receive the assigned treatment, but not when they receive no treatment; and immune $\{Y_{X=x} = 0, Y_{X=0} = 0\}$, which consists of subjects who never experience the event, regardless of whether they receive the assigned treatment. In the definition, $x = 2$ for the test treatment group ($R = 2$) and $x = 1$ for the control group ($R = 1$). Similar to Section 4.1.2, Assumption 2.1 implies that no preventive subject exists, and Assumption 2.2 implies that no causative subject exists.

Under this definition of principal strata, alternative assumptions of Assumptions 2.1 and 2.2 are as follows:

ASSUMPTION 3.3

$$\Pr(Y_{X=x} = 1, Y_{X=0} = 0 \mid X = R = x) \geq \Pr(Y_{X=x} = 0, Y_{X=0} = 1 \mid X = R = x) \textit{ for } x = 1, 2.$$

ASSUMPTION 3.4

$$\Pr(Y_{X=x} = 1, Y_{X=0} = 0 \mid X = R = x) \leq \Pr(Y_{X=x} = 0, Y_{X=0} = 1 \mid X = R = x) \textit{ for } x = 1, 2.$$

Assumption 3.3 implies that the number of causative subjects is not less than the number of preventive subjects, and Assumption 3.4 implies that the number of causative subjects is not more than the number of preventive subjects, within both assigned groups. Thus, these Assumptions are weaker than assumptions 2.1 and 2.2. Nevertheless, they can give the same bounds as those under Assumptions 2.1 and 2.2.

The MTS and RMTS (Assumptions 4.1 and 4.2) can also be applied to the case of noncompliance by receiving no treatment. For example, for $(s, t) = (2, 0)$ and $r = 2$, Assumption 4.1 is $E(Y_{X=x} \mid X = 2, R = 2) \geq E(Y_{X=x} \mid X = 0, R = 2)$, which means that subjects who received the assigned test treatment (i.e., compliers) tend to have larger outcome values than those who received no treatment (i.e., non-compliers) for the test treatment group. Under Assumptions 1 and 4.1, the upper bound of $E(Y_{X=x})$ becomes $E(Y_{X=x}) \geq E_{xx}$ ($E(Y_{X=x}) \leq E_{xx}$ under Assumptions 1 and 4.2) for $x = 1, 2$. Thus, the combination with inequality (5.1) derives bounds on ACE of:

$$(E_{22}p_{2|2} + K_0p_{0|2}) - E_{11} \leq \text{ACE} \leq E_{22} - (E_{11}p_{1|1} + K_0p_{0|1}).$$

When both MTR and MTS hold, the bounds on ACE are:

$$E(Y \mid R = 2) - E_{11} \leq \text{ACE} \leq E_{22} - E(Y \mid R = 1),$$

because $E(Y \mid R = x) \leq E(Y_{X=x}) \leq E_{xx}$ for $x = 1, 2$. When both RMTR and RMTS hold, these signs of inequalities for $E(Y_{X=x})$ are reversed.

Finally, we note that the MC and RMC (Assumptions 5.1 and 5.2), which derive the same bounds as those under the MTS and RMTS (Assumptions 4.1 and 4.2), are changed as follows for the case of noncompliance by receiving no treatment:

ASSUMPTION 5.3: Monotone confounding (MC)

Both $E(Y \mid X = R = x, Z = z)$ *and* $\Pr(X = x \mid R = x, Z = z)$ *are non-decreasing or non-increasing in* z *for* $x = 1, 2$ *and all* r*, and the components of* Z *are independent of each other.*

ASSUMPTION 5.4: Reverse monotone confounding (RMC)

One of E(Y | X = R = x, Z = z) *and* Pr(X = x | R = x, Z = z) *is non-decreasing and the other is non-increasing in z for x* = 1, 2 *and all r, and the components of Z are independent of each other.*

In some actual situations, assumptions presented in this section may hold for one of the test treatment and control groups but not for the other. In such cases, the assumptions can be applied only to one group. This example is introduced in the next sub-section.

5.3 Application

We apply the assumptions and bounds presented in Section 5.2 to the CDP trial introduced in Section 1 (Table 1). R represents the assigned group (R = 2 for the clofibrate group and R = 1 for the placebo group), and X is the compliance status (X = 2 for compliers in the clofibrate group, X = 1 for compliers in the placebo group, and X = 0 for non-compliers). Here, compliers and non-compliers are patients receiving more or less than 80% of the assigned treatment, respectively. Y is the incidence of deaths (Y = 1 for dead and Y = 0 for alive). Again, we note that ITT and PP analyses yielded ITT = 194/1065 – 523/2695 = –1.19% and PP = 106/708 – 274/1813 = –0.14%, respectively.

As in Section 4.3, it is necessary to discuss whether the assumptions hold. There may be a placebo effect, but it is not thought that the proportion of deaths will increase by receiving the placebo. Thus, Assumptions 2.2 (RMTR) and 3.4 can be assumed for (s, t) = (1, 0) and x = 1. However, a preventive effect of clofibrate may not be present (i.e., these assumptions may not be assumed for (s, t) = (2, 0) and x = 2) because of side-effects. The World Health Organization (WHO) has reported that in a large randomized trial, there were 25% more deaths in the clofibrate group than in the comparable high serum cholesterol control group (WHO, 1980). Because it is not clear whether the clofibrate has a positive or negative effect, we cannot assume the MTR or RMTR (and Assumption 3.3 or 3.4) for the clofibrate group.

Relating to the patients in this trial, health-oriented subjects might tend not to die and be more likely to comply with the assigned treatment, compared with subjects not concerned about their health. Under this observation, the RMTS (Assumption 4.4) would hold for both assigned groups. However, we note that some researchers may criticize this because some patients might not receive the treatment due to side-effects. In such a case, the RMTS may not hold for the clofibrate group. Nevertheless, we assume the RMTS for both assigned groups for illustrative purposes. Assumption 1 would hold because this trial was a double-blinded trial.

The arguments presented above demonstrate that the RMTR and RMTS can be assumed for the placebo group. Therefore, the bounds of $E(Y_{X=1})$ are $E_{11} \le E(Y_{X=1}) \le E(Y \mid R = 1)$, which yield 15.11% $\le E(Y_{X=1}) \le$ 19.41%. For the clofibrate group, the RMTS is assumed and then the bounds of $E(Y_{X=2})$ are $E_{22} \le E(Y_{X=2}) \le E_{22}p_{2|2} + K_1 p_{0|2}$ for $K_1 = 1$, which yields 14.97% $\le E(Y_{X=2})$ $\le$ 43.47%. In conclusion, the bounds on ACE are −4.43% ≤ ACE ≤ 28.36%. Unfortunately, we cannot conclude whether clofibrate is effective. However, the bounds improve those under Assumption 1 only: −32.94% ≤ ACE ≤ 33.31%, especially the lower bound.

6. Monotone instrumental variable

Sections 3-5 assumed the IV assumption (Assumption 1). As mentioned in Section 2, however, this assumption often may not hold in unblinded trials, in which subjects are aware of the assigned treatment and this knowledge may affect the potential outcomes. In the MRFIT (Section 4.3), subjects would have been aware of their assigned group because it was an unblinded trial, and thus the intervention itself might have evoked a psychological response. Furthermore, in addition to smoking cessation counseling, the intervention consisted of dietary advice to reduction blood cholesterol and hypertension medication. These interventions might also have influenced the incidence of CHD independent of smoking status. Thus, in this section, we relax the IV assumption to the following monotone instrumental variable (MIV) assumption (Manski & Pepper, 2000, 2009):

ASSUMPTION 6.1: Monotone instrumental variable (MIV)

$$E(Y_{X=x} \mid R = 2) \geq E(Y_{X=x} \mid R = 1).$$

The MIV assumption is only the replacement of equality in the IV assumption with inequality, and means that the values of potential outcomes for subjects assigned to $R = 2$ are overall larger than those assigned to $R = 1$. For example, consider an unblinded trial to compare a new treatment with a standard treatment, where the outcome is a measure such that a larger value is better for the subject's health. In such a trial, subjects may think that the new treatment is more effective than the standard treatment, and this thinking may give rise to better results for subjects assigned to the new treatment than those assigned to the standard treatment; this indicates that the MIV holds.

We can also consider the following reverse MIV (RMIV) assumption:

ASSUMPTION 6.2: Reverse monotone instrumental variable (RMIV)

$$E(Y_{X=x} \mid R = 2) \leq E(Y_{X=x} \mid R = 1).$$

We discuss the bounds on ACE under Assumptions 6.1 and 6.2 instead of Assumption 1. Noncompliance by switching the treatment (as in Sections 4) is discussed in Section 6.1, and noncompliance by receiving no treatment (as in Section 5) is discussed in Section 6.2. The derivations of inequalities in this section are outlined in Section 8.3.

6.1 Noncompliance by switching the treatment

The bounds introduced in Section 4 are extended to those under the MIV and RMIV (Assumptions 6.1 and 6.2). Under the MIV and RMIV, the bounds on ACE are:

$$(E_{21}p_{2|1} + K_0p_{1|1}) - (E_{12}p_{1|2} + K_1p_{2|2}) \leq \text{ACE} \leq (E_{22}p_{2|2} + K_1p_{1|2}) - (E_{11}p_{1|1} + K_0p_{2|1}), \quad (6.1)$$

$$(E_{22}p_{2|2} + K_0p_{1|2}) - (E_{11}p_{1|1} + K_1p_{2|1}) \leq \text{ACE} \leq (E_{21}p_{2|1} + K_1p_{1|1}) - (E_{12}p_{1|2} + K_0p_{2|2}). \quad (6.2)$$

These inequalities correspond to inequalities when a or b in max{a, b} and min{a, b} in inequality (4.1) are used. Therefore, the MIV and RMIV assumptions yield bounds on ACE with the same or broader width in comparison with the bounds under the IV assumption.

Even under the MIV (or RMIV) assumption, but not IV assumption, we can derive bounds on ACE with narower widths by applying assumptions in Section 4.2 (Chiba, 2010c). Each combination of the MIV or RMIV and the MTR or RMTR derives the improved lower or upper bounds on ACE in Table 3. Likewise, each combination of the MIV or RMIV and the MTS or RMTS derives the improved lower or upper bounds on ACE in Table 4.

Assumptions	Improved bound on ACE
MIV + MTR	ACE ≥ max{−ITT, 0}
RMIV + MTR	ACE ≥ max{ITT, 0}
MIV + RMTR	ACE ≤ min{ITT, 0}
RMIV + RMTR	ACE ≤ min{−ITT, 0}

Table 3. Improved bound on ACE under the MIV or RMIV and the MTR or RMTR, where ITT ≡ $E(Y \mid R = 2) - E(Y \mid R = 1)$.

Assumptions	Improved bound on ACE
MIV + MTS	ACE ≤ E_{22} - E_{11}
RMIV + MTS	ACE ≤ E_{21} - E_{12}
MIV + RMTS	ACE ≥ E_{21} - E_{12}
RMIV + RMTS	ACE ≥ E_{22} - E_{11}

Table 4. Improved bound on ACE under the MIV or RMIV and the MTS or RMTS.

Eight lower or upper bounds in Tables 3 and 4 yield the same or broader bounds as those under the IV assumption. Note that we can use Assumptions 3.1 and 3.2 instead of the MTR and RMTR (Assumptions 2.1 and 2.2), respectively, and Assumptions 5.1 and 5.2 instead of the MTS and RMTS (Assumptions 4.1 and 4.2), respectively. Further combinations of the above bounds can derive further improved bounds; for example, max{−ITT, 0} ≤ ACE ≤ PP under the MIV, MTR and MTS assumptions.

For illustration, we apply the bounds presented here to the MRFIT (Table 2), in which the IV assumption may not hold, as discussed above. Because the intervention consisted of dietary advice and hypertension medication as well as the therapy itself that might have evoked a psychological response, the potential incidence of CHD for subjects assigned to the test group might have been reduced, compared with subjects assigned to the control group. This observation shows that Assumption 6.2 (RMIV: $E(Y_{X=x} \mid R = 2) \leq E(Y_{X=x} \mid R = 1)$) is reasonable. Additionally, as discussed in Section 4.3, the RMTR (or Assumption 3.2) and RMTS are reasonable assumptions in this trial. In conclusion, the RMIV, RMTR and RMTS can be assumed, and then bounds on ACE become PP ≤ ACE ≤ min{−ITT, 0}, which yield −0.92% ≤ ACE ≤ 0%. In comparison with the IV (plus RMTR and RMTS) in Section 4.2 (−0.92% ≤ ACE ≤ −0.13%), the lower bound is the same but the upper bound is larger.

6.2 Noncompliance by receiving no treatment

The bounds introduced in Section 5 are extended to those under the MIV and RMIV (Assumptions 6.1 and 6.2). Under these assumptions, the bounds on ACE are:

$$K_0 - K_1 \leq \text{ACE} \leq (E_{22}p_{2|2} + K_1 p_{0|2}) - (E_{11}p_{1|1} + K_0 p_{0|1}), \tag{6.3}$$

$$(E_{22}p_{2|2} + K_0 p_{0|2}) - (E_{11}p_{1|1} + K_1 p_{0|1}) \leq \text{ACE} \leq K_1 - K_0, \tag{6.4}$$

respectively. The upper bound in inequality (6.3) is equal to that in inequality (5.1) and the lower bound in inequality (6.4) is equal to that in inequality (5.1). Unfortunately, the respective lower and upper bounds in inequalities (6.3) and (6.4) do not give any information.

As discussed in the above sub-section, by combining the MTR (or RMTR) and MTS (or RMTS), the bounds on ACE can be improved. Table 5 summarizes the bounds under the MIV or RMIV and the MTR and RMTR, and Table 6 summarizes those under the MIV or RMIV and the MTS and RMTS. The bounds in Tables 5 and 6 include K_0 or K_1, which is the finite range of Y. Specifically, in Table 6, the lower or upper bounds are not improved even when the MTS or RMTS is added. Thus, the bounds may not be greatly improved. However, further combinations of these assumptions can remove K_0 and K_1 from one of the lower and upper bounds. Such bounds are summarized in Table 7.

Assumptions	Bounds on ACE
MIV + MTR	$E(Y \mid R=1) - (E_{22}p_{2\mid 2} + K_1p_{0\mid 2}) \leq ACE \leq (E_{22}p_{2\mid 2} + K_1p_{0\mid 2}) - E(Y \mid R=1)$
RMIV + MTR	$E(Y \mid R=2) - (E_{11}p_{1\mid 1} + K_1p_{0\mid 1}) \leq ACE \leq K_1 - (E_{02}p_{0\mid 2} + K_0p_{2\mid 2})$
MIV + RMTR	$K_0 - (E_{02}p_{0\mid 2} + K_1p_{2\mid 2}) \leq ACE \leq E(Y \mid R=2) - (E_{11}p_{1\mid 1} + K_0p_{0\mid 1})$
RMIV + RMTR	$(E_{22}p_{2\mid 2} + K_0p_{0\mid 2}) - E(Y \mid R=1) \leq ACE \leq E(Y \mid R=1) - (E_{22}p_{2\mid 2} + K_0p_{0\mid 2})$

Table 5. Bounds on ACE under the MIV or RMIV and the MTR or RMTR[2].

Assumptions	Bounds on ACE
MIV + MTS	$K_0 - K_1 \leq ACE \leq E_{22} - (E_{11}p_{1\mid 1} + K_0p_{0\mid 1})$
RMIV + MTS	$(E_{22}p_{2\mid 2} + K_0p_{0\mid 2}) - E_{11} \leq ACE \leq K_1 - K_0$
MIV + RMTS	$K_0 - K_1 \leq ACE \leq (E_{22}p_{2\mid 2} + K_1p_{0\mid 2}) - E_{11}$
RMIV + RMTS	$E_{22} - (E_{11}p_{1\mid 1} + K_1p_{0\mid 1}) \leq ACE \leq K_1 - K_0$

Table 6. Bounds on ACE under the MIV or RMIV and the MTS or RMTS.

Assumptions	Bounds on ACE
MIV + MTR + MTS	$E(Y \mid R=1) - (E_{22}p_{2\mid 2} + K_1p_{0\mid 2}) \leq ACE \leq E_{22} - E(Y \mid R=1)$
RMIV + MTR + MTS	$E(Y \mid R=2) - E_{11} \leq ACE \leq K_1 - (E_{02}p_{0\mid 2} + K_0p_{2\mid 2})$
MIV + RMTR + RMTS	$K_0 - (E_{02}p_{0\mid 2} + K_1p_{2\mid 2}) \leq ACE \leq E(Y \mid R=2) - E_{11}$
RMIV + RMTR + RMTS	$E_{22} - E(Y \mid R=1) \leq ACE \leq E(Y \mid R=1) - (E_{22}p_{2\mid 2} + K_0p_{0\mid 2})$

Table 7. Bounds on ACE under some combinations of assumptions[3].

For illustration, we apply the bounds presented here to the CDP trial (Table 1). Although the IV (Assumption 1) would hold in this trial because it was a double-blinded trial, we here relax this assumption to the MIV and RMIV (Assumptions 6.1 and 6.2), and yield bounds on ACE under both assumptions. As discussed in Section 5.3, we assume the RMTS for the clofibrate group and the RMTR and RMTS for the placebo group. Then, under the MIV, the bounds of $E(Y_{X=2})$ and $E(Y_{X=1})$ are $K_0 \leq E(Y_{X=2}) \leq E_{22}p_{2\mid 2} + K_1p_{0\mid 2}$ and $E_{11} \leq E(Y_{X=1}) \leq E_{02}p_{0\mid 2} + K_1p_{2\mid 2}$, respectively, where $K_0 = 0$ and $K_1 = 1$ because Y is binary. These bounds yield bounds on ACE of $-74.74\% \leq ACE \leq 28.36\%$. Likewise, under the RMIV, the bounds on ACE become $-4.43\% \leq ACE \leq 90.05\%$, because $E_{22} \leq E(Y_{X=2}) \leq K_1$ and $E_{22}p_{2\mid 2} + K_0p_{0\mid 2} \leq E(Y_{X=1}) \leq E(Y \mid R = 1)$. Unfortunately, these bounds have a very broad width, and thus they do not provide enough information about treatment effects of clofibrate.

7. Conclusion

This chapter has presented bounds on ACE in randomized trials with noncompliance. Although the results presented here are relevant to the causal differences, they can also be readily applied to the causal risk ratio when the outcome is binary.

[2] If $(s, t) = (2, 1)$ in the MTR and RMTR (Assumptions 2.1 and 2.2) is used, the lower bound is 0 under the MTR and the upper bound is 0 under the RMTR.

[3] If $(s, t) = (2, 1)$ in the MTR and RMTR (Assumptions 2.1 and 2.2) is additionally used, a candidate of the lower bound is 0 under the MTR and that of the upper bound is 0 under the RMTR.

It is generally thought that the ITT analysis is likely to yield a downwardly biased estimate of causal effects (Sheiner & Rubin, 1995), whereas the PP analysis is likely to yield an upwardly biased estimate (Lewis & Machine, 1993). Thus, the ACE probably exists between the results of the ITT and PP analyses. As shown in Section 4.1, this is true under IV + MTR + MTS or under IV + RMTR + RMTS for noncompliance by switching the treatment. However, as shown in Sections 5 and 6, we cannot be certain that this is true when noncompliance is due to receiving no treatment and/or the IV assumption does not hold. Thus, investigators should not simply conclude that the ACE exists between the results of the ITT and PP analyses. Unfortunately, no standard method currently exists for estimating the ACE in randomized trials with noncompliance issues. Investigators should consider whether the assumptions presented in this chapter are valid and then yield bounds on ACE using the methodology described herein.

The needs from further methodologies in this field are three-fold. The first is to find weaker assumptions than those given here, which nevertheless can derive the same bounds. The second is to make assumptions that can derive the bounds with a narrower width, which are still reasonable in some situations. The ideal is to make a reasonable assumption that can give a point estimator. The third and final need is to extend the discussions in this chapter to more complex situations: for example, two types of noncompliance in this chapter may occur simultaneously, and more than two arms may be compared (Cheng & Small, 2006).

The other recent interest in causal inference is statistical analysis concerning the role of an intermediate variable between a particular treatment and outcome (Rubin, 2004; Joffe et al., 2007; VanderWeele, 2008b). Investigators are often interested in understanding how the effect of a treatment on an outcome may be mediated through an intermediate variable. For example, in the MRFIT, this implies that investigators are interested in how the effect of a multifactor intervention program on CHD mortality may be mediated through the smoking status 1 year after entry, rather than the effect of the smoking status 1 year after entry on CHD mortality. Such statistical analyses are closely related to issues of inference with a surrogate marker and issues of post-randomization selection bias and truncation-by-death (Zhang & Rubin, 2003; Chiba & VanderWeele, 2011). Further methodological research is needed to answer these issues.

8. Appendix: Derivations of equations and inequalities

This section outlines the derivations of the equations and inequalities presented in Sections 3, 4 and 6, which are outlined in Sections 8.1, 8.2 and 8.3, respectively.

8.1 Derivations of equations in Section 3

Equation (3.1) can be derived as follows:

$$\begin{aligned}
\mathrm{E}(Y_{X=2}) &= \mathrm{E}(Y_{X=2} \mid R=r) \\
&= \sum_{x=1,2} \mathrm{E}(Y_{X=2} \mid X=x, R=r)\Pr(X=x \mid R=r) \\
&= (E_{2r}-\alpha_r)p_{1|r} + E_{2r}p_{2|r} \\
&= E_{2r} - \alpha_r p_{1|r}.
\end{aligned}$$

The first equation holds by Assumption 1, and the third equation is derived by substituting $\mathrm{E}(Y_{X=2} \mid X=1, R=r) = \mathrm{E}(Y_{X=2} \mid X=2, R=r) - \alpha_r$ and applying the consistency assumption: $\mathrm{E}(Y_{X=2} \mid X=2, R=r) = \mathrm{E}(Y \mid X=2, R=r)$ (= E_{2r}). A similar calculation derives equation (3.2).

To derive equation (3.3), we consider the difference between $E(Y|R = 2)$ and $E(Y_{X=2})$ and between $E(Y|R = 1)$ and $E(Y_{X=1})$. The former difference derives:

$$\begin{aligned} E(Y \mid R=2) - E(Y_{X=2}) &= \sum_{x=1,2} E_{x2} p_{x|2} - (E_{22} - \alpha_2 p_{1|2}) \\ &= (E_{12} + \alpha_2) p_{1|2} - E_{22}(1 - p_{2|2}) \\ &= \{\alpha_2 - (E_{22} - E_{22})\} p_{1|2}. \end{aligned}$$

By a similar calculation, the latter difference becomes $E(Y|R = 1) - E(Y_{X=1}) = \{\beta_1 - (E_{21} - E_{11})\}p_{2|1}$. The difference between these equations derives equation (3.3).
The derivation of equation (3.5) is as follows. Simple algebra, $p_{2|r}$ × equation (3.1) plus $p_{1|r}$ × equation (3.2), yields $p_{2|r}\text{ACE} + E(Y_{X=1}) = E(Y|R = r) - (a_r - \beta_r)p_{1|r}p_{2|r}$. The difference between this equation with $r = 2$ and that with $r = 1$ is:

$$(p_{2|2} - p_{2|1})\text{ACE} = E(Y|R = 2) - E(Y|R = 1) - (a_2 - \beta_2)p_{1|2}p_{2|2} + (a_1 - \beta_1)p_{1|1}p_{2|1}.$$

This equation implies equation (3.5) for $p_{2|2} \neq p_{2|1}$.

8.2 Derivations of inequalities in Section 4

Inequality (4.1) can be derived as presented below. By substituting $K_0 \le E(Y_{X=x}|X = x^*, R = r) \le K_1$ for $x \neq x^*$ and $E(Y_{X=x}|X = x^*, R = r) = E(Y|X = x, R = r)$ (= E_{xr}) for $x = x^*$ (consistency assumption) into:

$$E(Y_{X=x} \mid R=r) = \sum_{x^*=1,2} E(Y_{X=x} \mid X = x^*, R=r)\Pr(X = x^* \mid R=r), \tag{8.1}$$

we obtain:

$$E_{xr}p_{x|r} + K_0 p_{x^*|r} \le E(Y_{X=x} \mid R = r) \le E_{xr}p_{x|r} + K_1 p_{x^*|r} \tag{8.2}$$

for $x \neq x^*$. Because $E(Y_{X=x}) = E(Y_{X=x}|R = r)$ by Assumption 1, the bounds of $E(Y_{X=x})$ become:

$$\max\begin{Bmatrix} E_{x1}p_{x|1} + K_0 p_{x^*|1} \\ E_{x2}p_{x|2} K_0 p_{x^*|2} \end{Bmatrix} \le E(Y_{X=x}) \le \min\begin{Bmatrix} E_{x1}p_{x|1} + K_1 p_{x^*|1} \\ E_{x2}p_{x|2} + K_1 p_{x^*|2} \end{Bmatrix}$$

for $x \neq x^*$. The difference between the lower and upper bounds of this inequality for $x = 1, 2$ is inequality (4.1).
Inequality (4.3) can be also derived using equation (8.1). Assumption 2.1 implies that $E(Y_{X=2}|X = x, R = r) \ge E(Y_{X=1}|X = x, R = r)$. Thus, by substituting this inequality with $x = 1$ into equation (8.1), we obtain:

$$\begin{aligned} E(Y_{X=2}) &= E(Y_{X=2} \mid R=r) \\ &\ge \sum_{x=1,2} E(Y_{X=x} \mid X = x, R=r)\Pr(X = x \mid R=r) \\ &= \sum_{x=1,2} E(Y \mid X = x, R=r)\Pr(X = x \mid R=r) \\ &= E(Y \mid R=r), \end{aligned} \tag{8.3}$$

and thus $E(Y_{X=2}) \ge \max\{E(Y|R = 1), E(Y|R = 2)\}$. Similarly, $E(Y_{X=1}) \le \min\{E(Y|R = 1), E(Y|R = 2)\}$ by substituting $E(Y_{X=2}|X = 2, R = r) \ge E(Y_{X=1}|X = 2, R = r)$ into equation (8.1). The difference between them is inequality (4.3).

In the case of a binary outcome variable, inequality (4.3) can also be derived under Assumption 3.1. By adding $\Pr(Y_{X=2} = 1, Y_{X=1} = 1 \mid X = x, R = r)$ on both sides of the inequality in Assumption 3.1: $\Pr(Y_{X=2} = 1, Y_{X=1} = 0 \mid X = x, R = r) \geq \Pr(Y_{X=2} = 0, Y_{X=1} = 1 \mid X = x, R = r)$, we obtain $\Pr(Y_{X=2} = 1 \mid X = x, R = r) \geq \Pr(Y_{X=1} = 1 \mid X = x, R = r)$. Because this inequality is a binary outcome version of $E(Y_{X=2} \mid X = x, R = r) \geq E(Y_{X=1} \mid X = x, R = r)$, inequality (4.3) is derived.
Inequality (4.4) can be derived as follows. Substituting $E(Y_{X=2} \mid X = 2, R = r) \geq E(Y_{X=2} \mid X = 1, R = r)$ ($x = 2$ and $(s, t) = (2, 1)$ in Assumption 4.1) into equation (8.1) yields:

$$\begin{aligned} E(Y_{X=2}) &= E(Y_{X=2} \mid R = r) \\ &\leq \sum_{x=1,2} E(Y_{X=2} \mid X = 2, R = r)\Pr(X = x \mid R = r) \\ &= E(Y \mid X = 2, R = r)(= E_{2r}), \end{aligned} \tag{8.4}$$

and thus $E(Y_{X=2}) \leq \min\{E_{21}, E_{22}\}$. Similarly, $E(Y_{X=1}) \geq \max\{E_{11}, E_{12}\}$ by substituting $E(Y_{X=1} \mid X = 2, R = r) \geq E(Y_{X=1} \mid X = 1, R = r)$ ($x = 1$ and $(s, t) = (2, 1)$ in Assumption 4.1) into equation (8.1). The difference between them is inequality (4.4).
Inequality (4.4) can also be derived under Assumption 5.1. To prove this, we need the following lemma (Esary et al., 1967):

LEMMA 1

Let f and g be functions with n real-valued arguments such that both f and g are non-decreasing or non-increasing in each of their arguments. If $Z = (Z_1, \ldots, Z_n)$ is a multivariate random variable with n components such that each component is independent of the other components, then $\mathrm{Cov}\{f(Z), g(Z)\} \geq 0$.

Let $f_r(Z) = E(Y \mid X = 2, R = r, Z = z)$, $g_r(Z) = \Pr(X = 2 \mid R = r, Z = z)$ and $F_{Z|R=r}$ denote the cumulative distribution function of Z conditional on $R = r$. Then, by Lemma 1, we obtain:

$$E_{F_{Z|R=r}}\{f_r(Z)g_r(Z)\} - E_{F_{Z|R=r}}\{f_r(Z)\}E_{F_{Z|R=r}}\{g_r(Z)\} = \mathrm{Cov}_{F_{Z|R=r}}\{f_r(Z), g_r(Z)\} \geq 0,$$

if both $f_r(Z)$ and $g_r(Z)$ are non-decreasing or non-increasing in z and the components of Z are independent. Thus, using the assumption that $Y_{X=x}$ is independent from X given R and Z, the following inequality is derived:

$$\begin{aligned} E(Y_{X=2} \mid X = 1, R = r) &= \sum_z E(Y_{X=2} \mid X = 1, R = r, Z = z)\Pr(Z = z \mid X = 1, R = r) \\ &= \sum_z \frac{E(Y \mid X = 2, R = r, Z = z)\Pr(X = 1 \mid R = r, Z = z)\Pr(Z = z \mid R = r)}{\Pr(X = 1 \mid R = r)} \\ &= E_{F_{Z|R=r}}[f_r(Z)\{1 - g_r(Z)\}]/\Pr(X = 1 \mid R = r) \\ &\leq E_{F_{Z|R=r}}\{f_r(Z)\}E_{F_{Z|R=r}}\{1 - g_r(Z)\}/\Pr(X = 1 \mid R = r) \\ &= E_{F_{Z|R=r}}\{f_r(Z)\} \\ &= E_{F_{Z|R=r}}\{f_r(Z)\}E_{F_{Z|R=r}}\{g_r(Z)\}/\Pr(X = 2 \mid R = r) \\ &\leq E_{F_{Z|R=r}}\{f_r(Z)g_r(Z)\}/\Pr(X = 2 \mid R = r) \\ &= \sum_z \frac{E(Y \mid X = 2, R = r, Z = z)\Pr(X = 2 \mid R = r, Z = z)\Pr(Z = z \mid R = r)}{\Pr(X = 2 \mid R = r)} \\ &= E(Y \mid X = 2, R = r). \end{aligned}$$

The second equation holds because $E(Y_{X=2} | X = 1, R = r, Z = z) = E(Y_{X=2} | X = 2, R = r, Z = z) = E(Y | X = 2, R = r, Z = z)$ by the independency and consistency assumptions. The fourth inequality holds because $1 - g_r(Z)$ is non-increasing when $g_r(Z)$ is non-decreasing. The fifth and sixth equations hold because:

$$E_{F_{Z|R=r}}\{g_r(Z)\} = \sum_z \Pr(X = 2 | R = r, Z = z)\Pr(Z = z | R = r) = \Pr(X = 2 | R = r).$$

A similar calculation derives $E(Y_{X=1} | X = 2, R = r) \geq E(Y | X = 1, R = r)$. The inequalities derived here are the same as those in Assumption 4.1. Therefore, inequality (4.4) can be derived under Assumption 5.1.

8.3 Derivations of inequalities in Section 6

$E(Y_{X=x})$ can be expressed as $E(Y_{X=x}) = E(Y_{X=x} | R = 1)\Pr(R = 1) + E(Y_{X=x} | R = 2)\Pr(R = 2)$. Therefore,

$$E(Y_{X=x} | R = 1) \leq E(Y_{X=x}) \leq E(Y_{X=x} | R = 2) \quad (8.5)$$

under Assumption 6.1 (MIV: $E(Y_{X=x} | R = 1) \geq E(Y_{X=x} | R = 0)$). All bounds under the MIV are derived based on inequality (8.5), while those under the IV (Assumption 1) are based on $E(Y_{X=x}) = E(Y_{X=x} | R = r)$. This is why inequality (6.1) corresponds to it when a or b in $\max\{a, b\}$ and $\min\{a, b\}$ in inequality (4.1) is used. This is also similar under the RMIV (Assumption 6.2), and then inequality (6.2) and the bounds in Tables 3 and 4 also correspond to those when a or b in $\max\{a, b\}$ and $\min\{a, b\}$ in the bounds presented in Section 4.1 are used. Therefore, the derivations of bounds in Section 6.1 are simple. Inequality (6.1) is derived by the combination of inequalities (8.2) and (8.5).

In Table 3, ACE $\geq \max\{-\text{ITT}, 0\}$ under the MIV and MTR is derived as follows. Because $E(Y_{X=2}) \geq E(Y_{X=2} | R = 1)$ from inequality (8.5), $E(Y_{X=2}) \geq E(Y | R = 1)$ from inequality (8.3) with $r = 1$. Likewise, $E(Y_{X=1}) \leq E(Y | R = 2)$ by $E(Y_{X=1}) \leq E(Y_{X=1} | R = 2)$ and the MTR (Assumption 2.1). The difference between these inequalities derives ACE $\geq -$ITT. Additionally, the MTR derives ACE $= E(Y_{X=1}) - E(Y_{X=0}) \geq 0$ directly. The other bounds in Table 3 can be derived in a similar way.

In Table 4, ACE $\leq E_{22} - E_{11}$ under the MIV and MTS is derived as follows. Because $E(Y_{X=2}) \leq E(Y_{X=2} | R = 2)$ from inequality (8.5), $E(Y_{X=2}) \leq E_{22}$ from inequality (8.4) with $r = 2$. Likewise, $E(Y_{X=1}) \geq E_{11}$ by $E(Y_{X=1}) \geq E(Y_{X=1} | R = 1)$ and the MTS (Assumption 4.1). The difference between these inequalities derives ACE $\leq E_{22} - E_{11}$. The other bounds in Table 4 can be derived in a similar way.

The inequalities in Section 6.2 can be derived in straightforward manner as the derivations of those in Section 6.1 by replacing $x = 1, 2$ in Section 6.1 to $x = 0, 1$ and $x = 0, 2$, although they may be somewhat complex.

9. Acknowledgment

This work was supported partially by Grant-in-Aid for Scientific Research (No. 23700344) from the Ministry of Education, Culture, Sports, Science, and Technology of Japan.

10. References

Angrist, J.D.; Imbens, G.W. & Rubin, D.B. (1996). Identification of causal effects using instrumental variables (with discussions). *Journal of the American Statistical Association*, Vol.91, No.434, (June 1996), pp.444-472, ISSN 0162-1459

Balke, A. & Pearl, J. (1997). Bounds on treatment effects from studies with imperfect compliance. *Journal of the American Statistical Association*, Vol.92, No.439, (September 1997), pp.1171-1176, ISSN 0162-1459

Brumback, B.A.; Hernán, M.A.; Haneuse, S.J.P.A. & Robins, J.M. (2004). Sensitivity analyses for unmeasured confounding assuming a marginal structural model for repeated measures. *Statistics in Medicine,* Vol.23, No.5, (March 2004), pp.749–767, ISSN 1097-0258

Cai, Z.; Kuroki, M. & Sato, T. (2007). Non-parametric bounds on treatment effects with non-compliance by covariate adjustment. *Statistics in Medicine,* Vol.26, No.16, (July 2007), pp.3188-3204, ISSN 1097-0258

Cheng, J. & Small, D.S. (2006). Bounds on causal effects in three-arm trials with non-compliance. *Journal of the Royal Statistical Society, Series B,* Vol.68, No.5, (November 2006), pp.815-836, ISSN 0964-1998

Chiba, Y. (2009a). The sign of the unmeasured confounding bias under various standard populations. *Biometrical Journal,* Vol.51, No.4, (August 2009), pp. 670-676, ISSN 0323-3847

Chiba, Y. (2009b). Bounds on causal effects in randomized trials with noncompliance under monotonicity assumptions about covariates. *Statistics in Medicine,* Vol.28, No.26, (November 2009), pp.3249-3259, ISSN 1097-0258

Chiba, Y. (2010a). Bias analysis of the instrumental variable estimator as an estimator of the average causal effect. *Contemporary Clinical Trials,* Vol.31, No.1, (January 2010), pp.12-17, ISSN 1551-7144

Chiba, Y. (2010b). An approach for estimating causal effects in randomized trials with noncompliance. *Communications in Statistics – Theory and Methods,* Vol.39, No.12, (January 2010), pp.2146-2156, ISSN 0361-0926

Chiba, Y. (2010c). The monotone instrumental variable in randomized trials with noncompliance. *Japanese Journal of Biometrics,* Vol.31, No.2, (December 2010), pp.93-106, ISSN 0918-4430

Chiba, Y. (2011). An alternative assumption for assessing the sign of causal effects. *Oriental Journal of Statistical Methods, Theory and Applications,* in press, ISSN Awaited

Chiba, Y.; Sato, T. & Greenland, S. (2007). Bounds on potential risks and causal risk differences under assumptions about confounding parameters. *Statistics in Medicine,* Vol.26, No.28, (December 2007), pp. 5125-5135, ISSN 1097-0258

Chiba, Y. & VanderWeele, T.J. (2011). A simple method for principal strata effects when the outcome has been truncated due to death. *American Journal of Epidemiology,* Vol.173, No.7, (April 2011), pp.745-751, ISSN 0002-9262

Coronary Drug Project Research Group (1980). Influence of adherence to treatment and response of cholesterol on mortality in the coronary drug project. *New England Journal of Medicine,* Vol.303, No.18, (October 1980), pp.1038-1041, ISSN 0028-4793

Cuzick, J.; Edwards, R. & Segnan, N. (1997). Adjustment for non-compliance and contamination in randomized clinical trials. *Statistics in Medicine,* Vol.16, No.9, (May 1997), pp.1017-1029, ISSN 1097-0258

Esary, J.D.; Proschan, F. & Walkup, D.W. (1967). Association of random variables, with applications. *Annals of Mathematical Statistics,* Vol.38, No.5, (October 1967), pp.1466-1474, ISSN 0003-4851

Fisher, L.D.; Dixon, D.O.; Herson, J.; Frankowski, R.; Hearron, M. & Peace, K.E. (1990). Intention to treat in clinical trials, In: *Statistical Issues in Drug Research and Development*, K.E. Peace (Ed.), 331-350, Marcel Dekker, ISBN 0-8247-8290-9, New York, USA

Frangakis, C.E. & Rubin, D.B. (2002). Principal stratification in causal inference. *Biometrics* Vol.58, No.1, (March 2002), pp.21-29, ISSN 0006-341X

Greenland, S. (2000). An introduction to instrumental variables for epidemiologists. *International Journal of Epidemiology*, Vol.29, No.4, (August 2000), pp.722-729, ISSN 0300-5771

Greenland, S. & Robins, J.M. (1986). Identifiability, exchangeability and epidemiologic confounding. *International Journal of Epidemiology*, Vol.15, No.3, (June 1986), pp.413-419, ISSN 0300-5771

Hernán, M.A. & Robins, J.M. (2006). Instruments for causal inference: An epidemiologist's dream? *Epidemiology*, Vol.17, No.4, (July 2006), pp.360–372, ISSN 1044-3983

Holland, P.W. (1986). Statistics and causal inference (with discussions). *Journal of the American Statistical Association*, Vol.81, No.396, (December 1986), pp.945-970, ISSN 0162-1459

Joffe, M.; Small, D. & Hsu, C.-Y. (2007). Defining and estimating intervention effects for groups that will develop an auxiliary outcome. *Statistical Science*, Vol.22, No.1, (February 2007), pp.74-97, ISSN 0883-4237

Lee, Y.; Ellenberg, J.; Hirtz, D. & Nelson, K. (1991). Analysis of clinical trials by treatment actually received: Is it really an option? *Statistics in Medicine*, Vol.10, No.10, (October 1991), pp.1595-1605, ISSN 1097-0258

Lewis, J.A. & Machine, D. (1993). Intention to treat - who should use ITT? *British Journal of Cancer*, Vol.68, No.4, (October 1993), pp.647-650, ISSN 0007-0920

Manski, C. F. (1990). Nonparametric bounds on treatment effects. *American Economic Review*, Vol.80, No.2, (May 1990), pp.319-323, ISSN 0002-8282

Manski, C.F. (1997). Monotone treatment response. *Econometrica*, Vol.65, No.6, (November 1997), pp.1311-1334, ISSN 0012-9682

Manski, C.F. (2003). *Partial identification of probability distributions*, Springer-Verlag, ISBN 0-387-00454-8, New York, USA

Manski, C.F. & Pepper, J.V. (2000). Monotone instrumental variables: With an application to the returns to schooling. *Econometrica*, Vol.68, No.4, (July 2000), pp.997-1010, ISSN 0012-9682

Manski, C.F. & Pepper, J.V. (2009). More on monotone instrumental variables. *Econometrics Journal*, Vol.12, No.S1, (January 2009), pp.S200-S216, ISSN 1368-4221

Mark, S.D. & Robins, J.M. (1993). A method for the analysis of randomized trials with noncompliance information: An application to the multiple risk factor intervention trial. *Controlled Clinical Trials*, Vol.14, No.2, (April 1993), pp.79-97, ISSN 1551-7144

Matsui, S. (2005). Stratified analysis in randomized trials with noncompliance. *Biometrics*, Vol.61, No.3, (September 2005), pp.816-823, ISSN 0006-341X

Multiple Risk Factor Intervention Trial Research Group (1982). Multiple risk factor intervention trial: Risk factor changes and mortality results. *Journal of the American Medical Association*, Vol.248, No.12, (September 1982), pp.1465-1477, ISSN 0098-7484

Piantadosi, S. (1997). *Clinical Trials: A Methodologic Perspective*, Wiley, ISBN 0-471-16393-7, New York, USA

Pearl, J. (1995). Causal inference from indirect experiments. *Artificial Intelligence in Medicine,* Vol.7, No.6, (December 1995), pp.561-582, ISSN 0933-3657

Pearl, J. (2000). *Causality: Models, Reasoning, and Inference,* Cambridge University Press, ISBN 0-521-77362-8, Cambridge, USA

Robins, J.M. (1989). The analysis of randomized and non-randomized AIDS treatment trials using a new approach to causal inference in longitudinal studies, In: *Health Service Research Methodology: A Focus on AIDS,* L. Sechrest, H. Freeman & A. Mulley (Eds), 113-159, DHHS Publication No.(PHS)89-3439, U.S. Public Health Service, Washington DC, USA

Robins, J.M. & Greenland, S. (1994). Adjusting for differential rates of PCP prophylaxis in high- versus low-dose AZT treatment arms in an AIDS randomized trial. *Journal of the American Statistical Association,* Vol.89, No.427, (September 1994), pp.737-749, ISSN 0162-1459

Robins, J.M. & Tsiatis, A.A. (1991). Correcting for non-compliance in randomized trials using rank preserving structural failure time models. *Communications in Statistics – Theory and Methods,* Vol.20, No.8, (January 1991), pp.2609-2631, ISSN 0361-0926

Rubin, D.B. (1974). Estimating causal effects of treatments in randomized and nonrandomized studies. *Journal of Educational Psychology,* Vol.66, No.5, (October 1974), pp.688-701, ISSN 0022-0663

Rubin, D.B. (1978). Bayesian inference for causal effects: The role of randomization. *Annals of Statistics,* Vol.6, No.1, (January 1978), pp.34-58, ISSN 0090-5364

Rubin, D. B. (1990). Formal models of statistical inference for causal effects. *Journal of Statistical Planning and Inference,* Vol.25, No.3, (July 1990), pp.279-292, ISSN 0378-3758

Rubin, D.B. (2004). Direct and indirect effects via potential outcomes. *Scandinavian Journal of Statistics,* Vol.31, No.2, (June 2004), pp.161-170, ISSN 1467-9469

Sato, T. (2006). Randomization-based analysis of causal effects, In: *Handbook of Clinical Trials: Design and Analysis,* T. Tango & H. Uesaka (Eds.), 535-556, Asakura Publishing, ISBN 978-4-254-32214-9, Tokyo, Japan (in Japanese)

Schwartz, D. & Lellouch, J. (1967). Explanatory and pragmatic attitudes in therapeutic trials. *Journal of Chronic Diseases,* Vol.20, No.8, (August 1967), pp.637-648, ISSN 0021-9681

Sheiner, L. & Rubin, D.B. (1995). Intention-to-treat analysis and the goals of clinical trials. *Clinical Pharmacology and Therapeutics,* Vol.57, No.1, (January 1995), pp.6-15, ISSN 0009-9236

VanderWeele, T.J. (2008a). The sign of the bias of unmeasured confounding. *Biometrics,* Vol.64, No.3, (September 2008), pp.702-706, ISSN 0006-341X

VanderWeele, T.J. (2008b). Simple relations between principal stratification and direct and indirect effects. *Statistics and Probability Letters,* Vol.78, No.17, (December 2008), pp.2957-2962, ISSN 0167-7152

World Health Organization (1980). W.H.O. cooperative trial on primary prevention of ischaemic heart disease using clofibrate to lower serum cholesterol: Mortality follow-up: Report of the committee of principal investigators. *Lancet,* Vol.316, No.8191, (August 1980), pp.379-385, ISSN 0140-6736

Zhang, J.L. & Rubin, D.B. (2003). Estimation of causal effects via principal stratification when some outcomes are truncated by "death." *Journal of Educational and Behavioral Statistics,* Vol.28, No.4, (December 2003), pp.353-368, ISSN 1076-9986

19

Design of Scoring Models for Trustworthy Risk Prediction in Critical Patients

Paolo Barbini and Gabriele Cevenini
Department of Surgery and Bioengineering, University of Siena
Italy

1. Introduction

Prediction of an adverse health event (AHE) from objective data is of great importance in clinical practice. A health event is inherently dichotomous as it either happens or does not happen, and in the latter case, it is a favourable health event (FHE).

In many clinical applications, it is relevant not only to predict AHEs happening (diagnostic ability) but also to estimate in advance their individual risk of occurrence using ordered multinomial or quantitative scales (prognostic ability) such as probability. An estimated probability of a patient's outcome is usually preferred to a simpler binary decision rule. However, models cannot be designed by optimising their fit to true individual risk probabilities because the latter are not intrinsically known, nor can they be easily and accurately associated with an individual's data. Classification models are therefore usually trained on binary outcomes to provide an orderable or quantitative output, which can be dichotomised using a suitable cut-off value.

Model discrimination refers to accurate identification of actual outcomes. Model calibration, or goodness of fit, is related to the agreement between predicted probabilities and observed proportions and it is an important aspect to consider in evaluating the prognostic capacity of a risk model (Cook, 2008). Model calibration is independent of discrimination, since there are risk models with good discrimination but poor calibration. A well-calibrated model gives probability values that can be reliably associated with the true individual risk of outcomes.

Many models have recently been proposed for diagnostic purposes in a wide range of medical applications and they also provide reliable estimates of individual risk probabilities. Two different approaches have been used to predict patient risk. The first approach is based on estimation of risk probability by sophisticated mathematical and statistical methods, such as logistic regression, the Bayesian rule and artificial neural networks (Dreiseitl & Ohno-Machado, 2002; Fukunaga, 1990; Marshall et al., 1994). Despite their great accuracy, these models are unfortunately not widely used because they are hard to design and call for difficult calculations, often requiring dedicated software and computing knowledge that doctors do not welcome, besides being difficult to incorporate in clinical practice. The second approach creates scoring systems, in which the predictor variables are usually selected and scored subjectively by expert consensus or objectively using statistical methods (den Boer et al., 2005; Higgins et al., 1997; Vincent & Moreno, 2010).

Despite their lower accuracy, scoring models are usually preferred to probability models by clinicians and health operators because they allow immediate calculation of individual patient scores as a simple sum of integer values associated with binary risk factors, without the need for any data processing system. It has also been demonstrated that in most cases, where a considerable amount of clinical information is available, their diagnostic accuracy is similar to that of probability models (Cevenini & P. Barbini, 2010, as cited in Cevenini et al., 2007). Computation facility of score models should be carefully evaluated in conjunction with their predictive performance. Too many simple models can lead to misleading estimates of a patient's clinical risk, which can be useless, counterproductive or even dangerous.

Any risk model, even if sophisticated and accurate in the local specific condition in which it was designed, loses much of its predictive power when exported to different clinical scenarios. Locally customized scoring models generally provide better performances than exported probability models. This reinforces the clinical success and effectiveness of scoring systems, the design and customisation to local conditions and/or institutions of which are usually much easier.

A limit of many scoring systems is their complex, involuted and even arbitrary design procedure that often involves contrivances to round off parameters of more sophisticated probability models to integer values. This can make their design even more complicated than that of probability models. Scoring often involves dichotomisation of continuous clinical variables to binary risk factors by identifying cut-off values from subjective clinical criteria not based on suitable optimisation techniques. However, whatever the design procedure, the main weakness of scoring models regards the interpretation of individual scores in terms of prognostic probabilities (model calibration), the reliability of which depends on the availability of a sufficient proportion of adverse outcomes and of a design procedure that provides precise individual risk estimation (Cevenini & P. Barbini, 2010). The Hosmer-Lemeshow test is commonly used to assess the calibration of probability models and therefore to manage their learning, but its results are unreliable when applied to models with discrete outputs, such as scoring systems (Finazzi et al., 2011).

This chapter provides an initial brief overview of general issues for the correct design of predictive models with binary outcomes. It broadly describes the main modelling approaches, then illustrates in more detail a method for creating score models for predicting the risk of an AHE. The method tackles and overcomes many of the above-mentioned limits. It uses a well-founded numerical bootstrap technique for appropriate statistical interpretation of simple scoring systems, and provides useful and reliable diagnostic and prognostic information (Carpenter & Bithell, 2000; DiCiccio & Efron, 1996). The whole design procedure is set out and validated by a simulation approach that mimics realistic clinical conditions. Finally, the method is applied to an actual clinical example, to predict the risk of morbidity of heart surgery patients in intensive care.

2. Model issues

Various pattern recognition approaches can be used to design models for separating and classifying patients into the two independent classes of adverse or favourable health outcome, AHE and FHE. The approaches fall into two main categories.

1. Probability models estimate a class-conditional probability, $P(AHE\,|\,x)$, of developing the adverse outcome AHE, given a set of chosen predictor variables or features x

(Bishop, 1995; Dreiseitl & Ohno-Machado, 2002; Fukunaga, 1990; Lee, 2004). A probability threshold value, P_t, is identified for classification, over which AHE is recognized to occur, that is when P(AHE | x)>P_t; the choice of P_t depends on the clinical cost of a wrong decision and influences model classification performance (E. Barbini et al., 2007).

2. Score models evaluate risk by a discrete scale of n positive integer values s_i (i = 0, 1, 2, ..., n) which includes zero to represent null risk, but rarely provides a threshold value for classification purposes (Cevenini & P. Barbini, 2010; Vincent & Moreno, 2010).

2.1 Discrimination and calibration

Whatever the risk model, its prediction power is generally expressed by discrimination and calibration (Cook, 2008; Diamond, 1992).

Discrimination is the capacity of a classification model to correctly distinguish patients who will develop an adverse outcome from patients who will not. It must be optimized during model design by ascertaining that the model learns all the discrimination properties valid for the population, correctly from the training sample and therefore shows similar performance in different samples (generalisation ability) (Dreiseitl & Ohno-Machado, 2002; Vapnik, 1999). Though many criteria exist for evaluating model discrimination capacity (Fukunaga, 1990), sensitivity (SE) and specificity (SP), which measure the fractions of correctly classified sick and healthy patients, respectively, are commonly used for statistical evaluations of binary diagnostic test performance. SE end SP are combined in the receiver operating characteristic (ROC) curve which is a graphic representation of the relationship between the true-positive fraction (TPF = SE) and false-positive fraction (FPF = 1-SP) obtained for all possible choices of P_t. The area under the ROC curve (AUC) is the most widely used index of total discrimination capacity in medical applications (Lasko et al., 2005).

Calibration, or goodness of fit, represents the agreement between model-predicted and true probabilities of developing the adverse outcome (Hosmer & Lemeshow, 2000). Retrospective training data only provides dichotomous responses, that is presence or absence of the AHE, so true individual risk probabilities cannot intrinsically be known. The only way to derive them directly from sample data is to calculate the proportion of AHEs in groups of patients, but this obviously becomes less accurate as group size decreases. Nevertheless, from a health or clinical point of view, it is often useful to have an estimation of the level at which each event happens, using a continuous scale, such as probability. For probability models with dichotomous outcomes, calibration capacity can be evaluated by the Hosmer-Lemeshow (HL) goodness-of-fit test, based on two alternative chi-squared statistics, $\hat{H}$ and $\hat{C}$ (Hosmer & Lemeshow, 2000). The first formulation compares model-predicted and observed outcome frequencies of fixed deciles of predicted risk probability; the second compares by partitioning observations into ten groups of the same size (the last group can have a slightly different number of cases) and calculating model-predicted frequencies from average group probabilities. The $\hat{C}$-statistic is generally preferred because it avoids empty groups, although it depends heavily on sample size and grouping criterion (den Boer et al., 2005). The HL test cannot really be applied to models with discrete outputs, such as score systems, because group sizes should themselves be adjusted on the basis of discrete values (Finazzi et al., 2011).

Calibration can be improved, without changing discrimination capacity, by suitable monotonic mathematical transformations of model predicted probabilities (Harrell et al., 1996). The mean squared error between model predicted probability and observed binary outcomes is sometimes calculated as a global index of model accuracy, and has been demonstrated to incorporate both discrimination and calibration capacities (Murphy, 1973).

2.2 Generalisation, cross-validation and variable selection

Generalisation is defined as the capacity of the model to maintain the same predictive performance on data not used for training, but belonging to the same population. A high generalisation power is of primary importance for predictive models designed on a sample data set of correctly classified cases (training set). Many different procedures, which involve different correctly classified data sets for testing model performance (testing sets), have been used to control model generalisation (Bishop, 1995; Fukunaga, 1990; Vapnik, 1999). A model generalises when differences between errors of testing and training sets are not statistically significant.

Theoretically, the optimal model is the simplest possible model designed on training data and has the highest possible performance on any other equally representative set of testing data. Excessively complex models tend to overfit, i.e. give significantly lower errors on the training data than on the testing data. Overfitting produces data storage rather than learning of prediction rules. Models must be designed to avoid overfitting and improve generalisation through efficient control of the training process. This control often includes suitable techniques for the selection of predictor variables (Guyon & Elisseeff, 2003).

Computer algorithms for properly controlling overfitting are known as cross-validation or rotation techniques and make efficient use of all available data to train and test the model (Vapnik, 1999). The most common type of cross-validation procedure is k-fold, where the original sample is randomly partitioned into k subsamples, one of which is used as testing set and the other k–1 as training set. The process is then repeated k times, changing the testing set each time so that all subsamples are used for testing. A convenient variant, more appropriate in dichotomous classification, selects each subsample to contain approximately the same proportion of cases in the two classes. When k is equal to sample size, n, the procedure is called leave-one-out. One case is tested at a time at each of the n training sessions using n–1 training cases. Resampling methods also exist, and include bootstrap methods that produce different data samples by randomly extracting cases with replacement from the original dataset (Chernick, 2007).

Cross-validation can be used to compare the performance of different predictive modelling procedures and, specifically, to select different sets of predictor variables with the same model. In fact, it is convenient to select the best minimum subset of predictor variables to control generalisation and to avoid information overlap due to correlation between variables. Computer-aided stepwise techniques are usually used to obtain optimal nested subsets of variables for this purpose. To train the model, a variable is entered or removed from the predictor subset on the basis of its contribution to a significant increase in discrimination performance (typically the AUC for dichotomous classification) at each step of the process. The stepwise process stops when no variable satisfies the statistical criterion for inclusion or removal (Guyon & Elisseeff, 2003).

3. Probability models

We now provide an overview of four approaches for estimating AHE risk probability: the Bayesian classification rule (Lee, 2004), k-nearest neighbour discrimination (Beyer et al., 1999), logistic regression (Dreiseitl & Ohno-Machado, 2002; Hosmer & Lemeshow, 2000), and artificial neural networks (Bishop, 1995; Dreiseitl & Ohno-Machado, 2002). Linear and quadratic discriminant analyses and related Fisher discriminant functions were not considered because they are strictly classification methods, and although they also enable easy derivation of prediction probabilities, they have been demonstrated to be equivalent to Bayesian methods (Fukunaga, 1990).

3.1 Bayesian classifiers

Bayes's rule allows the posterior conditional probability of AHEs to be predicted as follows (Lee, 2004):

$$P(AHE\,|\,x)=\frac{P(AHE)\,p(x\,|\,AHE)}{P(AHE)\,p(x\,|\,AHE)+P(FHE)\,p(x\,|\,FHE)} \tag{1}$$

where P(AHE) and P(FHE) = 1–P(AHE) are the prior probabilities of the adverse and favourable health events, respectively, p(x | AHE), and p(x | FHE) are the corresponding class-conditional probability density functions (CPDFs) of selected features x. Posterior probability of class FHE is simply P(FHE | x) = 1–P(AHE | x).

Setting the posterior class-conditional probability threshold P_t at 0.5, the Bayes decision rule gives minimum error. It amounts to assigning patients to the class with the largest posterior probability. A higher/lower value of P_t gives rise to a smaller/larger number of patients classified at risk.

Lack of knowledge about prior probability P(AHE), i.e. the prevalence of AHE, does not affect the discrimination performance of the Bayesian classifier since it can be counterbalanced by different choices of P_t. On the contrary, a reliable estimate of prognostic probability P(AHE | x) can be obtained only if all prior probabilities and CPDFs are correctly known.

Statistical assumptions are usually made about whether CPDFs have parametric or non parametric structure. In many cases they are assumed to be of the parametric Gaussian type, because this has been proven to provide good discrimination performance, especially if a subset of predictors can be optimally selected from a large set of clinically available variables (E. Barbini et al., 2007; Fukunaga, 1990).

3.2 K-nearest neighbour algorithms

The k-nearest neighbour algorithm is among the simplest non parametric methods for assigning patients based on closest training examples in the space of features x (Beyer et al., 1999). Euclidean distance is usually used to measure between-point nearness but other metrics must be introduced if non continuous variables are considered.

In our binary classification scheme, the training phase simply consists in partitioning feature space into the two regions or classes, AHE and FHE, based on the positions of training cases. Each new patient is assigned to the region in which the greatest number of its k neighbours occurs, where k is of course a positive integer.

With two classes, it is convenient to choose an odd k to avoid situations of equality. Typically, the choice of neighbourhood size depends on the type and size of the training set;

larger values of k generally reduce the effect of noise on classification at the expense of distinction between classes.
Heuristic techniques are used to obtain the optimal value of k. A common choice is to take k equal to the square root of the total number of training cases, but cross-validation methods, such as bootstrap, are often preferred.
Although k-nearest neighbour is not strictly a probability method, it has been demonstrated that the fraction of k neighbourhood training cases falling in the AHE region is a good estimate of class-conditional risk probability (Beyer et al., 1999).

3.3 Logistic regression

Logistic regression is perhaps the most popular method for estimating risk probabilities in the medical field (Hosmer & Lemeshow, 2000). Logistic regression is a variation of ordinary regression: it belongs to the family of methods called generalized linear models, which include a linear part followed by some associated function. It can be considered a predictive model to use when the dependent response variable is dichotomous and the independent predictor variables are of any type, i.e. continuous, categorical, or both. In d-dimensional feature space, the form of the model is:

$$\log\frac{P(AHE|x)}{1-P(AHE|x)}=c_0+c_1x_1+c_2x_2+...+c_dx_d \quad (2)$$

where "log" is the natural logarithm function, x_k (k = 1, 2, …, d) the observation data set and c_k (k = 0, 1, 2, ..., d) regression coefficients estimated from training data using maximum likelihood criteria.
The inverse of eq. 2 allows the posterior probability of AHE risk, P(AHE | x), to be modelled by a continuous S-shaped curve, even if all predictor variables are categorical. The argument of the logarithm of eq. 2 defines the probability of the outcome event occurring divided by the probability of the event not occurring and is known as the odds ratio. When it is specifically associated with dichotomous predictor variables (risk factors), it is a useful measure of the relative risk due to single risk factors. The reliability of logistic regression results is affected by linear correlations and interaction effects between predictor variables, dependence between error terms, and especially outliers.

3.4 Artificial neural networks

Artificial neural networks (or simply neural networks) are mathematical models miming the physiological learning functions of the human brain. They can be designed and trained to create optimal input-output maps of any physical or statistical phenomenon, the relationships of which may even be complex or unknown. They do not require sophisticated statistical hypotheses and account for all possible interrelations between predictor variables in a natural way. In this sense, neural networks can be considered universal approximators (Bishop, 1995).
A preliminary definition of network architecture is needed and should include number of neurons, number of layers, number and type of connections among neurons, type of neuronal activation functions and so on. Learning is the trickiest phase of neural networks: it consists of estimating network parameters (connection weights and activation thresholds) iteratively from training data, to minimize error between actual and model-estimated outputs. Feed-forward neural networks can be designed to directly estimate class-

conditional posterior probabilities from predictor variables, without requiring sophisticated statistical hypotheses. Their architecture can be variably complex, but should provide one output neuron with a logistic sigmoid activation function, generating an output between 0 and 1. Neural networks have been demonstrated to provide reliable estimates of class-conditional posterior probabilities, such as the AHE risk probability, P(AHE | x), that is (Bishop, 1995):

$$P(AHE \mid x)=\frac{1}{1+\exp(-f)} \qquad (3)$$
$$f=b+w_1u_1+w_2u_2+...+w_nu_n$$

where f is a linear function of n neuron inputs u_k (k = 0, 1, 2, ..., n), originating from the outputs of n preceding connected neurons, the parameters of which are connection weights, w_k, and neuron activation bias, b.

Under-learning can lead to high prediction errors, whereas over-learning can cause overfitting which produces loss of generalisation. Artificial neural network design is therefore anything but simple. Experience is necessary to manipulate heuristic procedures for suitable definition of network architecture and to correctly use iterative numerical training techniques that stop learning when the network begins to overfit.

4. Direct score model

A scoring model is a formula that assigns points based on known information, in order to predict an unknown future outcome. Many integer score systems have been designed for clinical application to critical patients. The most popular were derived from simplification of any of the above probability models by rounding their parameters to integer values. In particular, many approximate the coefficients of logistic regression models to the nearest integer values (Higgins et al., 1997). We do not dwell on the methodology of these score models here, directing readers to the specialised literature (Vincent & Moreno, 2010). Our main interest is to identify score values that give reliable probabilities of individual risk for prognostic purposes. We discuss on the design of a very simple score system that we call a "direct score model". We also provide a correct and useful statistical interpretation of model prognostic capacity, which can easily be extended to any other score model, even more sophisticated ones (Cevenini & P. Barbini, 2010).

4.1 Model design

Only binary predictor variables (risk factors) are used in this score model. The automatic computer procedure and model training is described by the following steps:

- All quantitative predictor variables are dichotomised by ROC curve analysis, identifying cut-off values giving equal sensitivity and specificity in relation to adverse outcomes.
- Risk factors over or under the cut-off value are coded 0 or 1, depending on whether the risk of AHE decreases or increases, respectively.
- The odds ratio of each binary variable is evaluated on the basis of the corresponding confidence interval (CI) (Agresti, 1999): variables with odds ratios not significantly greater than 1 are discarded.

- A forward iterative procedure is applied to a data sample (training set) which sums selected binary variables stepwise.
- All binary factors are reconsidered at each step, so that multiple selection of one factor gives rise to a multiple integer contribution to the score.
- At each step the risk factor providing the highest increment to AUC is included.
- Training is stopped when the cumulative increment in AUC obtained in five consecutive steps is less than 1%. This rather soft stopping criterion is used instead of well-established statistical methods (Zhou et al., 2008) to avoid selecting too few predictors, which reduces the possibility of associating an effective probability of AHE with each integer score.
- A testing dataset of the same size as the training set is used to evaluate model generalisation and to guide conclusive selection of the optimal predictor set.

Backward sessions and cross-validation trials cannot be applied because the model is non-parametric. Optimal model selection is carried out by a step-by-step analysis of model prognostic and diagnostic power. At each step w, the conditional probability of the adverse outcome (prognostic risk probability), $P_w(AHE|S_k)$, associated with each kth integer score value S_k, is estimated from sample data as the ratio of adverse events to the total number of events determining a model score S_k.

The bias-corrected and accelerated bootstrap method is applied to estimate 95% CIs of $P_w(AHE|S_k)$ using 2000 bootstrapped samples. This method makes it possible to infer complex statistics that are difficult or even impossible to represent mathematically and have proven to be theoretically and practically more accurate than other bootstrap methods (Cevenini & P. Barbini, 2010; DiCiccio & Efron, 1996). By graphic inspection of results, the convenience of grouping close scores having large 95% CI because of excessively low data frequencies is considered. The model is chosen to correspond to the iteration providing the largest number of score values or classes having sufficiently narrow and separate 95% CIs with respect to the training data, and at the same time giving testing-data probabilities falling within their 95% CIs.

Once the model is created, the score, S, associated with a generic patient is simply given by:

$$S=\sum_{i=1}^{d} p_i s_i \tag{4}$$

where d is the number of predictors in the model, p_i the binary value of the ith predictor, and s_i, its model-identified associated score. Finally, model discrimination and calibration performance are compared with a logistic regression model designed on the same training data.

All statistical procedures are evaluated at a significance level of 95%.

4.2 Simulation

Many realistic simulation experiments are carried out to validate and optimise model design. Predictor variables are all taken in binary form, skipping the dichotomisation of continuous variables. In particular, we consider d dichotomised binary predictors, obtaining $n = 2^d$ different combinations of these predictors. Each combination identifies one value of a discrete variable $x_j = j/n$ ($j = 0, 1, 2, ..., n-1$) ranging from 0 to 1. In this way two different beta probability density functions can be associated with adverse and favourable outcomes.

Beta distribution is particularly suitable for representing multinomial phenomena, such as that described by the above n discrete values. In detail, we refer to the discrete probability distribution of a multinomial variable x, the probability values of which are calculated using a beta probability density function.

Figure 1 shows an example with two different choices of the beta probability density function shape parameters, α and β, to simulate healthy and sick subjects. When the class-conditional probability density functions of a two-class classification problem are known, the highest achievable discrimination level is related to the areas of overlap. The lowest error probability of classification, ε, is given by:

$$\varepsilon = \int_{-\infty}^{+\infty} \min\{P(C_1)p(x \mid C_1), P(C_2)p(x \mid C_2)\}dx \tag{5}$$

where $P(C_h)$ and $p(x \mid C_h)$ are the prior probability and the class-conditional probability density function for class C_h ($h = 1, 2$), respectively. Prior probability of an adverse outcome, P(AHE), is also known as prevalence, π, and prior probability of favourable outcome, P(FHE), is $1-\pi$. Because of the discrete nature of variable x, in our simulation study, eq. 5 can be approximated as:

$$\begin{aligned} \varepsilon &= \frac{1}{n}\sum_{j=0}^{n-1} \min\left[\pi \times p(x_j \mid AHE), (1-\pi) \times p(x_j \mid FHE)\right] \\ p(x_j \mid AHE) &= B(x_j, \alpha_{AHE}, \beta_{AHE}) \\ p(x_j \mid FHE) &= B(x_j, \alpha_{FHE}, \beta_{FHE}) \end{aligned} \tag{6}$$

where α_{AHE}, β_{AHE}, α_{FHE} and β_{FHE} are the corresponding shape parameters of beta functions, $B_{AHE} = B(x_j, \alpha_{AHE}, \beta_{AHE})$ and $B_{FHE} = B(x_j, \alpha_{FHE}, \beta_{FHE})$, related to adverse and favourable outcomes, respectively.

Eq. 6 shows that ε depends on prevalence and beta parameters. At any iteration w of the above-mentioned stepwise procedure, for any k^{th} integer value of score S_k, the simulated "true" conditional risk probability, $P_w^t(AHE \mid S_k)$, can be calculated using the Bayes theorem, considering AHE prevalence, π, and the class-conditional score probabilities, $P_w^t(S_k \mid AHE)$ and $P_w^t(S_k \mid FHE)$, of adverse and favourable outcomes, respectively:

$$P_w^t(AHE \mid S_k) = \frac{\pi\, P_w^t(S_k \mid AHE)}{\pi\, P_w^t(S_k \mid AHE) + (1-\pi)\, P_w^t(S_k \mid FHE)} \tag{7}$$

By assuming mutually exclusive x_j events, the true class-conditional probabilities are simply obtained from the two simulated beta distributions as the sum of all the discrete probabilities corresponding to the x_j values giving the score S_k, that is:

$$\begin{aligned} P_w^t(S_k \mid AHE) &= \frac{1}{n}\sum_{x_j \in S_k} B(x_j, \alpha_{AHE}, \beta_{AHE}) \\ P_w^t(S_k \mid FHE) &= \frac{1}{n}\sum_{x_j \in S_k} B(x_j, \alpha_{FHE}, \beta_{FHE}) \end{aligned} \tag{8}$$

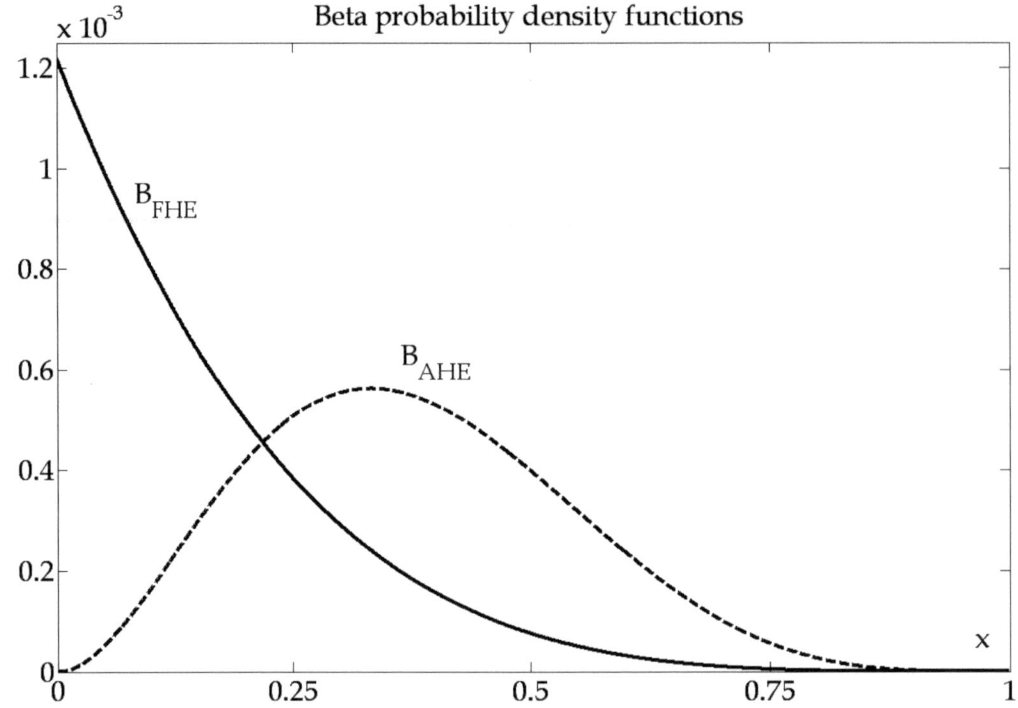

Fig. 1. Simulated probability density functions, B_{FHE} and B_{AHE}, for favourable and adverse outcomes, respectively: example with beta parameters $\alpha_{FHE} = 1$, $\alpha_{AHE} = 3$, $\beta_{AHE} = \beta_{FHE} = 5$

4.2.1 Simulation experiments

Simulation experiments are performed by randomly extracting $N = N_{AHE} + N_{FHE}$ data items from beta distributions of adverse and favourable outcomes, B_{AHE} and B_{FHE}, respectively, to form two samples of size $N_{AHE} = \pi \cdot N$ and $N_{FHE} = (1-\pi) \cdot N$. Each extracted item x_j ($j = 1, 2, ..., N$) is represented as a d-dimensional point in the discrete space of binary variables.

We use $d = 12$ binary variables and simulate nine different conditions corresponding to the combinations of three prevalence values and three levels of separation between event classes, obtained by changing the parameters of beta distributions. Low, medium and high separation between AHEs and FHEs are reproduced by increasing only the values of parameter α_{AHE}, specifically equal to 2, 3 and 5, respectively. The other three beta parameters are kept constant at $\alpha_{FHE} = 1$, $\beta_{AHE} = \beta_{FHE} = 5$. Prevalence values of 5%, 20% and 40% are tried. For each condition, six samples with progressively doubled sizes, namely N = 250, 500, 1000, 2000, 4000 and 8000, are extracted for a total of 54 simulation experiments covering a wide range of actual clinical situations (see also Table 1). Training data is not used because the simulation process enables the true probabilities, described above, to be evaluated exactly.

All computations are performed using MATLAB code.

4.2.2 Simulation results

The method is illustrated in detail by describing the results of a simulation of the 54 experiments performed. The experiment corresponding to N = 1000, π = 20% and $\alpha_{AHE} = 3$ is illustrated, because it is similar to an actual clinical condition that will be shown below.

Figure 2 shows the AUC values obtained using the forward selection of model features from simulated training data described above. The stopping criterion arrested the stepwise algorithm at the eleventh step, after 5 out of 12 predictor variables had been selected. In fact, the cumulative increment in AUC was about 0.8% in the last five steps (nos. 7-11). The variables are numbered in order of decreasing discrimination power. The most discriminating variable, no. 1, was entered five times ($s_1 = 5$) in the model, variable no. 2 three times ($s_2 = 3$) and variables nos. 3-5 only once each ($s_{3\text{-}5} = 1$).

Figure 3 shows the 95% confidence interval of score-associated risk probabilities identified by the bias-corrected and accelerated bootstrap method applied to simulated sample data, from step no. 2 to step no. 9. For each integer score value, the estimated 95% CI is plotted together with the corresponding true probability of AHE (calculated from the beta distribution) and the percentage of cases. The discrimination capacity of the model can be detected at every step by observing the growth of estimated AHE probability with the score, whereas calibration is demonstrated by true risk probabilities (stars), which fall in the corresponding 95% confidence interval of the training data, with the sole exception of certain high scores, where there may be too few cases.

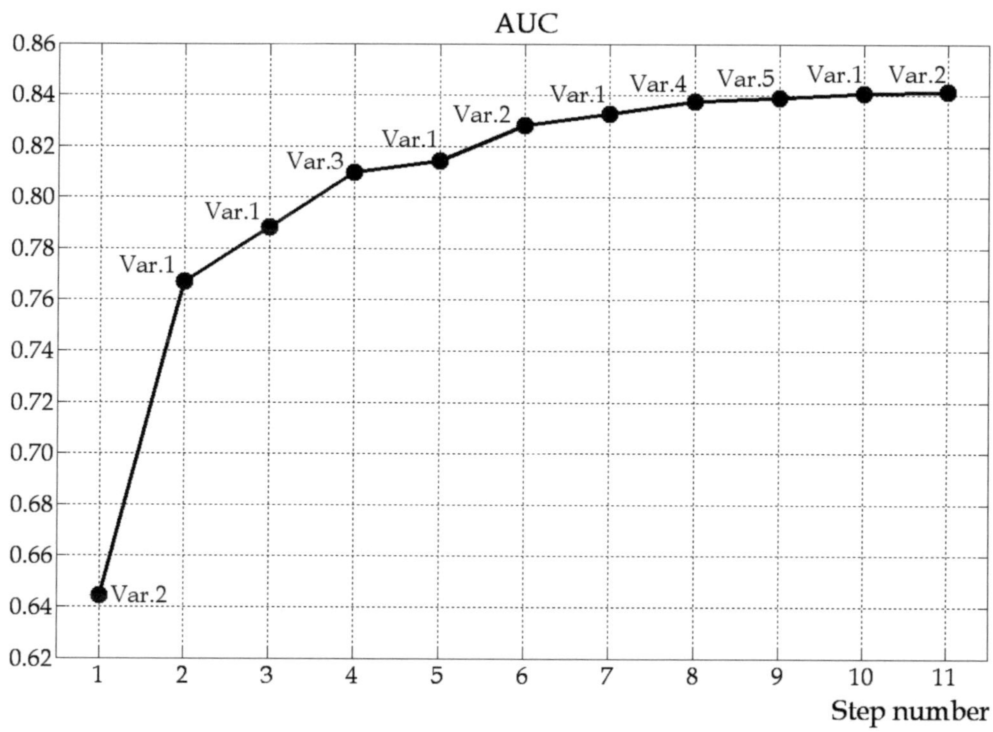

Fig. 2. Area under the ROC curve (AUC) during stepwise selection of model features from simulated data. The predictor variables entered are also indicated

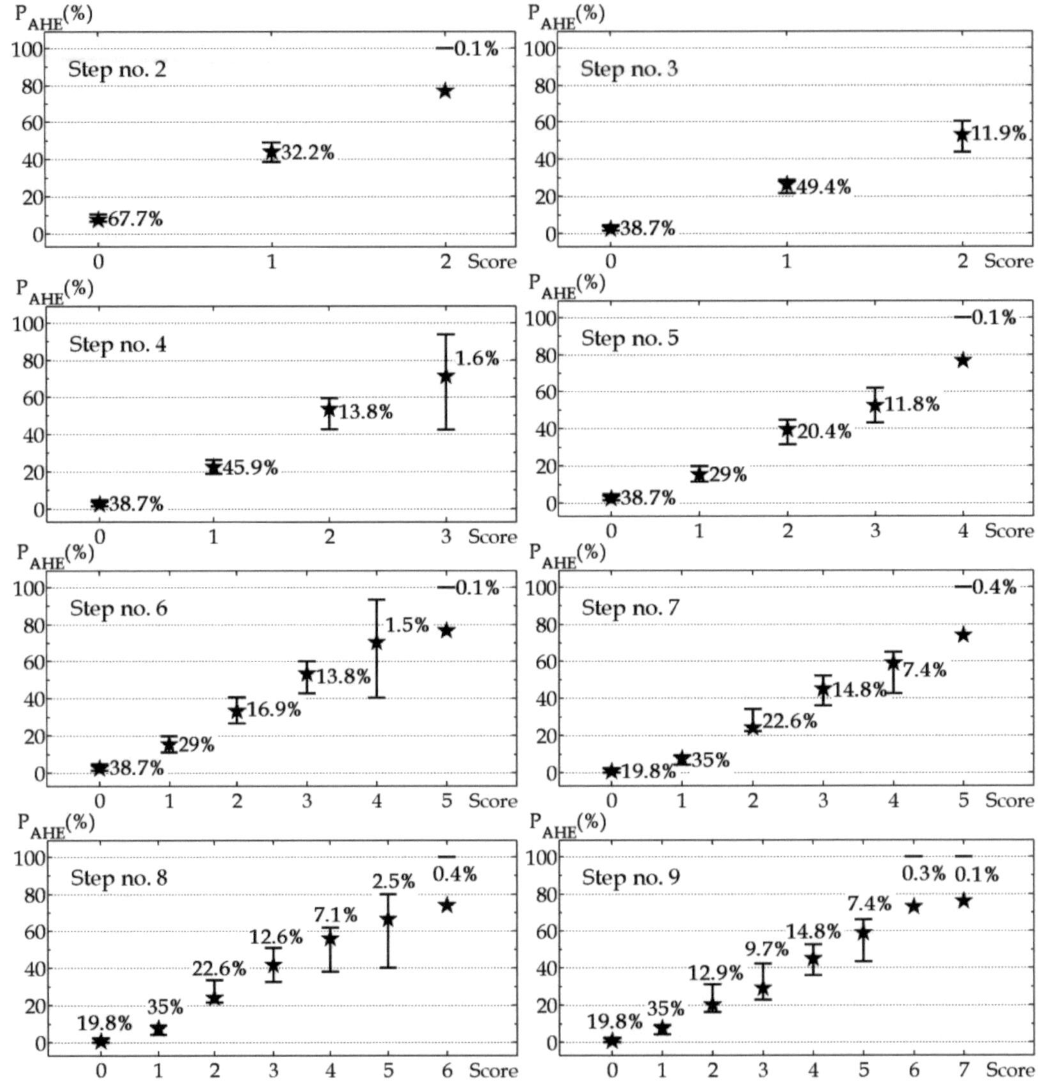

Fig. 3. 95% confidence intervals of AHE score probability, estimated from simulated training data, percentages of score cases and true probabilities (stars)

Now it is necessary to identify a model that reconciles calibration and discrimination. Excessively simple score models (few steps) have low discrimination power (low AUC) and give inopportunely separated 95% CIs. This can be observed at steps nos. 2 and 3 of Fig. 3 where only three score values (0, 1 and 2) are obtained: CIs between scores have very large gaps, suggesting that finer partitioning of the score axis can be achieved with a larger number of steps. Figure 2 indicates poor discrimination capacity of the scoring system at these initial steps.

On the contrary, if too many scores are used, as in steps nos. 7-9, the CIs are either too wide or overlap, worsening calibration accuracy. The width of score CIs increases significantly with decreasing observed frequency. For example, at step no. 4, score of 3 has only 16 cases (1.6%) and the corresponding 95% CI is so large that it completely overlaps with the previous score of 2. When the number of cases is even lower, as in step no. 9, where the highest scores of 6 and 7 have four and one cases, respectively, the bootstrap method fails to correctly estimate the CIs and the corresponding scores are totally unreliable in prognostic terms. Hence the need to combine neighbouring scores with too few cases. It is particularly convenient to pool the highest scores, which often have few cases, into a single class having a sufficient data frequency to significantly narrow the 95% CIs. For example, at step no. 6 it is useful to pool the last two scores of 4 and 5 into a single class. The pooling of adjacent scores with small data frequency enhances model prognostic reliability, usually with an insignificant reduction in discrimination capacity.

From the simulated experiment of Fig. 3, five score classes were identified as a suitable compromise between calibration and discrimination. At any step from no. 6 to no. 9, it is worthwhile combining scores greater than or equal to 4 and leaving the lower scores of 0-3 ungrouped, so as to form five score classes: 0, 1, 2, 3 and ≥ 4.

Figure 4 shows the results of pooling the three highest scores of step no. 8, which is preferred to the previous steps no. 6 and no. 7, because besides having higher discrimination capacity, the pooled class contains a greater number of cases, which narrows the related 95% CI to a greater extent. Just a small gap and a slight overlap can be observed in Fig. 4 between scores of 1 and 2, and between scores of 3 and the class of scores ≥ 4, respectively. Step no. 9 and subsequent steps not reported in Fig. 3 are discarded because no improvement can be obtained with respect to step no. 8 and CI overlap increases. Indeed, to improve the accuracy of estimates of individual probability of AHE, it could be worthwhile increasing the number of classes, tolerating a greater CI overlap. This can be done by analysing and selecting a step beyond the eighth, where the observed frequency in each class is of course significantly reduced, especially for high scores.

Comparison of the results of the three-step model with those of the eight-step pooled model shown in Fig. 4 indicates that the scoring system with five classes effectively fills the gaps between adjacent CIs of the simpler score model. At step no. 8, pooling of the highest scores does not significantly influence the discrimination capacity of the scoring system: the estimated AUC decreases slightly from 0.838 (95% CI, 0.781-0.885) to 0.827 (95% CI, 0.777-0.869).

Stepwise logistic regression applied to the training data used for the simulation example, set at statistical significance levels of 95% and 90% to enter and remove variables, respectively, selected the first five binary variables. Figure 5 compares ROC curves of the logistic model and the score model of Fig. 4. The ROC curve of true probability values, calculated from training data using beta distributions and the Bayes theorem, is also plotted (dashed line). AUCs of true data and the logistic model were 0.845 and 0.849, respectively.

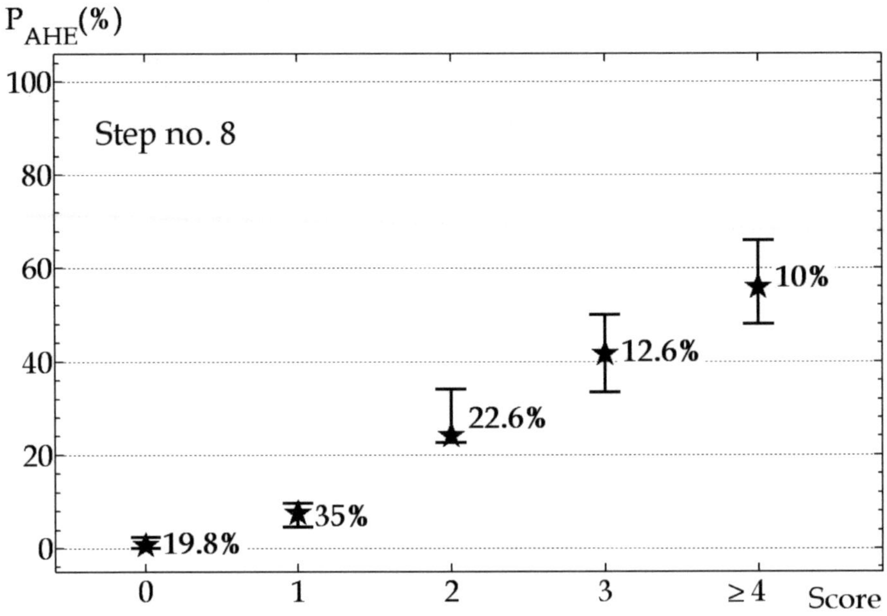

Fig. 4. 95% confidence intervals of AHE score probabilities estimated from simulated training data, percentages of score cases and true probabilities (stars) for the model identified at step no. 8

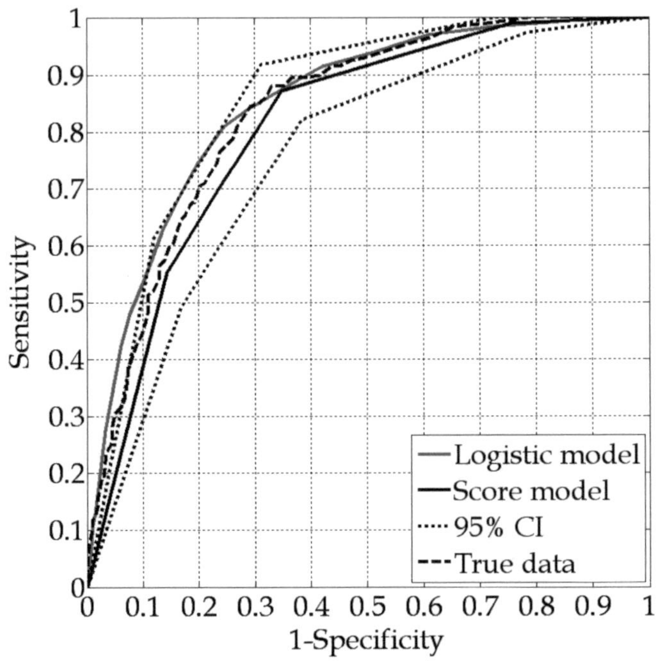

Fig. 5. ROC curves from simulated sample data. 95% CI refers to score model

When comparing model discrimination power by AUC, we have to consider that the ROC curve of the score model (continuous line) is drawn by connecting only 5 discrete points (score classes), whereas the logistic model curve (gray line) is based on more probability values. Figure 5 shows that the score model is close enough to the logistic and true ROC curves. Clearly, discretisation leads to a lower AUC, resulting in underestimation of score-model discrimination capacity. In addition, the true and logistic curves are to a large extent within the 95% CI of the score curve. Finally, in real clinical applications, logistic regression often includes continuous variables that may improve discrimination performance.

The HL goodness-of-fit test (Hosmer & Lemeshow, 2000) showed good calibration performance of the logistic model ($p = 0.751$). However, 95% of the training-data errors between model-estimated and true percentage risk probabilities were from about -10.5% (underestimation) and +12.0% (overestimation), revealing similar uncertainty to that of the score model.

Table 1 gives the number of score values or classes identified by the same procedure, for each of the 54 simulation experiments. It shows that the number of score classes increases with increasing sample size, prevalence and separation between event classes (decreasing error ε). The importance of estimating uncertainty suggests to keep 95% CIs of between-class probabilities separate, or slightly overlapping. This limits the identifiable number of score classes and provides reliable probability estimates. Enlargement and overlapping of 95% CIs and consequent loss of prognostic probability information depends heavily on the data frequency of score values or classes and their rate of AHEs influenced by prevalence. Small samples and/or low prevalence make it necessary to pool neighbouring scores to form classes with a sufficient number of cases to ensure a reliable estimate (narrow CI) of class probabilities.

	Low separation $\alpha_{AHE} = 2$			Medium separation $\alpha_{AHE} = 3$			High separation $\alpha_{AHE} = 5$		
Π%	5	20	40	5	20	40	5	20	40
ε% / N	5.0	20.0	32.9	5.0	17.7	23.9	4.6	11.4	13.7
250	2	3	3	3	4	4	3	4	4
500	3	4	4	4	5	5	4	5	5
1000	4	4	4	4	5	5	4	5	6
2000	4	5	5	5	5	6	5	6	6
4000	5	5	5	5	6	6	5	6	6
8000	5	6	6	6	6	7	6	7	7

Table 1. Simulation experiments: largest number of score classes having sufficiently narrow and separate 95% confidence intervals of prognostic probability. αAHE = shape parameter of AHE beta distribution; Π = prevalence; ε = lowest error probability of classification; N = sample size

Simulation experiments suggests grouping scores into classes when frequencies are less than about 3% and 10% of the whole sample for N = 8000 and N = 250, respectively. Only two classes are recognised in the worst condition of minimum sample size (N = 250), minimum prevalence (Π = 5%) and low separation between health events (α_{AHE} = 2). A maximum of seven score-classes is identified in conditions of large sample size (N = 8000), high prevalence and high separation between event classes. Although more score classes could be achieved with greater CI overlap, the cost would be unreliable estimates.
The discrimination of the different simulation experiments is assessed by AUC of true simulated probability calculated using beta functions. Conditions of large overlap between areas of beta functions (α_{AHE} = 2) lead to values of true AUC ranging from 0.72 to 0.75; medium overlap (α_{AHE} = 3) gives AUC values in the range 0.82-0.85 and the conditions of greatest separation (α_{AHE} = 5) produce AUCs between 0.92 and 0.95.

4.3 Clinical example

The approach was applied to actual clinical data of critical patients in the intensive care unit to evaluate their risk of morbidity after heart surgery.
We used a sample of 1040 adult patients younger than 80 years, who underwent coronary artery bypass grafting and were admitted to the intensive care unit of the Department of Surgery and Bioengineering of Siena University. 212 patients developed at least one serious postoperative complication (cardiovascular, respiratory, neurological, renal, infectious or hemorrhagic), corresponding to a morbidity of 20.4% (Cevenini & P. Barbini, 2010, as cited in Cevenini et al., 2007). The data was split randomly into a training and a testing set of the same size (520 cases), with the same number of patients with morbid conditions in each set (106 cases) to avoid misleading bias in the results.
Table 2 describes the 15 clinical variables used for score model design, six of which were binary in origin. The other nine continuous variables were dichotomised using cut-off values associated with the point of equal sensitivity and specificity on the respective ROC curves. Three of the resulting 15 binary variables were discarded because their odds ratios of morbidity were not significantly greater than 1. This left a total of 12 variables for training the score model, as in the simulation experiments.
This real clinical situation was similar to the simulation experiment with N = 500 and Π = 20% (see Table 1). Consulting Table 1, we expected to develop a score model with 4 or 5 classes, depending on the level of data separation between normal and morbid patients.
Figure 6 shows the stepwise procedure used to select the model variables. After step no. 8, AUC values of testing data (dashed line with stars) decreased and diverged from training data AUCs (continuous line with dots). This indicated overfitting that was possible because the criterion used to stop the training procedure was deliberately soft, to allow inclusion of more steps than needed for generalisation. In fact, as previously illustrated in the simulation results, investigation of extra steps can be useful to optimise model prognostic power through score pooling. Steps nos. 6, 7 and 8 gave similar prognostic performance, so we chose step no. 8, thus obtaining higher discrimination (greater AUC). A convenient class was formed by pooling scores greater than 3, as shown in Fig. 7. All 95% CIs of adjacent scores or classes were well-separated and all testing score probabilities (stars) fell within their corresponding CIs, thereby ensuring high prognostic reliability of the model. The pooling of the highest scores of the eight-step model led to a

slight but not statistically significant reduction in discrimination performance: the estimated training and testing AUCs decreased from 0.851 (95% CI, 0.781-0.909) to 0.835 (95% CI, 0.764-0.895) and from 0.841 (95% CI, 0.775-0.900) to 0.816 (95% CI, 0.743-0.879), respectively.

Variable description	Acronym	Type	Cut-off	Steps
Inotropic heart drugs	IHD	Binary		1,4,10 (LR)
O_2 delivery index	DO_2I	Continuous	< 280 ml/min/m^2	2 (LR)
Peripheral vascular disease	PVD	Binary		3,9 (LR)
O_2 extraction ratio	O_2ER	Continuous	≥ 38%	5 (LR)
Emergency	EM	Binary		6
CO_2 production	VCO_2	Continuous	< 180 ml/min	7
Pulmonary artery hypertension	PAH	Binary		8 (LR)
Cardio-pulmonary bypass time	CPB	Continuous	≥ 2 hours	11 (LR)
Intra aortic balloon pump	IABP	Binary		12 (LR)
Creatinine	Cr	Continuous	≥ 1 mg/l	NE (LR)
Potassium	K	Continuous	≥ 4.1 mEq/l	NE (LR)
Haemoglobin	Hb	Continuous	< 9.6 g/dl	NE
Cardiac index	CI	Continuous	< 2.4 l/min/m^2	NS (LR)
Mean arterial pressure	MAP	Continuous	> 95 mmHg	NS
Previous heart surgery	Re-do	Binary		NS

Table 2. Clinical variables, cut-off values for the dichotomisation of continuous variables and score-model entry steps. NE = not entered; NS = not statistically significant; LR = variable selected by stepwise logistic regression

Two logistic regression models were designed to compare the score model results on the same training data with the 15 clinical variables of Table 2. The first model, named LogCV, used the original continuous variables and the second (LogBV) dichotomised them (see Table 2). The stepwise regression procedure selected ten clinical variables (see Table 2) and provided training-data AUC values of 0.906 (HL test, p = 0.135) and 0.871 (HL test, p = 0.557) for LogCV and LogBV, respectively. Figure 8 compares the ROC curves. The LogCV ROC curve (continuous gray line) showed the greatest discrimination performance, mainly because the model selected many continuous variables (6 out of 10). Except for the highest specificity values, where the discretisation effect of scoring was more evident, the score model ROC curve (continuous black line) did not differ significantly from that of LogBV (dashed gray line), which was inside the respective 95% CI and close enough to the score-model points. Model scores computed using the testing data gave a ROC curve (dashed black line) not significantly different from the training data curve. Finally, it should be noted that the discrimination performance of logistic models decreased considerably when applied to testing data (ROC curves not reported in Fig. 8): AUCs of logCV and logBV were reduced to 0.879 and 0.826, respectively, thus suggesting a possible overfitting.

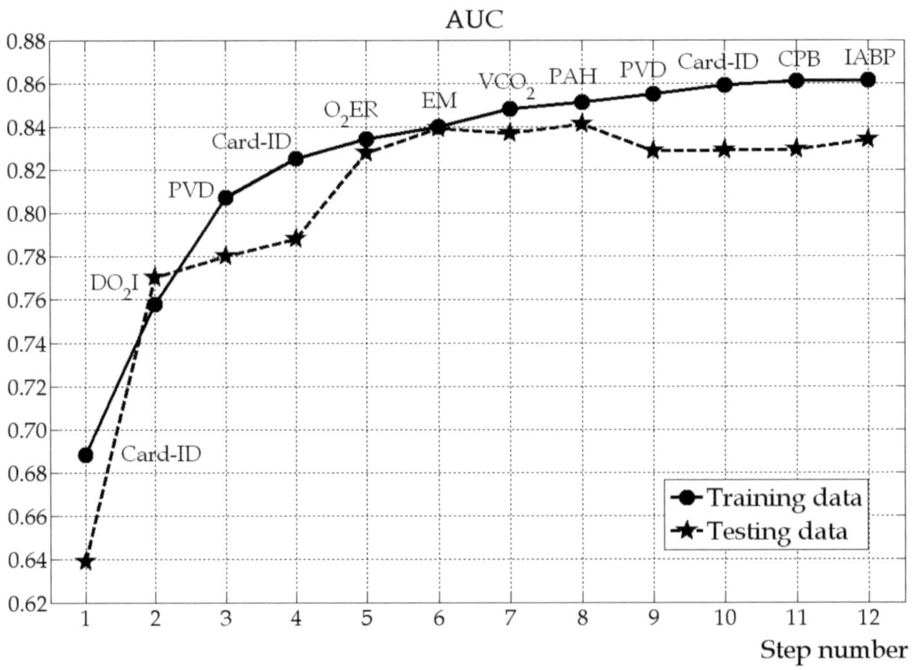

Fig. 6. Area under the ROC curve (AUC) during the stepwise selection of model features from clinical data. The predictor variables entered are also indicated

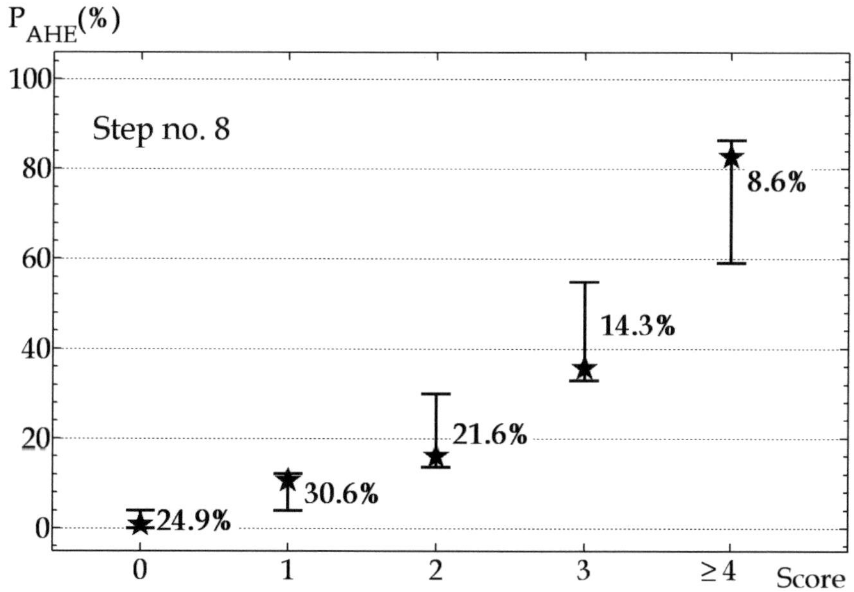

Fig. 7. Estimated 95% confidence intervals of AHE score probabilities from clinical training data, percentages of score cases and testing-data probabilities (stars) for the eight-step model chosen

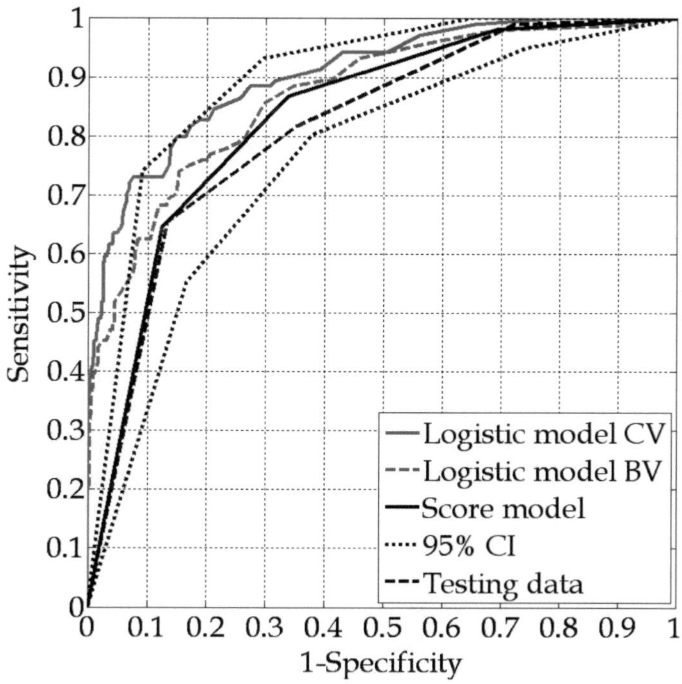

Fig. 8. ROC curves from clinical data. 95% CI refers to the score model. CV = also with continuous variables; BV = with binary variables only

5. Discussion

Many quantitative methods for assessing the health risk of critical patients have been developed in past and recent literature (E. Barbini et al., 2007; den Boer et al., 2005; Vincent & Moreno, 2010). They aim to provide objective and accurate information about patient diagnosis and prognosis. Experience has shown that simplicity of use and effectiveness of implementation are the most important requirements for their success in routine clinical practice. Scoring systems respond well to these requirements because their outcomes are accessible in real time without the use of advanced computational tools, thus allowing decisions to be made quickly and effectively. Many clinical applications can profit from their simplicity. For example, they are often used to suggest alternative treatments and organize intensive care resources, where surveillance of vital functions is the primary goal.

Other important benefits of score models are their easy updating and customisation to local institutions. In fact, because the standardisation of local practices is difficult and patient populations may differ, it is now accepted that predictive models must be locally validated, tuned and periodically updated to provide correct risk-adjusted outcomes. All models suffer from the limitation of foreseeing better future treatments and improving prognosis (den Boer et al., 2005). Even very accurate predictive models, when exported to clinical contexts different from those in which they were designed, have often proved unreliable (Murphy-Filkins et al., 1996). Appropriate design and local customisation of excessively sophisticated models is often easier said than done, especially in health centres where there is little technical expertise in developing models that can generalise, i.e. preserve their predictive performance on future data. On the contrary, simple score models can easily and frequently be updated to learn from new correctly-classified cases and are quite tolerant to missing data. This is very useful in clinical practice where data is usually scarce and training on as much available data as possible is of fundamental importance (Cevenini & P. Barbini, 2010, as cited in P. Barbini et al., 2007).

A major problem with score models is that they are difficult to calibrate, i.e. associate reliable estimates of prognostic risk probability with each score. Nevertheless, correct estimation of individual probability of adverse outcome for hospitalized critical patients is useful for prevention, treatment and quantification of health problems and costs. It can help experienced physicians to improve clinical management by optimizing the monitoring of patient status and enhancing the quality of care, and allow new generations of doctors to be better trained during postgraduate specialization and internship. Moreover, reliable knowledge of risk factors and their impact on clinical course and future quality of life can encourage public health policy for risk reduction (Hodgman, 2008).

The proposed method offers a simple risk-assessment system that associates a reliable estimate of the individual probability of developing an adverse event with predicted scores. The model is a very simple score of risk factors chosen, one or more times, by a stepwise procedure based on maximising discrimination through ROC analysis. No hypotheses or statistical models are involved. Since conventional methods for evaluating calibration, such as the Hosmer-Lemeshow test (Hosmer & Lemeshow, 2000), are unreliable for scoring systems, we analysed the 95% confidence interval of sample-estimated risk probabilities associated with each score step by step. The experimental score probability is easily evaluated by calculating the sampling rate of adverse outcomes having that score.

Unfortunately, the statistics of the sampling error are not simple to derive. We therefore preferred to use bootstrap resampling, a method commonly used in statistical inference to estimate confidence intervals (Carpenter & Bithell, 2000; DiCiccio & Efron, 1996). The bootstrap method is simpler and more general than conventional approaches; it requires no great expertise in mathematics or probability theory and is based on assumptions that are less restrictive and easier to control. The method can be used to evaluate statistics that are difficult or impossible to determine by conventional methods. We used an elaboration of the simplest bootstrap method of percentile intervals, known as bias-corrected and accelerated intervals, which avoids estimate bias and offers substantial advantages over other bootstrap methods, both in theory and practice (Chernick, 2007). Our simulation experiments confirmed the method's accuracy in estimating 95% CI of prognostic probabilities: when true probabilities were related to score values, or classes, with a sufficient number of sampled training data, they always fell within bootstrap-estimated 95% CIs (see Fig. 3). Bootstrap techniques are not too complex in a clinical environment, since nowadays many available packages for data processing include them for calculating confidence intervals. In any case, they are used exclusively during model design.

As shown in Fig. 3, step by step graphical inspection of probability CIs made it possible to choose the best model to compromise between calibration and discrimination, also suggesting convenient pooling of adjacent scores that gave large and overlapping CIs due to an insufficient number of cases or adverse events. The controlled simulation experiments showed that good calibration was achieved with a limited number of score classes, up to a maximum of seven in experiments with the biggest sample size, and high prevalence and separation between event classes (see Table 1). More classes could be identified if greater overlap of close scores were allowed, but when the number of classes became excessive, there were problems of overfitting. We also saw that a logistic model designed on the same training data provided nearly continuous probability estimates, the uncertainty of which was similar to that achieved by the score model. Significant improvement of discrimination performance could only be appreciated when continuous variables were also included in the logistic model, as in the clinical example described. This analysis can enable medical staff to select the best scoring system for any specific clinical context.

6. Conclusion

In critical care medicine, scoring systems are often designed exclusively on the basis of discrimination and generalisation characteristics (diagnostic capacity), at the expense of reliable individual probabilities (prognostic capacity). Our proposed approach that weighs both these capacities is validated by suitable simulation experiments, which also allow design conditions and application limits of scoring systems to be investigated for correct prediction of critical patient risk in a real clinical context.

The bias-corrected and accelerated bootstrap method for evaluating the 95% confidence interval, CI, of individual prognostic probabilities provides reliable estimates of true simulated probabilities. CIs are calculated for each score and at each step of scoring-system design. By increasing the number of steps, model discrimination power (greater AUC) and prognostic information (greater number of different score values) increases but widening and overlap of 95% CIs soon occurs, so that it becomes convenient to pool adjacent scores into score classes. The maximum number of different score classes giving distinct prognostic

information, that is having narrow and less overlapping 95% CIs, increases with increasing sample size and prevalence of adverse outcome and decreasing error probability of classification. It is strongly limited by reduced frequency of score cases and the respective rate of adverse events: in our simulated experiments, which covered a wide range of real conditions, it varied from 2 to 7.
Application of the method to a real clinical situation demonstrated that the technique can be a simple practical tool, providing useful additional prognostic information to associate with classes of scores, and enabling doctors to choose the best risk score model to use in their specific clinical context.

7. Acknowledgment

This work was partly financed by the University of Siena, Italy.

8. References

Agresti, A. (1999). On Logit Confidence Intervals for the Odds Ratio with Small Samples. *Biometrics,* Vol.55, pp. 597-602, ISSN 0006-341X

Barbini, E.; Cevenini, G.; Scolletta, S.; Biagioli, B.; Giomarelli, P. & Barbini, P. (2007). A Comparative Analysis of Predictive Models of Morbidity in Intensive Care Unit after Cardiac Surgery - Part I: Model Planning. *BMC Medical Informatics and Decision Making,* Vol.7, No.35, (22 November 2007), pp. 1-16, ISSN 1472-6947, Available from http://www.biomedcentral.com/1472-6947/7/35

Beyer, K.; Goldstein, J.; Ramakrishnan, R. & Shaft, U. (1999). When is Nearest Neighbor Meaningful?, *Proceedings of the 7th International Conference on Database Theory,* pp. 217-235, ISBN 3-540-65452-6, Jerusalem, Israel, January 10-12, 1999

Bishop, C.M. (1995). *Neural Networks for Pattern Recognition,* Oxford University Press, ISBN 0-19-853864-2, Oxford, UK

Carpenter, J. & Bithell, J. (2000). Bootstrap Confidence Intervals: When, Which, What? A Practical Guide for Medical Statisticians. *Statistics in Medicine,* Vol.19, No.9, pp. 1141-1164, ISSN 0277-6715

Chernick, M.R. (2007). *Bootstrap Methods: A Guide for Practitioners and Researchers*, Wiley, ISBN 978-0-471-75621-7, New York, USA

Cevenini, G. & Barbini, P. (2010). A Bootstrap Approach for Assessing the Uncertainty of Outcome Probabilities when Using a Scoring System. *BMC Medical Informatics and Decision Making,* Vol.10, No.45, (26 August 2010), pp. 1-9, ISSN 1472-6947, Available from http://www.biomedcentral.com/1472-6947/10/45

Cook, N.R. (2008). Statistical Evaluation of Prognostic versus Diagnostic Models: Beyond the ROC Curve. *Clinical Chemistry,* Vol.54, pp. 17-23, ISSN 1339-1348, Available from http://www.clinchem.org/cgi/content/full/54/1/17

den Boer, S.; de Keizer, N.F. & de Jonge, E. (2005). Performance of Prognostic Models in Critically Ill Cancer Patients - A Review. *Critical Care,* Vol.9, pp. R458-R463, (8 July 2005), ISSN 1364-8535, Available from http://ccforum.com/content/9/4/R458

Diamond, G.A. (1992). What Price Perfection? Calibration and Discrimination of Clinical Prediction Models. *Journal of Clinical Epidemiology,* Vol.45, No.1, pp. 85-89, ISSN 0895-4356

DiCiccio, T.J. & Efron, B. (1996). Bootstrap Confidence Intervals. *Statistical Science,* Vol.11, pp. 189-228, ISSN 0883-4237

Dreiseitl, S. & Ohno-Machado, L. (2002). Logistic Regression and Artificial Neural Network Classification Models: A Methodology Review. *Journal of Biomedical Informatics,* Vol.35, no.5-6, pp. 352-359, ISSN 1532-0464

Finazzi, S.; Poole, D.; Luciani, D.; Cogo, P.E. & Bertolini, G. (2011). Calibration Belt for Quality-of-Care Assessment Based on Dichotomous Outcomes. *PLoS One,* Vol.6, No.2, (23 February 2011), e16110, ISSN 1932-6203, Available from http://www.plosone.org/article/info%3Adoi%2F10.1371%2Fjournal.pone.0016110

Fukunaga, K. (1990). *Introduction to Statistical Pattern Recognition,* Academic Press, ISBN 978-0-12-269851-4, Boston, USA

Guyon, I. & Elisseeff, A. (2003). An Introduction to Variable and Feature Selection. *Journal of Machine Learning Research,* Vol.3, No.7-8, pp. 1157-1182, ISSN 1532-4435

Harrell, F.E. Jr; Lee, K.L. & Mark, D.B. (1996), Multivariable Prognostic Models: Issues in Developing Models, Evaluating Assumptions and Adequacy, and Measuring and Reducing Errors. *Statistics in Medicine,* Vol.15, No.4, pp. 361-387, ISSN 0277-6715

Higgins, T.L.; Estafanous, F.G.; Loop, F.D.; Beck, G.J.; Lee, J.C.; Starr, N.J.; Knaus, W.A. & Cosgrove III, D.M. (1997). ICU Admission Score for Predicting Morbidity and Mortality Risk after Coronary Artery Bypass Grafting. *The Annals of Thoracic Surgery,* Vol.64, No.4, pp. 1050-1058, ISSN 0003-4975

Hodgman, S.B. (2008). Predictive Modeling & Outcomes. *Professional Case Management,* Vol.13, pp. 19-23, ISSN 1932-8087

Hosmer, D.W. & Lemeshow, S. (2000). *Applied Logistic Regression,* Wiley, ISBN 0-4716-1553-6, New York, USA

Lasko, T.A.; Bhagwat, J.G.; Zou, K.H. & Ohno-Machado, L. (2005). The Use of Receiver Operating Characteristic Curves in Biomedical Informatics. *Journal of Biomedical Informatics,* Vol.38, No.5, pp. 404-415, ISSN 1532-0464

Lee, P.M. (2004). *Bayesian Statistics - An Introduction,* Arnold, ISBN 0-340-81405-5, London, UK

Marshall, G.; Shroyer, A.L.W.; Grover, F.L. & Hammermeister K.E. (1994). Bayesian-Logit Model for Risk Assessment in Coronary Artery Bypass Grafting. *The Annals of Thoracic Surgery,* Vol.57, No.6, pp. 1492-1500, ISSN 0003-4975

Murphy, A.H. (1973). A New Vector Partition of the Probability Score. *Journal of Applied Meteorology,* Vol.12, No.4, pp. 595-600, ISSN 0021-8952, Available from http://journals. ametsoc.org/toc/jam/12/4

Murphy-Filkins, R.; Teres, D.; Lemeshow, S. & Hosmer, D.W. (1996). Effect of Changing Patient Mix on the Performance of an Intensive Care Unit Severity-of-Illness Model: How to Distinguish a General from a Specialty Intensive Care Unit. *Critical Care Medicine,* Vol.24, No.12, pp. 1968-1973, ISSN 0090-3493

Vapnik, V.N. (1999). *The Nature of Statistical Learning Theory,* Springer-Verlag, ISBN 0-387-98780-0, New York, USA

Vincent, J.L. & Moreno, R. (2010). Clinical Review: Scoring Systems in the Critically Ill. *Critical Care,* Vol.14, No.2 (207), pp. 1-9, ISSN 1364-8535

Zhou, X.H.; Li, S.M. & Gatsonis, C.A. (2008). Wilcoxon-Based Group Sequential Designs for Comparison of Areas Under Two Correlated ROC Curves. *Statistics in Medicine,* Vol.27, No.2, pp. 213-223, ISSN 0277-6715

20

Human Walking Analysis, Evaluation and Classification Based on Motion Capture System

Bofeng Zhang[1], Susu Jiang[1], Ke Yan[1] and Daming Wei[1,2]
[1]*School of Computer Engineering and Science, Shanghai University*
[2]*Professor Emeritus, The University of Aizu, Fukushima,*
[1]*P. R. of China*
[2]*Japan*

1. Introduction

Gait analysis is the systematic study of human walking. It is helpful in the medical management of those diseases which affect the locomotion systems. Recently, the gait motion capture systems are becoming widely used by doctors and physical therapists for kinematics analysis and biomechanics and motion capture research, sports medicine and physical therapy, including human gait analysis and injury rehabilitation. This chapter describes some new progress on human walking analysis that our group made in the past few years based on motion capture system.

Generally, ageing causes many changes to neuromuscular system of a human being, for an example, his walking capabilities degenerate by ageing. Because these changes sometimes result in an increase the number of falls during daily walking, especially after the age of 75, it is very important to study the age related changes in the walking gait of elderly subjects. Many researchers studied stability of human walking gait and it was quoted that human walking gait stability decreases with age increasing the risk of falls in elderly people.

Many studies have been reported about the change in the kinematics parameters with age (Arif et al., 2004). This paper only focuses on the progress of walking modeling and walking stability. Especially, in order to simplify the method of data acquisition, this paper suggests process of reduction on dynamic stability features through feature selection. That will help us analyze stability in a more clear way.

1.1 Background of walking model

Various methods are used to overcome the difficulties imposed by the extraction of human gait features. Two approaches are being used for human gait analysis: model-based and non-model-based methods.

The non-model-based method is applied in image-based gait analysis (marker-less analysis). Feature correspondence between successive frames is based upon prediction, velocity, shape, texture and colour. Small motion between consecutive frames is the main assumption, whereby feature correspondence is conducted using various geometric constraints.

For the first one, a priori shape model is established to match real data to this predefined model, and thereby extracting the corresponding features once the best match is obtained. Stick models and volumetric models are the most commonly used methods. The model-

based approach is the most popular method being used for human motion analysis due to its advantages. It can extract detailed and accurate motion data.
Nash (Nash et al., 1998) proposed a parametric gait model consisting of a pair of articulated lines, jointed at the hip to extract moving articulated objects from a temporal sequence of images. Pendulum model was used to extract and describes human gait for recognition automatically (Cunado et al., 2003). The human leg was modelled as two pendulums joined in series. Zhang (Zhang et al., 2004) proposed a model-based approach to gait recognition by employing a 5-link biped locomotion human model. Akita (Akita, 1984) proposed a model consisting of six segments comprising of two arms, two legs, the torso and the head. Lee (Lee, 2003) suggested a 7-ellipse model, to describe a representation of gait appearance for the purpose of person identification and classification. A 2D stick figure model, which composed of 7 segments, was used to represent the human body, and joint angles and angular velocities are calculated to describe the gait motion (Yoo et la., 2002). Guo (Guo et al., 1994) represented the human body structure in the silhouette by a stick figure model which had 10 sticks articulated with six joints. Cheng (Cheng & Moura, 1998) represented the human body as a stick figure which was considered to be composed of 12 rigid parts. Dockstader (Dockstader et al, 2002) suggested the use of a hierarchical, structural model of the human body which had 15 points. Rohr (Rohr, 1994) proposed a volumetric model for the analysis of human motion, using 14 elliptical cylinders to model the human body. Karaulova (Karaulova et al., 2000) have used the stick figure model to build a novel hierarchical model of human dynamics represented using hidden Markov models.

1.2 Background of walking stability

Theoretically, human walking has rigid periodicity so the next step should repeat the first step strictly. That is to say, all steps must be consistent completely and have no any deference at all. In fact, there is no normal walking pattern and the walking pattern varies from person to person. These walking patterns are considered to be stable until and unless there is an evidence of fall of the person. During walking, human tries to generate periodic series of motions. But due to the physiological limitations, these motions do not re-main exactly periodic but contains some variability or randomness in it. He/she does not try to correct this variability or randomness of these motions if it remains within stability limits. This variability present in the walking patterns is due to not only internal perturbation but also due to external perturbations. The amount of variability present in the walking pattern reflects the quality of neuromuscular control of the human being.
There are many researches which are related to human walking stability. Corriveau et al compare the postural stability of elderly stroke patients with those of healthy elderly people using the distance between the centre of pressure (COP) and the centre of mass (COM) in terms of root mean square. Statistical significance of the COP-COM variable was larger in the stroke group than in healthy subjects, in both the anteroposterior (AP) and mediolateral (ML) directions (Corriveau et al., 2004).
Effect of age on the variability or irregularity of the acceleration of COM in ML, vertical and AP directions is analyzed by Arif et al, using approximate entropy technique for young and elderly subjects of subjects (Arif et al., 2004).
Literature (Hylton et al., 2003) tried to evaluate acceleration patterns at the head and pelvis in young and older subjects when walking on a level and an irregular walking surface. The subjects are two groups, 30 young people aged 22–39 years (mean 29.0, SD 4.3), and 30 older people with a low risk of falling aged 75–85 years (mean 79.0, SD 3.0).

The maximum Floquet multipliers (FM) are used to measure orbital stability of upper body in difference walking speed (Marin et al., 2006). Orbital stability changed very little with speed. The general purpose of (Kavanagh, 2006) is to examine factors that may influence acceleration features of the upper body during walking.

Balance in quiet upright stance, which was studied by (Stirling & Zakynthinaki, 2004), does not imply motionless stability, in fact a ML and AP body sway occurs. Almost 95% of the anterior-posterior sway happens around the ankle and the hip axis.

Sutherland et al investigated the development of mature walking in children of age from one to seven years old (Sutherland et al., 1980). The objective of literature (PH. Chou, 2003) was to investigate the gait maturation of Taiwan children. Elderly subjects exhibits gait pattern characterized by reduced velocity, shorter step length and increased step timing variability (Hylton et al., 2003). It is mentioned that elderly people reduce their walking speed to improve their walking stability in the literature.

While many walking stability indices have been proposed, there is still no commonly accepted way to define, much less quantify, locomotors stability.

1.3 Background of walking symmetry

The concept of gait symmetry itself is no acceptable unified definition, more often many people's research assumes that the normal gait is symmetric, which is to simplify data collection and analysis of gait. In fact gait symmetry was only evaluated with a small number of biomechanical studies that used quantitative data of the two lower limbs. In addition, the gait symmetry was not actually carried out enough exploration. It is because there is no participation of a considerable more number of test objects. One hand, the gait parameter of information provided is the effects of the movement not the reasons of the movement. This may also affect explaining the behaviour of the lower limbs. The other hand, the gait symmetry is not clearly defined, and the use only single gait parameters or a simple statistical method to compare which has made study of gait symmetry been more limited.

Maybe it stands to reason that a healthy man or woman has left leg and right leg symmetrically, and normal gait seems symmetric with ones right-side and left-side. What about the walking stability or dynamic balance if there is not so symmetric? Can we get some quantity or relationship of symmetry and balance?

Gait symmetry is multifaceted. Normal walking seems right-left symmetry because normal people walk with their right foot and left foot. The ability of maintaining balance is essential to keep normal walking. Poor balance is an independent risk factor for falling, so anything that improves balance can have a positive effect on safety and function after stroke. Balance is described as the ability to maintain or move within a weight-bearing posture without falling. We have not found any trends study relating to walking stability and symmetry of human gait. And the trends indicated what meanings.

Yang in his doctoral thesis paper (Yang, 2001) proposed the symmetry indicators of step length and stride length, to describe the step in the role of gait symmetry. But phase symmetry and the step length symmetry are not fully reflects the characteristics of gait, especially the joint angle in the role of symmetry.

2. Modeling assumptions and theoretical framework

Walking is a complex dynamic activity. A good human model for gait analysis should be simple, but extensive enough to capture the dynamics of most walkers.

Almost existing models, which have from 2 segments to more than 15 segments, have two pitfalls. Firstly, they paid more attention to the sagittal plane, and overlook the other two planes, transverse plane and frontal plane. Secondly, it is not enough to describe the particularity of the feet. Most of them regarded the foot as a point. Thus, it is difficult to decide the gait cycle, such as initial heel contact, heel rise, and toe off. So a new walking model, so called Fourteen-Linkage (FL) model, is proposed.

2.1 Fourteen-linkage model

DEFINITION 1. (Fourteen-Linkage Model) We suggest a walking model, which is a collection of 19 points, 14 segments and 12 joints, used to specify the position and the configuration of a human body, as shown in Fig. 1.

Position describes the location of a body segment or joint in space, measured in meters. In FL model, the 19 points can be decided by the 30 markers we measured from motion capture system. The relationships between the model and markers are also shown in Fig. 1(a).

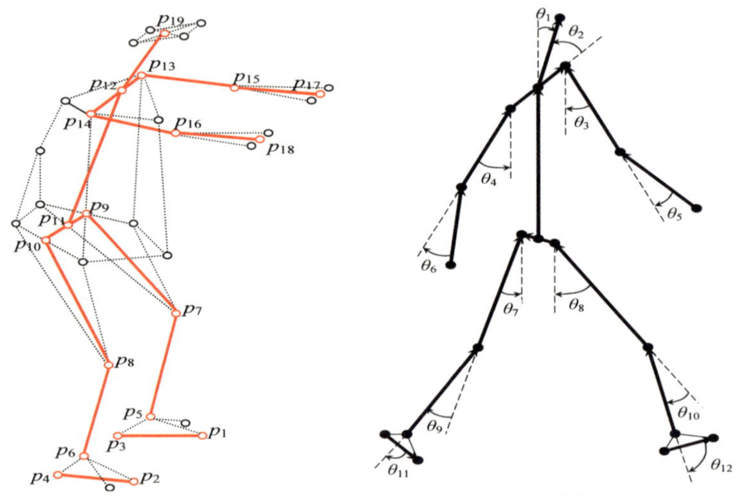

Fig. 1. Fourteen-linkage (FL) Model

Body segments are considered to be rigid bodies for the purposes of describing the motion of the body. 14 segments are composed of these points, such as head (S_1), shoulder (S_2), left and right upper-arms (S_3, S_4), left and right forearms (S_5, S_6), trunk (S_7), pelvis (S_8), left and right thighs (S_9, S_{10}), left and right shanks (S_{11}, S_{12}), and left and right feet (S_{13}, S_{14}).

12 joints between adjacent segments are composed of these segments, such as head-trunk (θ_1), head-shoulder (θ_2), shoulder (θ_3, θ_4), elbows (θ_5, θ_6), hips (θ_7, θ_8), knees (θ_9, θ_{10}), ankles (θ_{11}, θ_{12}), see Fig. 1(b).

2.2 Definitions of walking stability

In human movement, kinematics is the study of the positions, angles, velocities, and accelerations of body segments and joints during motion.

FL model M consists of displacement P, segment angle Φ, joint angle Θ, and their velocity V and acceleration A, angular velocity Ω and angular acceleration Λ at time t, represented as 9-tuple as Equation (1).

$$M = [P(t), \Phi(t), \Theta(t), \\ V(t), \Omega_{\Phi}(t), \Omega_{\Theta}(t), \\ A(t), \Lambda_{\Phi}(t), \Lambda_{\Theta}(t)] \tag{1}$$

where

$$P(t) = [p_1, p_2, p_3, \cdots, p_{19}]^T$$

$$\Phi(t) = [\varphi_1, \varphi_2, \varphi_3, \cdots, \varphi_{14}]^T$$

$$\Theta(t) = [\theta_1, \theta_2, \theta_3, \cdots, \theta_{12}]^T$$

$$V(t) = [v_1, v_2, v_3, \cdots, v_{19}]^T$$

$$\Omega_{\Phi}(t) = [\omega_{\varphi 1}, \omega_{\varphi 2}, \omega_{\varphi 3}, \cdots, \omega_{\varphi 14}]^T$$

$$\Omega_{\Theta}(t) = [\omega_{\theta 1}, \omega_{\theta 2}, \omega_{\theta 3}, \cdots, \omega_{\theta 12}]^T$$

$$A(t) = [a_1, a_2, a_3, \cdots, a_{19}]^T$$

$$\Lambda_{\Phi}(t) = [a_{\varphi 1}, a_{\varphi 2}, a_{\varphi 3}, \cdots, a_{\varphi 14}]^T$$

$$\Lambda_{\Theta}(t) = [a_{\theta 1}, a_{\theta 2}, a_{\theta 3}, \cdots, a_{\theta 12}]^T$$

Segment angle, as shown in Equation (2), is the angle of the projections of segment with the coordinate axes. It consists of the angles between projections in transverse plane, frontal plane and sagittal plane with axis X, Y and Z respectively, see Fig. 2.

$$\varphi = (\varphi_x, \varphi_y, \varphi_z) \tag{2}$$

Note that it is an absolute measure, meaning that it changes according to the orientation of the body.

Joint angle is the angle between the two segments on either side of the joint. It is defined as Equation (3).

$$\theta = (\theta_{xoy}, \theta_{yoz}, \theta_{zox}, \theta_s) \tag{3}$$

where θ_s is the joint angle in space, and θ_{xoy}, θ_{yoz}, θ_{zox} are the projections of joint angle in transverse plane, frontal plane and sagittal plane respectively. Since joint angle θ_s is relative to the segment angles, it doesn't change with the body orientation.

Velocity may be linear (change in displacement) or angular (change in angle). Normally, velocity is derived from displacement or angle data by the process of differentiation. Acceleration is change in velocity. Again, it may be linear (change in linear velocity) or angular (change in angular velocity). Acceleration, too, is usually calculated from the displacement data by differentiating twice. It can also be measured directly by an accelerometer.

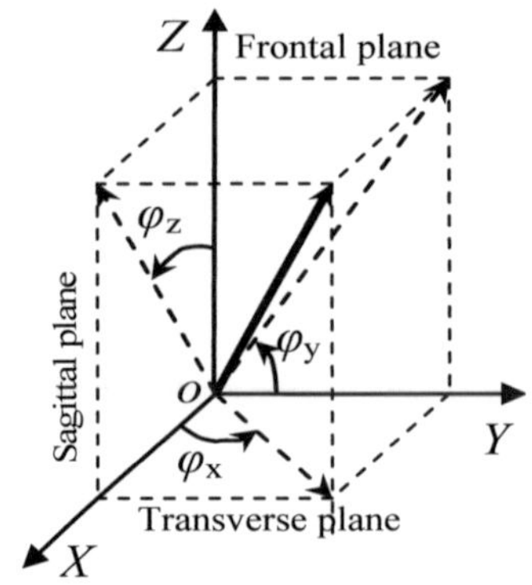

Fig. 2. Segment angle

2.3 Definitions of walking symmetry

For walking symmetry, only consider the bilateral of positions, segments and joints on both sides of human body. In FL-Model, there are 8 points, 5 segments and 5 joint angles unilateral met this condition. These attributes are all three-dimensional data. They are motion data and its velocity and acceleration of {Knee, Ankle, Heel, Toe, Shoulder, Elbow, Wrist, Hip}, Segment Angle and its velocity and acceleration of {Thigh, Shank, Foot, Upper-arm, Forearm}, Joint Angle and its velocity and acceleration of {Hip, Knee, Ankle, Shoulder, Elbow}. These attributes can also be expressed with $p_{1\sim10}$, $p_{13\sim18}$, $\varphi_{3\sim6}$, $\varphi_{9\sim14}$, $\theta_{3\sim12}$, as shown in Fig. 1.

3. Walking data preprocessing

Data preprocessing is an important issue for data analysis, as real-world data tend to be incomplete, noisy, and inconsistent. Data preprocessing includes data cleaning, data integration, data transformation, and data reduction. Although numerous methods of data preprocessing have been developed, data preprocessing remains an active area of research, due to the huge amount inconsistent or dirty data and the complexity of the problem. Before we talk about the methods of walking data preprocessing, let us have a look at walking data measuring.

3.1 Walking data measuring

There are many measurements of human gait, such as basic data (spatial and temporal data), kinematics (displacement, velocity and acceleration data), kinetics (force and moment data), electromyography (electrical activity of lower limb muscles), and image and graphics (individual silhouette images, monocular, image sequence, video). We adopt the kinematical approach in modeling the human movements.

Two kinds of data, motion data and acceleration data are measured using two different systems. The Motion data are gotten from motion capture system (Vicon MX System by OMG Plc), while acceleration data are obtained by a 3-axis accelerometer.

The providers walk along 5m straight line in level plane 3 times at them natural normal walking speeds. 30 markers are attached to the body, as shown in Fig. 3. Fig. 4 shows a snapshot of data acquisition using a motion capture system in the University of Aizu, Fukushima, Japan. The highlights show markers on human body.

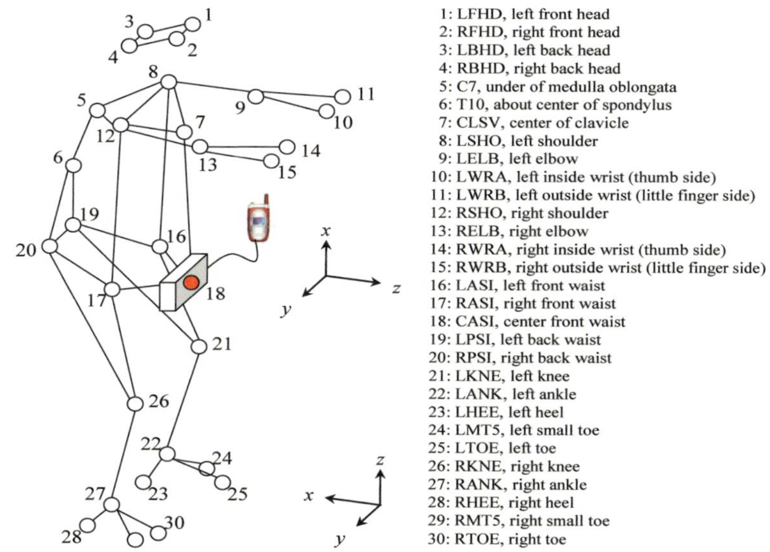

Fig. 3. Markers attached to the body

The motion capture system can detect the three dimensions displacement data at tree directions: anterior-posterior, left-right, and superior-inferior. The sampling rate of motion data is 120Hz. At the same time, a tri-axial accelerometer unit is mounted with CASI, the same point as marker 18, see Fig. 3. The accelerometer is connected with a mobile phone to save the acceleration data. After that the data can be transferred to computer. Acceleration data are also collected in three dimensions as same as motion data, including the gravity acceleration. But the directions are not same. The sampling rate of acceleration data is 90Hz. To calibrate the accelerometer, before each testing session, it was placed with each of the orthogonal axes vertically, to estimate the ±1g values.

By the way, a movie is taken by a video camera while he/she is walking. 44 normal persons from 20 to 69 year old are measured. These subjects are classified into 5 groups (20+, 30+, 40+, 50+, and 60+) by the age.

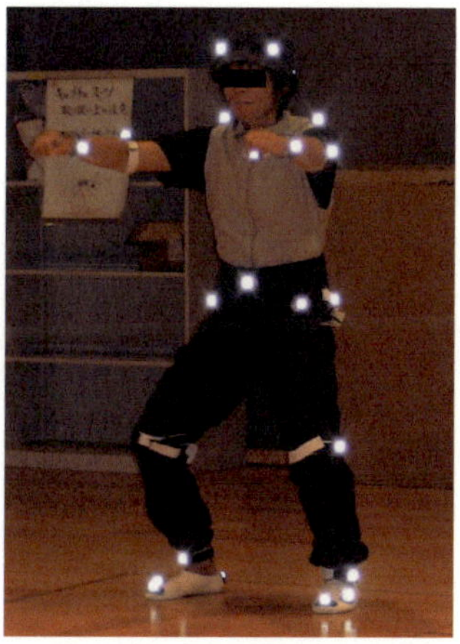

Fig. 4. A snapshot of data acquisition using a motion capture system

3.2 Data cleaning

Data cleaning attempts to fill in missing values, smooth out noise, and correct inconsistencies in the data.

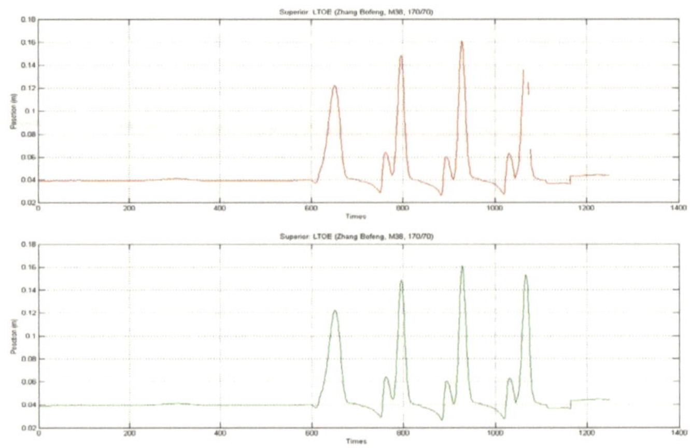

Fig. 5. Interpolation of missing data in left toe

3.2.1 Missing data

In the walking data measured by the motion capture systems, there are some missing data because the system can not detect the markers at a moment. Many interpolation methods could be used, such as nearest neighbor interpolation, linear interpolation, cubic spline interpolation, piecewise cubic Hermite interpolation and N-th degree polynomial interpolation. We choose the spline method to interpolate the missing data because the cubic spline interpolation is a piecewise continuous curve, passing through each of the values in the source data. An example is shown in Fig. 5.

3.2.2 Noisy data

In acceleration data, there are many noisy data, as shown in Fig. 6. We should try to identify and cut these noisy data from the source data.

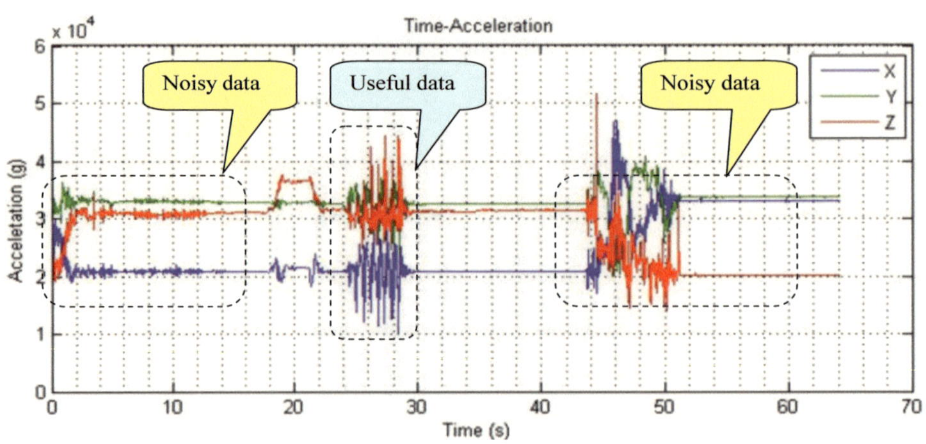

Fig. 6. The noisy data in acceleration data

And there are some noisy data in motion data caused by vibration. Since the walking signal resides in the low frequency range, it is easily affected by interference from other signal and noise sources. Butterworth low-pass filter is used to reduce noise by passing signal which frequency below twice walking cadence. Some examples are shown in Fig. 7 to Fig. 8.

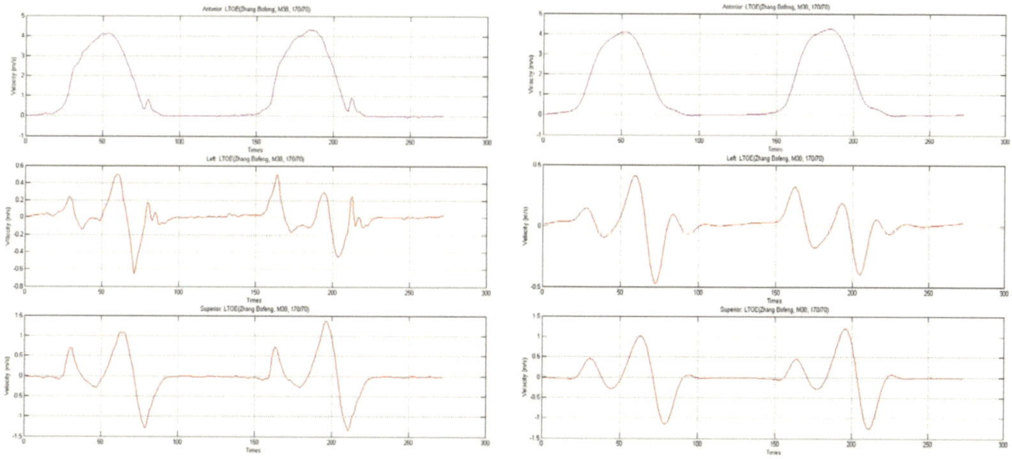

Fig. 7. Velocity data of left toe (No filtering & Filtering)

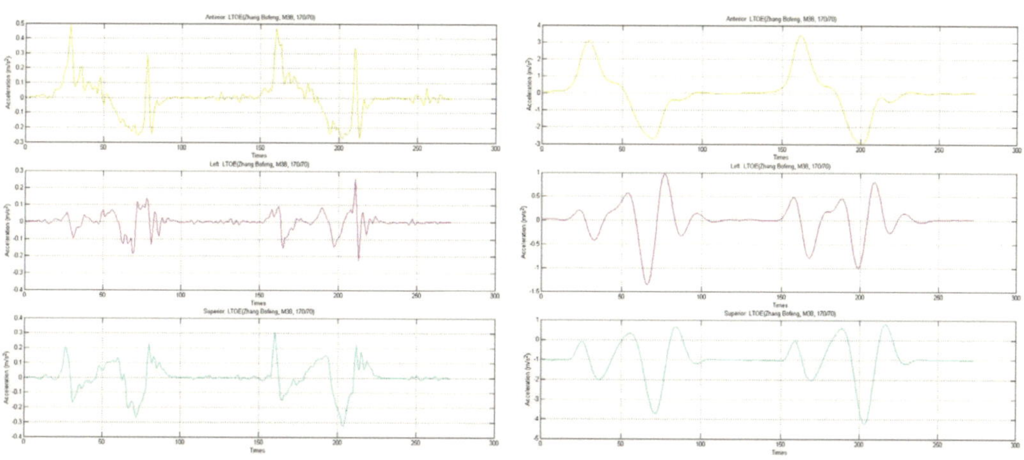

Fig. 8. Acceleration data of left toe (No filtering & Filtering)

3.2.3 Inconsistent data

Because of the faults of the measure systems, one marker can be identified as two or more. In the source file, there is more than one column to store them. So these inconsistent data must be processed by the mean methods, see Equation (4).

$$\begin{cases} \overline{x} = \dfrac{1}{N}\sum_{i=1}^{N} x_i \\ \overline{y} = \dfrac{1}{N}\sum_{i=1}^{N} y_i \\ \overline{z} = \dfrac{1}{N}\sum_{i=1}^{N} z_i \end{cases} \tag{4}$$

3.3 Data transformation

Data transformation converts the data into appropriate forms for analysis further. The coordinate of acceleration data is not parallel the space coordinate because the accelerometer is set up obliquely, so we need to normalize the coordinate.

3.3.1 Calibration

The aim of calibration is to transform raw data to acceleration of gravity (g). The standard of vibration amplitude is maintained in terms of electrical output of reference accelerometer corresponding to a known value of displacement. Acceleration singles are sampled at 90Hz using purpose-written software and saved on computer for subsequent analysis. To calibrate the accelerations before each testing session, they ware placed with each of the orthogonal axes vertically, first pointing up, then down, which enabled the device to be statically calibrated to estimate the ±1g values. An example is shown in Fig. 9.

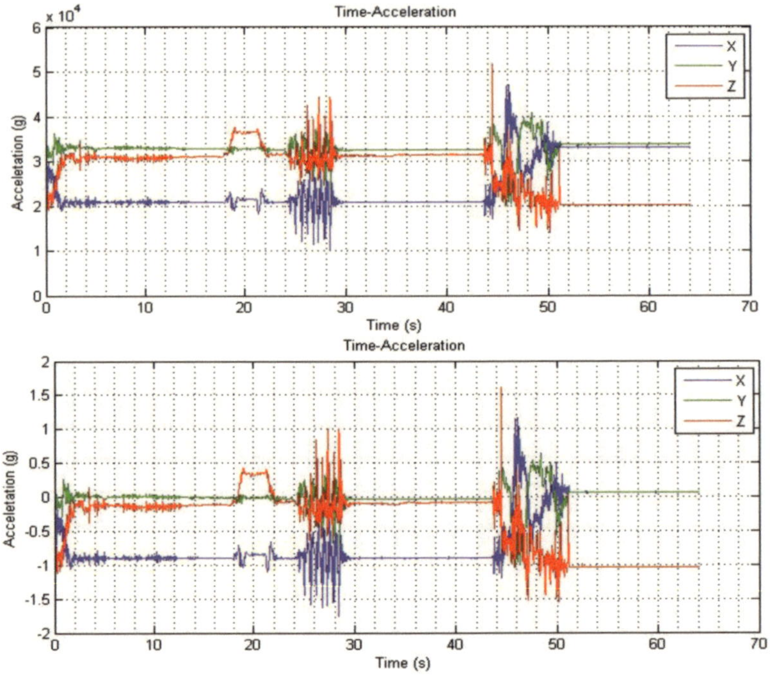

Fig. 9. Calibration of acceleration data

3.3.2 Adjusting acceleration data

Theoretically, the means of X and Y should be '0', that of Z should be '-1'. But actually, it is not true. The coordinate of acceleration data is not parallel with the space coordinate because the accelerometer is set up in gradient, see Fig. 10 so we need to adjust the coordinate.

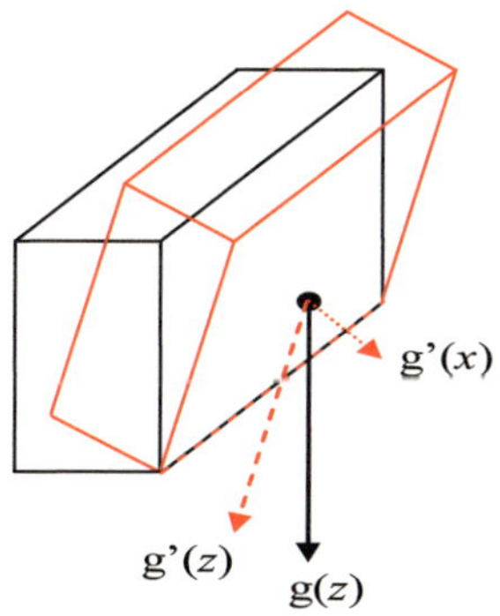

Fig. 10. The accelerometer set up in gradient

The method of adjusting is to rotate the accelerometer in correct position, as shown in Fig. 11. Adjusting rule is that the means of X and Y should be '0'. Firstly, calculate rotation matrix R with Homogeneous Coordinate used Equation (5), and then adjust the acceleration data to vertical position by Equation (6).

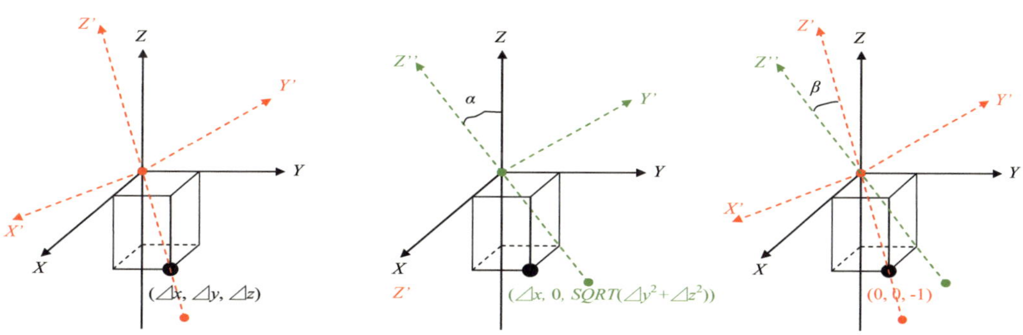

Fig. 11. Title of figure, left justified

$$R = R_x \times R_y = \begin{bmatrix} 1 & 0 & 0 & 0 \\ 0 & \cos(\alpha) & \sin(\alpha) & 0 \\ 0 & -\sin(\alpha) & \cos(\alpha) & 0 \\ 0 & 0 & 0 & 1 \end{bmatrix} \times \begin{bmatrix} \cos(\beta) & 0 & -\sin(\beta) & 0 \\ 0 & 1 & 0 & 0 \\ \sin(\beta) & 0 & \cos(\beta) & 0 \\ 0 & 0 & 0 & 1 \end{bmatrix} \quad (5)$$

$$A' = A \times R \quad (6)$$

An example of adjusting is shown in Fig. 12.

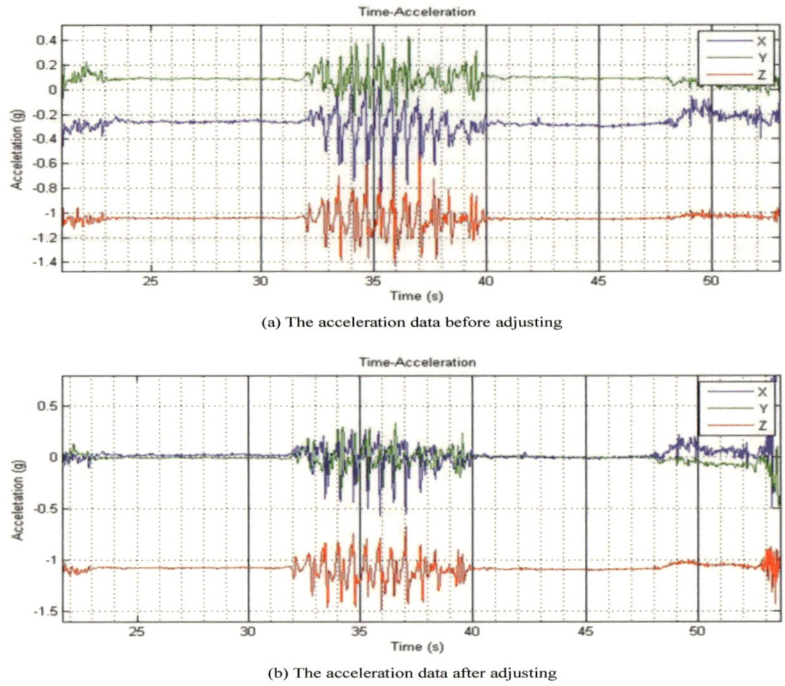

Fig. 12. An example of adjusting result

3.4 Data integration

Data integration combines data from multiple sources to form a coherent data store. Metadata, correlation analysis, data conflict detection, and the resolution of semantic heterogeneity contribute toward smooth data integration.

3.4.1 Converting the coordinates

The coordinate of acceleration data is different from that of motion data, so we should match the acceleration data and motion data in the same coordinates. We define the coordinates, as shown in Fig. 13, x: anterior, y: left, z: superior.

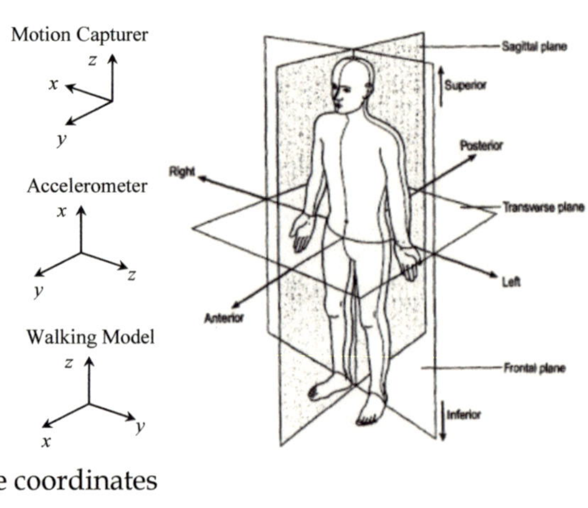

Fig. 13. Converting the coordinates

3.4.2 Aligning the acceleration data with the motion data

The acceleration data and motion data come from different systems, the sampling rates are different, the time of starting measurement are not same, as shown in Fig. 14

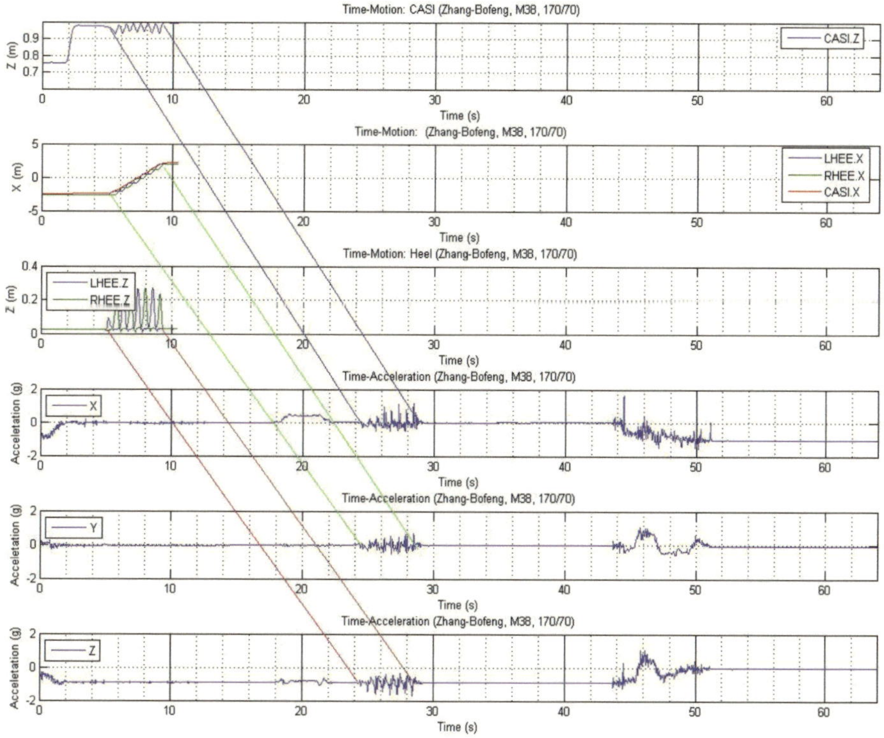

Fig. 14. Title of figure, left justified

so we must find which point of motion data is correlative with which point in acceleration data. The aligning method has two steps.

1. Computing the acceleration with motion data by Equation (7), as shown in Fig. 15.

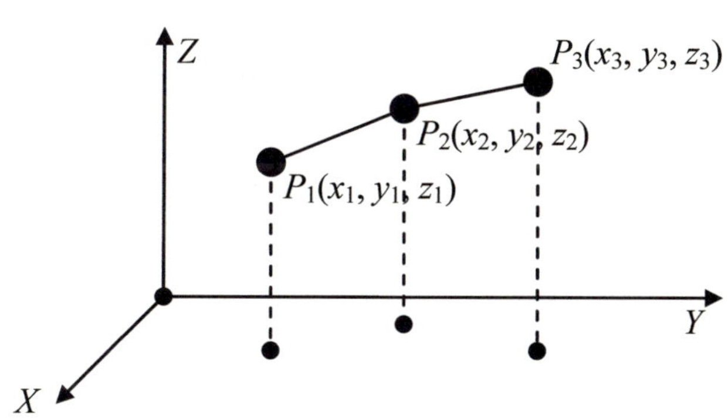

Fig. 15. Computing acceleration with motion data

$$\begin{cases} a_i(x) = \dfrac{x_{i+2} - 2x_{i+1} + x_i}{\Delta t^2} \\ a_i(y) = \dfrac{y_{i+2} - 2y_{i+1} + y_i}{\Delta t^2} \quad (i = 1, N-2) \\ a_i(z) = \dfrac{z_{i+2} - 2z_{i+1} + z_i}{\Delta t^2} \end{cases} \tag{7}$$

2. Comparing the acceleration between the computing data and accelerometer data by minimum of relativity. The result of aligning is shown in Fig. 16.

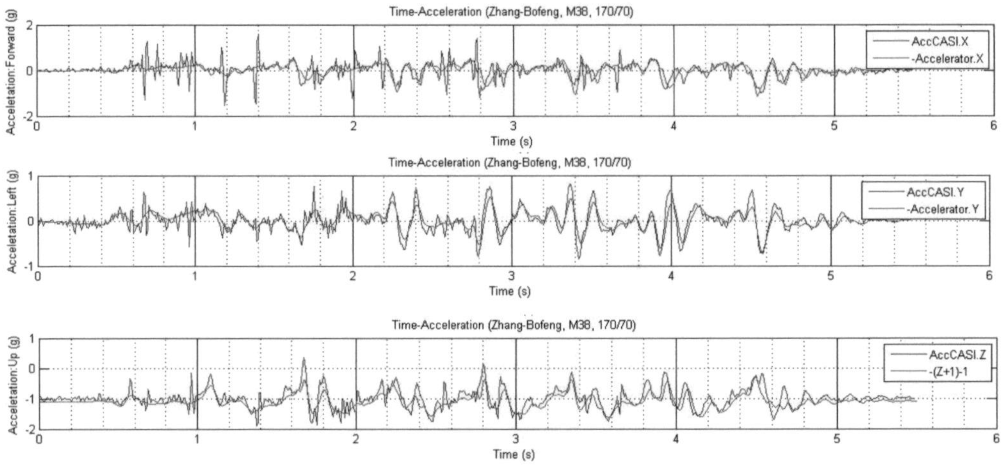

Fig. 16. The result of aligning motion data and acceleration data

3.5 Data reduction

Data reduction techniques can be used to obtain a reduced representation of the data while minimizing the loss of information content. To obtain a reduced representation of the data set, such as speed, average span, frequency, and so on, data reduction techniques can be applied, for examples, aggregation operations and conception hierarchy generation. We propose a hierarchical structure shown in Fig. 17.

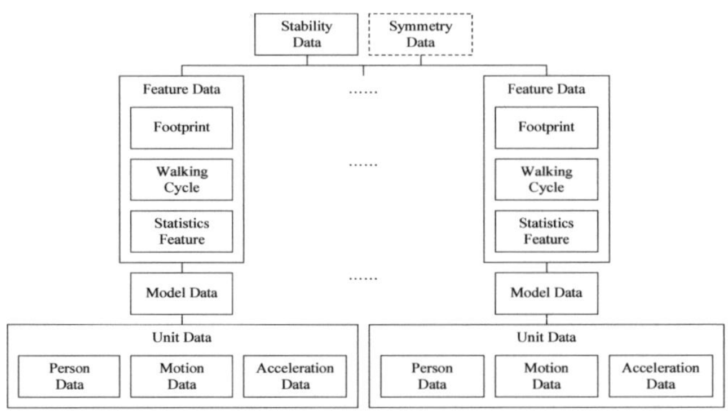

Fig. 17. The hierarchical structure of walking data

4. Walking stability analysis

Although there is now a wealth of literature pertaining to the maintenance of stability when standing, there is a relative paucity of information regarding the biomechanics and physiology of walking stability. Various models are currently in development, but a unified model of walking stability does not exist yet. Unlike standing, the balance of walking is a kind of dynamic balance (Menz, 2000).

Standard deviation is used to define the variability or randomness of the walking pattern. Less the amount of variability means better neuromuscular control and walking stability. We extract a set of hierarchical features from FL model, such as walking cycle features, footprint features.

4.1 Footprint stability

Footprint analysis is a typical method of walking research as shown in Fig. 18.

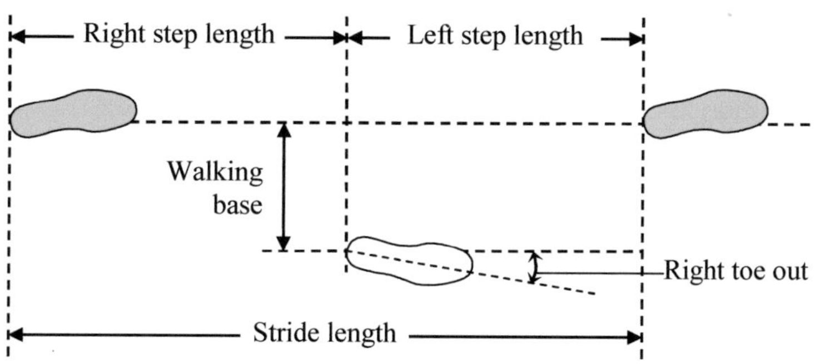

Fig. 18. Features of footprint stability

4.1.1 Definition of footprint stability

DEFINITION 2. (Footprint Stability) Footprint stability is described by the variability of the footprint stability features. We extract some of the stability features of footprint $F_S(F)$, such as the variability of cycle time f1, left step length f2, right step length f3, speed f4, walking base f5, left toe out f6, and right toe out f7, as shown in Equation (8).

$$F_S(F) = \sum_{i=1}^{7} \delta(f_i) / \mu(f_i) \tag{8}$$

where $\delta(f_i)$ is the standard deviation of the feature f_i, and $\mu(f_i)$ is the mathematical expectation of the feature f_i.

4.1.2 Effects of aging on footprint stability

Now, the variability of the footprint features per decade of age is calculated, as shown in Table 1.

The footprint variability in last row of Table 1 is sum of the above items. It can be seen that the variability is increasing with the age, see Fig. 19. That is to say, the footprint stability is declined with the age, and especially there is a dramatic increasing over 50 years old. But the twenties are exceptional, maybe because the twenties walk more springily than the elders.

Age	20+	30+	40+	50+	60+
CycleTime	0.0437	0.0293	0.0333	0.0464	0.0716
LStepLength	0.0825	0.0779	0.0568	0.0766	0.0811
RStepLength	0.0645	0.0790	0.1099	0.0586	0.0645
Speed	0.0833	0.0736	0.0819	0.0709	0.0880
WalkingBase	0.1783	0.1721	0.1495	0.1269	0.1343
LToeOut	0.4047	0.1579	0.2407	0.2383	1.3606
RToeOut	0.3246	0.2175	0.3473	0.5013	1.0242
$F_S(F)$	1.1817	0.8073	1.0195	1.1190	2.8243

Table 1. Variability of footprint features

4.2 Cycle stability

The gait cycle is defined as the time interval between two successive occurrences of one of the repetitive events of walking. The detection of the human gait period can provide important information to determine the positions of the human body.

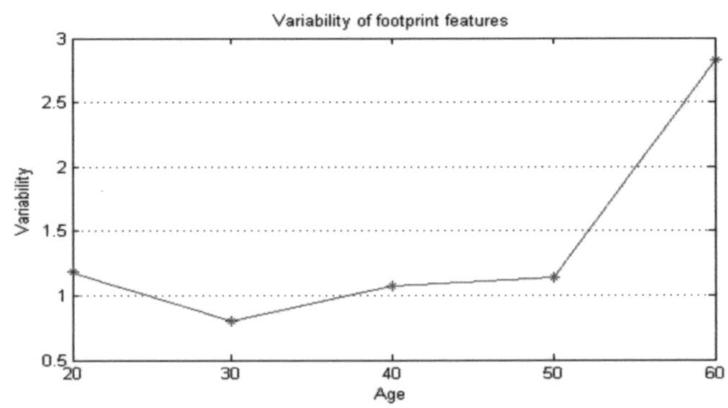

Fig. 19. Footprint stability with age

4.2.1 Definition of cycle stability

DEFINITION 3. (Cycle Stability) Cycle stability is described by the variability of the cycle stability features. The cycle stability $F_S(C)$ is defined as Equation (9).

$$F_S(C) = \sum_{i=1}^{7} \delta(c_i) / \mu(f_4) \tag{9}$$

where $\delta(c_i)$ is the standard deviation of the time when event i occurs, c_i = {LTO, LFA, LTV, LIC, RTO, RFA, RTV}, and $\mu(f_4)$ is the mathematical expectation of the speed f_4.

Generally, 7 events are used to identify major events during the walking cycle (Whittle, 2007). For the symmetry of left side and right side, 10 events are employed in this paper, as shown in Fig. 20.

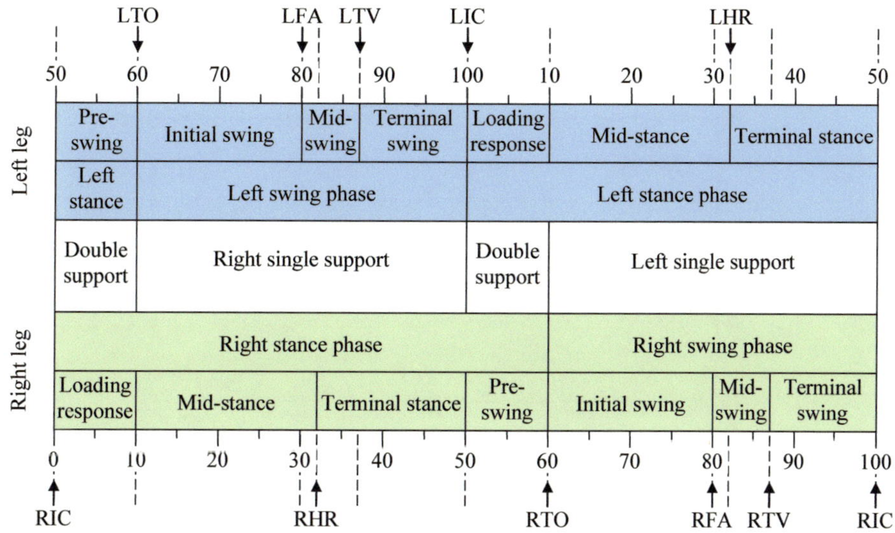

Fig. 20. Walking cycle in normal gait

Such as
RIC = right foot initial contact;
LTO = left toe off;
LFA = left foot adjacent to right foot;
RHR = right heel rise;
LTV = left tibia vertical;
LIC = left foot initial contact;
RTO = right toe off;
RFA = right foot adjacent to left foot;
LHR = left heel rise;
RTV = right tibia vertical.

4.2.2 Effects of aging on cycle stability

Table 2 shows the variability of walking cycle features per decade of age.

Age	20+	30+	40+	50+	60+
RIC	0.0000	0.0000	0.0000	0.0000	0.0000
LTO	1.6664	1.2287	1.2272	0.9334	1.2268
LFA	1.2846	1.7323	1.3302	1.0199	1.1198
LTV	1.6354	1.8543	1.4046	1.2759	0.9008
LIC	1.2822	1.0320	1.0900	0.9751	0.7036
RTO	1.3563	1.2323	1.2866	0.7376	0.8605
RFA	0.9731	1.3764	1.4480	1.0737	0.8847
RTV	1.0459	1.2067	1.3846	1.3705	1.0909
$F_S(C)$	9.2440	9.6627	9.1713	7.3861	6.7870

Table 2. Variability of walking cycle features

Fig. 21 shows that the cycle variability is declined with the age almost. This is not same as a common assumption. The reason is that the elder walking more rigidly and inflexibly.

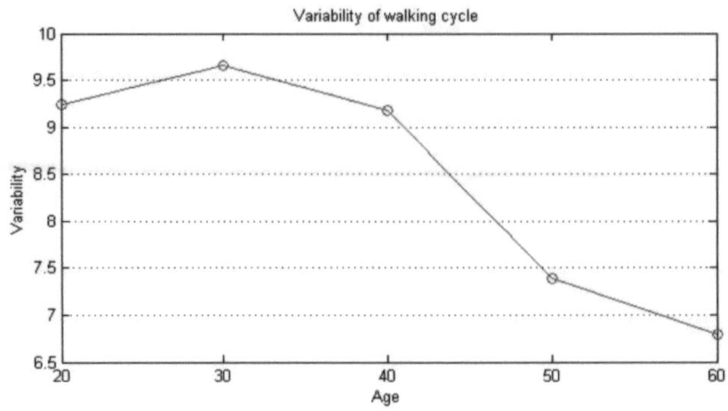

Fig. 21. Cycle stability with age

4.3 Orbital stability

Orbital stability defines how purely periodic systems respond to small perturbations discretely after one complete cycle (i.e. one stride) and may be better suited to study strongly periodic movements like walking (Marin, 2006).

4.3.1 Definition of orbital stability

DEFINITION 4. (Orbital Stability) Orbital stability is described by the variability of the orbital stability features. The orbital stability $F_S(O)$ of lower limbs is composed of three parts, position stability $F_S(P)$, segment stability $F_S(S)$ and Joint stability $F_S(J)$, as shown in Equation (10).

$$F_S(O) = F_S(P) + F_S(S) + F_S(J) \tag{10}$$

where position stability $F_S(P)$ is defined by standard deviation of the maximums and minimums of displacement, velocity and acceleration (knees, heels, and toes), as shown in Equation (11).

$$\begin{aligned} F_S(P) = {} & \delta[\vee(p_i(Z))] + \delta[\vee(v_i(Z))] + \delta[\vee(A_i(Z))] \\ & + \delta[\wedge(p_i(Z))] + \delta[\wedge(v_i(Z))] + \delta[\wedge(A_i(Z))] \\ & (i = 1 \sim 4,7,8) \end{aligned} \tag{11}$$

$\vee(x)$ and $\wedge(x)$ are the maximum and minimum value of x respectively.

Segment stability $F_S(S)$ is defined by standard deviation of the maximums and minimums of segment angle, angular velocity and angular acceleration (thighs, shanks and feet), as shown in Equation (12).

$$\begin{aligned} F_S(S) = {} & \delta[\vee(\varphi_i(Z))] + \delta[\vee(\omega_{\varphi i}(Z))] + \delta[\vee(\alpha_{\varphi i}(Z))] \\ & + \delta[\wedge(\varphi_i(Z))] + \delta[\wedge(\omega_{\varphi i}(Z))] + \delta[\wedge(\alpha_{\varphi i}(Z))] \\ & (i = 9 \sim 14) \end{aligned} \tag{12}$$

Joint stability $F_S(J)$ is defined by standard deviation of the maximums and minimums of displacement, velocity and acceleration (hips, knees and ankles), as shown in Equation (13).

$$F_S(J) = \delta[\vee(\theta_i(Z))] + \delta[\vee(\omega_{\theta i}(Z))] + \delta[\vee(\alpha_{\theta i}(Z))] \\ +\delta[\wedge(\theta_i(Z))] + \delta[\wedge(\omega_{\theta i}(Z))] + \delta[\wedge(\alpha_{\theta i}(Z))] \\ (i = 7 \sim 12) \tag{13}$$

Thus, the orbital stability of lower limbs includes 108 indexes. For examples, Fig.22 and Fig. 23 show the joint angles of hips (θ_7, θ_8), knees (θ_9, θ_{10}) and ankles (θ_{11}, θ_{12}) in sagittal plane during a single walking cycle, their angular velocity ($\omega_{\theta 9}$, $\omega_{\theta 10}$, $\omega_{\theta 11}$, $\omega_{\theta 12}$) and angular acceleration ($a_{\theta 9}$, $a_{\theta 10}$, $a_{\theta 11}$, $a_{\theta 12}$) respectively.

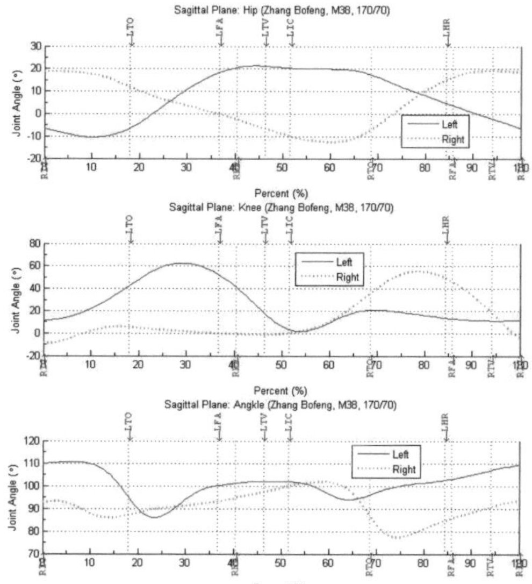

Fig. 22. Joint angles

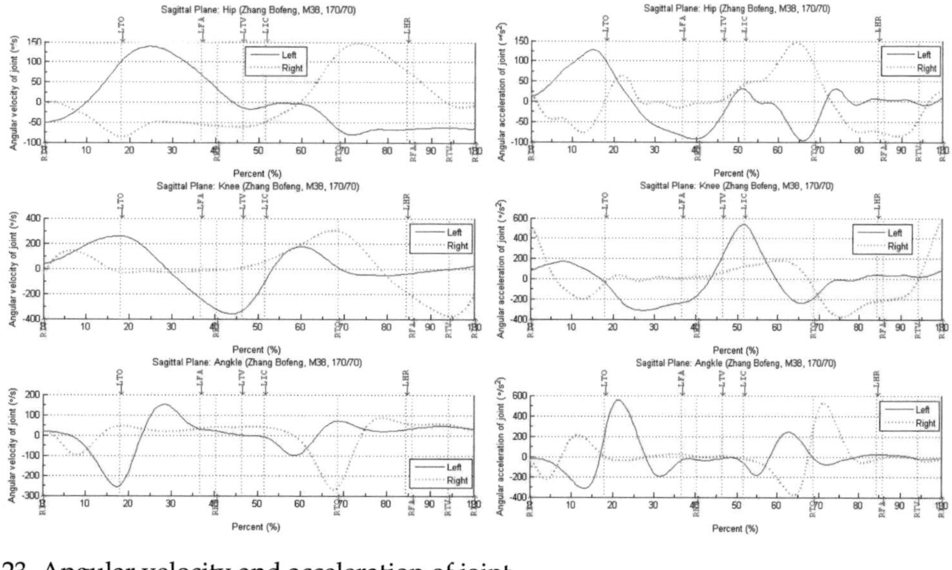

Fig. 23. Angular velocity and acceleration of joint

4.3.2 Outlier analysis in orbital stability

Because of the errors of computing, maybe there are few outliers in the features of orbital stability. For an example, the last 3 cycles of the displacement of right hip (p10) at vertical is shown in Fig. 25. There is an outlier in the last cycle, the left maximum point should be found instead of the right maximum point.

There are a variety of outlier detection approaches from several areas, including statistics, machine learning, and data mining. A kind of proximity-based outlier detection approach, called distance to k-nearest neighbor, is used to find the outliers in orbital stability. This approach is more general and more easily applied than statistical approached, since it is easier to determine a meaningful proximity measure for a data set than to determine its statistics distribution.

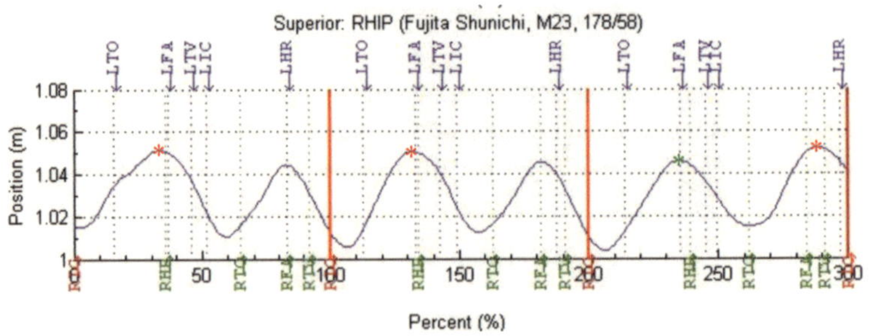

Fig. 24. Last 3 cycles of the displacement of right hip (p10) at vertical

Fig. 25 shows the outliers in the displacement of right hip (p10). The points with a circle are the outlier point. The outlier score of an object is given by the distance to its k-nearest neighbor, using a value of k = 5.

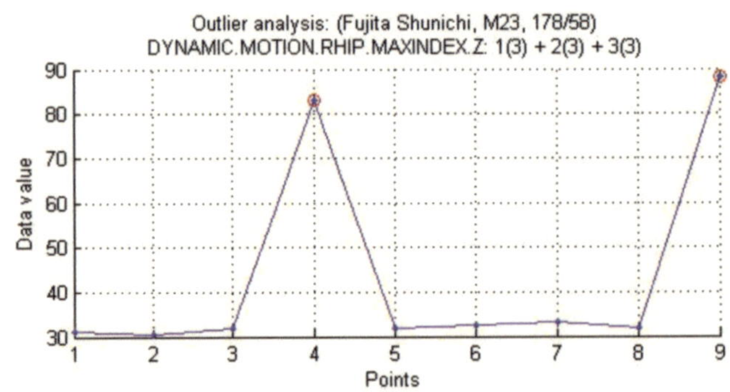

Fig. 25. Outliers in the displacement of right hip

4.3.3 Effects of aging on orbital stability

After analysis all subjects between 20 to 70 years old, the item results of orbital stability are shown in Fig. 26. The position stability $F_S(P)$, segment stability $F_S(S)$, joint stability $F_S(J)$ and the whole orbital stability are in shown in Fig. 27. It is observed that, although each of orbital variability does not increase strictly with age, the variability of orbital features increases with age generally. As persons grow old, the orbital stability is becoming weakly.

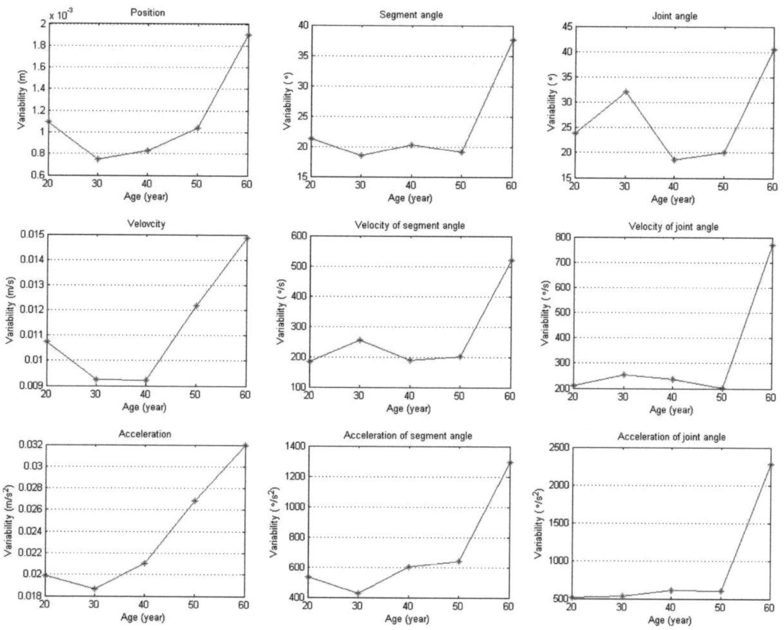

Fig. 26. Each item of orbital stability with age

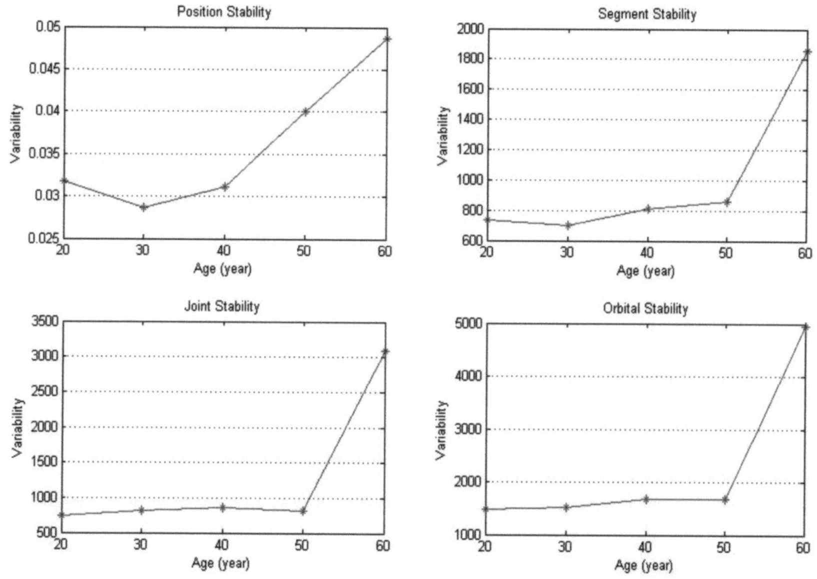

Fig. 27. Position stability, segment stability and joint stability, and orbital stability with age

4.4 Dynamic stability based on dynamic time warping (DTW)

Dynamic stability is the main reason for leading to falls for people, especially for elders. This section discusses age influence on dynamic stability based on dynamic time warping.

4.4.1 Definition of dynamic stability

Subject's walking is one kind of periodic movements and the same events will happen during different walking cycles, so the similarity of the data between adjacent cycles to assess subject's walking stability.

This paper used dynamic time warping (DTW) to calculate this similarity, which is a method for flexible pattern-matching scheme. It translates, compress and expands a pair of patterns so similar features within the two patterns are matched (Li, 2003). Fig. 28 and Equation (14) show details.

$$D(S_i) = \frac{\sum_{j=1}^{n-1} DTW(\theta_j, \theta_{j+1})}{n-1} \quad (n > 1) \tag{14}$$

where D is the number of walking cycles, $D(S_i)$ is the average of similarity at feature S_i.

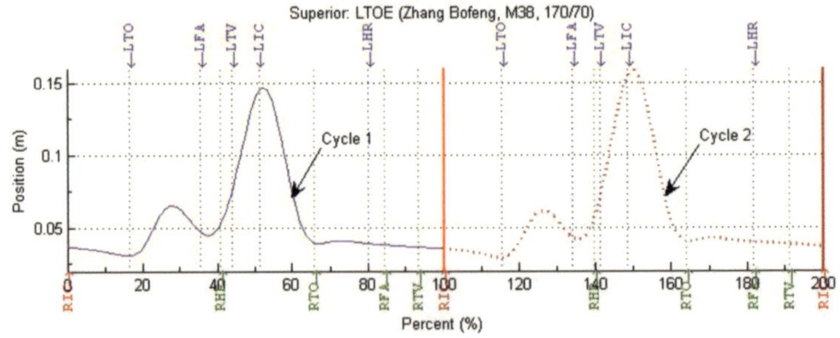

(a) The source data of left toe at superior

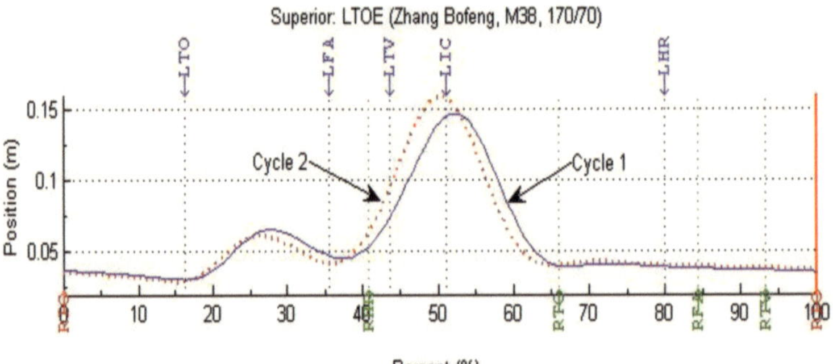

(b) Compare between two adjacent cycles

Fig. 28. Similarity between two adjacent cycles by DTW

4.4.2 Extracting of dynamic stability features

According to FL model, it's easy to get corresponding position, velocity and acceleration motion data of 19 points. Therefore, 19×3=57 features are extracted to describe human dynamic stability.

4.4.3 Effects of aging on dynamic stability

Equation (15) calculates the sum of single feature value by age.

$$S(A_k, S_i) = \frac{1}{m \times l_k} \sum_{j=1}^{m} D_j(S_i) \tag{15}$$

where m is the number of subjects in the same age class, l_k is the average leg length of subjects in the same age class, $D_j(S_i)$ is similarity value of the selected feature i by Equation (14), is a single stability value of the same feature i in the same age class A_k, and k is the number of age class.

According to Equation (14), similarity value of all selected features in the same age group was calculated by age.

$$F(A_k) = \sum_{i=1}^{p} S(A_k, S_i) \tag{16}$$

where p is the number of features, in this case, p is equal to 32, and k is equal to 5.

Fig. 29 shows trend on the change of dynamic stability.

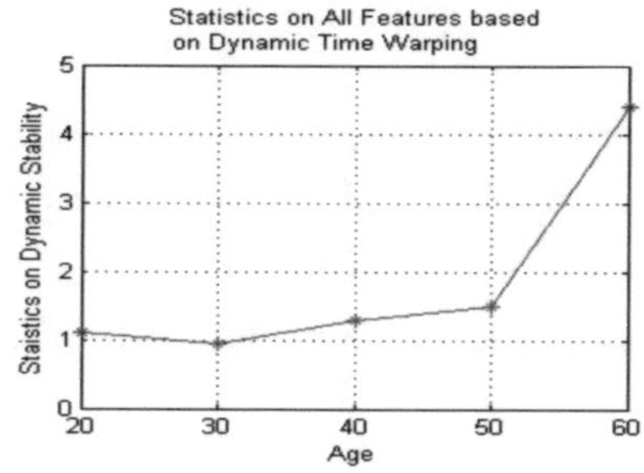

Fig. 29. Statistic on stability of all dynamic features

This figure tells us that if all dynamic features are employed to do statistics on such kind of stability, the dynamic stability is decreasing with ageing except the twenties. It seems that all of those features are desirable.

4.5 Feature selection on dynamic stability

The previous section did statistic on all 57 dynamic stability. To reduce the computational complexity, and more importantly, to get more important and contributing features, this paper did feature selection on those 57 dynamic features. On the one hand, it could simplify the method of data acquisition; On the other hand, it is more persuasive by analyzing those selected features.

This section ties to find the best features reflecting the relationship between age and walking stability among those 57 ones, which include 2^{57}-1 different kinds of feature combination. A classic method of feature selection, which is the cooperation of adaptive genetic algorithm and support vector machine, was used to do it.

4.5.1 Improved crossover operation

In order to avoid that better solutions with high fitness disappear in a standard genetic algorithm although the algorithm is accommodated again and again. This paper proposed a formulation to adjust crossover probability (p_c) between average fitness and maximum fitness, as shown in Equation (17).

$$p_c^i = \begin{cases} p_c^{i-1} * \dfrac{f' - f_{avg}}{f_{\max} - f_{avg}}, f' \geq f_{avg} \\ p_c^{i-1} * \dfrac{f_{avg} - f'}{f_{\max} - f_{avg}}, f' \prec f_{avg} \end{cases} \tag{17}$$

where f_{max} is the maximum fitness of current population, f_{avg} is the average fitness of current population, f' is the larger fitness between two individuals in crossover operation.

4.5.2 Improved mutation operation

Just as crossover operation, there are the same problems with mutation operation.
If probability of mutation (p_m) is undersize, new individual can't be generated easily, inversely, genetic algorithm will be a pure searching process.
To solve this problem, this paper improved it as shown in Equation (18).

$$p_m^i = \begin{cases} p_m^{i-1} * \dfrac{f - f_{avg}}{f_{\max} - f_{avg}}, f \geq f_{avg} \\ p_m^{i-1} * \dfrac{f_{avg} - f}{f_{\max} - f_{avg}}, f \prec f_{avg} \end{cases} \tag{18}$$

where f is the fitness of individual going to mutate. All other parameters have the same meaning as Equation (17).

4.5.3 Improved support vector machine (SVM)

According to information of age classification, SVM was used to separate datasets and assess fitness of specific feature combination during feature selection. This paper improves SVM in two parts: classification balancing and evaluation.
A conventional SVM is to build a decision function $f_c(x)$ for each class C. Then use Equation (19) as the predicted class label.

$$d(x) = \arg\max(f_c(x)) \tag{19}$$

However, this equation may fail to work in some skewed inseparable distribution. Therefore, it's improved as Equation (20), which suggests a function $p_c(f)$ to balance values of $f_c(x)$ in Equation (19).

$$d(x) = \arg\max(p_c(f_c(x))) \tag{20}$$

Another problem is about evaluation. Generally, correctness is calculated by *correctNumber/totalNumber*, but it does not fit well to skewed distributions. It's improved as Equation (21) described.

$$F(M,b,\vec{w}) = 1-(1-b)\times\sum_{i=1}^{n}\frac{e_i}{m} - U \tag{21}$$

$$U = \begin{cases} 0, & \sum_{i=1}^{n} e_i = 0 \\ b \times \dfrac{\max\limits_{0 \le i \le n} \dfrac{e_i w_i}{c_i}}{\max\limits_{0 \le i \le n} w_i} \times \dfrac{\sum_{i=1}^{n} \left| \dfrac{e_i w_i}{c_i} - \varsigma \right|}{n\varsigma}, & otherwise \end{cases}$$

where M is the confusion matrix, b is a coefficient that balances the total correctness and the balance achievement, $\vec{w}$ is the importance weight between classes, n is the number of classes, e_i is the sum of non-diagonal entries of i-th row of M, m is the sum of all entries of M, namely total number of patterns, $\sum_{i=1}^{n} w_i = n$, ς is the average value of ${e_i w_i}/{c_i}$.

4.5.4 Selected stable features

After 18 generations of GA, 32 walking stability features were selected with classification correctness from 89.4% to 94.7%.

To compare number of markers between before and after feature selection, those 32 features are marked with 14 red markers, as shown in Fig. 30. It means that there is (30-14)/30=53.3% reduction on markers, which could simplify equipment to a large extent.

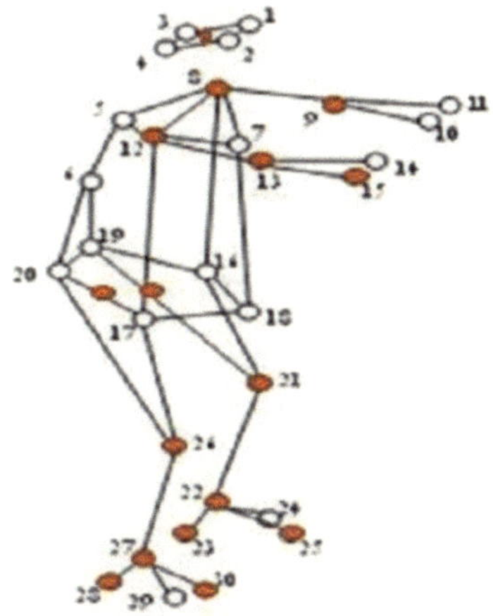

Fig. 30. Red markers corresponding to selected features

4.5.5 Effects of aging on dynamic stability after feature selection

Fig. 30 told us that the selected markers are almost symmetrical. To increase the symmetry, other three features are added, such as LHIP in position, RELB in velocity, RSHO and LELB in acceleration. Table 3 shows these fours features with gray background in details.

The difference between this method and previous one is the number of dynamic features. Therefore, the same statistic method will be applied on this one. Another, the similarity calculated by DTW is used to assess the stability of specific dynamic feature. Because DTW doesn't care about the data unite, all features from position, velocity and acceleration will be counted together.

Age	20+	30+	40+	50+	60+
Position					
LHIP	0.0001	0.0000	0.0001	0.0001	0.0003
RHIP	0.0001	0.0001	0.0001	0.0001	0.0003
CENT	0.0001	0.0000	0.0001	0.0001	0.0003
LKNE	0.0002	0.0005	0.0001	0.0006	0.0003
RKNE	0.0002	0.0002	0.0001	0.0004	0.0013
LANK	0.0012	0.0010	0.0001	0.0001	0.0009
RANK	0.0013	0.0006	0.0001	0.0001	0.0005
LHEE	0.0028	0.0027	0.0001	0.0002	0.0013
RHEE	0.0027	0.0018	0.0000	0.0001	0.0011
LTOE	0.0004	0.0001	0.0001	0.0001	0.0002
RTOE	0.0004	0.0002	0.0001	0.0001	0.0002
Velocity					
LELB	0.0125	0.0023	0.0122	0.0046	0.0055
RELB	0.0111	0.0030	0.0080	0.0039	0.0055
CENT	0.0021	0.0009	0.0016	0.0018	0.0024
LKNE	0.0109	0.0077	0.0038	0.0035	0.0066
RKNE	0.0109	0.0076	0.0024	0.0034	0.0054
LANK	0.0563	0.0405	0.0088	0.0091	0.0495
RANK	0.0678	0.0318	0.0594	0.0062	0.1520
LHEE	0.1522	0.1369	0.0055	0.0200	0.0775
RHEE	0.1447	0.0892	0.0073	0.0847	0.0662
LTOE	0.0336	0.0135	0.0067	0.0079	0.0158
RTOE	0.0400	0.0201	0.0129	0.0569	0.0204
Acceleration					
LSHO	0.0071	0.0030	0.0041	0.0061	0.0037
RSHO	0.0071	0.0033	0.0047	0.0054	0.0035
NECK	0.0062	0.0028	0.0038	0.0051	0.0031
LELB	0.0162	0.0046	0.0230	0.0080	0.0069
RELB	0.0137	0.0045	0.0094	0.0080	0.0077
CENT	0.0059	0.0029	0.0054	0.0349	0.0449
LKNE	0.0293	0.0179	0.0214	0.0119	0.0161
RKNE	0.0299	0.0187	0.0095	0.0136	0.0204
LANK	0.0765	0.0505	0.0342	0.0432	0.0562
RANK	0.0915	0.0544	0.4998	0.0270	2.2505
LHEE	0.1604	0.1196	0.0812	0.0901	0.0887
RHEE	0.1662	0.1154	0.0477	0.2507	0.0980
LTOE	0.1567	0.0687	0.0274	0.2517	0.0965
RTOE	0.2266	0.1225	0.0816	0.2483	0.1541
$F(A_k)$	**1.5449**	**0.9497**	**1.0028**	**1.0980**	**3.2639**

Table 3. Selected features in three types

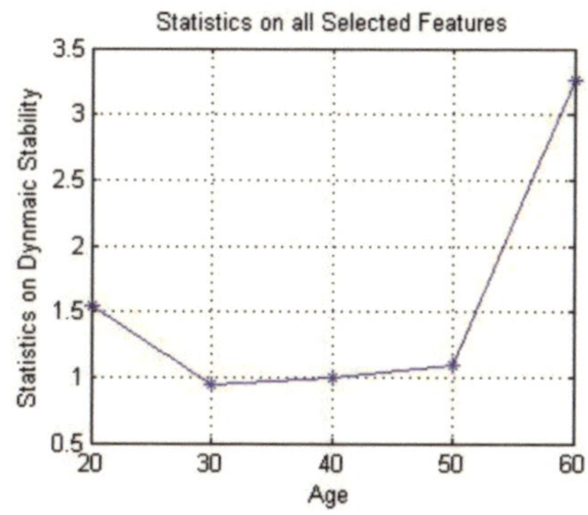

Fig. 31. Statistic on stability of selected dynamic features

As a response to the assumption that elder the person is, less stable his gait is. This method assesses walking stability by searching the best contributing features and doing statistics on them. The result shows that walking stability truly becomes worse as ageing except the group of twenties.

5. Walking symmetry analysis

Gait symmetry analysis is a part of normal gait analysis. Our research is based on the Fourteen-Linkage Walking Model of human. The detail of this model can be seen in chapter 2. We all know, gait symmetry reflects the general characteristics of human walk gait, and it is an important indicator to assess the function of the human walk. Especially in the human aging process the recession of brain and central nervous system and physiological function will affect the lower limb gait of left or right side, and lead gait mutation.

5.1 Footprint symmetry

Here, we mainly aim to investigate the footprint properties of the left and right foot. See Fig.32, the symmetric properties were step length and toe out angle of two feet.

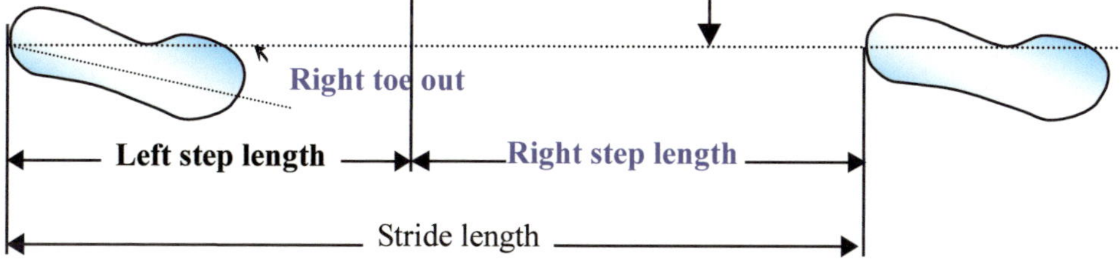

Fig. 32. Features of footprint for symmetry analysis

Besides step length and toe out angle, we also consider step factor and walk ratio.
Step factor is the value of step length divided by leg length.
Walk ratio is the value of step length divided by step rate and step rate is the number of steps per minute someone walks.

5.1.1 Definition of footprint symmetry

DEFINITION 5. (Footprint Symmetry) Footprint symmetry is described by the difference of the bilateral footprint features. We extract some symmetrical features of footprint as *S(F)*, which contains the difference of Step length about two feet, the difference of Toe out angle of right foot and left foot, the difference of bilateral Step factor and the difference of bilateral Walk ratio, as shown in Equation (22).

$$S(F) = \sum_{i=1}^{4} | \delta(LA_i) / \mu(LA_i) - \delta(RA_i) / \mu(RA_i) | \qquad (22)$$

Here $\delta(A_i)$ is the standard deviation of the feature A_i, and $\mu(A_i)$ is the mathematical expectation of the feature A_i. A_i is the element of {LStepLength, RStepLength; LToeout, RToeout; LStepFactor, RStepFactor; LWalkRatio, RWalkRatio}.
The δ/μ of footprint bilateral features per decade of age is calculated, shown as the upper part in Table 4. The last row of Table 4 is the *S(F)* of above items.

5.1.2 Effects of aging on footprint symmetry

It can be seen that the variation of footprint feature is mostly less than 0.02 excepted on feature *Toeout* as shown in Fig. 33.

Age	20+	30+	40+	50+	60+
S(StepLength)	*0.01818*	*0.00865*	*0.00238*	*0.01286*	*0.00210*
S(Toeout)	*0.01660*	*0.04051*	*0.04079*	*0.16155*	*0.05628*
S(StepFactor)	*0.01803*	*0.00859*	*0.00247*	*0.01157*	*0.00298*
S(WalkRatio)	*0.00814*	*0.01854*	*0.00939*	*0.00293*	*0.00638*
S(F)	**0.06095**	**0.0763**	**0.05504**	**0.18892**	**0.06774**

Table 4. Variation of footprint features

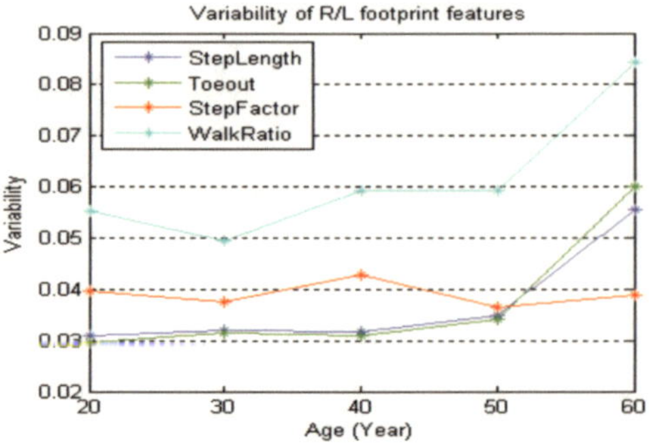

Fig. 33. Variation of footprint features

5.2 Cycle symmetry

This section shows the main characteristics of the symmetry of the gait cycles. As movement of two legs turns symmetrically, the ten tags of walking cycle (see Fig. 20) in fact is a symmetrical composition of 5 keywords in one side, they are TO, FA, TV, IC, HR.

5.2.1 Definition of cycle symmetry

DEFINITION 6. (Cycle Symmetry) Cycle symmetry is described by the variability of the cycle symmetric features. The cycle symmetry *S(C)* is defined as Equation (23).

$$\mathbf{S(C)} = \sum_{i=1}^{4} \left| \delta(LC_i) / \mu(LC_i) - \delta(RC_i) / \mu(RC_i) \right| / \mu(S_i) \qquad (23)$$

Here $\delta(C_i)$ is the standard deviation of the feature C_i and $\mu(C_i)$ is its mathematical expectation, and $\mu(S_i)$ is the mathematical expectation of the feature Speed. LC_i or RC_i is the element of {LTO, RTO; LHR, RHR; LFA, RFA; LTV, RTV}. Since the use of the relative value of sagittal plane, so the IC in here is meaningless.

5.2.2 Effects of aging on cycle symmetry

Here described left and right foot gait cycle symmetrical properties change with aging groups. We calculated the δ/μ on average speed of every decade of age, as shown in Table 5.

Age	20+	30+	40+	50+	60+
S(TO)	*0.05567*	*0.10183*	*0.04917*	*0.03336*	*0.05064*
S(FA)	*0.01323*	*0.01264*	*0.0179*	*0.01706*	*0.01161*
S(HR)	*0.03106*	*0.01222*	*0.03407*	*0.01832*	*0.02689*
S(TV)	*0.00201*	*0.03435*	*0.01366*	*0.01486*	*0.00648*
S(C)	**0.10198**	**0.16104**	**0.11479**	**0.08359**	**0.09562**

Table 5. Variation of cycle features

Also the last line of Table 5 is the different value of feet around the corresponding cycle time points. It can be seen that the variation of cycle feature of every group is less 0.20, but the variety has no obvious trend as shown in Fig. 34.

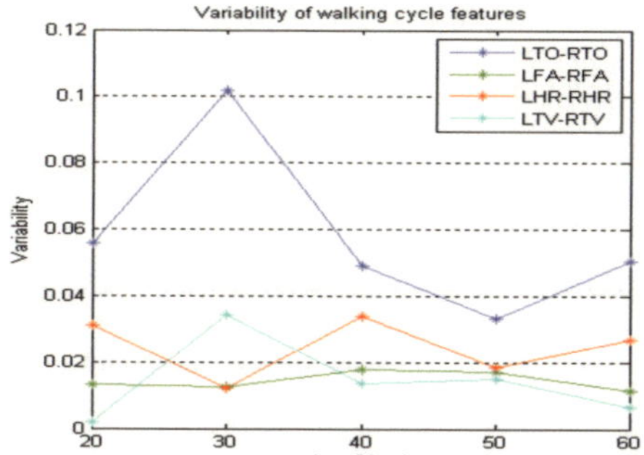

Fig. 34. Variation of cycle feature

5.3 Orbital symmetry

Orbital symmetry is described by the variability of the locus of symmetric points of body, in particular in the sagittal plane. Before doing calculation, we must do some adjustment about

dynamic data of right side and left side. Adjustment method is to move the left side data ahead about half stride cycle. That is, we let the LIC to match the RIC. The first removal data may put to last part according to stride cycle, or be doffed and then we got three steps bilateral data.
It is clearly that selected features of symmetry may as indicators for evaluation of a person's gait. According to our work, the indices of motion data may be an immediate measure for quantification dynamic gait symmetry. The indices of up-body even the arm can be used as a factor to qualify the symmetry of human walking. The symmetry of gait should include footprint, cycle and dynamic data.
Normal walking does not need consider anything, but walking is very complex control, including central command, physical balance and coordination control, involving segments about feet, ankle, knee, hip, torso, neck, shoulder, arm and joint coordination. Any aspect of the disorder may affect gait symmetry, and some abnormalities may be compensatory or conceal. Pathological gait is often characterized by asymmetry, the selected frequencies of the movements of the limbs may deviate considerably from their eigenfrequencies and symmetry may be abandoned (Murray, 1967).

5.4 Dynamic symmetry based on dynamic time warping

In theory, the dynamic symmetry of gait is described by the properties which dynamic changed. These dynamic properties consist of three parts: position point symmetry, segment angle symmetry and joints angle symmetry.

5.4.1 Definition of dynamic symmetry

Theoretically, dynamic symmetry is described by the variability of the walking symmetric bilateral features. The dynamic symmetry is also composed of three parts, position symmetry *S(Mo)*, segment symmetry *S(SA)* and Joint symmetry *S(JA)*, as Equation (24).

$$S(D) = S(Mo) + S(SA) + S(JA) \tag{24}$$

Here, $S(Mo)=\sum_{i=1}^{8}\Delta\left(LP(t)_i, RP(t)_i\right)$, $S(SA)=\sum_{i=1}^{5}\Delta\left(L\Phi(t)_i, R\Phi(t)_i\right)$, $S(JA)=\sum_{i=1}^{5}\Delta\left(L\Theta(t)_i, R\Theta(t)_i\right)$.

And LP(t)∈{ p1, p3, p5, p7, p9, p13, p15, p17 }, RP(t)∈{ p2, p4, p6, p8, p10, p14, p16, p18 }, LΦ(t)∈{ φ3, φ5, φ9, φ11, φ13 }, RΦ(t)∈{ φ4, φ6, φ10, φ12, φ14 }, LΘ(t)∈{ θ3, θ5, θ7, θ9, θ11 }, RΘ(t)∈{ θ4, θ6, θ8, θ10, θ12 }.
The symbol *Δ* in the formulas will be described in next section. It is the DTW algorithm used to calculate the distance of two sequences with different length of them. Here consider all the symmetry properties included on upper body and lower body is want given the general definition of gait dynamic symmetry.
Considering 3-dimension, add *d={x, y, z}* to Equation (24), then we got Equation (25).

$$S_d(D) = S_d(Mo) + S_d(SA) + S_d(JA) \tag{25}$$

Here *Mo* means motion data which has 8 attributes, *SA* means Segment Angle data and *JA* means Joint Angle data, they both have 5 attributes. There is a total of 18 attributes.
Actually, we use the index like $S_x(Mo)$, $S_y(Mo)$, $S_z(Mo)$ and $S_x(SA)$, $S_y(SA)$, $S_z(SA)$ and $S_x(JA)$, $S_y(JA)$, $S_z(JA)$, not the $S_d(D)$.
The dynamic walking symmetry also has velocity and acceleration data. We got attributes as follow: $VMo \subset V(t)$, $VSA \subset \Omega\Phi(t)$, $VJA \subset \Omega\Theta(t)$, $AMo \subset A(t)$, $ASA \subset \Lambda\Phi(t)$, $AJA \subset \Lambda\Theta(t)$.
Then, we also can do calculation with three velocity equations.

Similarly, it can easily be listed out three acceleration formulas. Thus, we have three sets of attributes, each containing 18 attributes. So, considering three directions, the dynamic symmetry may include 3×18×3=162 indexes.

5.4.2 Effects of aging on dynamic symmetry

We use DTW algorithm to calculate the discrepancy between right data and left data on all attributes of all tested persons. The example of calculated result is shown as Fig. 35. We can see that somebody was more asymmetry than others on this attribute, for example number 2 and number 11 in Z direction.

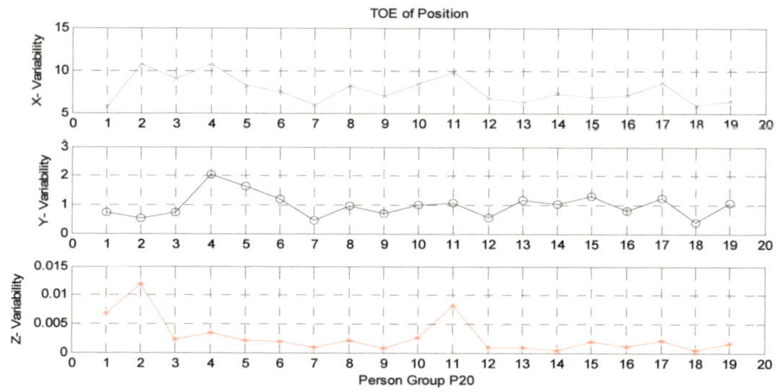

Fig. 35. Example of calculated result on one attribute

A total of 162 attribute needs for a similar calculation, to get the related discrepant values like Fig. 35. These results were used to do statistical analysis about gait symmetry.

5.5 Feature selection on dynamic symmetry

The dynamic symmetry is concerned with some direction features more meaningfully. Also some features did not reflect out gait characteristics goodly. Therefore, it is necessary in a large number of features to make a choice.

The existing gait symmetry indicators more used in accordance with the swing phase and stance phase, then neglected bilateral discrepancy of these phase while them were divided from cycles, thereby reducing the sensitivity of indicators.

We analyzed all results of the calculations and found that the dynamic symmetry is concerned with some direction indicators more meaningfully. Also some indicators did not reflect out gait characteristics goodly. Therefore, it is necessary in a large number of indicators to make a choice. In other words, it must do some feature selection.

Human walking is a complex procedure with both limb position variability and limb motion. When quantifying symmetry of walking gait, the used parameters and calculations should be chosen carefully (Karaharju-Huisnan, 2001)

5.5.1 Selected symmetric features

Although the tested persons are all healthy and walking with normal gait, but the individual may have a great difference in gait symmetry. So the general average method may result in larger bias, then it can think over use standard deviation.

Consider the three dimensional direction respectively, the gait symmetry data can available in three matrices. Then the rows of the matrix are the various attributes, and columns correspond

to the tested persons of gait symmetry data. In this way we get three $54 \times n$ matrices and n is person number. The original data come from the calculation results of bilateral discrepancy about symmetric attributes, and the calculation method was described in above sections.
For every attribute, that is the row of the matrix here, it can use the function *fa* to calculate the minimal rate of discrepant value.

$$fa = \frac{\bar{A} - A_{\min}}{A_{\max} - A_{\min}} \tag{26}$$

Here A also expresses the discrepant value on attribute A of all persons. So $\bar{A}$ is the average value of all tested persons on attribute A, the A_{min} is the minimum value of the row, and the A_{max} is the maximum value evidently.
It is clear, attribute A is the element of the set which includes all symmetric attributes about 8 position items, 5 segment angle items, 5 joint angle items and their velocity and acceleration data.
The following table shows the comparable rates on Z direction, or namely sagittal direction.

	SHO	ELB	WRI	HIP	KNE	ANK	HEE	TOE
Mo	0.166	0.157	**0.030**	**0.033**	0.113	**0.073**	0.151	0.180
VMo	0.408	0.177	**0.059**	**0.029**	0.453	**0.063**	0.289	0.292
AMo	0.266	0.305	**0.042**	**0.024**	0.262	**0.046**	0.292	0.176

Table 6. Position attributes with velocity and acceleration

	UPPERAR	FOREAR	THIGH	SHANK	FOOT
SA	0.191	**0.048**	**0.034**	**0.079**	0.132
VSA	0.147	0.109	**0.038**	**0.046**	0.225
ASA	0.220	**0.043**	**0.039**	**0.032**	0.168

Table 7. Segment angle attributes with velocity and acceleration

	SHOULDER	ELBOW	HIP	KNEE	ANKLE
JA	0.213	0.124	**0.031**	0.144	0.109
VJA	0.172	0.280	0.133	**0.069**	0.247
AJA	**0.046**	**0.042**	**0.037**	**0.048**	**0.031**

Table 8. Joint angle attributes with velocity and acceleration

There are 24 attributes in Table 6 to Table 8, and their rate less than 0.1 (see bold). In other words, these attributes have expressed better gait symmetry in this database. Also it can do same work on other two directions.
These attributes can be selected out for future testing a person whether or not symmetrical of his gait.

5.5.2 Clustering on symmetry features for classification

We use dynamic time warping (DTW) algorithm to calculate the similarity between bilateral symmetric attributes. Consider the three dimensional direction respectively, the gait symmetry data can available in three matrices. Then the rows of the matrix are the various attributes, and columns correspond to the tested persons of gait symmetry data. In this way we get three *54xn* matrices (assumed we have *n* valid test persons). The matrices data come from the calculation results of bilateral discrepancy about symmetric attributes.

Now we plan to do some clustering analysis, we need an algorithm which is no high cost on machine, but better on efficiency. Since there is a lot of clustering algorithms, for the sake of quickly carry out research and obtain some results, we have chosen the affinity propagation clustering algorithm APCLUSTER (Frey & Dueck, 2007). The reason for using this algorithm is that it not only can do clustering on data but also can pass the original information rather than random values into the clustering processing, and meanwhile the algorithm has good performance and efficiency.

Using the APCLUSTER algorithm, we have done all the attributes clustering analysis in collusion with age or height or weight and so on. But in order to facilitate description, the following example is mainly discussed on age and gait symmetric data of sagittal direction. In addition, here we had 48 valid test objects, that is to say $n=48$.

Before the data entry the clustering algorithm function for computing, we also need to normalize the data, so that the two vectors may in the same range, and then the output graphics could be easier to see clearly with the clustering results. The normalizing ways and means are as follows.

$$x_i' = \frac{x_i - \min A}{\max A - \min A} \tag{27}$$

In the Equation (27), the *A* is a vector and x_i is its element. The *minA* is the minimum element of the vector and evidently the *maxA* is the maximum element of the vector. We get normalized element data as x_i'. That is, the original vector is $A = (x_1, x_2, ..., x_n)$, and then the normalized vector is $A' = (x_1', x_2', ..., x_n')$.

Here are some examples of clustering of symmetric attributes. One clustering result is shown in Fig. 36. The inputs of the clustering algorithm are two vectors, one is the test person's gait kinetic data of Position Elbow and another is the corresponding age data.

In terms of our Fourteen-Linkage walking model, there are 54 symmetric attributes in one direction and they can be done clustering analysis. So there are 162 attributes in all for three directions. For each gait symmetric attribute to do clustering, the original symmetry data must be normalized to a vector. Take test person's age data to a vector, and take their gait data of one symmetric attribute to another vector. So the horizontal axis is normalized age data, and the vertical axis is normalized data of the symmetric attribute.

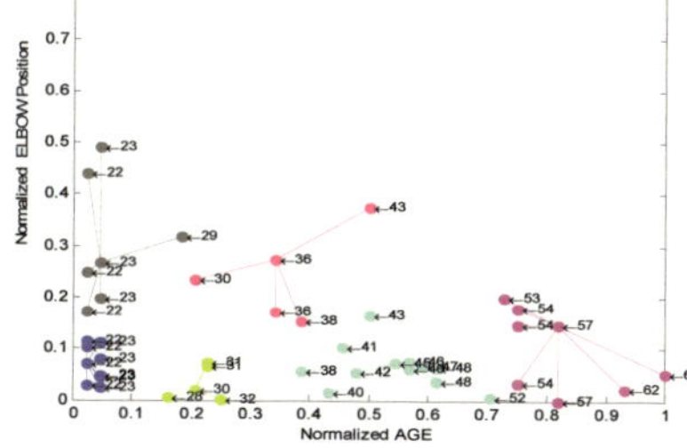

Fig. 36. Clustering on Position Elbow and Age

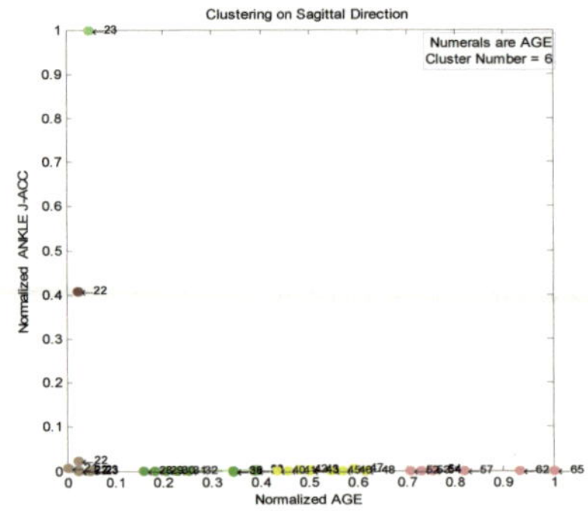

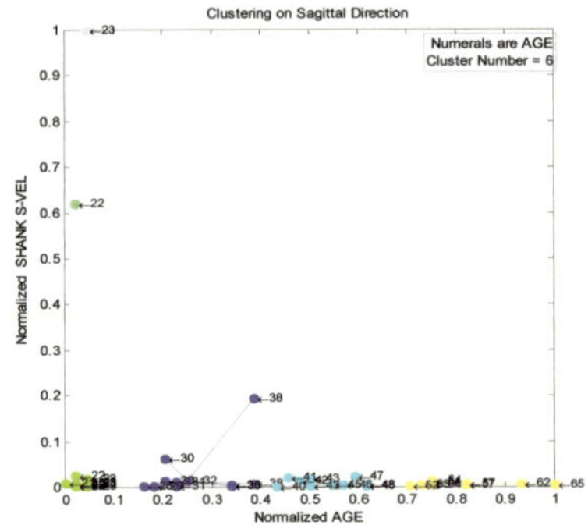

(a) Clustering on Acc of Joint Ankle and Age (b) Clustering on Vel of Segment Shank and Age

Fig. 37. More examples of clustering

For all the clustering results how to evaluate them. We used the following formula to calculate a mean square error. The formula is as follows.

$$SA = \frac{1}{m}\sum_{i=1}^{m}\left(\frac{1}{n_i}\sum_{j=1}^{n_i} D\left(G_i(j) - C_i\right)\right) \tag{28}$$

Here m is the number of clustering centres or number of clustering groups, n_i is the number of members of each group, and C_i is the clustering centre of group i, while $G_i(j)$ denoted the member-point of the group i.
The distance calculation in the Equation (28) can use the Euclid's, such as the Equation (36).

$$D_1\left(G_i(j) - C_i\right) = \sqrt[2]{\left(x_{G_i(j)} - x_{c_i}\right)^2 + \left(y_{G_i(j)} - y_{c_i}\right)^2} \tag{29}$$

Of course, the distance can be calculated using other methods, such as the absolute value of errors. This will be discussed later.
Use the Equation (28) with (29), we have calculated the values of all the clustering, choose the smallest ten values of the clustering attributes, and listed in Table 9.

Attributes of Z-dir	No.	SA using D_1	Clustering
THIGH S-ACC	1	0.035657274	6
HIP J-ACC	2	0.035669813	6
ANKLE J-ACC	3	0.035717594	6
THIGH S-VEL	4	0.035719691	6
HIP P-VEL	5	0.035746144	6
SHANK S-ACC	6	0.036075667	6
WRIST P-ACC	7	0.036825407	6
SHANK S-VEL	8	0.037846491	6
KNEE J-VEL	9	0.03882457	6
WRIST Posit	10	0.044141919	5

Table 9. Top ten minimum values of clustering results

From the Table 9, we can see that the smaller the SA value of 10 attributes has a relatively closer clustering results. In the Equation (28), if using other methods to calculate the distance, such as the Equation (30) and (31), we can compare their 10 minimum value of corresponds to the attributes and found that many of them are same, only individual attribute of exceptions, shown in Table 10. We followed the value of SA from small to large, listed from top to bottom.

$$D_2(G_i(j)-C_i)=abs(y_{G_i(j)}-y_{c_i}) \tag{30}$$

$$D_3(G_i(j)-C_i)=\left(y_{G_i(j)}-y_{c_i}\right)^2 \tag{31}$$

Although every time the results of clustering is not exactly the same, but in the course of dozens of experiments, the attributes of the top ten were similar broadly, only slightly changed before and after the order. The values of these attributes are the 10 smallest of SA which value was calculated by three different distance formula D_1, D_2, and D_3. So that you can more clearly see that most of these attributes are overlapped. This indicates that the relationship of that using any distance formula and the selection of attributes was not so great.

Attributes	**SA using D_1**	**Attributes**	**SA using D_2**	**Attributes**	**SA using D_3**
THIGH S-ACC	0.035657274	THIGH S-ACC	0.00017294	THIGH S-ACC	0.000000074
HIP J-ACC	0.035669813	HIP J-ACC	0.000523717	THIGH S-VEL	0.000001067
ANKLE J-ACC	0.035717594	THIGH S-VEL	0.000598035	HIP J-ACC	0.000003165
THIGH S-VEL	0.035719691	ANKLE J-ACC	0.000894828	ANKLE J-ACC	0.000006696
HIP P-VEL	0.035746144	HIP P-VEL	0.001258594	HIP P-VEL	0.000008664
SHANK S-ACC	0.036075667	SHANK S-ACC	0.001953265	SHANK S-ACC	0.000023426
WRIST P-ACC	0.036825407	HIP P-ACC	0.00276713	WRIST Posit	0.000090040
SHANK S-VEL	0.037846491	WRIST P-ACC	0.002879147	ANKLE P-VEL	0.000131324
KNEE J-VEL	0.03882457	WRIST Posit	0.005047818	WRIST P-ACC	0.000172132
WRIST Posit	0.044141919	SHANK S-VEL	0.00685193	HIP Joint	0.000225147

Table 10. Comparison of three distance calculation

We can see Fig. 36 and Fig. 37 are different in shape and the latter are not so beautiful shape. These clusters are very closer to the center of all its members. Perhaps because of the presence of a large offset values, so most of the clusters are compressed in a small range. We can find that clustering results displaying isolated points of the cluster, actually these points show these persons with bad gait symmetry. It is maybe the method to classify asymmetry gait and symmetry gait.

6. Conclusions and discussions

6.1 Main conclusions

In this paper, we have proposed a so-called FL model to analyze the walking stability and symmetry of different age subjects while walking on a normal pace. The most important finding is that human walking stabilities are not strictly monotone decreasing with age. Walking stability of human beings varies with age, but does not reduce in the elderly people always.

1. The variability of footprint increases with age for subjects over 30 years old, and it dramatically increases for the elderly over 60 years old, showing much less footprint stability.
2. The variability of walking cycle declines with age. That is to say, the elderly subjects have more cycle stability.
3. The variability of orbital increases with age for all subjects. In other words, the elderly has weaker orbital stability.
4. Human dynamic stability decreases with age except the twenties, which proves previous assumptions. This data mining technology not only gets the contributing dynamic stability features, but also makes the data acquisition simpler.

6.2 Discussions in clinic

Aging effects on motor control have been implicated as a key factor in adjusting posture during walking. Sensory feedback and muscular strength play important roles in maintaining stability against the presence of unpredictable external perturbations or internal variations of gait.

The footprint stability and walking stability of 20 years old subjects is less than that of over 30 years old. This cannot certify that 20 years old subjects have less quality of neuromuscular control. Nevertheless, they have much strength to control their walking pattern, so it shows a springily walking pattern. The orbital stability is strictly monotone decreasing with age. The orbital stability could express the ability of stability control more appropriately.

As we mentioned above, in most comprehensive opinions, walking stability will decrease with ageing. But the cycle stability increase with age. Why? It seems to be more confused to understand. In fact, in the three kinds of stability, only the cycle stability describes the relative stability of walking, which is the relative relationship among occurrence sequence of cycle events in a walking cycle, while the other two kinds of stability are absolute stability of posture. That indicates that the elderly subjects have a rigid and inflexible walking pattern. The elderly improves his/her walking stability by maintaining cycle stability more carefully, because it needs less strength to control cycle stability than the other two. That is to say, young subjects have more powerful muscles to control walking balance, while elderly subjects improve their walking stability by keeping their fixed walking patterns carefully. This is one of the most important findings of this paper.

One conclusion about gait symmetry is that, according to the attributes that selected out by APCLUSTER algorithm and our calculation analysis, we can classify some test objects in order to better meet the natural age groups. An appropriate grouping method to gait symmetry analysis will make the results of statistical analysis more meaningful.

Another conclusion is that, when the symmetry evaluation of normal walking gait, compared the trunk with the limbs, the latter gave larger contribution. Thus, if we have a device to measure gait symmetry of normal people, it may be wrong to wear it at the waist. It may very appropriate if we paste the device somewhere in the lower extremities (for example, shank or ankle), of course pair-wise and it will be more effective.

The next study is to further deepen the existing clustering classification, including gait symmetry attributes and the relationship between weight and height in order to obtain meaningful results. It is our goal that combining gait symmetry attributes with a number of individual characteristics may construct a simple approach to determine a test object should belong to which group.
Clinical gait analysis is aimed at revealing a key aspect of abnormal gait and impact factors, so as to assist the rehabilitation assessment and treatment, but also help to assist the clinical diagnosis, evaluation. We hope that we can evaluate the symmetry degree of a person gait accurately, not whether symmetry or asymmetry. In other words, it can't use one piece of value, but use a set of indices to evaluate. And then each index may indicate an aspect of gait symmetry.
Further research needs to determine how these gait symmetry is related to actual fall risk. At least to a certain extent, the symmetry between the low-body such as legs seems to codetermine the stability of walking.

7. Acknowledgment

This work is supported in part by the Fukushima Prefectural Foundation for the Advancement of Science and Education (No.F-18-10), Japan, Shanghai, and Shanghai Leading Academic Discipline Project (J50103), China, and Pujiang Program from Science and Technology Commission of Shanghai Municipality, China.
The basic part of this work was implemented in the Biomedical Information Technology Lab, the University of Aizu, Fukushima, Japan.

8. References

Akita, K. (1984). Image Sequence Analysis of Real World Human Motion, *Pattern Recognition*, 17(1),1984, pp. 73-83

Arif, M. Ohtaki, Y. Nagatomi, R. & Inooka, H. (2004). Estimation of the Effect of Cadence on Gait Stability in Young and Elderly People using Approximate Entropy Technique. *Measurement Science Review*, Volume 4, Section 2, 2004, pp.29-40

Cheng, J.C. & Moura, J. M.F.(). Automatic Recognition of Human Walking in Monocular Image Sequences, Journal of VLSI Signal Processing Systems, 20(1-2), 1998, pp. 107–120

Chou, PH.; Chou, YL; Su, FC.; Huang, WK & Lin, TS. (2003). Normal Gait of Children, *Biomedical Engineeringapplications, Basis & Communications,* Vol. 15 No. 4 August 2003, pp. 160-163

Corriveau, H.; Hébert R.; Raîche, M. & Prince, F. (2004). Evaluation of postural stability in the elderly with stroke, *Archives of Physical Medicine and Rehabilitation,* Vol 85, Issue 7, pp.1095-1101

Cunado, D.; Nixon, M.S. & Carter, J.N. (2003). Automatic Extraction and Description of Human Gait Models for Recognition Purposes, *Computer Vision and Image Understanding*, Vol.90, No.1, (April 2003), pp. 1-41, ISSN 1077-3142

Dockstader, S. L.; Bergkessel, K. A. & Tekalp A. M., Feature Extraction for the Analysis of Gait and Human Motion, *Proc. of 16th International Conference on Pattern Recognition,* Canada, 2002,pp.5-8.

Frey, B.J. & Dueck, D. (2007). Clustering by passing messages between data points, *Science,* Vol 315, No 5814, pp 972-976, February 2007

George, F. (2000). Falls in the Elderly, *American Family Physician,* Apr. 2000

Guo, Y.; Xu, G. & Tsuji, S. (1994). Understanding Human Motion Patterns, *Proc. The 12th IAPR International Conference on Pattern Recognition*. Vol.2, 1994, pp. 325-329

Hylton B.M.; Stephen, R. L. and Richard, C. F. (2003). Age-related differences in walking stability. *Age and Ageing* 2003, 32, pp.137-142

Karaharju-Huisnan, T.; Taylor, S.; Begg, R.; Cai, J. & Best, R. (2001). Gait symmetry quantification during treadmill walking, *The Seventh Australian and New Zealand Intelligent Information Systems Conference*, 18-21, Nov. 2001, pp. 203 - 206

Karaulova, I.A.; Hall, P.M. & Marshall, A.D.(2000). A Hierarchical Model of Dynamics for Tracking People with a Single Video Camera, *Proc of the 11th BMVC,* 2000, pp. 262-352

Kavanagh, J. (2006). Dynamic stability of the upper body during walking. *PhD thesis*, School of Physiotherapy and Exercise Science, Griffith Health, Griffith University, 2006.

Lee, L. (2003). Gait Analysis for Classification, *AI Technical Report* 2003-014, Massachusetts Institute of Technology-artificial Intelligence Laboratory, 2003.

Li, Y.; Wen, C.L.; Xie, Z. & Xu, X.H. (2003). Synchronization of batch trajectory based on multi-scale dynamic time warping, *Proceeding of the Second International Conference on Machine Learning and Cybernetics*, 2003.

Marin, L.C.; Kang, H.G. & Dingwell, J.B. (2006). Changes in the Orbital Stability of Walking Across Speeds, *Proceedings of the 30th Annual Meeting of the American Society of Biomechanics*, Blacksburg, VA, September 6-9, 2006.

Menz HB. (2002). Walking Stability in Young, Old and Neuropathic Subjects, *PhD thesis,* School of Physiology and Pharmacology, Faculty of Medicine, University of New South Wales, 2002.

Murray, M.P. (1967). Gait as A Total Pattern of Movement, *American Journal of Physical Medicine*, 46(1), 1967, pp. 290-332.

Nash, J.; Carter, J.N. & Nixon, M.S. (1998). Extraction of Moving Articulated Objects by Evidence Gathering, *Proc. of the 9th British Machine Vision Conference*, ISBN 9781901725049, Southampton, UK, September 14-17, 1998, pp. 609-618

Nichols, D.S. Balance retraining after stroke using force platform biofeedback. Phys Ther. 1997 May; 77(5), pp. 553-8

Rohr, K. (1994). Towards model-based recognition of human movements in image sequences", CVGIP: IU, 74(1), 1994, pp. 94-115

Stirling, J.R. & Zakynthinaki, M.S. (2004). Stability and the maintenance of balance following a perturbation from quiet stance, *Chaos: An Interdisciplinary Journal of Nonlinear Science,* March 2004, Volume 14, Issue 1, pp. 96-105

Sutherland, D.H.; Olshen, R.A.; Cooper, L. & Woo, SLY. (1980). The Development of Mature Walking, *Bone Joint Surg*, 1980,Vol. 62A, No. 3, pp 336-353

Whittle, M. W. (2007). *Gait Analysis: An Introduction*, (4th ed), Elsevier Health Sciences, ISBN 9780750688833, New York

Woollacott, M.H. & Tang, P.F. (1997). Dynamic Balance Control During Walking in the Older Adult: Research and its Implications, *Physical Therapy*, 7(6), 1997, pp. 646-660

Yang N.F. (2001). Coordination Analysis and Parametric Description of Human Movements, *doctoral thesis*, Tsinghua University, 2001

Yoo, J. H.; Nixon, M. S & Harris, C. J. (2002). Extracting Gait Signatures based on Anatomical Knowledge. *Proc. of BMVA Symposium on Advancing Biometric Technologies,* 2002.

Zhang, R.; Vogler, C. & Metaxas, D. (2004). Human Gait Recognition, *Proceedings of the 2004 IEEE Computer Society Conference on Computer Vision and Pattern Recognition Workshops* (CVPRW'04), 2004, pp.1-8

21

The Role of Mass Media Communication in Public Health

Daniel Catalán-Matamoros
University of Almería
Spain

1. Introduction

The mass media are intensively employed in public health. Vast sums are spent annually for materials and salaries that have gone into the production and distribution of booklets, pamphlets, exhibits, newspaper articles, and radio and television programs. These media are employed at all levels of public health in the hope that three effects might occur: the learning of correct health information and knowledge, the changing of health attitudes and values and the establishment of new health behavior.

Mass media campaigns have long been a tool for promoting public health (Noar, 2006) being widely used to expose high proportions of large populations to messages through routine uses of existing media, such as television, radio, and newspapers. Communication campaigns involving diverse topics and target audiences have been conducted for decades. Some reasons why information campaigns fail' is an early landmark in the literature. Exposure to such messages is, therefore, generally passive (Wakefield, 2010). Such campaigns are frequently competing with factors, such as pervasive product marketing, powerful social norms, and behaviours driven by addiction or habit.

Mass media campaigns have generally aimed primarily to change knowledge, awareness and attitudes, contributing to the goal of changing behaviour. There has not normally been a high expectation that such campaigns on their own would change people's behaviour. Theory suggests that, as with other preventive health efforts, mass media campaigns are most likely to reduce unhealthy attitudes if their messages are reinforced by other efforts. Reinforcing factors may include law enforcement efforts, grassroots activities, and other media messages.

There is a vast literature relating to public health information campaigns. Much theoretical literature is devoted to the topic of effectiveness of health communication strategies. Mass media campaigns have usually been one element of broader health promotion programmes with mutually reinforcing components:

1. Mobilising and supporting local agencies and professionals who have direct access to individuals within the target population.
2. Bringing together partnerships of public, voluntary and private sector bodies and professional organisations.
3. Informing and educating the public, but also setting the agenda for public debate about the health topic, thereby modifying the climate of opinion surrounding it.

4. Encouraging local and national policy changes so as to create a supportive environment within which people are more able to change their behaviour.

This book chapter will first focus on some key concepts such as communication campaigns *vs* mass media campaigns, advertising *vs* communication campaigns, the concept of risk and risk communication campaigns. Later on, the chapter will focus on the effectiveness of public health campaigns using mass media communication.

2. Communication campaigns *vs* mass media campaigns

There is often confusion between the labels campaign, communication campaign or program, media or mass media campaign, and intervention. No particular definition adequately covers current practice, and there are many local variations of what is meant by these labels. Indeed, a variety of definitions exists in the literature but the following elements of a *communication* campaign are essential (Rogers and Storey 1987).

Firstly, a campaign is purposive. The specific outcomes can be extremely diverse ranging from individual level cognitive effects to societal or structural change.

Secondly, a communication campaign is aimed at a large audience. Rogers and Storey (1987) note that 'large' is used to distinguish campaigns from interpersonal persuasive communications by one individual (or a few people) aiming to seek to influence only a few others.

Thirdly, communication campaigns have a specified time limit. This is not to state that all campaigns are short lived. For example, the initial Stanford Heart Disease Prevention Program ran for three years, however follow-up investigations were conducted over decades.

The fourth point is that a communication campaign comprises a designed set of organised activities. This is most evident in message design and distribution. Messages are organised in terms of both form and content, and responsibility is taken for selecting appropriate communication channels and media. As Rogers and Storey (1987) point out, even those campaigns whose nature or goal is emancipation or participation involve organised message production and distribution.

In summary, the term communication campaign implies that:

- it is planned to generate specific outcomes;
- in a relatively large number of individuals;
- within a specified time period; and
- uses an organised set of communication activities.

Rogers and Storey (1987) observe that in the modern communication campaign, modest changes in audience behaviour are frequently achievable, and it is important for the campaign planner to set modest and realistic expectations about what can be achieved. They argue that a health promotion campaign might be considered successful or effective if about five percent of the target (or segmented) audience does adopt measurable changes in health behaviour over the longer-term.

In this context, it is important to define a communication campaign. It should be noted that the word communication is used to highlight the fact that not all campaigns necessarily involve mass media messages, or mass media messages in isolation, and that communication campaigns may be small-scale in scope and audience reach.

3. Advertising and communication campaigns

Elliott (1987), one of Australia's leading communication practitioners, offers a particularly informative look at the differences between advertising and communication campaigns. His literature review and analyses of campaigns are especially relevant because they are based largely on experience. He defines a set of parameters for considering and planning for a campaign's realistic outcomes.

Elliott's (1987) basic premise is that the objectives and processes that are appropriate for commercial advertising are usually inappropriate for health promotion. The essential differences between advertising and health campaigns lie in the nature of the product, the processes involved in promotion and, of course, in the nature of audiences. Elliott argues that advertising by itself will not result in fundamental changes in behaviour: "Commercial products are regarded by many as trivial and superficial, not as central and ego-involving to the individual as ill health. They are positive and attractive and can be relatively easily obtained. By contrast, health publicity is largely negative: it preaches the avoidance of something negative (which is enjoyable), often involving short-term unpleasantness, for the sake of benefits that are long-term, probabilistic and not guaranteed".

Elliott (1987) draws on previous research to demonstrate once again that advertising does not have massive effects on potential consumers, as many might believe. However, he notes that small changes in market share for a particular product that are achieved as a consequence of advertising may result in greatly increased sales and profits. In this regard, it is useful to recall Rogers and Storey's (1987) assertion that a health promotion campaign might be considered successful if five percent of the target audience make long-term changes in overt health behaviour.

Commercial advertising techniques are but one element of a communication campaign using mass media. The following table is comparing communication campaigns and advertising.

Typical Communication Campaign	Typical Advertising Campaign
Persuasive focus involving response shaping, reinforcement attitude change; behavioural change.	Focus on feelings and perceptions toward product. Not attitude change.
Difficult to specify individual desires and wants.	Based on the idea of satisfying desires and wants.
Designed to meet societal or individual needs in face of risk.	May be designed to create desire and need.
May not be in line with prevailing attitudes and opinions.	Plays on prevailing attitudes and opinions.
Usually against the tide of public opinion.	Tries to stay with the tide of public opinion.
Not usually seen as a personal benefit as such and may be designed to create a social benefit.	Usually, if not exclusively, a personal benefit.

Typical Communication Campaign	Typical Advertising Campaign
Involves personal cost, sometimes even discomfort.	Cost is one of choice among competing brands.
Message is that all people should adopt or comply.	Products/services that are not accepted fail.
Often difficult to see short-term outcomes.	Easy to see, and outcomes can usually be quantified.
Reward difficult to see.	Reward easy to see.
People may express support for socially desirable behaviour but not adopt the behaviour.	
Experience is the best way to change attitudes - not mass media.	
Tries to define communication objectives as changes in individuals: • Increased salience; • Strengthening or attitude change; • More positive disposition to behave in a desired direction; • Adoption of behaviour either in the short or long term; • Awareness of unintended consequences.	Market objectives often confused with communication objectives. Focus on behavioural outcomes with intermediary objectives such as reinforcing loyal buyers' beliefs, creating consumer satisfaction, maintaining brand salience.
May be very sensitive, obtrusive, and emotional.	May not involve great emotional or affective attachment.
Many times involves an organisational bias - in the 'public service/interest'. Educational campaigns favoured even when evidence shows previous similar campaigns failed.	Campaigns that fail or result in loss lead to immediate action.
Sometimes, objectives confused with education or mere dissemination of information.	
Organisation may constrain budget, processes and structure of the campaign.	All about excitement, sexuality, self-indulgence, and even power.
Government equated to what ought to be done, what should be done, etc. It is the 'parental' mode.	Talks to the child in us.

Typical Communication Campaign	Typical Advertising Campaign
Information often perceived to be unreliable because: •Most groups perceive others as the problem or cause. •Many see themselves compliant with the attitudes or behaviour, when they are not •People seek justification for non-compliance and may give misleading information in any evaluation.	Easy to get information about products and services. Yet, advertising does not work in the way that most people believe. Advertising does not have massive effects on people.
Some people have pre-existing beliefs or ideas about 'communication'. Unrealistic expectations about what can be achieved.	Can be targeted to specific audiences or segments and expectations adjusted.
Often difficult to identify target audience. Audience could be everyone. Expectations should be low.	
Secondary audiences may be critical in facilitating change.	Secondary audiences rarely critical in mass advertising.
Usually a major objective related to a social concern.	Usually aiming at slight modifications.
Tends to be strategy based on modifications/change or slow down of undesirable attitudes/behaviours.	Tends to be strategy based on start or stop.
Slow processes involved over time.	May see instant results.
Television's commercial 'values' may be inappropriate to the campaign's message.	Commercial television is commercial television advertising; the program is designed to deliver an audience to an advertiser.

Table 1. Comparison of communication and advertising campaigns

4. The concept of risk

Most health communication campaigns involve risk, i.e. risks to people and societal risks. The concept of risk has been at the focus of contemporary thinking in recent years because of the salience and threat of environmental issues, which have received extensive public and media attention.

Giddens (1999) observes that most traditional cultures did not have a concept of risk and argues that it is a concept associated with modern industrialised civilisation, embodying ideas about controlling or conquering the future. People are forced to negotiate their lives around risks, and to rely increasingly on their own judgments about risks. Experts can assess the likelihood and magnitude of a given risk, however the public understanding of a given risk takes on meaning through our cultural practices.

One important cultural site for the production of meanings about risk is media content, including communication campaigns. The meaning of a particular health risk to various groups in society, for example, develops through the continuing and often changing representations of that risk in media content, and in scientific and medical discourses, as well as through other social and cultural practices. It is against this background of changing technical, media and public discourses that communication campaigns are planned.

Wynne (1996) argues that, just as expert opinion is central to ideas about risk, so too is lay criticism and comment. He observes that, while risks may be debated within scientific or 'public accountability' discourses, they are dealt with by most people as individuals in very specific situations, at the level of the local, the private, the mundane, the everyday, and intimate experiences. Wynne argues that it is essential to examine how perceptions of risks are constructed by local, or as he terms it 'situated', knowledge, as well as by expert knowledge. For example, there are profound differences across class, gender, race, ethnicity, age and other variables in the ways people understand, interpret and respond to health risks. Individualism might suggest a degree of choice in negotiating risk, but it is recognised that, within the power structures of our society, some people have more authority over the ways risks are identified, defined as public, and managed, than do other people. Anecdotally, it has been noted that a teenage boy will ask for the cigarette packet with the warning label 'Smoking is dangerous to pregnant women' because 'it doesn't apply to him'.

This risk perspective offers invaluable insights for communication campaign planners. This section of communication literature has one point of origin in the environmental sciences, and is particularly important to review because of its parallels to more general communication campaigns.

4.1 Risk communication campaigns

Risk communication campaigns offer the promise of resolving public conflict and diminishing fear about new large-scale technologies, such as nuclear power, as well as promoting safety campaigns concerned with science, technology and health. The concept of communication being 'in the public interest' was viewed as essential in fulfilling the public's need for information and education, or for promoting behavioural change and protective action, in the face of an anticipated disaster or hazard.

Brown and Campbell (1991) note that many western societies recognised the need for public information about science and technological risks. They link heightened interest in risk communication to the emergence of environmental impact legislation and the requirement to inform the public. The early risk communication campaign model involved 'experts'attempting to persuade the public of the validity of their scientific and technical risk assessments of a particular hazard. It is perhaps unsurprising that many such campaigns met with limited success, as the reviews outlined above would predict.

A fundamental change in campaign planning occurred with the recognition that public perceptions of various risks differed widely. This change is viewed historically as a turning point for risk communication research. As Hadden (1989) observes, old risk communication models, such as those involving scientific experts attempting to persuade lay people of the validity of their risk assessments and decisions, are impeded by lay risk perceptions, by lay people's difficulties in understanding mathematical probabilities, and by technical and scientific difficulty.

Leiss (1998) argues that the changed research direction is a shift in emphasis from 'risk' to 'communication' in the concept of risk communication. In other words, it involves 're-framing the issue of risk communication as a problem in communication theory and practice, rather than in the concept of risk'. Risks perceived as familiar, controlled, voluntary, beneficial, and fair are more likely to be acceptable to most people than risks perceived in opposite ways (Slovic, 1994). For example, the perceived health risks of chemical pollution from a local industrial factory are different from the perceived risks from exceeding the speed limit on a country road: the first is involuntary and unfamiliar, while the latter may be considered voluntary and familiar.

Risk perception research adds to the body of knowledge in this area by accounting for seemingly irrational responses by various publics to identified and potential hazards. It should be noted that the same risk might in fact produce very different perceptions in differing groups of people, depending upon the context in which the risk is understood and interpreted. These varied perceptions may produce differing policy or strategic decisions about risk 'management' and responses by 'experts'. Rowan (1996) puts forward the following argument about generalised perception factors: [The factors] are expressions of various types of power: informational, decisional and distributional. People who feel deprived of facts, unable to control their own lives, and forced to bear the costs but not the benefits are likely to be outraged by news of some new risk. To be effective risk communication must involve power sharing. Therefore, risk communication may not reduce conflict and smooth risk management. Empowerment can be destabilising in the short term, but it leads to more broadly based policy decisions, which can hold up over the long term.

As a consequence, contemporary risk communication campaigns attempt to be more individually reflexive and, as Hadden (1989) argued, the key to this approach lies in establishing dialogue or conversations with the public. The notion of one-way, top-down, expert-to-public campaigns is replaced with a more interactive process designed to empower various publics. Campaigns recognise that understanding the complexities of health issues, including technical knowledge, are not necessarily beyond ordinary people. They also highlight the potential importance of the interplay between scientific forms of knowledge and those that may be considered are more cultural. In other words, lay knowledge about health issues cannot be ignored in communication campaigns.

Hadden (1989) notes that campaigns that emphasise dialogue among parties and active participation in assessing and managing risk, are 'impeded by the lack of, or difficulty in establishing, participatory institutions'. Similarly, in a health context, Needleman (1987) notes that the goal of empowering those at risk to make an informed choice is laudable, however the risk communication intervention needs to be more than merely the dissemination of information:

The intervention must, somewhere along the line, stimulate individual and/or collective behavioural changes that reduce health risks. Otherwise, the risk communication becomes a kind of *ritualistic activity*, an end in itself in which the formal aspects of conveying risk information take precedence over their actual health impact.

The emergence of a participatory or dialogue model, which attempts to explore the disparity between expert information and a diverse public knowledge, has challenged both the 'scientific' approach to the problem of risk communication, and indeed the later perception research.

Brown and Campbell (1991) have placed risk communication models within a two by two matrix that categorises the underlying approach in terms of low and high power devolvement, and low and high community interaction. Older models of risk communication are low in terms of both power sharing and community interaction, in contrast to newer dialogue models that are high in power sharing and high in community interaction (see Table 2).

		Community Interaction	
Power sharing	Low	Low "Information" Leaflets Displays	High "Consultation" Public meetings Planning Inquiries
	High	"Canvassing" Surveys Groups Interviews	Conversation Searching focus Planning cells

Table 2. Risk Communication "Conversation Models"

The key message from Brown and Campbell's (1991) table to communication planners is to take full account of the day-to-day experiences, perceptions and cultural values of various audiences in the formative stages of any campaign. Formative research should go beyond simple quantitative measures to include more reflexive, cultural understandings of campaign messages and audiences. Of equal importance is the need to understand what various audiences bring to the reception process in their use of mass media, and their use of mass media in terms of understanding health issues.

British researcher Jenny Kitzinger, who has completed many studies on health issues, says (1994): We are none of us self-contained, isolated, static entities; we are part of complex and overlapping, social, familial and collegiate networks. Our personal behaviour is not cut off from public discourses and our actions do not happen in a 'cultural vacuum'. We make sense of things through talking with and observing other people, through conversations at home or at work; and we act (or fail to act) on that knowledge in a social context. When researchers want to explore people's understandings, or to influence them, it makes sense to employ methods, which actively encourage the examination of these social processes in action.

The notion of an active dialogue model may appear idealistic or impractical, however it should be contrasted with the failures of the dominant 'top-down' campaign strategies, which comprised the older risk communication approach. An active dialogue model examining expert and lay knowledge should not be viewed as ignoring technical health knowledge. The approach explicitly acknowledges the legitimacy of all sources of knowledge central to risk dialogue, including technical knowledge (Handmer 1995). It acknowledges the importance of investigating the interplay between various discourses, including scientific, medical, health, media, and lay discourses, in planning any communication campaign.

The key message from Brown and Campbell's (1991) table to communication planners is to take full account of the day-to-day experiences, perceptions and cultural values of various audiences in the formative stages of any campaign. Formative research should go beyond simple quantitative measures to include more reflexive, cultural understandings of campaign messages and audiences. Of equal importance is the need to understand what various audiences bring to the reception process in their use of mass media, and their use of mass media in terms of understanding health issues.

British researcher Jenny Kitzinger, who has completed many studies on health issues, says (1999): We are none of us self-contained, isolated, static entities; we are part of complex and overlapping, social, familial and collegiate networks. Our personal behaviour is not cut off from public discourses and our actions do not happen in a 'cultural vacuum'. We make sense of things through talking with and observing other people, through conversations at home or at work; and we act (or fail to act) on that knowledge in a social context. When researchers want to explore people's understandings, or to influence them, it makes sense to employ methods, which actively encourage the examination of these social processes in action. The notion of an active dialogue model may appear idealistic or impractical, however it should be contrasted with the failures of the dominant 'top-down' campaign strategies, which comprised the older risk communication approach. An active dialogue model examining expert and lay knowledge should not be viewed as ignoring technical health knowledge. The approach explicitly acknowledges the legitimacy of all sources of knowledge central to risk dialogue, including technical knowledge. It acknowledges the importance of investigating the interplay between various discourses, including scientific, medical, health, media, and lay discourses, in planning any communication campaign.

5. Content and delivery of mass media campaigns

Several aspects of mass media campaigns may influence their effectiveness. These can be categorized into variables related to message content and to message delivery.

5.1 Message content

One important aspect of message content involves the themes used to motivate the desired behavior change. Some common motivational themes in mass media campaigns to prevent unhealthy behabiours include:

- fear of legal consequences
- promotion of positive social norms
- fear of harm to self, others, or property
- and stigmatizing unhealthy behabiours as irresponsible and dangerous

The actions promoted by the campaigns also vary, ranging from messages related to abstinence or moderation to more specific behavioural recommendations. Decisions related to message content are generally made based on the opinions expressed by experts or focus groups rather than on evidence of effectiveness in changing behaviour (Randy et al., 2004).

Another aspect of message content relates to the optimal amount of anxiety produced (Witte & Allen, 2000; Tay, 2002). The effectiveness of "fear-based" campaigns is the subject of a long-standing controversy. Some level of anxiety arousal is generally seen as a desirable motivator. However, several authors have cautioned that generating intense anxiety by emphasizing the severity of a problem and the audience's susceptibility to it can cause some people to ignore or discount the campaign messages. Although this caution appears to be justified, increasing the strength of a fear appeal also increases the probability that the audience will change their attitudes, intentions, and behaviours. These changes are maximized, and defensive avoidance minimized, when the anxiety-arousing message is accompanied by specific information about actions that people can take to protect themselves. The degree of persuasion versus defensive avoidance produced may be influenced by interactions between the message content and characteristics of the recipient. For instance, strong fear appeals may be more effective for motivating a response among segments of the audience that initially do not view the problem addressed as being important or relevant to them. They may also be more persuasive to people who are already engaging in the desired behaviour.

5.2 Message delivery

A mass media campaign cannot be effective unless the target audience is exposed to, attends to, and comprehends its message. Two important aspects of message delivery are control over message placement and production quality. Control over message placement helps to ensure that the intended audience is exposed to the messages with sufficient frequency to exceed some threshold for effectiveness.

It also allows for the optimal timing and placement of those messages. This control can only be assured with paid campaigns. Those that rely solely on donated public service time may attain adequate exposure, but message placement and frequency are ultimately left to media schedulers and station management; paid advertising time always gets preferential placement. Assuming that the target audience is adequately exposed, high production quality of the campaign messages may maximize the probability that the audience will pay attention to them. High production quality may also improve the chances of eliciting the intended emotional impact.

5.3 Message pretesting

Pretesting of campaign themes and messages is also thought to be important for a successful outcome (Hornik & Woolf, 1999). Pretesting can help to assess which themes or concepts are most relevant to the target audience. It can also help to ensure that the target audience will attend to and comprehend the specific messages presented. The importance of pretesting is highlighted by an evaluation of a mass media campaign designed to prevent alcohol-related problems by encouraging drinking in moderation. No pretesting of ads was done for this campaign, and a survey conducted at midcampaign found that over a third of respondents thought that the ads were promoting alcohol consumption. Many mistook them for beer ads.

6. Effectiveness of the mass media campaigns

An Australian review of mass media health promotion campaigns in two areas, cardiovascular risk behavior and safety restraints (Redman, Spencer, and Sanson-Fisher, 1990) illustrates these moderate effects. The authors began with 24 studies but determined that only nine met their criteria for adequate evaluation methodologies. These nine were further divided into two models of media effects: media only and media as agenda-setting plus community programming. Not surprisingly, they concluded that media only campaigns had discouraging results but that most studies of media plus intensive community interventions reported significant changes in behavior. The authors, however, challenged these positive results by questioning how important the media component was to the success of such combined programs.

It is probably time to consider a fourth era and that one is characterized by the use of the internet and by paid media rather than relying on public service time. It is too early to have much data from this fourth era but the White Houses' Office of the Drug Czar's anti-drug campaign shows some promising results as do many of the state anti-smoking campaigns.

What has been missing from these previous reviews is a systematic analysis of the size of effects achieved for different types of objectives, e.g., awareness, knowledge, attitudes, and behaviors. It was addressed this gap by identifying and reviewing the extant empirical data from evaluations of mass mediated health campaigns.

Campaign Objective	Average Size of Change %
Awareness (N=16)	56
Knowledge change (N=15)	22
Attitude change (N-21)	8
Behavior change (N=29)	13

Table 3. Average changes achieved after mass-mediated health campaigns

6.1 Changing knowledge and awareness

Changing behaviour is the highest priority in any public health campaign, however, most of the mass media will change knowledge and awareness more easily than behaviour.

Theoretically, the mass media are supposed to be most effective in achieving awareness. This review supports that expectation. When measuring awareness as simple recognition of the message, up to 83% levels of awareness have been reported, with a median of 48%. Although, without a pre message measure, some of this (perhaps up to 9%) may be measurement error, e.g., a desire to please the interviewer.

Ceiling effects must also be considered. If awareness is moderately high before the campaign, there are ceilings on the increases possible and probably these increases are harder to achieve. If both pre and post levels of awareness are available, increases can be calculated based on the percent of audience possible to change. For example, if awareness of the seriousness of colon cancer was 11% prior to a campaign and 40% after it, the increase, instead of being 29% would be 29% of the possible change of 89% which is 33%.

Knowledge gain is clearly achievable using mass mediated health campaigns. When exposure is guaranteed, dramatic increases in knowledge (as large as 60%) have been observed. When exposure is not guaranteed but the campaign can saturate a community, knowledge gains around 25% seem feasible. The size of these knowledge gains decrease when the campaigns are national in scope and must compete with numerous other stimuli. Still, most of the campaigns were successful in achieving some knowledge gain, although around 10% appears to be a more achievable increase. Multi—channel campaigns appear to be much more successful than single channel, especially print only campaigns.

Below there is some evidence about changes in levels of knowledge and awareness during mass media public health campaigns:

Alcohol

- Awareness of 'sensible drinking message' unit - up from 39 to 76%, 1989–94
- Knowledge of units in popular drinks - up 300%, 1989–94
- People's accurate assessment of their own drinking - up 5%, 1990–94.

HIV/AIDS

- Changes in levels of tolerance: those in the general public who say that homosexual relations are always or mostly wrong - 74% in 1987; 44% in 1997

- Attitudes to people with HIV infection: those who think people with AIDS have only themselves to blame - 57% in 1987; 36% in 1996
- Belief that a condom protects against HIV: 66% in 1986; 95% in 1997
- Women aged 18–19 whose partners used condoms: 6% in 1986; 22% in 1993.

Folic acid

- Spontaneous awareness of folic acid - 9% in 1995; 39% in 1997
- Sales of folic acid supplements and prescription rates - up 50% in an eight-month period.

Immunisation - the Hib vaccine

- Awareness of the Hib vaccine: 5% in 1992; 89% in 1993.

Skin cancer

- Proportion of the public who thought a suntan was important -28% in 1995; 25% in 1996
- Proportion of people who say they use a sunscreen when sunbathing in this country - 34% in 1995; 41% in 1996.

Note

With complex interventions that are intended to work synergistically it is difficult to attribute impacts to particular intervention components. Also, factors external to interventions - particularly if they are about sensitive subjects - may add to or subtract from their impact.

6.2 Changing attitudes and behaviours

All but four of the 21 evaluations of these health communication campaigns showed significant attitude change. The actual amount of change varied considerably. These results suggest that if exposure is insured, considerable attitude change is possible. The greatest amount of change (+38% for an AIDS video shown in waiting rooms of STD clinics (Solomon & DeJong, 1986) a case of forced exposure. The ARTA campaign (Woods, Davis, & Stover, 1991) also demonstrated considerable attitude change, an average of 20% across five attitude items, however, it must be remembered that the ARTA camp has received unusually high exposure for a PSA campaign, and was only part of extensive media coverage of HIV/AIDS. Therefore, it is impossible to know how much of that change is attributable to the campaign itself. Some of the evaluations clearly suffered from ceiling effects and the results are difficult to interpret. The surveys measuring outcomes of one of the Cancer Prevention Awareness campaigns, for example, found pre—campaign levels of 90+% on some of the items leaving little room to measure change. In spite of more control over airing than the typical PSA, the single channel campaigns did not achieve as much attitude change.

Although behaviour is normally considered one of the most difficult objectives to achieve in mediated health campaigns, the campaigns reviewed here were quite successful. Only six of the 29 behavioral change campaigns identified failed to achieve some level of change. The average change reported was 13% should be noted that these results may be biased by the tendency toward not publishing non—significant findings.

The literature is beginning to amass evidence that targeted, well-executed health mass media campaigns can have small-to-moderate effects not only on health knowledge, beliefs, and attitudes, but on behaviours as well, which can translate into major public health impact given the wide reach of mass media. Such impact can only be achieved, however, if principles of effective campaign design are carefully followed.

There is renewed interest in the possibility of achieving policy goals through behaviour change. For example, a recent report commissioned for the Cabinet Office (Halpern and Bates, 2004) states that: 'Behaviourally based interventions can be significantly more cost-effective than traditional service delivery.' Interventions to change health-related behaviour may range from a simple, face-to-face consultation between professional and patient to a complex programme, often involving the use of mass media. This briefing looks first at the evidence on the effectiveness of interventions in changing behaviour generally; and second at the evidence concerning mass media campaigns.

A range of types of intervention aim to change 'risky' behaviours:

- Increasing knowledge and awareness of risks (through information and awareness-raising), or knowledge and awareness of services to help prevent risks
- Changing attitudes and motivations, eg through messages aimed at young people about the harm smoking does to skin and appearance
- Increasing physical or interpersonal skills, eg in using condoms, or deploying assertiveness skills to suggest that condoms be used
- Changing beliefs and perceptions, eg through interventions aimed at increasing testicular self-examination in men by raising their awareness of risk and 'normalising' self-examination
- Influencing social norms, eg by changing public perceptions of secondary smoking, or public acceptance of breastfeeding
- Changing structural factors and influencing the wider determinants of health, eg by implementing clean-air policies to decrease pollution and improve health
- Influencing the availability and accessibility of health services.

The evidence suggests that the following characteristics are the key elements for success in changing behaviour:

- Using theoretical models in developing interventions
- Intervening at multiple levels when appropriate
- Targeted and tailored (in terms of age, gender, culture, etc), making use of needs assessment or formative research
- Providing basic, accurate information through clear, unambiguous messages
- Using behavioural skills training, including self-efficacy
- Joining up services with other community provisions, eg providing transport links from community centres to clinics, or situating health services in accessible community settings
- Working with community members as advocates of appropriate services
- Providing alternative choices and risk reduction (eg promoting condom use), rather than simply telling people not to do something (eg don't take drugs, don't have sex)
- Addressing peer norms and social pressures.

Even though mass media health campaigns are used extensively, considerable debate continues over their effectiveness. This review differed from previous ones in that it included only those campaign evaluations that collected quantitative evidence of impact and it organized these data according to campaign objectives. In general, the results confirm Rogers and Storey's (1987) description of the era of moderate effects. As McGuire's (1989) hierarchy of effects model would predict, the size of the effects were greater at the earlier steps, i.e., awareness, and knowledge than the later stages of attitude change, and behavior change.

7. Lessons about implementing mass media campaigns

A report published by the National Health Services in UK (2004) on anti-smoking campaigns in the 1990s high-lighted lessons, some of which may be of general value:

- Campaigns need to contain a variety of messages – 'threatening' and 'supportive' styles of delivery can complement each other
- Anti-smoking advertising has to compete in a crowded media marketplace – a hook is needed to engage the emotions of the target audience
- Emotions can be engaged using humour, fear, sympathy or aspiration
- TV advertising, in particular, is better at jolting smokers than delivering encouraging or supportive messages
- Smokers want help and encouragement to quit
- Advertising should not tell people what they should do
- Smokers are motivated by knowing that they are not alone, and that support and help are available – they need reminding of the benefits of not smoking
- Content and style of delivery are of equal importance – smokers can accept unpalatable messages if the context is encouraging and supportive.

8. Conclusion

Mass media health campaigns clearly can be an effective tool for health promotion whether the effort is on a national or local scale. We should stop arguing whether they are more or less effective than other strategies or whether one channel is better than another. Instead we should carefully formulate our conceptual model of how we expect an intervention to work and then evaluate it accordingly. Health promotion interventions are not like pills – they are much more complex and indirect in the way they work. Therefore our evaluation designs may be very different allowing us to track a social influence process and document its effects on social and political institutions as well as on individuals.

8.1 When to use the media

It is apparent from the evidence that the media can be an effective tool in health promotion, given the appropriate circumstances and conditions. Some of the situations in which media have been found to be most appropriate are as follows.

1. When wide exposure is desired. Mass media offer the widest possible exposure, although this may be at some cost. Cost–benefit considerations are at the core of media selection.
2. When the timeframe is urgent. Mass media offer the best opportunity for reaching either large numbers of people or specific target groups within a short timeframe.
3. When public discussion is likely to facilitate the educational process. Media messages can be emotional and thought provoking. Because of the possible breadth of coverage, they can be targeted at many different levels, stimulating discussion and thereby expanding the impact of a message.
4. When awareness is a main goal. By their very nature, the media are awareness-creating tools. Where awareness of a health issue is important to its resolution, the mass media can increase awareness quickly and effectively.
5. When media authorities are 'on-side'. Where journalists, editors and programmers are on-side with a particular health issue, this often guarantees greater support in terms of space and editorial content.

6. When accompanying back-up can be provided on the ground. Regardless of whether media alone are sufficient to influence health behaviour, it is clear that the success of media will be improved with the support of back-up programmes and services.
7. When long-term follow-up is possible. Most changes in health behaviour require constant reinforcement. Media programmes are most effective where the opportunity exists for long-term follow-up. This can take the form of short bursts of media activity over an extended period, or follow-up activities unrelated to media.
8. When a generous budget exists. Paid advertising, especially on television, can be very expensive. Even media with limited reach, such as pamphlets and posters, can be expensive depending on the quality and quantity. For media to be considered as a strategy in health promotion, careful consideration of costs and benefits needs to be undertaken.
9. When the behavioural goal is simple. Although complex behaviour change such as smoking cessation or exercise adoption may be initiated through media programmes, the nature of media is such that simple behaviour changes such as immunisation or cholesterol testing are more easily stimulated through the media. In general, the more complex the behaviour change, the more back-up is required to supplement a media health programme.
10. When the agenda includes public relations. Many, if not most, health promotion programmes have an agenda which is not always explicit - maybe to gain public support or acknowledgement, to solicit political favour, or to raise funds for further programmes. Where public relations are either an explicit or implicit goal of a programme, mass media are effective because of their wide-ranging exposure.

8.2 Further research questions

1. *Evaluating message content effects:* What is the relative effectiveness and cost-effectiveness of various campaign themes (e.g., law enforcement, legal penalties, social stigma, guilt, injury to self and others) for reducing unhealthy behaviours? For influencing public support for stronger prevention activities?
2. *Evaluating message delivery effects:* What is the dose–response curve for varying levels of advertising exposure (e.g., none, light, moderate, and heavy)? Does the shape of this curve vary according to message content and the outcome evaluated? What is the relative effectiveness and cost-effectiveness of different media types (TV, radio, etc.)? Paid advertising and public service announcements? What is the optimal exposure schedule for public health mass media campaigns (e.g., intermittent waves of messages vs a steady flow)? How should mass media campaigns be adapted to the changing media environment (e.g., market segmentation, Internet, message filtering devices)?
3. *Evaluating message/recipient interactions:* To what extent are certain population groups more or less likely to be influenced by mass media campaigns? Are some themes more likely than others to influence "hard-to-reach" target groups (e.g., enforcement themes for "hard-core" drinking drivers)?
4. *Improving research design:* What measurement issues need to be addressed to improve assessment of media and message exposure? What research designs can best address problems in measuring exposure?

9. References

Brown, J. & Campbell, E. (1991). Risk communication: Some underlying principles. *Journal of Environmental Studies*, Vol. 38, 1991, 297-303.

Elliott, B.J. (1987). *Effective Mass Communication Campaigns: A Source Book of Guidelines*. Elliott & Shanahan Research, North Sydney.

Giddens, A. (1999). Risk and Responsibility. *Modern Law Review,* Vol. 62, No. 1, 1999, 1-10.

Hadden, S.G. (1989). Institutional Barriers to Risk Communication. *Risk Analysis,* Vol. 9, 1989, 301–308.

Halpern, D. and Bates, C. (2004) Personal responsibility and changing behaviour: the state of knowledge and its implications for public policy. London: Cabinet Office, Prime Minister's Strategy Unit. www.strategy.gov.uk/files/pdf/pr.pdf

Hornik, R., Woolf, K.D. (1999). Using cross-sectional surveys to plan message strategies. *Soc Marketing Q,* Vol. 5, 1999; 34–41.

Kitzinger, J. (1999). Researching risk and the media. *Health, risk & Society,* Vol. 1, No. 1, 1999, 55-69.

Leiss, W. (1998). Risk Communication and public knowledge. In: *Communication Theory Today,* Crowley, D. &. Mitchell, D. (Eds.), Polity Press, Oxford.

McGuire, W.J. (1989). Theoretical Foundations of Campaigns. In: *Public Communication Campaigns,* Rice, R.E. & Atkin, C. (Eds.), 43-65, Newbury Park, Sage Publications, CA.

Needleman, C. (1987). Ritualism in communicating risk information. *Sci Tech Hum Values,* Vol. 12, 1987, 20-25.

Noar, S.M. (2006). A 10-Year Retrospective of Research in Health Mass Media Campaigns: Where Do We Go From Here?. *Journal of Health Communication: International Perspectives,* Vol. 11, No. 1, 2006, 21 - 42, 1087-0415.

Randy, W.E., Shults, A., Sleet, D., Faahb, J.L., Thompson, R.S. & Rajab, W. (2004). Effectiveness of Mass Media Campaigns for reducing drinking and driving and alcohol-involved crashes. Am J Prev Med, Vol. 27, No. 1, 2004, 57-65.

Redman, S., Spencer, E.A., & Sanson-Fisher, R.W. (1990). The role of mass media in changing health-related behavior: a critical appraisal of two models. *Journal of Health Promotion of Australia,* Vol. 7, No. 2, 1990, 91-99.

Rogers, E.M. & Storey, J.D. (1987). Communication campaigns. In: *Handbook of communication science,* C. Berger & S. Chaffee (Eds.), 817-846, Newbury Park, Sage, CA.

Rowan, F. (1996). The high stakes of risk communication. *Preventive Medicine,* Vol. 25, 1996, 26-29.

Slovic, P. (1994). Perceptions of risk: Challenge and paradox. In: *Future and risk management,* Brehmer, B. & Sahlin, N.E. (Eds.), 63-78, Kluwer Academic Publishers, NY.

Solomon, D.S. (1982). Health campaigns on television. In: *Television and behavior*. Pearl, D., Bouthilet, L. & Lazar, J. (Eds.). NIMH Technical Reviews, Washington, DC.

Szerzynski, B., & Wynne, B. (1996). *Risk, Environment and Modernity. Towards a new Ecology,* SAGE Publications, London.

Tay, R. (2002). Exploring the effects of a road safety advertising campaign on the perceptions and intentions of the target and nontarget audiences to drink and drive. *Traffic Inj Prev,* Vol. 3, 2002, 195–200.

Wakefield, M.A., Loken, B. & Hornik, R.C. (2010). Use of mass media campaigns to change health behaviour. The Lancet, Vol. 376, No. 9748, Oct 2010, 1261-71, 0140-6736.

Witte, K., Allen, M. (2000). A meta-analysis of fear appeals: implications for effective public health campaigns. *Health Educ Behav,* Vol. 27, 2000, 591–615.

Woods, D.R., Davis, D., & Westover, B.J. (1991). "American Responds to AIDS": Its content, development process, and outcome. *Public Health Reports,* Vol. 106, No. 6, 1991, 616-622.

22

The Unresolved Issue of the "Terminal Disease" Concept

Sergio Eduardo Gonorazky
Hospital Privado de Comunidad de Mar del Plata, Argentina

1. Introduction

1.1 Prefatory emarks

"I have already told you with what care they look after their sick, so that nothing is left undone that can contribute either to their case or health; and for those who are taken with fixed and incurable diseases, they use all possible ways to cherish them and to make their lives as comfortable as possible. They visit them often and take great pains to make their time pass off easily; but when any is taken with a torturing and lingering pain, so that there is no hope either of recovery or ease, the priests and magistrates come and exhort them, that, since they are now unable to go on with the business of life, are become a burden to themselves and to all about them, and they have really out-lived themselves, they should no longer nourish such a rooted distemper, but choose rather to die since they cannot live but in much misery; being assured that if they thus deliver themselves from torture, or are willing that others should do it, they shall be happy after death: since, by their acting thus, they lose none of the pleasures, but only the troubles of life, they think they behave not only reasonably but in a manner consistent with religion and piety; because they follow the advice given them by their priests, who are the expounders of the will of God. Such as are wrought on by these persuasions either starve themselves of their own accord, or take opium, and by that means die without pain. But no man is forced on this way of ending his life; and if they cannot be persuaded to it, this does not induce them to fail in their attendance and care of them: but as they believe that a voluntary death, when it is chosen upon such an authority, is very honourable, so if any man takes away his own life without the approbation of the priests and the senate, they give him none of the honours of a decent funeral, but throw his body into a ditch."[1] Sir Thomas More (1516)

In 1977, Leon Eisenberg suggested a distinction should be made between the terms "disease" and "illness" (Eisenberg, 1977): *"The dysfunctional consequences of the Cartesian dichotomy have been enhanced by the power of biomedical technology. Technical virtuosity reifies the mechanical model and widens the gap between what patients seek and doctors provide. Patients suffer "illnesses"; doctors diagnose and treat "disease". Illnesses are experiences of discontinuities in states of being and perceived role performances. Diseases, in the scientific paradigm of modern medicine, are abnormalities in the function and/or structure of body organs and systems. Traditional healers also redefine illness as disease: because they share symbols and metaphors consonant with lay beliefs, their healing rituals are more responsive to the psychosocial context of illness…When physicians dismiss illness because ascertainable "disease" is absent, they fail to meet their socially assigned responsibility. It is essential to reintegrate "scientific" and "social" concepts of disease and illness as a basis for a functional system of medical research and care."*.

---

[1] Direct quotations appear in italics.

Allan Young (Young, 1982) draws a further distinction between "disease", "illness" and "sickness": *"DISEASE retains its original meaning (organic pathologies and abnormalities). ILLNESS is essentially the same, referring to how disease and sickness are brought into the individual consciousness. SICKNESS (...) is redefined as the process through which worrisome behavioral and biological signs, particularly ones originating in disease, are given socially recognizable meanings, i.e. they are made into symptoms and socially significant outcomes. Every culture has rules for translating signs into symptoms, for linking symptomatologies to etiologies and interventions,and for using the evidence provided by interventions to confirm translations and legitimize outcomes. The path a person follows from translation to socially significant outcome constitutes his sickness. Sickness is, then, a process for socializing disease and illness"*. These ideas were later reinstated by other authors and publications, such as The Hastings Center Report: The Goals of Medicine. Setting New Priorities (Callahan et al., 1996). In this document, "disease" is defined as a physical or mental dysfunction, based on a deviation from the statistical standard, which causes impairment or increases the probability of an early death; "illness" is understood as an individual's subjective perception that his or her physical or mental wellness is either altered or absent, affecting the ability to perform normal daily activities as a consequence; "sickness" is the social perception of an individual's health status, usually, an external perception that this individual has physical or mental difficulties.

The different realities of patients, their families, physicians and society at large, which will be discussed below, lead us to consider an anthropological perspective in which the medical point of view of **terminal disease** is integrated with another that takes into account the suffering patients and their families undergo (**terminal illness**) and with the polymorphous interpretation made by the family and society (**terminal sickness**).

If we consider that the meaning of a word is made up of the set of relations (both situational and paradigmatic) reflected in that word, and that those relations are built all through the history of mankind and each individual's own history, we should understand that it is not possible to provide univocal answers in the case of such an expression as "terminal disease", which carries multiple meanings with it.

The medical description of terminal disease, the suffering patients and their families undergo, and the view society holds are often mutually and internally contradictory. The situation arising out of this is both complex and dynamic, hence the need for a dialogue focused on the suffering endured by the "protosufferers" (patients and next of kin) when it comes to making decisions involving them.

The meaning of terminal disease should ultimately be a single, non-reproducible, contextualized construction, one which embodies the dialectic contribution made by the various agents involved.

The purpose of this paper is to question the pretended univocity of the definition of terminal disease as it is understood from an exclusively unidimensional approach (the medical one), definition which, from a functional point of view, turns out to be a rigid concept that imposes itself over the needs of patients, their families, and even healthcare workers.

It should be borne in mind that the definition of terminal disease is not intended to be solely descriptive, but, as it is later observed, it has a determining functional nature. Based on it, it could be determined whether a particular treatment is futile or not, or if therapeutic obstinacy or neglect is evidenced, or whether those who are close to the patient (next of kin, caregivers and therapists) are respectful of the patient's dignity.

It could be said that decision-making from a functional perspective frequently fails to overtly specify whether a given disease is terminal or not. However, an in-depth look into the matter reveals that it does so implicitly, in so far as it considers whether the implementation of measures which will unnecessarily prolong life and/or the suffering of patients and their families is unsubstantial or not.

The concept of terminal disease will be discussed all through this paper; however, it is convenient to clarify *ad initio* that, in fact, there are no terminal diseases but terminal patients, and this is precisely the main guiding principle behind this work. Reification of the concept of terminal disease, disregarding the terminal patient, frees many from the burden of disentangling the complex, dynamic nature of each situation in particular and the commitment which that entails.

2. Terminal disease, terminal illness and terminal sickness

2.1 Terminal disease or the medical point of view

The definition of terminal disease is seemingly simple, clear and univocal. The Spanish Society of Palliative Care (Sociedad Española de Cuidados Paliativos [SECPAL, n.d.]), for example, provides the following definition:

"In the case of terminal diseases, a number of elements should be present. These elements are important not only to consider a terminal disease as such but also to determine the most suitable therapy.

The key elements are:

1. *Presence of advanced, progressive, incurable disease.*
2. *Reasonable unresponsiveness to the specific treatment.*
3. *Presence of multiple, changing, severe symptoms or problems of multifactorial origin.*
4. *Great emotional impact on the patient, the family and healthcare workers, closely related to the implicit or explicit immediacy of death.*
5. *Life expectancy of six months or less.*

This complex situation requires the uninterrupted provision of appropriate care and support.

End-stage CANCER, AIDS, motor neuron disease, specific organ system failure (kidney, heart, liver failure, etc.) meet these criteria to a greater or lesser extent. Traditionally, providing adequate care to end-stage cancer patients has been the raison d'etre of Palliative Care.

It is ESSENTIAL not to consider a potentially curable patient as terminally ill."

Some of the controversial aspects of this definition will be discussed below. It is worth pointing out, however, that this definition is not to be rejected entirely. In fact, it could be accepted as a guideline, but not as a dogma that should be asserted over concrete decisions.

2.1.1 How advanced, incurable and progressive a disease should be to be considered terminal

2.1.1.1 Advanced disease and life expectancy

An 84-year-old male patient has a 10-year history of dementia. For the last three years, he has been bedridden, unable to walk, with incontinence of bowel and bladder. His ability to communicate is nearly lost (he occasionally answers "yes" or "no" to questions), he does not react to simple commands, and he rarely recognizes loved ones. He does not present swallowing difficulties but is unable to feed himself (he requires help from a caregiver). Could this patient be considered terminally ill?

In his statement for the Association of Alzheimer Disease, SG Post expresses that *"the advanced stage of dementia includes a loss of all or nearly all ability to communicate by speech, inability to recognize loved ones in most cases, loss of ambulation without assistance, incontinence of bowel and/or bladder, and some weight loss due to swallowing difficulties. The advanced stage is generally considered terminal, with death occurring on average within two years."* (Post, 2007).

The preceding definition extends life expectancy from the maximum of six months, as stated by the Spanish Society of Palliative Care, to an average of two years. This evident inconsistency of criteria shows us that the definition of the concept from the medical perspective is not univocal.

At the age of 42, Stephen Jay Gould, the famous paleontologist, was diagnosed with an abdominal mesothelioma and was informed that the median mortality after discovery was 8 months. In his article "The Median isn't the Message", Gould explains why it is the variance more than the mean, or the median in his case, what should be taken into account to establish a disease prognosis. The reason he gives is that the most common statistical measures of central tendency (either the mean or the median) are useful only to define a Platonic state but not the hard reality of the dispersion of results (Gould, 1985). Gould died at the age of 62.

Defining how advanced a disease is by establishing a period of time which is not only arbitrary but dubious as an estimate seems to be far from functional when it comes to making the kind of decisions we are concerned with. In other words, as it was once expressed by Sir William Osler (Osler, n.d.), *"Medicine is a science of uncertainty and an art of probability"*.

2.1.1.2 Incurable, untreatable and disease-modifying drugs

In medicine, it is well-known that incurable is not synonymous with untreatable. Also, for certain diseases, there are therapies which, without being necessarily palliative, modify disease progression without curing it. In other words, disease progression in a group of subjects receiving a new drug may be statistically better relative to a particular aspect when compared to an untreated group.

The fact that a disease is incurable but its progression may be slowed down creates a grey area between "curable and incurable". Disease-modifying drugs are useful but they do not cure.

Furthermore, certain measures considered therapeutic or even curative in some cultures are not accepted in others. A clear example is the rejection of blood transfusion by Jehovah's Witnesses.

2.1.1.3 Lack of primary injury progression is not synonymous with lack of disease progression

Non-progressive secondary injuries may put a patient at such a risk that, in the event of complications, they may cause his or her death.

Patients with severe sequelae, such as irreversible permanent vegetative state following anoxic or traumatic brain injury, who exhibit no progression of their primary brain injury, may be maintained in that state through intensive care procedures. These procedures are usually implemented to prevent the occurrence of complications or to reverse them if they occur. Yet, in settings with less sophisticated means, patients are expected to progress towards death. Anencephaly could be mentioned as another example of nonviable disease, possibly comparable to an irreversible vegetative state; it is terminal but it does not meet the progressiveness criteria required in the definition.

In spite of the lack of primary injury progression, there could be modifications which may improve or worsen the clinical condition, thus challenging the univocal definition of the term "progressive disease".

Furthermore, there are dimensions in the progression of a disease which cannot be seen from an exclusively biological perspective, such as the social and psychological impact that failure of recovery has on patients, their families and even the community (and this impact can certainly be progressive). In other words, there may not be an "unfavourable" progression in biological terms but there could be one from a psychological and/or social point of view.

2.1.2 Discussion

While a two-valued logic provides us with safe, clear definitions (advanced vs. not advanced, progressive vs. non-progressive, incurable vs. curable), our patients' individual situations, seen from a medical perspective, challenge us to adhere to a multi-valued, even fuzzy, logic, in which "things are to the extent they are, and things are not to the extent they are not", and in which "nothing exists by itself but in relation to other things".

If we understand that there are no diseases but patients, that there are no absolute, timeless realities but concrete, historical circumstances in which individuals live, get sick and die, the criteria to define a disease as advanced, progressive or incurable vary, and, as we have already mentioned, they need to be specified by medical professionals considering each individual case.

2.2 Terminal illness or the patient's perspective

Recently published news articles in Argentina (Carbajal, 2011a, 2011b, 2011c, 2011d, 2011d), described the situation of a 19-year-old girl (MG) who had been diagnosed with neurofibromatosis type I (Von Recklinghausen disease). The girl considered she had an "advanced" form of the disease. She was bedridden and had severe shortness of breath; however, she was in full possession of her mental faculties. *"It is not fair to live like this. Nearly all of my body is numb, and whatever I feel is painful. I can't even hold a cup in my hand, and I'm forced to lie down all the time. I choke, I can't breathe. This is not a life worth living; I don't want to go on like this. But they don't understand, they think one can always pull through. But I can't bear it any longer, I simply can't"*, one of the articles transcribed. Despite her medical condition, MG was lucid and was very clear when expressing her position. Physicians considered that hers was not a terminal disease; nonetheless, the patient wanted to be given sedatives to induce unconsciousness and stop feeling pain.

The case became known to the public. Melina, that was her name, was apparently sedated in the end, and died a few days after the media published her case (Carbajal, 2011e, 2011f).

Ramón Sampedro was a patient who was not considered terminal from a medical point of view. He was quadriplegic due to a traumatic cervical spine injury, and was bedridden for more than 30 years as a consequence of this. In his "Letters from Hell", where he claimed to be living in, he expressed (Sampedro, 2004), (translation is mine):

"To no avail, I say to them: No!, I am dead!,

I tell them I can't speak like them
Because it is absurd to speak as human beings do
And they don't let me be, either dead or alive
These crazy, freaked-out nuts"

A different situation is that of Stephen Hawking's, who could find his purpose in life despite having a progressive disease and being severely disabled. Yet, no comparison between these two patients' moral values is intended, this last example has been introduced to show that personal experiences with a particular medical condition vary greatly.

In his 1845 short story, "The Facts in the Case of Mr. Valdemar" (Poe, 1845), Edgar Allan Poe presents a visionary metaphor of today's intensive care units with their intervened deaths which is worth commenting on. Mr. Valdemar, who is *"in articulo mortis"*, accepts to undergo an experimental hypnotic technique and he is suspended between life and death for a period of seven months. During that time, he is not allowed to die but he cannot be awakened either. The objective of the investigator carrying out the experiment is to find out up to what extent or for how long, the hypnotic process would be able to prevent death from occurring. During the 7-month experiment, Mr. Valdemar is visited by physicians and friends and receives continuous nursing care. All through this process, however, Mr. P (the mesmerist) is unable to make decisions. It is Mr. Valdermar himself who, given the investigator's inability, begs: *"For God´s sake! -quick!-quick!–put me to sleep-or, quick!– waken me!–quick!–I say to you that I am dead."*.

In light of a helpless but grandiose medicine, which does not allow either to live or to die, it is the undead who demands changing the status quo.

JV, a 38-year old male patient who suffered from amyotrophic lateral sclerosis, was fully aware of his disease and its prognosis. Percutaneous gastrostomy for enteral feeding was suggested when he was still able to undergo the procedure, but he rejected it. He also expressly refused in writing to receive invasive or non-invasive ventilatory support of any kind. He was later hospitalized due to an infectious complication. At that moment, he was unable to express himself orally (he communicated what he wanted to say by pointing at letters on a sign with his right index finger). To our surprise, when his wife asked him whether he still rejected ventilatory support, despite not being dyspneic at that time, he reproached her for such a question because it seemed to suggest she wanted him to die. Then, he indicated that he obviously wanted to be provided with ventilatory support if it was required. A few days later, it was necessary to implement the support. The patient survived 4 months in the intensive care unit and finally died.

In 2008, the case of a 13-year-old girl named Hannah Jones became known to the public. She had previously suffered from leukemia and refused to have a heart transplant to treat a chemotherapy-induced cardiomyopathy (BBC News, 2008). Her attending physicians sought court intervention to force her to undergo surgery. The media informed that physicians recommended the transplant as the only solution available, but they could not guarantee survival after the surgery. And, if she survived, her leukemia could relapse and her new heart would last ten years at the most. Hannah decided that she had suffered long enough and told her physicians that she preferred to spend the rest of her life without having to go through another traumatic treatment. Her parents were supportive of her decision, but the hospital where she was being treated in Herefordshire interfered with Hannah's decision. Physicians warned Hannah's mother, Kirsty (a nurse), that they would apply for a court order at the High Court in London to remove the child's custody from them. The following day a child protection officer visited Hannah at home. Nobody knows what Hannah said to the officer, but, a few hours later, the Hospital Legal Department withdrew the legal action. *"The girl is firm in her decision to refuse surgery"*, said the child protection officer. *"It is incredible that such a young person who has gone through so many things has the courage to defend her rights"*, her father Andrew proudly said.

Hannah did not have what in medical terms would be considered a terminal disease; however, she made the decision to refuse the suggested treatments with apparent autonomy and competence. She had already decided that her illness was terminal. She could have been wrong, but so could have been her physicians thus prolonging her suffering.

Dr Tony Calland, chairman of the British Medical Association's ethics committee, is quoted in the same BBC News article: *"a child of Hannah's age was able to make an informed decision to refuse treatment". Dr Calland said he understood why a doctor might have taken this action. He said: "I think some doctors take the view that they must intervene and they are making that decision in what they see as the best interests of the patient. But of course best interests of patients is not just the best medical interests - it's the overall holistic interests of the person in general." He added: "I think obviously a child of 13 with these circumstances should be perfectly capable of making the decision and particularly when supported by the parents.".*

In the city of Mar del Plata, Argentina, a patient was admitted to the General Acute Care Hospital (Hospital Interzonal de Agudos) with a history of diabetes and gangrene in the right foot. Above-knee leg amputation was performed on August 9, 1995 after obtaining consent from the patient (he had denied consent previously). On August 16, 1995 he was diagnosed with necrosis of the left first and fourth toes, cellulitis and edema involving the entire foot were also observed. On August 23, 1995 he was diagnosed with vascular ischemia of the left lower limb. Below-knee amputation was indicated, but the patient refused to undergo this procedure. The following was documented with respect to his refusal: *"The patient refuses to receive treatment, his decision being entered into his medical record. Considering that the patient is lucid, we deem it advisable to notify the Direction in the event of a legal issue."*. The patient was perfectly lucid and fully aware that he was putting his life at risk. The Hospital Ethics Committee stated that patient autonomy should be respected. However, court intervention was sought, and the judgment was granted in favour of the patient and his decision (Hooft, 1995).

As we have already mentioned, a typical example in which the concept of "terminality" differs between patients and physicians is that of Jehovah's Witnesses. A Jehovah's Witness patient who presents with hemorrhage caused by a treatable condition prefers to refuse blood transfusion and die rather than violate his or her religious beliefs for a treatment not considered as such.

Autonomous and competent patients who refuse a particular treatment and put their lives at risk when making such a decision provide their own concept of "terminality", different from their physicians' concept.

The poet (Victor Jara) expresses *"life is eternal in five minutes"*. A few days or hours stolen from death may be enough for some patients to reconcile with their loved ones or to say goodbye to them. Conversely, a few minutes or hours, or sometimes months or years, may be tormentous for other patients because of the physical, mental and/or moral suffering they have to endure during that time. Those who find meaning in the agony of the last moments of life are no better than those who no longer find a reason to go on living.

2.2.1 Discussion

In any case, patients themselves are the ones who have to endure suffering. Our role as family members, friends and healthcare providers is to cooperate with them in the construction of their own meaning of life and death, as long as they allow us to do so.

2.3 Terminal sickness or the perspective of the family, caregivers, next of kin, society and the state

There is a large number of well-known cases published in the medical literature or by the media in which patients and/or their families have spent long years in distress struggling to have an illness recognized as terminal in order to allow the sufferer to die with dignity and loved ones to mourn their loss.

The hegemonic line of thought, however, considers death as a failure that should be delayed as long as possible. Sufferers (patients and/or their families) are thus severed from the decision-making process, and medicine, the courts and religious institutions are allowed to exercise their power over other people's bodies even if, after a long pilgrimage, sufferers are granted what they have asked for.

We have already commented on situations in which patients refused treatments which they considered futile or required measures to be taken so that they could die with dignity. We also examined the case of a patient who, having an illness which his physicians considered had reached its end-stage, first refused and then asked for support measures.

Greater is the complexity of the cases in which patients are unable to express themselves and it is their family who ask for withdrawal of life-sustaining measures in the absence of the patients' explicit statement of their will to do so.

Patients in an irreversible permanent vegetative state are not considered terminally ill in the applicable definitions. Due to their brain injury, these patients have neither self-awareness nor awareness of the surroundings. They do not feel pain but they are able to breathe autonomously. They may have some reflex activity, including eye movements, grimacing and grunting. They are unable to take food or fluids by mouth and they require tube feeding for nutrition and hydration. The sleep-wake cycle is preserved and, if they are provided with adequate care, they do not look critically ill at first sight. A distinction should be made, however, between the irreversible permanent vegetative state and the potentially reversible persistent vegetative state. After coming out of a coma due to brain injury, a patient progresses to a vegetative state if sufficient sparing of the brain stem allows for preservation of his or her autonomic functions. Recovery from a vegetative state is unlikely after three months if brain damage is anoxic or a year if brain damage is traumatic; in those cases, the vegetative state is said to be permanent. "Vegetative" does not mean that the patient is a vegetable but that the so-called vegetative functions are preserved (breathing, heart rate, body temperature control, blood pressure, gastrointestinal motility, etc.) (The Multi-Society Task Force on PVS, 1994a, 1994b). The vegetative state must be distinguished from the minimally conscious state, in which the patient shows minimal self-awareness and awareness of the surroundings.

Our purpose is to show that these medical conditions are seen from different perspectives by families, physicians, the courts and society at large. Some of them consider that these patients are terminally ill and that they are being subjected to futile treatments, whereas others see them as living patients who are comparable to other disabled individuals and whose life should be sustained regardless of their families' wish or the wish they may have expressed when they were competent.

In 1975, 21-year-old Karen Ann Quinlan suffered a cardiopulmonary arrest after ingesting a combination of alcohol and tranquilizers. She subsequently went into a permanent vegetative state and was placed on mechanical ventilatory support. Hers was the first case in which parents requested withdrawal of the ventilator. Physicians turned down the request, so Mr. and Mrs. Quinlan resorted to the courts. New Jersey Supreme Court authorized the family's request relying on the substituted judgment standard, which is intended first to determine the individual's own needs and wishes and then to decide on how to proceed once his or her personal value system is known. In Quinlan's case, the court sought to protect the autonomy of an individual who was unable to defend it on her own by honouring her parent's opinion (Beauchamp, Childress, 1999). Additionally, as Annas clearly recalls: "*Since the court believed that the physicians were unwilling to withdraw the ventilator because of the fear of legal liability, not precepts of medical ethics, it devised a mechanism to grant the physicians prospective legal immunity for taking this action. Specifically, the New Jersey Supreme Court ruled that after a prognosis, confirmed by a hospital ethics committee, that there is "no reasonable possibility of a patient returning to a cognitive, sapient state," life-sustaining treatment can be removed and no one involved, including the physicians, can be held civilly or criminally responsible for the death.*" (Annas, 2005).

Once ventilatory support was withdrawn, Karen continued breathing on her own and lived for another 9 years (10 years since she had suffered the cardiopulmonary arrest) still sustained by tube feeding. Her parents did not consider requesting discontinuation of artificial feeding (Kinney et al, 1994), which could mean that Karen's parents considered that the need for ventilatory support indicated that her condition was terminal, while the other life-sustaining measures placed her in a different situation.

Nancy Cruzan's case provides us with another context. Nancy was in a permanent vegetative state as a result of a car accident she had had in 1983 (Annas, 1990). She required tube feeding but not ventilatory support. When her parents were certain that she would not recover, they requested discontinuation of the treatment stating that this was Nancy's desire as expressed by her in the past. Physicians did not accept treatment withdrawal, but the trial court authorized it. On appeal, the Supreme Court of Missouri reversed the trial court judgment and so did the U.S. Supreme Court (it was the first time that the U.S. Supreme Court had heard a case like this). Among the reasons provided, it was stated that even though a patient had the right to refuse treatment, the same decision made by surrogates on behalf of a previously competent patient could not be accepted. It was also expressed that the State should in principle favour the preservation of life and that the patient's decision as to the withdrawal of treatment should be practically indubitable (halfway between what society considers in that situation and what the law considers beyond any reasonable doubt). This last requirement limited the decision-making capacity of Nancy's parents, who loved her beyond doubt.

A new petition was submitted to the Supreme Court of Missouri, and the court rejected it again stating that there was no clear and convincing evidence that Nancy would have refused tube feeding had she been alive. It was also added that artificial nutrition and hydration were considered ordinary treatment procedures which should be provided under any circumstances, and that the State's interest in preserving life was absolute and unconditional. The State Court also expressed that although the patient is in an irreversible vegetative state, "***She is not dead. She is not terminally ill. Medical experts testified that she could live another***

thirty years"[2] (Cruzan vs. Hamon, 1989). The U.S. Supreme Court, in turn, pointed out that tube feeding was **an extraordinary treatment procedure which could be discontinued** and that if there was enough evidence of the patient's wishes, artificial feeding could be removed. It also expressed that even though the State of Missouri should set the standard to discern what the patient's wishes were, it did not have the absolute right to deny refusal of treatment. In light of new evidence provided by Nancy's friends and acquaintances with respect to what her wishes would have been in her situation, the Court of Missouri authorized the removal of artificial nutrition and hydration. The treatment was discontinued on December 15, 1990 and Nancy died 12 days later (Cruzan vs. Director, 1990).

Although the definition of terminal disease was not the main discussion in this case, as seen above, it is explicitly mentioned by the Supreme Court of Missouri: "***She is not terminally ill***".

Dissenting opinions as regards Nancy's state were expressed by the U.S. Supreme Court Justices and the President of the Supreme Court of Missouri, which are worth transcribing (Cruzan vs. Director, 1990).

Justice Brennan from the U.S. Supreme Court, with whom Justices Marshal and Blackmun joined, expressed the following (bold emphasis is mine):

"*Medical technology has effectively created a* ***twilight zone of suspended animation where death commences while life****, in some form, continues. Some patients, however, want no part of a life sustained only by medical technology. Instead, they prefer a plan of medical treatment that allows nature to take its course and permits them to die with dignity.*"

"*Nancy Cruzan has dwelt in that twilight zone for six years... The Court would make an exception here. It permits the State's abstract, undifferentiated interest in the preservation of life to overwhelm the best interests of Nancy Beth Cruzan, interests which would, according to an undisputed finding, be served by allowing* ***her guardians to exercise her constitutional right to discontinue medical treatment****. Ironically, the Court reaches this conclusion despite endorsing three significant propositions which should save it from any such dilemma. First, a competent individual's decision to refuse life-sustaining medical procedures is an aspect of liberty protected by the Due Process Clause of the Fourteenth Amendment.* ***Second, upon a proper evidentiary showing, a qualified guardian may make that decision on behalf of an incompetent ward****. Third, in answering the important question presented by this tragic case, it is wise "'not to attempt, by any general statement, to cover every possible phase of the subject.'". Together, these considerations suggest that Nancy Cruzan's liberty to be free from medical treatment must be understood in light of the facts and circumstances particular to her. A grown woman at the time of the accident, Nancy had previously expressed her wish to forgo continuing medical care under circumstances such as these. Her family and her friends are convinced that this is what she would want. A guardian ad litem appointed by the trial court is also convinced that this is what Nancy would want. Yet the Missouri Supreme Court, alone among state courts deciding such a question, has determined that an irreversibly vegetative patient will remain a passive prisoner of medical technology -- for Nancy, perhaps for the next 30 years.*"

Justice Stevens, in turn, extensively quotes Judge Blackmar from the Supreme Court of Missouri who explained that decisions about the care of chronically ill patients were traditionally private: "*I would not accept the assumption, inherent in the principal opinion, that, with our advanced technology, the state must necessarily become involved in a decision* ***about using extraordinary measures to prolong life. Decisions of this kind are made daily by the patient***

[2] Hereinafter bold emphasis is mine.

or relatives, on the basis of medical advice and their conclusion as to what is best. Very few cases reach court, and I doubt whether this case would be before us but for the fact that Nancy lies in a state hospital. *I do not place primary emphasis on the patient's expressions, except possibly in the very unusual case, of which I find no example in the books, in which the patient expresses a view that all available life supports should be made use of. Those closest to the patient are best positioned to make judgments about the patient's best interest."*

"Judge Blackmar then argued that Missouri's policy imposed upon ***dying individuals*** *and their families a controversial and objectionable view of life's meaning: "****It is unrealistic to say that the preservation of life is an absolute, without regard to the quality of life.*** *I make this statement only in the context of a case in which the trial judge has found that there is no chance for amelioration of Nancy's condition. The principal opinion accepts this conclusion.* ***It is appropriate to consider the quality of life in making decisions about the extraordinary medical treatment.*** *Those who have made decisions about such matters without resort to the courts certainly consider the quality of life, and balance this against the unpleasant consequences to the patient. There is evidence that Nancy may react to pain stimuli. If she has any awareness of her surroundings, her life must be a living hell. She is unable to express herself or to do anything at all to alter her situation.* ***Her parents, who are her closest relatives, are best able to feel for her and to decide what is best for her. The state should not substitute its decisions for theirs. Nor am I impressed with the crypto-philosophers cited in the principal opinion, who declaim about the sanctity of any life without regard to its quality.*** *They dwell in ivory towers.""*

"Finally, Judge Blackmar concluded that the Missouri policy was illegitimate because it treats life as a theoretical abstraction, severed from, and indeed opposed to, the person of Nancy Cruzan, adding that "the Cruzan family appropriately came before the court seeking relief. The circuit judge properly found the facts and applied the law. His factual findings are supported by the record and his legal conclusions by overwhelming weight of authority. The principal opinion attempts to establish absolutes, but does so at the expense of human factors. In so doing it unnecessarily subjects Nancy and those close to her to continuous torture which no family should be forced to endure."

Justice Stevens, in turn, pointed out that *"It is perhaps predictable that courts might undervalue the liberty at stake here. Because death is so profoundly personal, public reflection upon it is unusual. As this sad case shows, however, such reflection must become more common if we are to deal responsibly with the modern circumstances of death.* ***Medical advances have altered the physiological conditions of death in ways that may be alarming: Highly invasive treatment may perpetuate human existence through a merger of body and machine that some might reasonably regard as an insult to life rather than as its continuation. But those same advances, and the reorganization of medical care accompanying the new science and technology, have also transformed the political and social conditions of death: People are less likely to die at home, and more likely to die in relatively public places, such as hospitals or nursing homes****(…).The trial court's order authorizing Nancy's parents to cease their daughter's treatment would have permitted the family that cares for Nancy to bring to a close her tragedy and her death. Missouri's objection to that order subordinates Nancy's body, her family, and the lasting significance of her life to the State's own interests. The decision we review thereby interferes with constitutional interests of the highest order(...).It seems to me that the Court errs insofar as it characterizes this case as involving "judgments about the 'quality' of life that a particular individual may enjoy. "* ***Nancy Cruzan is obviously "alive" in a physiological sense. But for patients like Nancy Cruzan, who have no consciousness and no chance of recovery, there is a serious question as to whether the mere persistence of their bodies is "life" as that word is commonly understood, or as it is used in both the Constitution and the Declaration***

of Independence. The State's unflagging determination to perpetuate Nancy Cruzan's physical existence is comprehensible only as an effort to define life's meaning, not as an attempt to preserve its sanctity(...).”

In their words, these judges forestall several of the theses put forward in this document: the irreducibility of life to its mere biological nature, the need to consider such aspects as quality of life, the ability to stop the progression of a severe medical disease through technology (a disease which would be otherwise terminal) but, at the same time, the inability to reverse the condition, the fact that these cases are usually settled in a different way when decision-making occurs within the family circle (Nancy's case reached the U.S. Supreme Court because she was hospitalized in a state hospital).

A very different case (the reverse of the preceding one) is that of Helga Wanglie, an 86-year-old patient who died after being in a vegetative state for more than a year (Miles, 1991). At the age of 85, she was hospitalized with symptoms of shortness of breath caused by chronic bronchiectasis. She required emergency intubation. During hospitalization, she acknowledged discomfort and occasionally recognized her family. Five months later, she was referred to a chronic care facility after several unsuccessful attempts to withdraw ventilatory support. A week later, she experienced a cardiopulmonary arrest, from which she was successfully resuscitated. She was then transferred to an intensive care unit, where she was diagnosed with hypoxic-ischemic encephalopathy. Physicians suggested removing the ventilator first a month and then two months after diagnosis. They did not believe that ventilatory support would benefit the patient in any way. The family, however, rejected this suggestion saying that doctors should not play God and that Helga would not be better off dead. They also added that she had not expressed any decisions with respect to such a situation. Ten months after her first admission and five months after the cardiopulmonary arrest, Helga was still unconscious and supported by a ventilator. A medical consultant whose opinion was requested at that time considered that the patient was at the end of her life, and that mechanical ventilation was not beneficial for the patient, that it would not cure her lung condition and that she would not survive without it. However, because ventilation could prolong life, it could not be considered futile. The conflict between the family and the hospital, which held that it was not obliged to provide non-beneficial medical treatment, was finally taken to court. It was first determined that the hospital had no financial interesting in withdrawing treatment since expenses were covered by Medicare for the first hospitalization and by a private insurance for the second one. The trial court also appointed the patient’s husband as the person who could best represent her interests. In the light of uncertainty about its legal obligation, the hospital decided to continue providing the treatment. However, Mrs. Wanglie died of septicemia three days after the court ruling.

The debate that followed was largely focused on discussing that while there is general agreement that patients may refuse treatment, it is arguable whether they or their families have the right to claim for any kind of medical treatment, regardless of its efficacy, additionally bringing up the issue of fair distribution of healthcare resources into the discussion.

What was interesting about the court decision was that it asserted the family’s right to make decisions on behalf of an incompetent patient (Angell, 1991). However, it did not bring into consideration the discussion about the contents of their decision and its eventual futility.

From the physicians’ point of view, Helga was terminally ill. The family, however, did not seem to consider the concept of terminality as a point of discussion. What mattered to them was that the patient was alive and that her state was better than being dead.

"For the first time in the history of the United States, Congress met in a special emergency session on Sunday, March 20, to pass legislation aimed at the medical care of one patient – Terri Schiavo. President George W. Bush encouraged the legislation and flew back to Washington, D.C., from his vacation in Crawford, Texas, so that he could be on hand to sign it immediately. In a statement issued three days earlier, he said: "The case of Terri Schiavo raises complex issues(. . . . Those who live at the mercy of others deserve our special care and concern. It should be our goal as a nation to build a culture of life, where all Americans are valued, welcomed, and protected – and that culture of life must extend to individuals with disabilities." (Annas, 2005) This is how Annas describes the shock produced by the decision of the courts of Florida to authorize withdrawal of artificial nutrition and hydration from Terri Schiavo, a patient who was in a permanent vegetative state.

In 1990, when she was 27 years-old, Terri had a cardiac arrest, which was probably caused by hypokalemia induced by an eating disorder. She progressed to a permanent vegetative state due to the resulting hypoxic-ischemic encephalopathy and she required tube feeding placement. Eight years later, her husband requested legal authorization to discontinue tube feeding. A judge found that there was clear and convincing evidence that Terri was in a permanent vegetative state and that had she been able to decide on her own, she would have chosen to discontinue the treatment. The Appellate Court affirmed the judgment and the Supreme Court of Florida declined to review it. The situation was somehow similar to that after the final decision in Nancy Cruzan's case.

However, the case became more complex and sparked nationwide debate and international attraction when Terri's parents claimed that there was evidence of treatment which would help her recover from her condition. This claim was refuted by three of the five experts asked to examine the patient (two appointed by Terri's husband, two by her parents and one by the trial court judge). The Supreme Court of Florida refused to hear an appeal again on the grounds that the parents had no standing to bring it. The State Legislature, in turn, passed a bill which gave Governor Jeb Bush the authority to order the reinsertion of the feeding tube (it had been removed after the court decision), which was reinserted as ordered. The Supreme Court of Florida declared that the law was unconstitutional and the U.S. Supreme Court refused to hear an appeal brought by the Governor. The trial court judge finally ordered the tube to be withdrawn on March 18, at 1 p.m.

Amidst death threats against one of the judges, and after another unsuccessful attempt by the Florida Legislature to pass a new bill aimed at restoring Terri's tube feeding, the U.S. Congress met in an emergency session, interrupting their Easter recess, in order to pass a bill which would allow Terri's parents to bring an appeal. In spite of this, Terri's parents could not modify the court decision and Terri finally died on March 25, 2005.

In this particular case, the concept of terminal disease was not openly discussed. However, it could be said that it was implicitly present in more than one aspect of the debate. The possibility of maintaining a patient in a permanent vegetative state, "suspended" for an indefinite period of time as opposed to an advanced cancer patient, led some people to consider Terri as a terminally ill patient whose life was being artificially sustained, while others believed that she was not actually terminally ill. In the first case, tube feeding was considered futile, a measure which undermined the patient's dignity and whose withdrawal would allow for her condition to follow its natural course; in other words, it would allow the patient to die. In the second case, the treatment was deemed vital since its discontinuation would lead to the patient's death (she would be killed instead of being allowed to die). Those who argued for the withdrawal believed that the patient's wishes, or the wishes of those who represented her interests, would be violated if treatment was withheld; while those who opposed discontinuation considered treatment withdrawal as an offense against life.

In the debate held in the U.S. House of Representatives, several of its members showed crass ignorance of what an irreversible vegetative state is. Furthermore, some members who are also physicians offered their opinions about Terri's condition without conducting their own examinations (Quill, 2005).

The media, in turn, showed people, some of them were children, trying to bring Terri a glass of water, claiming that she was being starved to death and dehydrated (this shows that most people ignored the patient's real condition — she was unable to swallow and feel hunger or thirst).

A similar case was debated in Argentina, though it did not have the same impact as Terri's case in the United States. A female patient (MdelC) had been in a permanent vegetative state under her husband's care for two years. She progressed to that state after suffering heart failure when giving birth to her fourth child (all the children were under the father's care after that tragic event). In 2000, the patient's husband (AMG) petitioned the court for withdrawal of tube feeding, but her parents objected to the request.

In his critical review of the decision adopted by the courts of the Province of Buenos Aires (Argentina) with regard to this case, Dr. Carlos Gherardi clearly shows how ignorance and prejudice may lead to unfounded decisions (Gherardi, 2007). It is worth quoting what he wrote in the introduction to his review: *"We should start by transcribing the description of the patient provided by the Counsel for Minors and Incompetent Persons, which was repeatedly quoted in the relevant judgments: "I was really surprised because I did not find what I had expected. Based on the diagnosis, I thought I would find a physically impaired person, who would be completely unable to move, asleep, dishevelled, and connected to a mechanical respirator and machines controlling her heart rate, but the truth is that I found a woman with a very good physical appearance. She was breathing on her own and there were no machines controlling her. She only has a feeding tube which provides her with nutrition and hydration. I was really shocked to see her blink, she looked towards different places, she coughed and moved when doing so, and she made some facial gestures." The Counsel requested the petition to be dismissed "in limine" on the grounds of the defense of the right to life and because he considered that if the petition were sustained, it would eventually constitute neglect followed by death or aggravated homicide. In his argumentation, the Counsel makes reference to the Creator and the Parable of the Talents. He concludes that: "the hope for a Miracle should never be abandoned. Love and faith will always dwell in a heroic heart. And, waiting for God's time, which we know is different from man's time, is an act of heroism.".*

This unusual account, made by the only court officer who actually saw the patient, seems to be referring to an individual in a nearly normal condition when, in fact, the patient is a person who has tragically and irreversible lost all cognitive activity, and who does not exhibit the essential communicative skills and affective expression inherent to a person's identity. It is quite clear that this account had an impact on the judges and that it was considered reliable by them, since it was frequently quoted by the Court Attorney and some of the judges when providing the reasons for their votes. The probably erroneous perception of those who had to decide on such a complex and debatable issue may have been enhanced by the fact that none of them actually saw the patient and that they did not take into account the evidence provided by the various witnesses (family members, professionals, priests). Even though there was no procedural obligation, nothing prevented the judges from hearing the witnesses' statements, which would have contributed to their knowledge of the case. It is hard to believe that none of the judges felt the moral obligation to see the patient or meet her husband and children to evaluate the situation of the family."

Dr. Gherardi adds that *"the patient's husband expressed that he did not know what her preferences were with respect to life-sustaining measures. However, two people who were close to the patient, one of them was a psychologist, stated that the patient had previously told them that if she had been in such a condition, she would not have wished to be kept alive. These statements were not taken into account by the judges and they were not accepted as witnesses, and neither were others who offered their testimony."*.

The courts not only rejected the evidence provided by a psychologist and one of the patient's friends about her preferences, but it also based its considerations on an erroneous interpretation of the purpose of medicine ("to defend life at all costs"), the patient's medical condition, the situation the family was going through, and the suffering endured by those who took care of the patient, especially her husband. One of the judges (who never actually saw the patient) reveals an absolute lack of respect for the patient and her caregivers when he appeals to a possible miracle and calls for heroism while waiting for God's time. Should not therapeutic obstinacy be considered as an example of man's challenge to God's time?

Regardless of technological advances and the development of new goals, just as before, today's medicine will seldom cure, will often provide relief and will always have to comfort. It is not its objective to defeat death, because human beings are doomed to die. It should try to avoid early death but it should also allow patients to die in peace. And, it should not defend life at all costs since, in doing so, it would fall into such a negative value as therapeutic obstinacy. Allowing a dying person to die is not the same as killing him or her. By showing respect for a dignified death, we are also dignifying life. We dignify others when we consider them as persons, when we respect them, listen to them, watch them, talk to them. In the abovementioned case, regardless of the adopted decision, the judges showed a clear lack of respect for the patient's dignity in their failure to see or listen. With their behaviour, they ultimately showed the opposite side of therapeutic obstinacy: neglect.

3. Conclusion

We usually define "terminal disease" as a pathological condition that cannot be cured and, in spite of the treatments applied, it will end up in the death of the patient in a short period of time, i.e. 6 months. We consider that this definition is unilateral (made up by physicians). We propose that the real meaning should come up as a construction based on the dialogue between patients, their families, caregivers and healthcare workers. In addition, this process should be developed by incorporating the cultural concepts of the society in which each individual lives. The aim of this construction is to show that the meaning of "terminal disease" is not unique but multidimensional, since it can change depending on the circumstances.

4. Acknowledgement

The author would like to express his gratitude to the Ethics Comitte of the Hospital Privado de Comunidad de Mar del Plata (Private Hospital of the Community of Mar del Plata) for letting me be a member of it, to Dr Jorge Manzini for his teachings and his critical review of the manuscript, and to Anna Banchik for her providing me part of the bibliography. This work was financially supported by the Fundación Médica Mar del Plata (Mar del Plata Medical Foundation).

5. References

Angell, M. (1991). The case of Helga Wanglie. A new kind of "right to die" case. *N Engl J Med.*, Vol.325, No.7, (August 1991), pp 511-2, ISSN 0028-4793

Annas, GJ. (1990). Nancy Cruzan and the right to die. *N Engl J Med.*, Vol.323, No.10, (September 1990), pp. 670-673, ISSN 0028-4793

Annas, GJ. (2005). "Culture of life" politics at the bedside--the case of Terri Schiavo. *N Engl J Med.* Vol.352, No.16, (April 2005), pp. 1710-1715, ISSN 0028-4793

BBC News. (2008) Girl wins right to refuse heart (11 November 2008). Available from http://news.bbc.co.uk/2/hi/uk_news/england/hereford/worcs/7721231.stm (accessed 05 March 2011)

Beauchamp, TL. & Childress, JF. (1999). *Principios de Ética Médica*, Masson, S.A., ISBN 84-458-0480-4, Barcelona, Spain

Callahan, D. et al. (1996) The goals of medicine. Setting new priorities. *Hastings Cent Rep.*, Vol.26, No.6, (November-December 1996), pp.S1-27,1996. ISSN 0093-0334

Carbajal, M. (2011a). Pagina 12. La niña que pelea por una muerte digna. Edition 19 february 2011. Available from http://www.pagina12.com.ar/diario/sociedad/3-162653-2011-02-19.html (accessed 8 March de 2011)

Carbajal, M. (2011b).Pagina 12 El dictamen del Comité de bioética. Edition 28 february 2011. Available from http://www.pagina12.com.ar/diario/elpais/subnotas/163187-52260-2011-02-28.html (accessed 8 March de 2011)

Carbajal, M. (2011c).Pagina 12 Quiero transitar lo último que me queda en paz. Edition 28 february 2011 Available from http://www.pagina12.com.ar/diario/elpais/1-163187-2011-02-28.html (accessed 8 March 2011)

Carbajal, M. (2011d).Pagina 12. Una visión desde la bioética. Edition 28 february 2011. Available from http://www.pagina12.com.ar/diario/elpais/subnotas/163187-52259-2011-02-28.html (accessed 8 March de 2011)

Carbajal, M. (2011e).Pagina 12 La chica que peleó por una muerte digna. Edition 2 march 2011. Available from http://www.pagina12.com.ar/diario/sociedad/3-163303-2011-03- 02.html (accessed 8 March de 2011)

Carbajal, M. (2011f).Pagina 12 La espera de Melina. Edition 2 march 2011. Available from http://www.pagina12.com.ar/diario/sociedad/subnotas/163303-52292-2011-03-02.html (accessed 8 March 2011)

Cruzan v. Harmon (1989), 760 S.W.2d 408, 411 (Mo. 1989) in Cruzan, By Her Parents And Co-Guardians V. Director, Missouri Department Of Health Supreme Court Of The United States 497 U.S. 261 June 25, 1990, Decided. Available from http://law2.umkc.edu/faculty/projects/ftrials/conlaw/cruzan.html (accessed 19 March 2011)

Cruzan, By Her Parents And Co-Guardians V. Director (1990), Missouri Department Of Health Supreme Court Of The United States 497 U.S. 261 June 25, 1990, Decided. Available from http://law2.umkc.edu/faculty/projects/ftrials/conlaw/cruzan.html (accessed 19 March 2011)

Eisenberg, L. (1977). Disease and illness. Distinctions between professional and popular ideas of sickness. *Cult Med Psychiatry*. Vol.1, No.1, (April 1977), pp. 9-23, ISSN (electronic): 1573-076X

Gherardi, CR. (2007) *La Ley* Actualidad . Vol. LXXI, No.245, (December 2007), pp. 1-3, ISSN 0036-1636

Gould, S. (1985) The Median isn´t the Message. Available from http://www.phoenix5.org/articles/GouldMessage.html (accessed 27 march 2011)

Hooft, P. (1995). Juzgado de Primera Instancia en lo Criminal y Correccional N° 3, Mar del Plata, setiembre 18 de 1995.-"Dirección del Hospital Interzonal General de Agudos (HIGA) de Mar del Plata s/ Presentación" (firme), In: Cuestiones bioéticas en torno a la muerte, T Zamudio (Ed), *Cuadernos de Bioética*. Ed. Ad Hoc. ISSN 0328-8390. Buenos Aires, Argentina. Available from http://www.muerte.bioetica.org/juris/fallos5.htm (accessed 08 November 2009)

Kinney, HC.; Korein, J.; Panigrahy, A.; Dikkes, P. & Goode, R. (1994) Neuropathological findings in the brain of Karen Ann Quinlan. The role of the thalamus in the persistent vegetative state. *N Engl J Med.*, Vol.330, No.21, (May 1994), pp. 1469-1475, ISSN 0028-4793

Miles SH. (1991). Informed demand for "non-beneficial" medical treatment. *N Engl J Med.*, Vol.325, No.7, (August 1991), pp. 512-515, ISSN 0028-4793

More, T. (1516) *"Utopia"*. Transcribed from the 1901 Cassell & Company Edition by David Price, Project Gutenberg Ebook Utopia Available from http://www.gutenberg.org/files/2130/2130-h/2130-h.htm (accessed 27 March 2011)

Osler, W. (n.d.). Available from http://en.wikiquote.org/wiki/William_Osler (accessed 27 March 2011)

Poe, EA. (1845). The Facts in the Case of M. Valdemar. From *The Works Of Edgar Allan Poe*, Vol. II A.C. Armstrong & Son, New York, 1884. Available from http://www.taalfilosofie.nl/bestanden/bar_analyse_valdemar_eng_poe_tekst.pdf (accessed 27 March 2011)

Post, SG. (2007), The Aging Society And The Expansion Of Senility: Biotechnological And Treatment Goals, In: *The Oxford Handbook of Bioethics*, B.P. Steinbock (Ed), 304-323, Oxford University Press Inc, ISBN 978-0-19-927335-5, New York, USA

Quill, TE. (2005). Terri Schiavo--a tragedy compounded. *N Engl J Med.*, Vol.352, No.16, (April 2005), pp. 1630-1633, ISSN 0028-4793

Sampedro Ramón (2004). *Cartas desde el Infierno*. Editorial Planeta, S.A, ISBN: 9788408056324, Barcelona, Spain

SECPAL (n.d.) *Guía de Cuidados Paliativos*. Available http://www.secpal.com/guiacp/index.php?acc=dos (accessed 6 March 2011)

The Multi-Society Task Force on PVS. (1994a) Medical aspects of the persistent vegetative state (1). *N Engl J Med.*, Vol.330, No.21, (May 1994), pp. 1499-1508, ISSN 0028-4793

The Multi-Society Task Force on PVS. (1994b) Medical aspects of the persistent vegetative state (2). *N Engl J Med.*, Vol.330, No.22, (June 1994), pp. 1572-1579, ISSN 0028-4793

Young, A. (1982) The Anthropologies of Illness and Sickness. *Annual Review of Anthropology*, Vol.11, (1982), pp. 257-285, ISSN: 0084-6570

23

Prolactin and Schizophrenia, an Evolving Relationship

Chris J. Bushe[1] and John Pendlebury[2]
[1]*Eli Lilly and Company Ltd, Basingstoke,*
[2]*Ramsgate House, Manchester*
UK

1. Introduction

Prolactin is a polypeptide hormone originally discovered from the crop glands of pigeons in 1933 (Riddle et al, 1933; Bushe and Pendlebury, 2010), however there was some scepticism that prolactin even existed in humans until the 1970s as human prolactin was considered identical to growth hormone (GH). During the 1970s, the development of radioimmunoassay techniques allowed the isolation of prolactin and its subsequent measurement (Kohen and Wildgust, 2008). Since that time, awareness of the consequences of hyperprolactinaemia in psychiatry has been less than rapid despite clear evidence that many psychotropic agents, in particular antipsychotics, elevate prolactin levels to some degree in many patients. As a result, prolactin monitoring is not commonplace and many clinicians remain unsure of its utility. In part, this may relate to lack of knowledge regarding pathological endpoints caused by hyperprolactinaemia.

In the last decade, however, awareness has begun to emerge of the potential consequences of untreated hyperprolactinaemia including short-term adverse events of sexual dysfunction, amenorrhoea and infertility and longer term consequences that may include bone fractures and breast cancer. This has been due in part to a number of reviews focussing on the potential consequences of hyperprolactinaemia and the relatively high prevalence of this adverse event (Haddad and Wieck, 2004; Bostwick et al, 2009; Bushe and Pendlebury, 2010),). In 2008 the first set of prolactin monitoring guidelines was published and more recent data have begun to evaluate the use of specific polypharmacy to reduce prolactin levels (Peveler et al, 2008). There remain, however, many unanswered questions; most relate to the need to establish the true incidence of longer term sequelae of hyperprolactinaemia and to the simple question- what level of prolactin actually carries consequences and when? When one considers that prolactin has at least 300 biological actions it may be that this diversity of function will lead to research that further defines the precise role of and subsequent pathology induced by hyperprolactinaemia (Fitzgerald and Dinan, 2008).

2. Prolactin – What do we know about the hormone?

2.1 Structure and release

Prolactin, a polypeptide hormone that binds to prolactin receptors, is considered part of the Class 1 cytokine receptor family present in various organs including pancreas, liver, uterus and prostate and consequently may have some immunological activity. It is predominantly synthesised and secreted from the lactotroph cells of the anterior pituitary (Fitzgerald and Dinan, 2008). Lactotrophs form around 20-50% of the cellular population of the pituitary with those in the more inner zones being more responsive to dopamine. Structurally, prolactin is a single chain of 199 amino-acids containing six cysteine residues and three disulfide bonds with 40% homology between the genes encoding prolactin and GH (Fitzgerald and Dinan, 2008).

Prolactin is released from the anterior pituitary in a pulsatile manner and has a half life of around 50 minutes (Citrome, 2008). It peaks around 10 times per day in young adults (Holt, 2008) with a marked circadian rhythm highest during sleep and reaching a nadir during waking hours. Time of measurement is thus important to standardise and is best undertaken before drug dosing in a fasting state in the morning, although this is not always pragmatic in schizophrenia due to the nature of the illness. Measurement of levels during the day needs to be relatively precise as stress factors, exercise and eating can alter levels. In addition, there appears to be an annual circadian variation though with little clinical relevance. Garde et al (2000) reported that prolactin was highest in healthy female subjects in March-May (153 mIU/L) and lowest in September-November (98 mIU/L) (Garde et al, 2000).

Increasingly other confounding factors are being recognised that potentially also affect prolactin levels and any clinical interpretation of abnormality. For example, fluctuating prolactin levels have been found to be greater over the 24-hour period after dosing with perospirone than with either risperidone or olanzapine, despite the magnitude of hyperprolactinaemia being greater with risperidone (Yasui-Furukori et al, 2010). Recent data are supportive of current smokers taking antipsychotics having both a lower mean prolactin level (odds ratio [OR] 2.3, 95% confidence interval [CI] 1.2-4.7, p=0.002) and a lower prevalence of hyperprolactinaemia (Mackin et al, 2010) and other data are supportive at a minimum that is true in females (Ohta et al, 2011). This may be a critical confounder in schizophrenia where almost all patients smoke and indeed smoke more cigarettes than smokers in the general population. Other confounders are much better recognised with a study of 154 schizophrenia patients taking 6mg risperidone reporting that prolactin levels correlate with gender (higher in females), age (lower in older patients) and smoking status (p<0.01) based on a multiple regression analysis (Ohta et al, 2011).

Control of prolactin secretion from the anterior pituitary is predominantly under the control of dopamine released via hypothalamic dopaminergic neurons, the tuberoinfundibular and tuberohypophyseal dopaminergic neurones (Holt, 2008). Dopamine is transported from the hypothalamus to the anterior pituitary via the long hypophyseal portal vessels and inhibits the high basal secretory tone of the lactotroph. This high basal secretory activity is unique amongst endocrine cells. The released prolactin regulates the dopamine synthesis from the hypothalamus via a feedback loop.

The mechanism whereby prolactin is elevated by D2 blockade remains undetermined. However, the most likely explanations relate to speed of D2 dissociation and the ability of the antipsychotic to cross the blood brain barrier (Bushe et al, 2010), with drugs dissociating slowly being associated with greater prolactin elevation. In contrast, quetiapine, an example of an antipsychotic with fast dissociation, has low rates of prolactin elevation being associated with central D2 occupancy that falls from initial blockade of 60-70% at 2 hours post-dosing to around 30% at 24 hours.

3. Measurement of prolactin and definition of hyperprolactinaemia

Units of measurement have the potential to cause some confusion as US and EU data are often presented in ng/ml whereas most UK data are in mIU/L. Conversion rates from ng/ml to mIU/L are not standardised and vary between 21.2 and 36 dependent on the assay employed (Bushe et al, 2008). Furthermore, clinical reports do not always report either the normal range utilised or sometimes the units of measurement (McEvoy et al, 2007).

Definitions of hyperprolactinaemia vary depending upon the upper limit of normal (ULN) for the local assay. Normal ranges for females tend often to be around 30% higher than males, with some laboratories also reporting separate ranges for premenopausal and postmenopausal females. In the psychiatric literature, some of the highest ULNs for females are around 700 mIU/L and, for males, 500 mIU/L (Bushe and Shaw 2007), with lowest ULN at 300 mIU/L for females (Meaney et al, 2004). The Maudsley guidelines 10th edition (Taylor et al, 2009) gives fairly specific advice on blood sampling (1 hour after waking or eating) and cites normal ranges in both ng/ml and mIU/L. In their view, the ULN for females is <530 mIU/L and for males is <424 mIU/L; re-testing is advised if the prolactin level is between 530-2120 mIU/L.

There is currently also no specific definition for an elevated prolactin level that may be regarded as clinically non-significant and when we published our original data set there was no specific guidance to either diagnose or grade level of severity of hyperprolactinaemia (Bushe/Shaw 2007). Thus, we created three specific grades of hyperprolactinaemia: slightly elevated (<1000 mIU/L), significant elevation (1001-2000 mIU/L) and severe elevation (>2000mIU/L). This was based on empirical judgement and not with relation to specifically defined outcomes. In general terms, prolactin levels <2000 mIU/L may be due to a medication effect but other causes can include microprolactinoma, pituitary stalk compression, renal failure or hypothyroidism (Holt, 2008). The literature currently reports that macroprolactinomas are the most common cause of prolactin levels >2120 mIU/L in the general population (Bushe et al, 2010) although other authors propose higher levels (3180 mIU/L) at which hyperprolactinaemia can be assumed to be caused by a macroprolactinoma (Holt, 2008).

When evaluating hyperprolactinaemia it is also critical to understand the incidence or prevalence of hyperprolactinaemia from the patient perspective as opposed to a mean level from a cohort. Recent data are now tending to more commonly include both variables (Mackin et al, 2011) whereas in our 2008 review of this topic we reported that though 60% of studies reporting prolactin data included some degree of categorical analysis, this was seen mainly in the naturalistic studies (88%) rather than the randomised controlled trials (42%) (Bushe et al, 2008).

4. Consequences of hyperprolactinaemia

Many of the longer term definitive outcomes associated with elevated prolactin remain unknown. Recent findings of prolactin receptors in atherosclerotic plaques in coronary arteries of healthy subjects indicate a possible role of prolactin even in coronary artery disease (Reuwer et al, 2009). There are, however, three areas of pathology that would seem to be closely linked to elevated prolactin, sexual function, bone loss and cancer and these can be considered as short- and longer term potential adverse events.

4.1 Short term consequences of hyperprolactinaemia

4.1.1 Sexual function

Sex hormone dysregulation may be the underlying cause of both acute and longer term adverse events associated with hyperprolactinaemia as prolactin has a significant effect on sex hormone regulation and prolactin levels in patients treated with antipsychotics are inversely related to steroid sex hormone concentrations (Smith, 2002). However, the absolute link between prolactin and sexual dysfunction is complex. The relative short-term consequences of hyperprolactinaemia are well described and, in addition, to sexual dysfunction include menstrual disturbances, acne, infertility, galactorheoa and gynaecomastia although prevalence rates were until recently not well reported. In 2011, the European First Episode Schizophrenia Trial (EUFEST) study of first episode schizophrenia patients reported that sexual dysfunction was very common at baseline (Malik et al, 2011) and although often attributed to antipsychotics this is not the complete picture as smoking, physical illness, depressive and negative symptoms may also be relevant (Malik et al, 2011). Over the 1-year study, changes in prevalence of sexual dysfunction were small and varied little between antipsychotics despite hyperprolactinaemia being very common and moderately severe (Kahn et al, 2008). The authors concluded that their data emphasized that schizophrenia the illness was a key influence on sexual dysfunction although hyperprolactinemia undoubtedly plays an additional role (Malik et al, 2011). There is also an important investigational aspect to consider. In most antipsychotic studies previous medication prior to study entry is either inadequately or incompletely described, which makes interpretation of variables such as prolactin and sexual dysfunction complex. It is possible that changes measured during the trial may relate to the removal of a previous antipsychotic. As such the only data that can give a true baseline are data in treatment-naïve subjects from studies such as EUFEST. Not all data, however, are consistent with this view that prolactin may play a smaller role in sexual dysfunction than expected (Knegtering et al, 2008). For example, in a 6-week, open label study including 264 patients treated with antipsychotics, prolactin-raising antipsychotics were linked with significantly more sexual-related adverse events than patients treated with prolactin-sparing antipsychotics. The authors concluded that around 40% of emerging sexual adverse events in schizophrenia are attributable to prolactin (Knegtering et al, 2008). The importance of seeking overt symptomatology however is that it offers the opportunity to measure prolactin as many guidelines have previously not suggested prolactin measurements until the presence of relevant symptoms. The literature is fairly conclusive that sexual dysfunction is not always regarded as an important aspect to discuss with patients in routine clinical practice.

4.2 Longer term consequences of hyperprolactinaemia

4.2.1 Bone

Data on hyperprolactinaemia and bone loss have appeared during the last decade predominantly due to the work of Veronica O'Keane. Her group systematically followed the link between hyperprolactinaemia and sex hormones (males and females) and then between hyperprolactinaemia and bone loss. Some studies suggest that even relatively short periods of hyperprolactinaemia can have significant adverse effects on bone density (Meaney and O'Keane, 2007; O'Keane, 2008). Young women may be particularly susceptible to hyperprolactinaemia, and osteoporosis and osteopenia may develop in the first 8 years of antipsychotic treatment (Meaney and O'Keane, 2007; O'Keane, 2008). Of more concern is the finding that deterioration can be measured over a single year and essentially cannot be prevented (Meaney and O'Keane, 2007; O'Keane, 2008). A second set of key epidemiological studies evaluating fractures in large UK cohorts was published suggesting that hip and other bone fractures are a sequelae of mental illness and its treatment. Howard reported that hyperprolactinaemia and prolactin-elevating antipsychotics have been associated with a doubling of the risk of hip fracture in schizophrenia patients in a large UK study (OR 2.6, CI 2.43-2.78) (Howard et al, 2007). A second study also using the UK General Practice Research Database (GPRD) reported that in women the highest relative risk of fracture in a mentally ill population were in the youngest cohorts, whereas in males the greatest risks were seen in older age (Abel et al, 2008). The results showed that the relative risk (RR) of any fracture was increased more than double in females with psychotic disorders (RR 2.5: CI 1.5-4.3) but that even greater risk was measured in the cohort aged 45-74 years with psychotic disorders, with a relative risk in women of RR 5.1 (CI 2.7-9.6) and in males RR 6.4 (CI 2.6-16.1) when looking specifically at hip fractures (Abel et al, 2008). This risk may be seen to an even greater extent in males than females (Howard et al, 2007) and is present after adjusting for the other risk factors for osteoporosis highly prevalent in a cohort of patients with severe mental illness (poor diet, low exercise rates, increased alcohol consumption and decreased sunlight exposure). Other data however are needed for other fracture sites (radius and vertebrae) together with some indication as to whether it is the cumulative length of hyperprolactinaemia that is crucial (a sort of area under the curve measurement) or the effect of a critical peak level of prolactin. Recent data in non-schizophrenic males with prolactinoma reported that using DEXA scanning of the lumbar spine vertebral fractures were diagnosed in 37.5% of patients compared with 7.8% of controls ($p<0.001$) (Mazziotti et al, 2011) and that these developed independently of hypogonadism.

4.2.2 Possible association with cancer

A recent systematic review concluded that breast cancer is significantly increased in females with schizophrenia but the data have simply not been published to establish the degree of the putative role of prolactin in this increased risk (Bushe et al, 2009). A number of epidemiological studies have reported data over the last 25 years but it is only in the last few years that clarity has emerged. The importance of systematic review in addressing a clinical question is clear. In this case, when studies with adequate powering and follow up undertaken in an age group where cancer developed (>50 yrs for breast cancer predominantly) are considered, the results were clear. The specific relevance of breast cancer is that it is the most common cancer in women in the UK, it accounts for 23% of all female cancer cases worldwide, there is a lifetime risk of 1 in 9 in the general population and this risk is increasing (Bushe et al, 2010). A recent meta-analysis that included fewer studies than our systematic review (Catts et al, 2008) reported a 12% increased risk (Standardised Incidence Ratio [SIR] 1.12, 95% CI 1.02-1.23) with a more recent UK study reporting an increased risk of 52% in schizophrenia adjusting for recognised confounders such as poverty (Hippisley-Cox et al, 2007). One can only speculate over the role of prolactin and mammary carcinogenesis, however in animal toxicity and molecular studies, it has been recognised over many years (Harvey 2008) that there is a very strong association. The US Nurses' Health Study evaluated prolactin samples from 32,826 patients with normal prolactin levels during the period 1989 to 1990 and these subjects have been extensively followed over 20 years, providing conclusive evidence linking prolactin and breast cancer in the general population. Many of their study reports suggest prolactin levels to be linked to the risk of breast cancer development both in pre- and postmenopausal women (Tworoger and Hankinson, 2006; Tworoger et al, 2007). An example of these data found prolactin levels in the upper quartile of normal to be associated with an increased risk compared to the lower quartile of normal (OR 1.34, 95% CI 1.02-1.76) (Tworoger et al, 2007). Any definitive link, however, has yet to be established in schizophrenia and bipolar disorder.

A large retrospective cohort study of 52,819 females receiving antipsychotics and 55,289 control women reported a 16% increased risk of breast cancer (Wang et al, 2002) with a dose response relationship suggesting a greater risk of breast cancer with increased doses of antipsychotic. Regardless of relationship with prolactin, identical breast cancer screening should be encouraged in all schizophrenia subjects as in the general population. Screening rates for schizophrenia patients are very low compared with the general population for an illness that is very common (lifetime prevalence 1 in 9 and rising) and often curable (Bushe et al, 2010).

Hyperprolactinaemia has also been linked to pituitary adenomas and adenocarcinomas and putatively to prostate cancer (Harvey et al, 2008). The US Food and Drug Administration Adverse Event Reporting System pharmacovigilance database study strongly linked risperidone (adjusted reporting ratio 18.7) with the highest frequency of pituitary adenomas compared with haloperidol (5.6), ziprasidone (3.0) and olanzapine (2.3) (Szarfman et al, 2006). A recent case series is suggestive that amisulpride may also be associated with the development of prolactinomas mediated via hyperprolactinaemia (Akkaya et al, 2009).

The multiple actions of prolactin and relative lack of research into hyperprolactinaemia suggest that additional potential long-term effects may be discovered potentially in glands such as the thyroid. Recent data suggest there may be an association with autoimmune thyroiditis and in 75 schizophrenia patients, the prevalence of hyperprolactinaemia was higher in patients with thyroid autoantibodies (p=0.045) (Poyraz et al, 2008).

5. Relationship between serum prolactin concentration and adverse events

This is a complex question that remains totally unanswered for the potential longer term sequelae but can be partially addressed for short-term adverse events. There would seem to be two potential associations. Firstly, a chronic prolactin elevation that reaches a cumulative threshold over a longer term and secondly, a peak prolactin level that requires a trigger threshold to initiate pathology. Levels <1000 mIU/L are associated with decreased libido and infertility, 1000-1600 mIU/L with oligomenorrhoea, and >2000 mIU/L with amenorrhea and hypogonadism (Peveler et al, 2008). Hypogonadism is the main driver for bone mineral density loss and fractures although the possibility exists that prolactin may have a direct osteoclastic effect. Data on longer term prolactin levels tend not to report the associated changes in sex hormones making interpretation complex. The topic has, however, been reviewed (Bushe et al, 2008) and in cross-sectional prevalence studies that report bone mineral density loss in association with typicals or risperidone over 8-21 years, the mean cohort values ranged 908-3024 mIU/L (Bushe et al, 2010). These levels are common and are reached quickly in patients treated with risperidone and amisulpride (Bushe and Shaw 2007; Bushe et al, 2008). A small case series of patients receiving paliperidone reported hyperprolactinaemia within 3 weeks with levels ranging from 1500-3996 mIU/L (Skopek et al, 2010). Prolactin levels related to breast cancer in schizophrenia and bipolar disorder are unknown, however data are supportive of levels as low as 500 mIU/L being associated with an increased risk of breast cancer in the general population over the medium term (Tworoger and Hankinson 2006, Tworoger et al, 2007). However, it is critical to understand that whereas there is a strong link between prolactin and breast cancer in the general population, there are no data to address this topic in schizophrenia and bipolar disorder. In addition, breast cancer has very many aetiological factors that include social demographics, education, obesity and family history and the role of prolactin is simply not known.

6. How common is hyperprolactinaemia in an antipsychotic-treated cohort?

6.1 Overview

There are few cohorts where prolactin levels have been obtained in a complete cohort and rates of hyperprolactinaemia will be dependent on many factors including medication choice, gender, age and length of follow up. Data derived from epidemiological databases is also confounded by selection bias. Without knowing how many subjects were tested there is little way to put perspective around these data (Montgomery et al, 2004). A true perspective requires a complete cohort to be tested. Many other confounders will remain, however, including gender, smoking status, adherence to treatment, age and time on treatment.

Olanzapine, for example, may give a transient elevation of prolactin that reduces over the first months in some patients but during chronic administration prolactin elevation may remain (Bushe et al, 2008). Naturalistic data may thus be informative as prolactin monitoring is not routine and prevalence rates in complete populations screened will reflect previous under-diagnosis. Two recent naturalistic analyses in which asymptomatic schizophrenia populations have been screened for prolactin report similar prevalence of hyperprolactinaemia: 38% and 39% in UK (n=194) and Norway (n=106), respectively (Bushe and Shaw 2007; Johnsen et al, 2008). The UK study measured prolactin in the total population of a catchment area in Halifax receiving antipsychotics for schizophrenia or bipolar disorder. The population was clinically asymptomatic prior to the study. Hyperprolactinaemia was more common in females than males (52 vs. 26%), consistent with most other data (Bushe et al, 2008), and significantly elevated levels (>1000 mIU/L) were measured in 21% of subjects. For 13% of females and 19% of males, prolactin levels were above the normal limit but below 1001 mIU/L. Categorical rates of hyperprolactinaemia in trials range from 33 to 69% and confirm that no antipsychotic is prolactin neutral (Bushe et al, 2008). Most studies report both a higher prevalence and severity of hyperprolactinaemia in females as was the case in the Halifax study which found 13% of females had levels >2000 mIU/L compared with 2% of males (Bushe and Shaw, 2007).

6.2 Rates of hyperprolactinaemia with individual antipsychotics

The ideal studies to evaluate prolactin would be a long-term, first episode study where the confounding factor of previous antipsychotic usage would not need addressing and which included multiple treatment arms and a longer term randomised study in chronic schizophrenia. There are few such studies with the exception of EUFEST (Kahn et al, 2008) and CATIE (Lieberman et al, 2005). EUFEST was a 1-year, first episode study and CATIE, an 18-month study with multiple treatment arms. Both these studies concluded that hyperprolactinaemia was common though EUFEST failed to find a direct link between prolactin and sexual dysfunction.

The totality of the data is convincing that there is no such entity as a "prolactin-sparing" antipsychotic, however, data are sometimes complex to interpret. There are numerous confounding factors but broadly psychotropic polypharmacy, the choice and the dose of medication are relevant factors as are often the lack of reported data on previous antipsychotic treatment. Adherence is also important as many typicals are now administered by long-acting depot formulations whereas rates of non-adherence to all forms of antipsychotic are high. When these factors are compounded with other confounders (gender, age and smoking), definitive statements regarding prolactin become less precise though some conclusions can be made with reasonable certainty.

Much of the reported data tend to come from relatively short-term clinical trials, often done for drug registration purposes, or cross-sectional prevalence data. Neither data set has properly established the long-term trajectory of hyperprolactinaemia and there are no data to support the concept of regression back to baseline.

There are, however, a number of disparate data on comparable rates of hyperprolactinaemia amongst antipsychotics and the largest data sets reporting prolactin include a 6-week paliperidone study in 628 schizophrenia patients (Kane et al, 2007) and a 1-year risperidone and haloperidol in first episode psychosis study in 555 patients (Schooler et al, 2005). Cohort sizes range from <50 to 2725 (Bushe et al, 2010). There is also surprisingly little dissonance amongst the data sets despite many of the confounders already discussed. .

In summary, for individual antipsychotics the prevalence of hyperprolactinaemia is highest in risperidone, paliperidone and amisulpride-treated patients and approaches 100% in female patients (72-100%) being significantly higher than in patients treated with conventional antipsychotics (33% in a UK cohort on depot antipsychotics) (Bushe et al, 2008; Bushe and Shaw 2007). The recently licensed paliperidone, which is 9-hydroxyl-risperidone, the active metabolite of risperidone, has similar prolactin elevation to risperidone (Berwaerts et al, 2010).

Clinicians have been aware for many years that risperidone is associated with hyperprolactinaemia, however there has been less clarity regarding whether hyperprolactinaemia with risperidone is more prevalent than with conventional antipsychotics. A key study was a long-term, randomised clinical trial (RCT) in first-episode psychosis with subjects randomised to risperidone or haloperidol and a median treatment-length of 206 days (Schooler et al, 2005). This study reported significantly higher rates of hyperprolactinaemia (74% vs. 50%) and mean prolactin levels in the risperidone cohort than the haloperidol cohort. CATIE also reported significantly greater prolactin elevation with risperidone than perphenazine (Lieberman et al, 2005) though only mean changes in individual drug cohorts were reported, not categorical numbers of patients with hyperprolactinaemia.

Although conventional antipsychotics were for a long time regarded as almost uniformly being associated with hyperprolactinaemia, the data are not supportive of this conclusion and recent data on conventional antipsychotics suggest significantly lower prevalence rates of 33-35% in a depot-treated population (Bushe and Shaw, 2007). In part, this may relate to dosing issues. For example, Asian populations using higher doses of haloperidol (15-16mg) than typically used in Europe, have prevalence rates of hyperprolactinaemia (60-66%) approaching those of risperidone and amisulpride (Bushe et al, 2010). Supportive of this dosing issue is the excellent study from Kleinberg in approximately 2000 patients which concluded that although risperidone was associated with higher rates of hyperprolactinaemia compared with 10 mg haloperidol, no comparative differences emerged with 20mg haloperidol (Kleinberg et al, 1999). Doses of haloperidol currently used are more reflective of studies such as EUFEST, in which the maximum permitted dose was 4 mg.

Our own naturalistic series concluded that hyperprolactinaemia with oral risperidone was indeed almost 100% in females and between 63-100% in males (Bushe et al, 2008). Similar levels of hyperprolactinaemia are measured with amisulpride though data in large cohorts is lacking other than from EUFEST (Bushe et al, 2008). Depot formulations of risperidone may have a lower prevalence of hyperprolactinaemia relating to dose (53-67%) (Bushe et al, 2008; Bushe and Shaw, 2007). Paliperidone is the major metabolite of risperidone (9-hydroxyl-risperidone) and prolactin values are either similar or greater than those of risperidone (Berwaerts et al, 2010).

Aripiprazole is associated with the lowest rates of hyperprolactinaemia with prevalence rates of 3-5% in RCTs that increase to incidence rates of 17% in naturalistic studies (Bushe et al, 2010) .Recent data have evaluated aripiprazole as a prolactin-lowering agent when combined with haloperidol or risperidone with some success. Although studies report rapid reductions in prolactin levels after commencing aripiprazole (Shim et al, 2007), this may partially relate to removal of a previously used prolactin-elevating drug. Aripiprazole, however, in a placebo controlled trial when added to high-dose haloperidol (20-25 mg/day) in a cohort of schizophrenia patients resulted in normalisation of prolactin in 85% of subjects by 8 weeks contrasting with 3.6% of the placebo group ($p<0.001$) (Shim et al, 2007). Further research is indicated into the dosage of aripiprazole that may give maximal benefit.

For the remaining antipsychotics, hyperprolactinaemia is sometimes reported though significantly less often than for risperidone and amisulpride. Our review of the data found that for quetiapine reported rates range from 0-29% and for olanzapine from 6-40% (Bushe et al, 2008) although most studies report rates at the lower end of the spectrum. In a recent 6-month study of schizophrenia, patients randomised to quetiapine or olanzapine, 33% had hyperprolactinaemia at baseline which normalised in almost all patients as early as 14 days (Bushe et al, 2009). There were no significant differences between the drugs in changes in prolactin.

The depot formulation of olanzapine has recently been trialled in a complex, non-inferiority study compared with oral olanzapine. The quality of the data and trial design has meant that aspects such as dose response with variables such as prolactin have been investigated (Hill et al, 2011). Significant dose-related changes in prolactin were measured over the 24-week study, however it should be noted that a small mean increase in prolactin was measured only in the cohort receiving 600 mg/month (oral equivalent estimated as 20 mg/day). In this 600 mg/month cohort, 7/21 of female subjects (33%) moved from a normal into a high range level (Table 1). This emphasises the importance of analysing prolactin data not only as mean changes in a cohort but also the categorical changes to provide data that are meaningful in terms of patient outcomes (Bushe et al, 2008). This concept is also well demonstrated in the 555 schizophrenia patient study, Schizophrenia Trial of Aripiprazole (STAR), in which subjects were randomised to either aripiprazole or standard of care treatment (Hanssens et al, 2008; Kerwin et al,2007). There was a mean decrease of 34.2 mg/dl in the aripiprazole-treated cohort, however using a categorical analysis, hyperprolactinaemia was reported in 16.8% of subjects.

	300 mg/month (N=140)	405 mg/month (N=318)	600 mg/month (N=141)
Mean change (micrograms/l) (SD)	-5.61 (12.49)	-2.76 (19.02)	3.58 (33.78)

Table 1. Prolactin changes over 24 weeks with depot olanzapine at various dosages in a randomised controlled trial (Hill et al, 2011)

7. What are the current views of EU guidelines on all aspects of prolactin?

Only one set of guidelines, published in 2008, is devoted to prolactin and it provides both advice and the data and rationale behind the consensus group's conclusions (Peveler et al, 2008). Prior to this many guidelines did not give specific recommendations (Citrome et al, 2008). In general terms, other guidelines and relevant Summaries of Product Characteristics do not provide a specific monitoring schedule and tend to advocate prolactin monitoring only when symptoms are detected.

In 2006, guidelines on bipolar disorder from the National Institute of Clinical Excellence recommended limited pre-treatment monitoring of prolactin levels for risperidone with further monitoring should symptoms develop. The only other guideline to recommend pre-treatment monitoring are the Maudsley guidelines (Taylor et al, 2009). These guidelines recommend baseline prolactin monitoring, followed up at 6 and 12 months. Furthermore, the guidelines advise switching medications if hyperprolactinaemia is symptomatic or, alternatively, adding aripiprazole. The guidelines also concur broadly that hyperprolactinaemia is associated with both short- and longer term adverse events that include bone mineral density loss and a possible increase in the risk of breast cancer. The 2005 recommendations from the World Federation Society of Biological Psychiatry (WFSBP) curiously conclude that whereas prolactin elevation was frequent with amisulpride and typicals (>10%), it was measured only "sometimes" (<10%) with risperidone (Falkai et al, 2006). Current data now seems to have clarified these frequencies rather differently (Bushe et al, 2010; Bushe et al, 2008). The 2008 UK prolactin guidelines recommend prolactin monitoring in all patients pre-treatment regardless of medication and after 3 months of treatment with a stable dose, in addition to further monitoring when there are relevant clinical symptoms (Peveler et al, 2008). With a normal prolactin level there is no further need for monitoring in the absence of clinical symptoms. Significant dose change should also lead to consideration of further monitoring. These UK guidelines give a clear strategy for investigating the aetiology of hyperprolactinaemia in patients receiving antipsychotics and warn against concluding too easily that antipsychotics are responsible. A differential diagnosis must be considered but must always include a pregnancy test in females and thyroid function tests. Prolactin levels can be elevated to levels in excess of >2000 mIU/L in patients taking antipsychotics, however in any patient with prolactin elevation greater than 3000 mIU/L, a prolactinoma should be considered and referral to an endocrinologist is warranted. In the Halifax cohort we measured prolactin levels >2000 mIU/L in 13% of all antipsychotic-treated females and 2% of males. Antipsychotic cessation even for short periods has not been clinically recommended due to risk of worsening of the mental state although in theory this could be considered a diagnostic tool for patients taking oral preparations (Peveler et al, 2008).

8. The management of treatment-emergent hyperprolactinaemia

The management of treatment-emergent hyperprolactinaemia is complex and many of the issues have been considered by the 2008 prolactin guidelines who referenced previous recommendations (Serri et al, 2003). However, newer data have since emerged allowing novel potential management strategies to be considered (Peveler et al, 2008). Levels <1000 mIU/L can simply be monitored but in the presence of symptoms that suggest sex hormone deficiency, it is suggested that such levels should not be allowed to continue long-term due to the potential risk of bone mineral density loss (Peveler et al, 2008). Persistent levels >1000 mIU/L need consideration for medication change or dose reduction, if appropriate. The consensus group concluded that the use of dopamine agonists should be considered only in exceptional circumstances due to the risk of worsening the psychosis (Peveler et al, 2008). This view however is challenged by the Maudsley guidelines (Taylor et al, 2009) which advocate use of dopamine agonists if patients need to remain on the specific prolactin-elevating antipsychotic. They make an interesting observation that although the three agents cited (amantadine, cabergoline and bromocriptine) have the potential to worsen psychosis, that this has not been shown in clinical trials. Although there are many reviews relating to prolactin in the context of severe mental illness, there are currently few, if any, systematic reviews and meta-analyses. A recent systematic review that incorporated a meta-analysis compared the effects of bromocriptine and cabergoline in treating hyperprolactinaemia due to idiopathic causes and prolactinomas (Dos Santos Nunes et al, 2011). They concluded that cabergoline was significantly superior to bromocriptine in normalising both prolactin levels and resuming normal ovulatory cycles. Thus, cabergoline may potentially be the dopamine agonist of choice should this be mandated.

What is currently emerging in an early research phase is the use of specific polypharmacy designed to reduce prolactin levels whilst maintaining treatment on the original antipsychotic. There is little doubt that aripiprazole may have the lowest potential for prolactin elevation, although as we have already stated, in the STAR study 17% of patients did have hyperprolactinaemia (Kerwin et al, 2007 ;Hanssens et al, 2008) although in RCTs, the prevalence rates of 3% seem consistent (Bushe et al, 2008). The combination of adding aripiprazole to risperidone results in significant reductions in plasma concentrations of prolactin of between 35-63%, with maximal benefit measured with aripiprazole doses around 6 mg (Yasui-Furukori, 2010) and possibly doses as low as 3 mg. In 2009, the Maudsley guidelines stated their view that in the presence of symptomatic hyperprolactinaemia options included changing antipsychotics or adding aripiprazole to the existing treatment. As a strategy it is clear that there may be benefit to some patients, however aripiprazole as a partial dopamine agonist has been shown to be associated with worsening of psychosis in some patients. The complete risk-benefit equation for use of aripiprazole in this manner will require further clinical trials. Other salient issues to consider include the reality that schizophrenia the illness, and its associated symptomatology, is the cause of some of the more overt sexual dysfunction (Malik et al, 2011). Reducing prolactin may not always lead to clinical improvement. The correlation between prolactin and sexual dysfunction however is thus complex. In a case series although all subjects had reduction in prolactin levels, only around half reported improved sexual function (Chen 2011). The reality of the situation is that individual patients will require individual solutions. A physician considering changing an antipsychotic in a stable patient must carefully balance the risks and benefits of continued treatment.

There will be patients who are clearly at high risk of prolactin-related adverse events for whom usage of potentially prolactin-elevating antipsychotics needs to be carefully considered,eg, patients with a history of breast cancer or osteoporosis. The other angle to management is to ensure high screening rates for patients at high risk of treatment-emegent osteoporosis and provision of relevant treatment to potentially reduce fracture incidence (Graham et al, 2011).

9. Hyperprolactinaemia in children and adolescents

There would seem to be an increasing usage of antipsychotic drugs in the treatment of many childhood psychiatric illnesses including attention deficit hyperactivity disorder, bipolar disorder and childhood schizophrenia. In general, it would seem that prolactin levels are elevated in children by the same antipsychotics that induce hyperprolactinaemia in adults (Rosenbloom, 2010). For example, in a recent review, 100% of a cohort of 34 children aged 5-14 years treated with risperidone had prolactin elevation(Rosenbloom, 2010). Prolactin levels were also assessed in a naturalistic study of children and adolescents receiving antipsychotics and in some cases concurrent stimulants (Penzner et al, 2009). This analysis revealed a number of interesting findings, however, the addition of a stimulant did not affect prolactin levels compared to no usage. It had been hypothesised that stimulant treatment may reduce any hyperprolactinaemia induced. Adolescents treated with olanzapine when compared to adults treated in clinical trials are also likely to have greater increases in prolactin levels.

The data on prolactin elevation and longer term outcomes in childhood is clearly complex to obtain. Data however do exist and broadly seem to mirror the findings in adults where hyperprolactinaemia is associated with decreased bone mineral density (O'Keane, 2008). A cross-sectional study of 83 boys aged 7-17 years treated for 3 years with the combination of selective serontonin reuptake inhibitors (SSRIs) and risperidone reported that after adjustments, a negative association was found between bone mineral density at the distal radius and serum prolactin level (Rosenbloom, 2010). The data furthermore was suggestive that this bone mineral density reduction may relate to a direct effect of prolactin on bone turnover as there was no relationship between testosterone levels and prolactin. The risk associated with longer term hyperprolactinaemia can be postulated to be a deleterious effect on peak bone mass attainment (Rosenbloom, 2010).

When considering their prolactin guidelines in 2008, the consensus group concluded that there were two groups in whom prolactin elevation should be avoided where possible. Firstly, in those when peak bone mass has not yet been attained, such as in children and young adults up to the age of 25 years (Peveler et al, 2008) with females being more vulnerable to the adverse effect of prolactin elevation than males. Risperidone is certainly being used in a variety of childhood psychiatric illnesses at young ages. A recent report in a small cohort of patients with conduct disorder (mean age 42 months) treated with risperidone at a mean dosage of 0.78mg/day and a maximum of 1.5mg/day (Ercan et al, 2011) found substantial increase in prolactin from a baseline mean of 5.3 ng/ml to 70 ng/ml at 8 weeks. Six of the eight children who completed the study had hyperprolactinaemia without clinical symptoms, as stated by the authors. Studies suggest that children are more sensitive to the prolactin elevating adverse effects of antipsychotics and care is needed to keep these to a minimum (Correll, 2011). The second high risk group would include those with a relevant strong family history of breast cancer or osteoporosis.

10. Further research. What are the unanswered questions?

1. **What are the longer term trajectories of prolactin levels for patients with elevated prolactin?** Research has firmly established that hyperprolactinaemia emerges within days as a consequence of treatment and, as we have shown in a large RCT, equally rapidly reverts to normal with removal of the prolactin-elevating antipsychotic (Bushe et al, 2009). What is less well established is the trajectory of prolactin levels over a longer term period. Do they remain at the same level? Short-term RCTs are unlikely to address this issue and current data that follow patients for 1 year have only reported baseline and endpoint data, not the trajectory of the prolactin response (Schooler et al, 2005). In the absence of a proven mechanism for how and why antipsychotics elevate prolactin differentially (Bushe et al, 2010), one can only speculate.
2. **What are the longer term outcomes for patients with elevated prolactin?** Over the last 10 years patients receiving biologics to treat rheumatoid arthritis have been entered into voluntary, long-term databases that have addressed, albeit in a naturalistic manner, incidence of potentially associated adverse events (cancers, reactivation of tuberculosis (TB), serious infections). There is a need to formally determine the longer term harm of untreated hyperprolactinaemia in psychiatry. The last decade has better defined potential longer term sequelae of hyperprolactinaemia and these clearly cannot be measured within formal RCTs. In 2011, the clear options involve using either large epidemiological databases, prospectively and retrospectively or creating prospective collections of clinical data such as through usage of registers. The challenge exists in creating appropriate databases that allow long-term follow up of both prolactin levels and clinical outcomes. Certainly the data on bone fractures (Howard et al, 2007; Abel et al, 2008) has shown us the potential. The World Health Organization (WHO) initiated a number of databases to measure cancer rates in schizophrenia in the 1970s (Bushe and Hodgson, 2010) and have the knowledge and ability to conduct similar projects worldwide relating to outcomes of hyperprolactinaemia.
3. **What is and how can we measure the true risk-benefit of switching antipsychotic treatments**? There is absolute agreement that usage of drugs such as dopamine agonists have significant potential to worsen schizophrenia illness (Peveler et al, 2008). This creates a dichotomy where the clinician can reduce the dose or change the antipsychotic, or do nothing. There is no single pragmatic endpoint that captures this risk. A relatively short-term RCT (1 year or less) looking at formal changes in rating scales, remission levels or relapse rates may be helpful. At a minimum, it may tell us the psychiatric outcome of switching patients from prolactin-elevating antipsychotics compared to maintaining the status quo. It is difficult to see any individual institution or pharmaceutical company undertaking such a complex and expensive study, and the only viable option would be for larger bodies, such as the European Medicines Agency, National Institute of Mental Health or potentially WHO to undertake this work.

4. **Can genetics help us predict individual responses to potentially prolactin-elevating antipsychotics?** Data allow us to predict which antipsychotics are more likely to elevate prolactin but not with any precision. Potentially any patient given any antipsychotic may have prolactin elevation ranging from small to large. In the future, one can imagine that genetics will better help us understand which patients are more at risk of adverse events associated with individual antipsychotics and also their likelihood of a clinical response. Genetic variation is likely to contribute substantially. Certainly this work is ongoing in the area of weight change with antipsychotic treatment and we can expect that pharmacogenetics may play a critical role (Reynolds, 2007).
5. **Can antipsychotic polypharmacy be a potential treatment option?** Aripiprazole is already cited as a potential treatment option as an additive treatment in the influential Maudsley guidelines (Taylor et al, 2009). With the increasing availability of generic antipsychotic options over the next decade one can envisage a greater degree of polypharmacy similarly designed to reduce or prevent specific adverse events. Prolactin is one area where at least five established antipsychotics are cited as not usually associated with hyperprolactinaemia (Taylor et al, 2009). Such experimental combinations have not been well researched to date and will require a solid trial base before definitive conclusions can be drawn.
6. **How important is the prolactin receptor in terms of cancer?** The prolactin signalling cascade may be important in the pathology of breast and prostate cancers. The antagonism of the prolactin receptor and its pathways may also be important. As we learn the molecular and genetic perspectives of the role of prolactin and its signalling pathways, we may learn more about any potential role of antipsychotic treatments and their relevance in these pathways (Jacobson et al, 2011).

11. Conclusion

Long-term antipsychotic treatment currently represents a usual outcome for patients with schizophrenia and bipolar disorder. Hyperprolactinaemia can be measured in between 33-69% of patients in antipsychotic studies and many antipsychotics significantly elevate prolactin with no suggestion of any longer term decline in prolactin levels. Hyperprolactinaemia can no longer be regarded in any sense as a benign abnormality and it may have significant potential short- and potential longer term consequences. Whereas the short-term adverse events are more easily detectable, the potential longer term consequences may remain hidden and undetectable until a bone fracture or cancer emerges. Over the last 10 years, patients receiving biologics to treat rheumatoid arthritis have been entered into voluntary, long-term databases that have addressed, albeit in a naturalistic manner, incidence of potentially associated adverse events (cancers, reactivation of TB, serious infections). There is a need to formally determine the longer term harm of untreated hyperprolactinaemia in psychiatry. In addition, future research needs to focus on the risk-benefit for the usage of prolactin-elevating antipsychotics.

12. References

[1] Abel KM, Heatlie HF, Howard LM, Webb RT. Sex- and age-specific incidence of fractures in mental illness: a historical, population-based cohort study. J Clin Psychiatry. 2008;69:1398-403

[2] Akkaya C, Kaya B, Kotan Z, et al. Hyperprolactinemia and possibly related development of prolactinoma during amisulpride treatment; three cases. J Psychopharmacol 2009;23:723-6
[3] Berwaerts J, Cleton A, Rossenu S, et al. A comparison of serum prolactin concentrations after administration of paliperidone extended-release and risperidone tablets in patients with schizophrenia. J Psychopharmacol. 2010 Jul;24(7):1011-8
[4] Bostwick JR, Guthrie SK, Ellingrod VL. Antipsychotic-induced hyperprolactinemia. Pharmacotherapy 2009;29:64-73
[5] Bushe C, Shaw M. Prevalence of hyperprolactinaemia in a naturalistic cohort of schizophrenia and bipolar outpatients during treatment with typical and atypical antipsychotics. J Psychopharmacol 2007; 21:768-73.
[6] Bushe C, Shaw M, Peveler RC. A review of the association between antipsychotic use and hyperprolactinaemia. J Psychopharmacol 2008;22(2 Suppl):46-55
[7] Bushe C, Sniadecki J, Bradley AJ, Poole Hoffman V. Comparison of metabolic and prolactin variables from a six-month randomised trial of olanzapine and quetiapine in schizophrenia. J Psychopharmacol. 2010 Jul; 24(7):1001-9.
[8] Bushe CJ, Bradley AJ, Wildgust HJ, Hodgson RE. Schizophrenia and breast cancer incidence. A systematic review of clinical studies. Schizophr Res 2009;114:6-16
[9] Bushe CJ, Hodgson R. Schizophrenia and cancer: in 2010 do we understand the connection? Can J Psychiatry. 2010 Dec;55(12):761-7
[10] Bushe CJ, Bradley A, Pendlebury J. A review of hyperprolactinaemia and severe mental illness: are there implications for clinical biochemistry? Ann Clin Biochem. 2010 Jul;47(Pt 4):292-300
[11] Catts VS, Catts SV, O'Toole BI, Frost AD. Cancer incidence in patients with schizophrenia and their first-degree relatives - a meta-analysis. Acta Psychiatr Scand 2008;117:323-36
[12] Chen CY, Lin TY, Wang CC, Shuai HA. Improvement of serum prolactin and sexual function after switching to aripiprazole from risperidone in schizophrenia: a case series. Psychiatry Clin Neurosci. 2011; 65(1):95-7.
[13] Citrome L. Current guidelines and their recommendations for prolactin monitoring in psychosis.J Psychopharmacol. 2008 Mar; 22(2 Suppl):90-7.
[14] Correll CU. Addressing adverse effects of antipsychotic treatment in young patients with schizophrenia. J Clin Psychiatry. 2011 Jan; 72(1):e01.
[15] Dos Santos Nunes V, El Dib R, Boguszewski CL, Nogueira CR. Cabergoline versus bromocriptine in the treatment of hyperprolactinemia: a systematic review of randomized controlled trials and meta-analysis. Pituitary. 2011 Jan 8. [Epub ahead of print]
[16] Ercan ES, Basay BK, Basay O, et al. Risperidone in the treatment of conduct disorder in preschool children without intellectual disability. Child Adolesc Psychiatry Ment Health. 2011 Apr 13;5(1):10. [Epub ahead of print]
[17] Falkai P, Wobrock T, Lieberman J, et al; WFSBP Task Force on Treatment Guidelines for Schizophrenia. World Federation of Societies of Biological Psychiatry (WFSBP) guidelines for biological treatment of schizophrenia, part 1: acute treatment of schizophrenia. World J Biol Psychiatry 2005;6:132-191
[18] Fitzgerald P, Dinan TG. Prolactin and dopamine: what is the connection? J Psychopharmacol 2008;22(2 Suppl):12-19

[19] Garde AH, Hansen AM, Skovgaard LT, Christensen JM. Seasonal and biological variation of blood concentrations of total cholesterol, dehydroepiandrosterone sulfate, hemoglobin A 1c), IgA, prolactin, and free testosterone in healthy women. Clin Chem. 2000;46:551-9 Erratum in: Clin Chem 2001; 47:1877

[20] Graham SM, Howgate D, Anderson W, et al. Risk of osteoporosis and fracture incidence in patients on antipsychotic medication.Expert Opin Drug Saf. 2011 Jul;10(4):575-602

[21] Haddad PM, Wieck A. Antipsychotic-induced hyperprolactinaemia: mechanisms, clinical features and management. Drugs 2004;64:2291-314

[22] Hanssens L, L'Italien G, Loze JY, et al. The effect of antipsychotic medication on sexual function and serum prolactin levels in community-treated schizophrenic patients: results from the Schizophrenia Trial of Aripiprazole (STAR) study (NCT00237913). BMC Psychiatry. 2008 Dec 22;8:95

[23] Harvey PW, Everett DJ, Springall CJ. Adverse effects of prolactin in rodents and humans: breast and prostate cancer. J Psychopharmacol 2008; 22(2 Suppl):20-7.

[24] Hill AL, Sun B, Karagianis JL, et al. Dose-associated changes in safety and efficacy parameters observed in a 24-week maintenance trial of olanzapine long-acting injection in patients with schizophrenia. BMC Psychiatry. 2011 Feb 15;11:28.

[25] Hippisley-Cox J, Vinogradova Y, Coupland C, Parker C. Risk of malignancy in patients with schizophrenia or bipolar disorder: nested case-control study. Arch Gen Psychiatry 2007; 64:1368-76.

[26] Holt RIG. Medical causes and consequences of hyperprolactinaemia. A context for psychiatrists. J Psychopharmacol 2008;22(2 Suppl):28-37

[27] Howard L, Kirkwood G, Leese M. Risk of hip fracture in patients with a history of schizophrenia. *Br J Psychiatry* 2007;190:129-34

[28] Jacobson EM, Hugo ER, Borcherding DC, Ben-Jonathan N. Prolactin in breast and prostate cancer: molecular and genetic perspectives. Discov Med. 2011 Apr;11(59):315-24.

[29] Johnsen E, Kroken RA, Abaza M, et al. Antipsychotic-induced hyperprolactinemia: a cross-sectional survey. J Clin Psychopharmacol 2008;28:686-90

[30] Kahn RS, Fleischhacker WW, Boter H, et al. Lancet. 2008 Mar 29;371(9618):1085-97.Effectiveness of antipsychotic drugs in first-episode schizophrenia and schizophreniform disorder: an open randomised clinical trial. Lancet. 2008 29;371(9618):1085-97.

[31] Kane J, Canas F, Kramer M et al. Treatment of schizophrenia with paliperidone extended-release tablets: a 6-week placebo-controlled trial. Schizophr Res 2007;90:147-61.

[32] Kerwin R, Millet B, Herman E et al. A multicentre, randomized, naturalistic, open-label study between aripiprazole and standard of care in the management of community-treated schizophrenic patients. Schizophrenia Trial of Aripiprazole: (STAR) study. Eur Psychiatry. 2007;22:433-43

[33] Kleinberg DL, Davis JM, De Coster R et al. Prolactin levels and adverse effects in patients treated with risperidone. J Clin Psychopharmacol 1999;19:57-61

[34] Knegtering H, van den Bosch R, Castelein S, et al. Are sexual side effects of prolactin-raising antipsychotics reducible to serum prolactin? Psychoneuroendocrinology 2008;33:711-17

[35] Kohen D, Wildgust HJ. The evolution of hyperprolactinaemia as an entity in psychiatric patients. J Psychopharmacol 2008;22(2 Suppl):6-11
[36] Lieberman JA, Stroup TS, McEvoy JP et al. Effectiveness of antipsychotic drugs in patients with chronic schizophrenia. N Engl J Med 2005; 353:1209-23
[37] Mackin P, Waton A, Nulkar A, Watkinson HM. Prolactin and smoking status in antipsychotic-treated patients. J Psychopharmacol. 2011;25(5):698-703.
[38] Mazziotti G, Porcelli T, Mormando M et al.. Vertebral fractures in males with prolactinoma. Endocrine. 2011 Jun;39(3):288-93.
[39] Malik P, Kemmler G, Hummer M et al, Sexual dysfunction in first-episode schizophrenia patients: results from European first episode schizophrenia trial. J Clin Psychopharmacol. 2011 Jun;31(3):274-80.
[40] McEvoy, JP, Lieberman, JA, Perkins DO et al. Efficacy and tolerability of olanzapine, quetiapine and risperidone in the treatment of early psychosis: A randomized, double-blind 52-week comparison. Am J Psychiatry 2007; 164:1050-60
[41] Peveler RC, Branford D, Citrome L, et al . Antipsychotics and hyperprolactinaemia: clinical recommendations. J Psychopharmacol 2008;22(2 Suppl):98-103
[42] Meaney AM, Smith S, Howes OD, et al.. Effects of long-term prolactin-raising antipsychotic medication on bone mineral density in patients with schizophrenia. B J Psychiatry 2004;184:503-8
[43] Meaney AM, and O'Keane V. Bone mineral density changes over a year in young females with schizophrenia; relationship to medication and endocrine variables. Schizophr Res 2007;93:136-43
[44] Montgomery J, Winterbottom E, Jessani M et al. Prevalence of hyperprolactinemia in schizophrenia: association with typical and atypical antipsychotic treatment.J Clin Psychiatry. 2004 Nov;65(11):1491-8
[45] National Institute for Health and Clinical Excellence (NICE). Bipolar disorder. The management of bipolar disorder in adults, children and adolescents, in primary and secondary care. NICE clinical guideline 38, 2006 [cited 2011 May 14]; Available from: www.nice.org.uk/CG038
[46] Ohta C, Yasui-Furukori N, Furukori H, et al. The effect of smoking status on the plasma concentration of prolactin already elevated by risperidone treatment in schizophrenia patients. Prog Neuropsychopharmacol Biol Psychiatry. 2011;35(2):573-6.
[47] O'Keane V, Meaney AM. Antipsychotic drugs. A new risk factor for osteoporosis in young women with schizophrenia? J Clin Psychopharmacol 2005;25:26-31
[48] O'Keane V. Antipsychotic-induced hyperprolactinaemia, hypogonadism and osteoporosis in the treatment of schizophrenia. J Psychopharmacol 2008;22 (2 suppl):70-75
[49] Penzner JB, Dudas M, Saito E ,et al. Lack of effect of stimulant combination with second-generation antipsychotics on weight gain, metabolic changes, prolactin levels, and sedation in youth with clinically relevant aggression or oppositionality.J Child Adolesc Psychopharmacol. 2009 Oct;19(5):563-73
[50] Poyraz BC, Aksoy C, Balcioğlu I. Increased incidence of autoimmune thyroiditis in patients with antipsychotic-induced hyperprolactinemia. Eur Neuropsychopharmacol 2008;18:667-72

[51] Reuwer AQ, Twickler MT, Hutten BA, et al. Prolactin levels and the risk of future coronary artery disease in apparently healthy men and women. Circ Cardiovasc Genet. 2009; 2(4):389-95.
[52] Reynolds G. The impact of pharmacogenetics on the development and use of antipsychotic drugs. Drug Discov Today. 2007 Nov;12(21-22):953-9
[53] Riddle O, Bates RW, Dykshorn SW. (1933). The preparation, identification and assay of prolactin - a hormone of the anterior pituitary. Am J Physiol 1933;105:191-216
[54] Rosenbloom AL. Hyperprolactinemia with antipsychotic drugs in children and adolescents. Int J Pediatr Endocrinol. 2010;2010. pii: 159402. Epub 2010 Aug 24.
[55] Schooler N, Rabinowitz J, Davidson M, et al. Risperidone and haloperidol in first episode psychosis: A long term randomised trial. Am J Psychiatry 2005;162:947-53
[56] Serri O, Chik CL, Ur E, Ezzat S. Diagnosis and management of hyperprolactinemia. Canadian Medical Association Journal 2003;169:575-581
[57] Shim JC, Shin JGK, Kelly DL et al. Adjunctive treatment with a dopamine partial agonist, aripiprazole, for antipsychotic-induced hyperprolactinemia: a placebo-controlled trial. Am J Psychiatry. 2007;164:1404-10
[58] Skopek M, Manoj P. Hyperprolactinaemia during treatment with paliperidone. Australas Psychiatry. 2010 Jun;18(3):261-3.
[59] Smith S, Wheeler MJ, Murray R, O'Keane V. The effects of antipsychotic-induced hyperprolactinaemia on the hypothalamic-pituitary-gonadal axis. J Clin Psychopharmacol 2008;22:109-14
[60] Szarfman A, Tonning JM, Levine JG, Doraiswamy PM. Atypical antipsychotics and pituitary tumours: a pharmacovigilance study. Pharmacotherapy 2006;26:748-58
[61] Taylor D, Paton C, Kapur S. The Maudsley prescribing guidelines. 10th ed. London: Informa Healthcare; 2009
[62] Tworoger SS, Eliassen AH, Rosner Bet al. Plasma prolactin concentrations and risk of postmenopausal breast cancer. Cancer Res 2004;64, 6814-19
[63] Tworoger S, Eliassen AH, Sluss P, Hankinson SE. A prospective study of plasma prolactin concentrations and risk of premenopausal and postmenopausal breast cancer. J Clin Oncol 2007;25:1-7
[64] Tworoger SS, Hankinson SE. Prolactin and breast cancer risk. Cancer Lett 2006; 243:160-9.
[65] Wang PS, Walker AM, Tsuang MT et al. Dopamine antagonists and the development of breast cancer. Arch Gen Psychiatry 2002;59:1147-54
[66] Yasui-Furukori N, Furukori H, Sugawara N, et al. Prolactin fluctuation over the course of a day during treatments with three atypical antipsychotics in schizophrenic patients. Hum Psychopharmacol. 2010 Apr;25(3):236-42
[67] Yasui-Furukori N, Furukori H, Sugawara N, et al.. Dose-dependent effects of adjunctive treatment with aripiprazole on hyperprolactinemia induced by risperidone in female patients with schizophrenia..J Clin Psychopharmacol. 2010 Oct;30(5):596-9.

24

Tolerance to Tick-Borne Diseases in Sheep: Highlights of a Twenty-Year Experience in a Mediterranean Environment

Elisa Pieragostini, Elena Ciani,
Giuseppe Rubino and Ferruccio Petazzi
University of Bari
Italy

1. Introduction

The European landscape is characterised by a range of diverse farming systems. These relate not only to varied geographical environments and animal genetic resources, but also to different social and cultural contexts for farming and food production. This diversity is unique to Europe and, among the European countries, Italy is the home for a great variety of native breeds because of its complex orography and its long boot shape with very different climatic conditions from north to south. In the 1980's, two of us moved from northern Italy to Apulia and soon came to appreciate the differences between the biotic and abiotic features of northern environment and the Apulian one. One of the most impressive differences were the enzootic tick borne diseases (TBD) and the related responses of the animals. As a consequence, much of our professional life has been devoted to the challenges posed by the diseases and to the study of the genetic peculiarities of native breeds both *per se* and in terms of their tolerance to TBD.

This report is a review of the results obtained in a 20-year experience investigating the haematological features and tolerance to tick-borne diseases in Mediterranean native sheep breeds - mainly Apulian native breeds - compared to exotic breeds under various experimental conditions. In the wake of William Thomson (Lord Kelvin), a pioneer in thermodynamics and electricity, who said in 1891 that when you can measure what you are speaking about, and express it in numbers, you know something about it, but when you cannot measure it, your knowledge is of a meager and unsatisfactory kind, the central concept or research theme that guided all our research efforts stems from the notion that direct measurement of disease phenotypes and/or physiological features such as the hematological pattern provides a direct assay for measuring disease changes and the attitude of a genetic pool in facing disease. The work is concerned with the following main issues:

- Haematological pattern of Apulian native sheep breeds
- Breeds and tolerance to TBD in Apulia
- Response to experimental anaemia
- Response to *Anaplasma ovis* infection in experimentally infected sheep.

2. Haematological pattern of Apulian native sheep breeds

In Apulia, the region covering the heel of the boot-shaped Italian peninsula, the rather harsh conditions of the soil and climate and the selective pressure of endemic haemotropic parasites have yielded genetic pools that are generally rustic and tolerant to the diseases caused by haemotropic parasites. An evaluation of the local genetic resources to explore their potential for sustainable and profitable genetic development programs is based on the knowledge of the physio-pathological features of blood according to species, breed and animal.

2.1 The Apulian sheep native breeds

Altamurana and Leccese, the latter also known as Moscia Leccese, are two ancient dairy breeds native to Apulia whose origins are not fully known. It is thought that they developed from an Asian breed, particularly from a Zackel type stock. They are rough wooled, well suited to life in harsh and semiarid conditions and they make good use of marginal pastures. Both breeds are seriously endangered. Though not as endangered as the former two breeds, Gentile di Puglia sheep may be considered, according to Alderson (2009), at risk of extinction because of their numerical scarcity and population trends. Yet, the Gentile di Puglia is classified as one of the main fine-wooled ovine breeds. The origin of the breed can be traced back to ancient Roman times when the soft fleece of an Apulian sheep, the Tarentine breed, was used to make the *togas* of important Roman citizens. According to William Youatt (1867), the Tarentine breed "had gradually spread from the coast of Syria and the Black Sea, and had now reached the western extremity of Europe. Many of them mingled with and improved the native breeds of Spain, while others continued to exist as a distinct race; and, meeting with a climate and a herbage suited to them, retained their original character and value, and were the progenitors of the Merinos of the present day."

2.2 Adult haematological pattern

Table 1 has been compiled from the existing repertoire of haematological values obtained analysing the blood of Apulian sheep; it reports least-square means (LSM) and standard error (SE) of haematological data obtained by analysing blood samples collected in population surveys of Gentile di Puglia and Leccese (Pieragostini et al., 1994; Pieragostini, 2006). Samples for Altamurana sheep were obtained from 58 purebred ewes ranging from 2-6 years of age and bred on an experimental farm near Bari (Pieragostini et al., 1999). Comparison with the literature (Jain, 1993), where range and medians are available, is also shown. On the basis of the normal probability plot, our data appear to follow a normal distribution where the median equals the mean.
When compared to normal blood values for sheep in the literature (Greenwood, 1977; Jain, 1993), the blood of Apulian sheep appears to be characterized by fewer erythrocytes that are normal in size and have higher haemoglobin content. This phenomenon typically seems to reflect a Mediterranean/North-African ovine blood picture (Pieragostini et al., 1994). The decreased PCV values correspond to lower blood viscosity and thus greater availability of water, which seems to be of particular adaptive significance in habitats characterized by an arid climate like Apulia (Ariely et al. 1986). The fact that some blood factors are related to the suitability of the breeds under particular environmental conditions was suggested long ago (Cresswell & Hutchings, 1962).

	Altamurana		Gentile di Puglia		Leccese		Jain (1993)	
Parameter	LSM±SE	N	LSM±SE	N	LSM±SE	N	range	median
RBC ($10^6/\mu l$)	8.3±0.13	58	9.4±0.06	263	8.3±0.14	145	9 - 15	12
Hb (g/dl)	9.8±0.11	58	10.4±0.25	263	9.3±0.32	996	9 - 15	11
PCV (g/dl)	30.6±0.33	58	30.6±0.16	263	29.5±0.11	996	26 - 45	34
MCV (fl)	37.9±0.52	58	32.8±0.13	263	36.4±0.59	145	28 - 40	34
MCH (pg)	12.2±0.15	58	11.2±0.05	263	11.6±0.21	145	8 - 12	10
MCHC (g/dl)	32.2±0.16	58	34.1±0.44	263	32.4±0.36	996	31 - 34	32
WBC ($10^3/\mu l$)	7.4±0.20	58	8.4±0.16	178	7.8±0.19	145	4 - 12	8

Table 1. Least-square means (LSM) and standard error (SE) of haematological data from adult animals belonging to native Apulian sheep breeds. RBC, Red Blood Cells; Hb, Haemoglobin; PCV, Packed Cell Volume; MCV, Mean Corpuscular Volume; MCH, Mean Corpuscular Haemoglobin, MCHC, Mean Corpuscular Haemoglobin Content; WBC, White Blood Cells; N, Number of animals.

Comparison of the data in table 1 shows that the haematological patterns in the three breeds are broadly the same. Gentile sheep seem to exhibit slight differences from the other two breeds, particularly as to the erythrocyte count, the mean corpuscular volume (MCV) and the mean corpuscular haemoglobin (MCH); in fact they are apparently the most European among the three. The traditional breeding sites of Gentile and Leccese differ substantially; one is in the southern part and the other in the northern part of Apulia, which is 500 Km long extending from the 39° to the 42° parallel. The Altamurana breeding site is in the Murgia uplands, in the central portion of Apulia. Its location in a rather harsh environment, together with the common origin of the two breeds, may account for the fact that Altamurana is closer to Leccese than to Gentile (Tab.1). However, a non-negligible point is that the physiological pattern characterizing the Altamurana and the Leccese breeds differs considerably from that of the Gentile di Puglia, as they belong to the group of dairy breeds while the Gentile is a fine wool and meat-producing sheep.

2.3 Lamb haematological pattern

Although the paucity of data in the literature concerning the haematological picture of lambs is scarce, general and particular information is available on the developmental pattern of their haematological values. The development of haematological picture of Altamurana lambs was investigated to assess the normal blood parameters and check the first occurrence in the blood smears of endemic endoerythrocytic parasites (Pieragostini et al., 2000). Standard haematological values were calculated for 22 Altamurana lambs controlled from birth to 18 months of age The values recorded in the neonatal period were strongly affected by birth weight. As clearly shown in table 2, the haemoglobin concentration (Hb), packed cell volume (PCV) and white cell count (WBC) exhibited significant age-dependent variations, particularly Hb % and PCV decreased while WBC increased.

Over weeks 1-5, red cell indices mainly followed the same trends as the Hb and PCV. Over the first four months, the RBC values on average remained unchanged at approximately 9 million/μl but then decreased. Starting from the fifth month, overall mean values were practically the same as in adults.

Age	Haematological parameters						
	RBC (10^6/μl)	Hb (g/dl)	PCV (g/dl)	MCV (fl)	MCH (pg)	MCHC (g/dl)	WBC (10^3/μl)
	LSM±SE	LSM±SE	LSM±SE	LSM±SE	LSM±SE	LSM±SE	LSM±SE
2 days	9.6±0.9	13.0±1.0	42.0±4.1	43.7±3.0	13.5±0.9	31.1±1.34	4.5±1.0
7 days	8.7±1.1	12.6±0.9	39.7±1.9	46.2±6.0	14.7±2.2	31.7±1.17	5.4±1.6
15 days	9.0±0.9	12.5±0.7	39.5±2.0	44.1±2.8	14.0±0.5	31.7±1.5	5.6±2.8
21 days	9.4±0.8	11.6±0.7	35.7±1.5	38.2±3.32	12.4±1.0	32.5±2.1	5.3±1.7
30 days	9.2±1.2	11.2±0.5	35.4±1.9	38.7±4.9	12.4±1.5	31.7±1.4	6.1±2.5
45 days	9.9±1.2	10.8±0.8	35.5±2.0	36.1±3.8	11.0±1.4	30.5±1.9	7.5±2.1
2 months	9.8±0.8	10.7±0.4	34.9±2.1	35.6±3.0	10.9±0.9	30.6±1.3	7.8±1.7
3 months	9.3±0.8	10.5±0.4	32.7±1.4	35.4±3.1	11.4±1.0	32.2±0.9	6.8±1.8
4 months	9.1±1.2	10.3±0.6	32.6±1.9	36.2±3.1	11.4±1.0	31.5±0.8	8.1±2.0
7 months	7.8±0.5	9.1±0.5	29.9±1.4	38.4±1.3	11.7±0.6	30.6±0.8	7.9±1.9
9 months	7.9±0.7	9.4±0.8	30.1±1.3	38.1±2.6	11.9±0.9	31.2±1.5	7.3±1.4
12 months	7.5±0.3	9.4±0.5	28.5±1.5	38.0±2.1	12.4±0.6	32.8±1.3	8.9±1.4
15 months	7.6±0.4	9.3±0.4	28.4±1.5	37.5±2.5	12.2±0.7	32.7±1.3	8.8±1.4
18 months	7.8±0.3	9.3±0.3	28.6±0.7	36.8±1.0	12.0±0.5	32.6±0.7	8.6±1.4

Table 2. Least-square means (LSM) and standard errors (SE) of haematological values recorded for 22 Altamurana lambs controlled from birth to 18 months of age. Modified from Pieragostini et al. (2000). RBC, Red Blood Cells; Hb, Haemoglobin; PCV, Packed Cell Volume; MCV, Mean Corpuscular Volume; MCH, Mean Corpuscular Haemoglobin, MCHC, Mean Corpuscular Haemoglobin Content; WBC, White Blood Cells.

Considering that reference data are mainly from breeds originally selected in northern European countries, when a comparison was made between 12 month-old Altamurana lambs and their northern counterparts, the erythrocytes of the Altamurana were fewer (7.5 *versus* 11.8 millions/μl) but bigger (38.0 ft *versus* 26.5 ft) and full of haemoglobin (12.4 pg *versus* 9.3 pg). This is the same phenomenon encountered in Mediterranean/North-African ovine blood picture as well as in the native Apulian adults.

The overall pattern is suggestive of erythrocyte physiological effectiveness, which was confirmed by the perfect physical development of the subjects examined in this study. In the blood smears obtained at seven months of age, namely in full spring when lambs start to graze pastures, endoerythrocytic enzootic parasites (*Theileria* spp. and *Anaplasma* spp.) were recorded and then became a constantly occurring phenomenon as will be documented in the following sections.

3. Breeds and tolerance to TBD in Apulia

Tick-borne diseases are of global importance to human and animal health and welfare. They are also responsible each year for dramatic economic losses which comprise direct losses from death of animals, loss of productivity and indirect losses due to the costs of control measures. In 1979, the amount of losses were estimated to be globally USD 7 billion (McCosker, 1979), but several reports on the economic costs of specific tick-borne diseases indicated that the earlier report is an underestimate (Jongejan & Uilenberg, 2004). There is a wide portfolio of measures which could be used to control tick-borne diseases among which both husbandry practices and host-related factors such as age, innate tolerance and breed are of great importance. Breeds whose historical breeding site is situated under the latitude of 41° show the ability to thrive in areas where tick borne diseases (TBD) are common. This trait, which can be defined as tolerance to TBD, is associated with the ability to resist the development of anemia in the face of infection.
A review on host resistance to tick borne diseases is documented in cattle (Correia de Almeida Regitano & Prayaga, 2010). As for other species, the case of the tolerance to tick-borne diseases shown by the sheep and horse native to Apulia is emblematic (Pieragostini & Petazzi, 1999; Rubino et al., 2006). In southern Italy, and particularly in Apulia, pyroplasmosis represents a longstanding and heavy burden for every type of livestock farm (Ceci & Carelli, 1999). Previous work performed on Gentile di Puglia sheep found that blood smears for parasite detection revealed an overall positivity rate of 93% for tick borne parasites (TBP) (Pieragostini et al, 2006). This high TBP positivity rate associated to normal blood values highlighted the tolerance of the native sheep towards TBP infection and accounted for endemic TBD.

3.1 Tick borne diseases in Apulian native sheep: A low income disease

According to Townsend & Thirtle (2001), studies of the rates of return to research have usually been based on the implicit assumption that if there were no research, then there would be neither growth nor decline in output or productivity. In the case of livestock, particularly in those areas characterized by a sub-tropical disease ecology, the assumption is especially unreasonable. It ignores the losses that would have occurred in the absence of livestock health research, resulting in an underestimation of the rates of return. The financial impact of a range of clinical and subclinical diseases and mortalities on farms is difficult to assess because there are insufficient accurate survey data on their prevalence causes or production losses on a national basis. Thus demonstration of the economic advantage of animal health is one of the relevant issues in animal production. Pieragostini et al. (1996) carried out a four year study to check the economic and zoonotic importance of TBD on sheep farms.
To this purpose sheep belonging to breeds tolerant to TBD systematically underwent one prophylactic treatment with diminazene aceturate (Berenil, Hoechst, AG, Germany) in full spring before the mating season. Table 3 shows the results obtained. The comparison between the reproductive values in the treated sheep and in an untreated control group highlighted significant differences in fertility and fecundity, with the group of treated sheep that were more fertile and fecund. Pyroplasmosis, even though unapparent, represents an important cause of perturbation of animal welfare. The authors estimated relevant ($\approx$30%) economic losses in non treated animals, thus defining pyroplasmosis as a "low income disease".

Parameter	Altamurana		Leccese		Total	
	T (N =149)	NT (N = 259)	T (N = 49)	NT (N = 89)	T (N = 198)	NT (N = 348)
Fertility (%)	93[a]	65[b]	86[a]	62[b]	91[A]	64[B]
Prolificacy (%)	139	131	144	142	138	134
Fecundity (%)	132[a]	89[b]	119[a]	90[b]	128[A]	89[B]

Table 3. Least-square means of the reproductive parameters in Altamurana and Leccese sheep and in the whole sample (Total), as a function of the prophylactic treatment against pyroplasmosis with diminazene aceturate (T = treated, NT = not treated). Modified from Pieragostini et al. (1996). Means within rows with different letters significantly differ: capital letters: P< 0.001; small letters: P<0.05.

3.2 Breed sheep and TBD

It is now generally acknowledged that importing exotic breeds can result in activities within the livestock sector that are uneconomic and/or have a negative impact on the environment. In many cases these activities are subsidized or otherwise provided for by development programs such as the case of Apulia which was documented in a study assessing attempts to introduce highly productive north European sheep breeds to Apulia (Pieragostini & Petazzi, 1999). The investigation analyzed data concerning the incidence and severity of pyroplasmosis in the five years spanning 1980-1984 on an experimental farm situated on the Murgia uplands in the province of Bari. The farm contained sheep belonging to gene pools of different geographical origin (Apulian, Italian island and north European breeds) or genotype classification (pure breeds or crossbreds) (Fig. 1).

The northern Finnish, Friesian and Romanov breeds were very susceptible to the disease; conversely, the native Apulian breeds showed very low rates of morbidity and mortality, followed in turn by breeds like Sardinian and Comisana, whose native areas have climatic and pedological characteristics similar to those of Apulia (Fig. 2). It is also worth noting that while the native and island breeds were regularly taken out to graze, the north European breeds were kept constantly under cover to reduce the likelihood of encountering ticks.

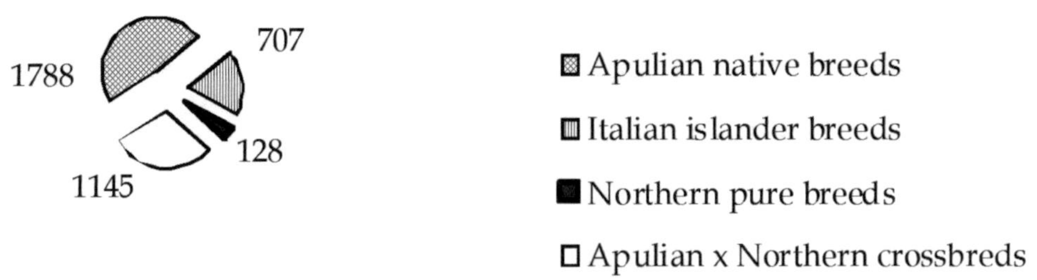

Fig. 1. Size of the investigated samples, clustered as sheep ecotypes. Modified from Pieragostini & Petazzi (1999).

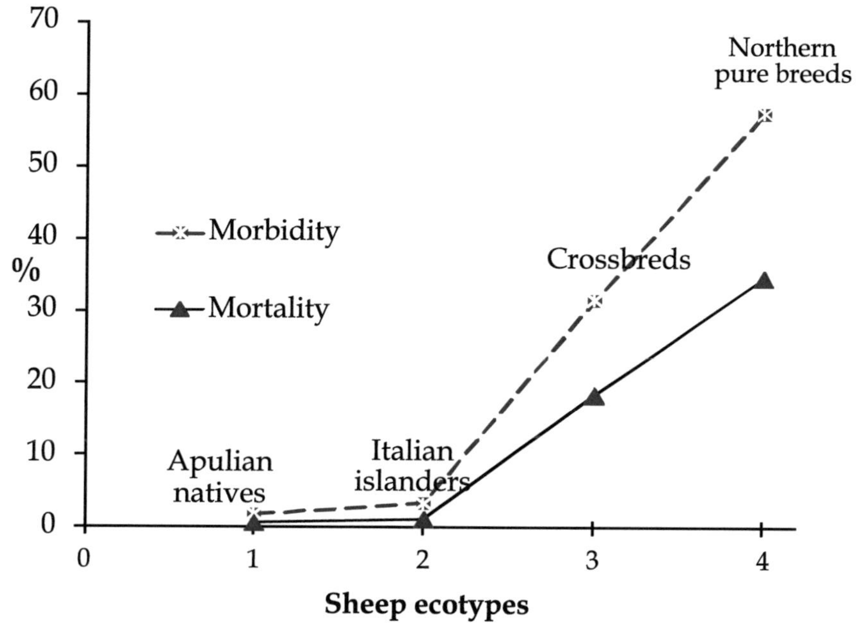

Fig. 2. Graphical representation obtained by processing morbidity and mortality data evidencing the influence of genotype on tolerance to pyroplasmosis in sheep living in Apulia. 1, Apulian native breeds (Altamurana, Gentile di Puglia and Leccese); 2, Italian islander breeds (Comisana and Sardinian); 3, Crossbreds (Finnish x Altamurana, Finnish x Leccese, Friesian x Altamurana, Friesian x Leccese; Romanov x Altamurana, Romanov x Leccese); 4, Northern pure breeds (Finnish, Friesian and Romanov). Modified from Pieragostini & Petazzi (1999).

A further element to consider is that attempts to improve the productivity of Apulian breeds by crossing them with the above exotic breeds failed because of the high mortality in generations F1 and F2, almost solely due to TBD. Though the mortality rates in crossbred animals were lower than those registered in the respective parental pure breeds, the number of individuals killed by the impact with endoerythrocytic pathogens was in any case too high (Fig. 2).

Pathogens were not accurately classified since the study analyzed data from farm records in which the veterinarians' diagnosis at death, due to TBD, always mentioned pyroplasmosis. The cases, which we were able to observe, concerned five Romanov sheep and seven Suffolk (occasionally found in the course of time and seriously ill prior to our visit). Examination of the animals always revealed classic symptoms of babesiosis and this was confirmed once the blood samples taken at the same time were analyzed. The haematological situation showed severe microcytic and hypochromic anaemia and *Babesia ovis (B. ovis)* was consistently identified in the blood smears.

By contrast, among the resilient breeds of sheep, the animals infected with pyroplasmosis showed only a state of discomfort which usually does not last more than few days and is characterized by a brief rise in temperature, slight dejection in the form of a tendency to move away from the flock, loss of appetite which might also be very transitory, translucent mucosae, slightly blueish against a pale background and in a few cases subicteric.

3.3 Piroplasmosis in naturally infected tolerant sheep

Resistance is a dynamic process of parasite regulation by the host. The pathogen must penetrate host cell barriers in sufficient numbers, attack target cells and replicate. Sub-clinical or clinical expression of the disease is dependent on the pathogen's virulence and the interaction between pathogen and host characteristics. Particularly, the phenomenon of tolerance to tick borne pathogens (TBP) is closely linked to a particular type of anaemia which is generally the symptom *par excellence* of the disease. In the tolerant animals, as shown in a study carried out on Altamurana sheep, this takes a benign macrocytic and hyperchromic form. A comparison of the haematological parameters of healthy sheep with those of sick sheep in table 4 showed that the latter presented a numerical deficiency of red blood cells that was compensated by the fact that the mean corpuscular volume (MCV) increased by about 50% as did the mean corpuscular haemoglobin (MCH). The results shown in table 4 did not stem from a dedicated investigation because the haematologic alterations were met with by chance when investigating on the functional effect of a rare alpha globin gene variant. At sampling, the affected sheep did not show any patent signs of the disease and thus only the haemocromocytometric parameters, the related observation of blood films and the results of the osmotic fragility test led to classifying the sampled animals in healthy and affected. Observation of blood films in this study and in other subsequent occasional analyses on Apulian sheep in similar conditions, highlighted that in most cases there were mixed infections in which *Anplasma* spp. and/or *Theileria* spp. and/or *Babesia* spp. occurred at the same time (Fig. 3). *B. ovis* was consistently present in the blood films of the affected animals with visible symptoms of haematuria. This fact, taken together with the evidence from tests on Romanov sheep infected and killed by babesiosis, convinced us that *B. ovis* was one of the causes of the pathogenetic activity in Apulian sheep, and certainly in non-native breeds. However, diseases often occur in clusters of time (years, seasons, production cycles, etc.) and space (herd, pasture, farm, region, etc.) and the prevalence of this pathogen was never the target of a dedicated epidemiological investigation.

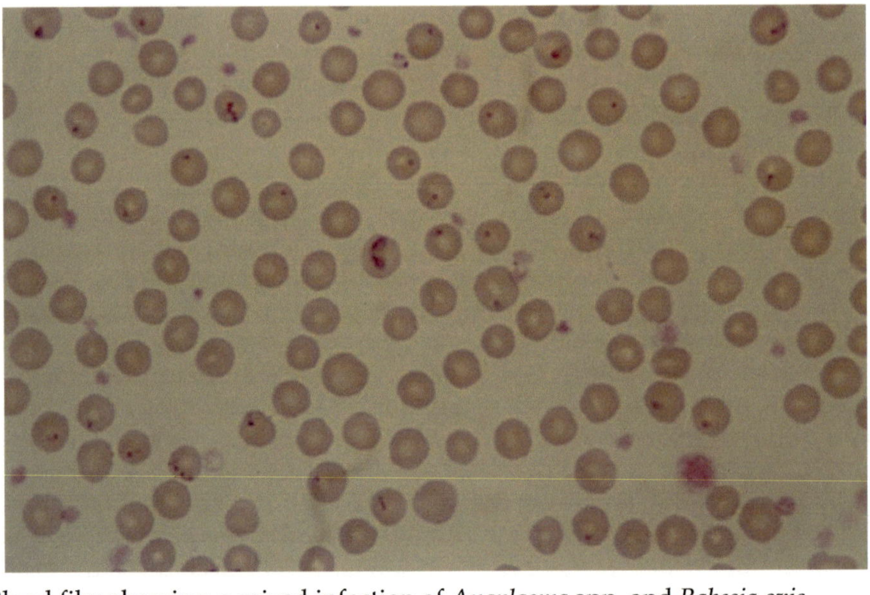

Fig. 3. Blood film showing a mixed infection of *Anaplasma* spp. and *Babesia ovis*.

Haematological parameters	Samples		Significance
	Healthy (N =22)	Affected (N =28)	
RBC ($10^6/\mu l$)	9.5±0.19	6.3±0.70	**
Hb (g/dl)	9.9±0.18	9.2±0.50	*
PCV (g/dl)	32.3±0.55	30.3±0.50	**
MCV (fl)	34.3±1.43	48.7±1.29	**
MCH (pg)	10.4±0.46	15.2±0.42	**
MCHC (g/dl)	30.5±0.44	31.2±0.40	n.s.
WBC ($10^3/\mu l$)	9.6±0.40	9.5±0.37	n.s.
MCF (g%NaCl for 50% haemolysis)	0.72±0.02	0.82±0.03	**

Table 4. Comparison of the haematological parameters recorded in healthy and affected Altamurana sheep (mean values ± standard errors). Modified from Pieragostini & Petazzi, 1999. (RBC=Red Blood Cells; Hb=Haemoglobin %; PCV= Packed Cell Volume; MCV= Mean Corpuscular Volume; MCH=Mean Corpuscular Haemoglobin, MCHC=Mean Corpuscular Haemoglobin Content; WBC=White Blood Cells; MCF=Mean Corpuscolar Fragility) *$P<0.05$;**$P<0.01$; n.s.= not significant.

3.4 Anaplasmosis in naturally infected splenectomized sheep

Anaplasmosis is one of the most important tick-borne diseases of ruminants worldwide. The disease is caused by infection of animals with the obligate intraerythrocytic bacteria *Anaplasma* spp. which is classified in the family *Anaplasmataceae*, order *Rickettsiales* (Dumler et al, 2001). This section includes some experiences with sheep splenectomy and describes disease onset and course in eight splenectomized TBD-tolerant sheep that were naturally infected with piroplasms. Though the trials had been performed in different time periods, the results obtained were very similar and the facts surrounding the experiments gave us both general and specific insights into the field of splenectomy of carrier sheep from areas where endoerythrocytic parasites are endemic.

Particularly in the first trial, the surgical operation had two purposes: a) to evaluate the rôle of the spleen as a filter-pad to check parasites and as modulator of the direct response to anemia; b) to obtain a high number of parasites in the blood to prepare a local specific antigen.

The following trials were mainly related to the need to obtain *A. ovis* which was isolated from splenectomized sheep allowed to be naturally infected pasturing in tick areas.

Splenectomy was slightly traumatic for all the subjects and 24 hours after the surgical operation the sheep showed normal functions. The sheep were identified with female names for easier checking. Clinical evaluation was done on a daily basis and rectal temperatures were recorded every morning for 12 weeks post splenectomy. Blood and serum samples were routinely collected twice a week during the observation period. Haematological variables were evaluated using a haematology analyzer. The erythrocyte fragility test was performed by exposing erythrocytes to hypotonic saline solutions decreasing by 0.02% starting from 0.86%. Parasites in the blood were checked by Giemsa staining every 3 days. During the acute phase of the disease, the most important haematological values, erythrocyte fragility and parasitaemia were monitored daily. In the case of Gilda, Lina and Zoppina, which were part of the experiment to check the response to *A. ovis* infection of different sheep breeds, described in section 5, parasite density was estimated on thin blood film and expressed as the percentage of parasitized red blood cells.

Fifteen days after the splenectomy, the general situation worsened and the animals became anorexic, staggering with a severe anaemia and dehydration. At the same time the RBC, Hb% and PCV values dropped (Tab. 5), and a number of organisms started appearing in the blood films (Rosalba showed a carpet of *A. ovis;* Stella a great deal of *A. ovis;* Lisa and Lola a great deal of *A. ovis* and a few *Babesia* spp.; Claretta a great number of *Theileria* spp.). Rosalba and Stella died of severe anaemia respectively 24 hours and 4 days after the diagnosis despite specific drugs and whole blood trasfusions with blood drawn from a donor subject. Claretta, Lisa and Lola showed less violent initial symptoms, the anaemic crisis was less severe and following a therapy with anti-protozoal drugs associated with desametazone they gradually began to eat and became clinically and haematologically healthy in 15-20 days. Since Lina, Zoppina, and Gilda, were included in the above cited experimental design to investigate the tolerance to *A. ovis,* they were constantly monitored and parasitaemia was recorded every two days after splenectomy. The cases of Lina and Zoppina allowed comparison between a mixed infection by *T. ovis* and *A. ovis* and an almost single infection by *A. ovis*. Interestingly, the two sheep coped differently with the infections. Though both animals were positive for *A. ovis* and *T. ovis* after splenectomy, the maximum of parasitized erythrocytes (MPE) by *T. ovis* peaked to 17% in Zoppina, while in Lina *T. ovis* caused a latent infection. Conversely, MPE by *A. ovis* in Zoppina was less than a half that of Lina (Tab. 5).

	Splenectomized sheep							
	Rosalba	Stella	Lisa	Lola	Claretta	Lina	Zoppina	Gilda
Year of splenectomy	1994	1994	1994	1994	1994	2009	2009	2010
Incubation Time (days)*	19	21	25	32	42	29	35	21
Max Temperature (C°)	39.80	39.80	39.60	39.40	39.20	39.40	39.20	39.60
Min PCV (g/dl)	7	7	10	10	11	10	11	10
PCV reduction (%)	75	74	56	55	57	61	75	60
Hb reduction (%)	73	74	58	53	52	55	72	54
Max parasitemia *A.ovis*(%)	>70	>60	n.e.	n.e.	n.e.	36	15	60
Max parasitemia *T.ovis* (%)	n.e.	n.e.	n.e.	n.e.	n.e.	3	17	2

Table 5. Summary of clinical findings recorded in eight sheep splenectomised in different time periods (n.e.=observed but not estimated; *Incubation Time=number of days from first observation of infected blood cells on stained blood smears to the peak of the disease).

Then, Lina developed the disease after an incubation period of 29 days and recovered within a month, exhibiting a slight decrease in PCV (less than 25%) on post-splenectomy day 90 due to a slight increase in parasitaemia by *A. ovis* (Fig. 4). The two sheep were transfused with blood from a healthy donor sheep and treated every two days for a week with oxytetracycline (Terramicina long acting 1000 mg) and dexamethasone (Desashock Fortdodge Animal Health S.p.a., 80mg single dose). Both Lina and Zoppina quickly recovered from the disease, reaching normal blood values within four weeks, but, one month after their recovery, they had a relapse which they coped with successfully.

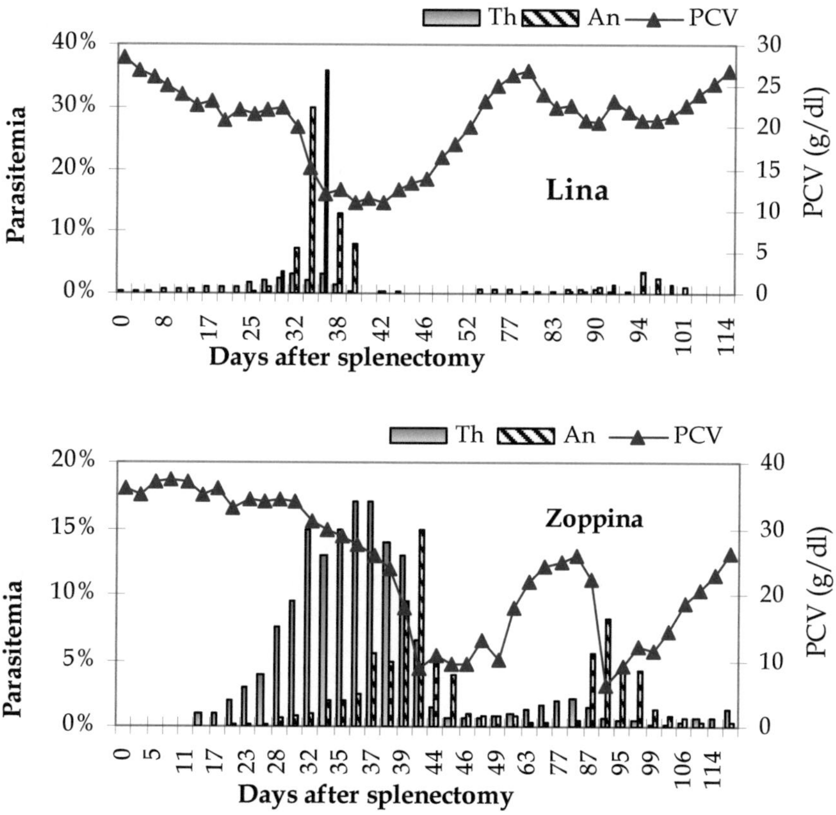

Fig. 4. Trend of PCV values and parasite densities (*An=Anaplasma ovis* and *Th=Theileria ovis*) expressed as percentage of red blood cells parasitized in Lina and Zoppina, the two splenectomized sheep monitored over a five week period after splenectomy.

During the recovery period, clinical examination revealed only pale mucous membranes. The pattern of evolution of the disease and recovery in Gilda was almost the same as in Lina except for a higher level of parasitaemia. In this instance *A. ovis* was the sole agent of the illness of our sheep. Secondly, the increase in *A. ovis* is apparently slowed down by the presence of *T. ovis* which seems to have a 'buffer effect' on the appearance of anaplasmosis but not in tempering its severity. Three points emerge from these results: i) in contrast to babesiosis and to the literature of some years ago (Radostits et al., 2000), hemoglobinuria did not occur in any of the seven severe cases of anaplasmosis; ii) treatment produced an immediate reduction in parasitaemia without leading to a complete clearance of the parasites; iii) disease relapse might be accounted for by the persistence of *A. ovis.*

Though not a novelty, in areas with enzootic erythrocytic parasitoses, even apparently healthy breeding animals may host pathogens and show tolerance and/or premunition to them without presenting with circulating parasites. This is a limit that should always be taken into account and may constitute a complication for any stress-associated situation. Anaemia secondary to anaplasmosis may evolve in a remarkably violent fashion probably due to the mechanism effected by the reticulo-endothelial system (RES) virtually with no haemolysis. In our small experience the use of desametazone had a beneficial effect as it reduced the general response to the stimulation of the pathogen and particularly macrophage activity and improved red blood cell membrane response. Several years have elapsed since the first experiment and Lola, Lisa and Claretta got back to 'normal life' and, before their death, caused by old age, they showed no signs of disease which might have been related to haematological parasitosis. As to Lina, Gilda and Zoppina, they are back in the flock following a normal breeding and reproductive cycle. With no doubt the spleen naturally acts as an immunologically active filter-pad countering even severe red blood cell deprivation; its activity is particularly prominent in the presence of antibodies given that even after splenectomy these animals were still able to resist local diseases. There are grounds to believe that the animals may have a genetically derived tolerance to such instances based on active, diffuse and efficient structural systems which do not relate to one sole organ.

4. Response to experimental anaemia

It is difficult to distinguish whether, in the case of native sheep, the slightness of the degree of anaemia should be considered the cause or the effect of tolerance. However, it is certain that these animals have an unquestionable ability to maintain a good level of homeostasis during TBD evidenced from the data shown in table 4, particularly those concerning PCV, Hb and MCHC.

To the purpose, four sheep belonging to a sensitive and non tolerant breed (Romanov), and four sheep to a sensitive but tolerant breed (Altamurana) underwent regular bleeding for seven days, stopping when the decrease of the packed cell volume ranged from 35 to 40%, the same as usually observed in clinical ovine babesiosis caused by *B. ovis* (Yeruham et al., 1998).

Over time the quantity and quality of the evolution of the haematological response were checked. The regression analyses performed to compare the two breeds with respect to the various data sets, gave the following results (Tab. 6):

- the intrabreed correlation coefficients recorded for PCV, Hb and RBC, were statistically significant only in the case of Romanov sheep, testifying to high difformity in the anaemization response between Romanov individuals, while Altamurana sheep behaved almost the same;
- the comparisons between the correlation coefficients obtained for PCV, Hb and RBC, in the two different breed groups were highly statistically significant.

Of these two points, while the latter might have been expected as the trial was based on the assumption of difference between the two breeds, the former result opens new vistas in the evaluation of the phenomenon. The low variability in the response to the anaemization exhibited by Altamurana sheep might be the result of the selection pressure acted by the constant presence of anaemizing parasites. Conversely the variability of the Romanov sheep could be taken as the individual response to the impact of an unusual stress.

As a general consideration, the two groups were composed by animals which were profoundly different and constantly on different levels from the haematological point of view. Both situations observed seemed to represent different aspects of normality, particularly the Altamurana sheep are constantly "poor" in the absolute levels of PCV, Hb and RBC and constantly "richer" regarding the derived parameters, MCV, MCH, MCHC, the latter being constantly those expressing haematological "efficiency" in the face of anaemia (Pieragostini & Petazzi, 1999). So if it is a matter of fact that from the numerical point of view, the two breeds' responses to anaemization are to a large extent not very dissimilar, the greater efficiency of the local breeds is beyond doubt. It is not to be excluded that this may be identified in their greater capacity to cope with anoxemic stress, both by the production of red globules enriched with haemoglobin and maybe also by accelerating the turnover of older and less efficient red blood cells.

Contrasts	**Haematological parameters**		
	RBC	Hb	PCV
Within Altamurana	n.s.	n.s.	n.s.
Within Romanov	***	***	***
Between Altamurana and Romanov	****	****	****

Table 6. Statistical significance of the differences between the correlation coefficients calculated by the regression analysis performed to compare the two breeds, Altamurana and Romanov, with respect to the hematological parameters RBC (Red Blood Cells), Hb (Haemoglobin) and PCV (Packed Cell Volume). ***$P<0.001$; ****$P<0.0001$; n.s., not significant.

The reading of these haematological aspects should be looked at without losing sight of the general aspect of the overall comparison between the two breeds. From this point of view, the considerable difference in absolute values, apparently almost negligible as regards the curve trends, becomes very striking in the comparison between the general situations of overall well-being of the two breeds compared. The Altamurana sheep continued to exhibit apparent good health when subjected to anaemization, at ease with their surroundings, ready to feed and drink. Conversely, the Romanovs exhibited a serious dulling of the senses and lack of reaction once anaemization was achieved; this necessitated support treatments with rehydrating solutions to allow them to overcome their state of anergy (Pieragostini & Petazzi, 1999). These results strongly support the hypothesis that, beyond the environmental factors such as stress, nutrition and other conditions, which in general facilitate infections (Agyemang et al., 1990; Bennison et al., 1998; Oppliger et al., 1998) and which are supposed to be particularly relevant in the case of non-native breeds, genetic predisposition plays a major role also in the pathogenesis of TBD.

5. Response to *Anaplasma ovis* infection in experimentally infected sheep

Animal well-being has become a significant concern among consumers who expect food animals to be well treated, raised in idyllic environments, and free of disease. Consumers also expect their meat products to be free of residual antibiotics and therapeutic drugs. For these reasons, new approaches or alternatives to addressing animal diseases are needed. One approach is genetic selection for animals resistant to disease, that is: an approach whose focus is on accepting certain constraints of the environment and using breeds that can cope with these constraints, as opposed to the earlier approach which focussed on changing the environment to create opportunities for exotic breeds to be productive. But identifying the phenotype for disease resistance is difficult.

As to TBD, the response is known to be under multi-factorial regulation (Horin, 1998; Aguilar-Delfin et al., 2001). As highlighted in the above section 4, the phenomenon of tolerance is a broad-based one and possibly not unrelated to the erythropoietic system in different sheep breeds or to the haemoglobin genetic systems (Pieragostini et al., 2003; Pieragostini et al., 2006).

Anyway, the success of selection for disease resistance is dependent on correctly identifying the disease agent and the phenotype for disease resistance. For example, as to TBP in small ruminants, there are several reports concerning the presence of *Babesia, Theileria,* and *Anaplasma* species infecting sheep and goats in many countries world-wide but, in many regions of the Old and the New World, the identity of the tick-borne disease agents of sheep and goats and of their vector ticks is uncertain. But perhaps, the biggest challenge of selecting for disease resistance is to accurately identify the phenotype for disease resistance and/or to have reliable genetic markers with high predictive values for a disease phenotype. Phenotypic variability induced by parasites is a matter of fact, as impressively exemplified by the high number of haemoglobinopathies in human populations living in malaria-endemic areas (Evans & Wellems, 2002).

Recalling Feynman's[1] saying that nature repeats itself at every scale, we suggested that the unusual haemoglobin polymorphism recorded in Apulian native sheep breeds and the related functional effects might have an adaptive significance, also being somehow related to the selective pressure of tick borne parasites (TBP) (Pieragostini et al., 1994; Pieragostini et al., 2003; Pieragostini et al., 2006). Based on these considerations, we aimed to define the phenotype of the tick borne diseases in different sheep breeds starting from the one caused by *A. ovis*, the most common parasite in our area as confirmed by a small survey on sheep TBP performed in 10 farms (throughout Apulia) on 240 individuals. *A. ovis* was identified in 58% of samples, followed by *T. ovis* (5.8%) and *T. annulata* (4.5%). *Theileria* spp. were present in mixed infections with *A. ovis, B. ovis* (0.9 %) or *Babesia* spp. (0.9 %). In particular the presence of *A. ovis* was confirmed by specific polymerase chain reactions (PCRs) for *Anaplasma* spp. (Stuen et al., 2003) and *A. ovis* (de la Fuente et al., 2005; de la Fuente et al., 2007). Then PCRs followed by reverse line blot hybridization of the amplified 18SrRNA gene from *Theileria* and *Babesia* species, was used to detect specific probes for *Theileria/Babesia catch all, Theileria sp1 china, Theileria sp2 chinal, T. buffely, T. annulata, T. velifera, T. taurotragi, T. mutans, T. lestoquardi, T. ovis, B. bovis, B. bigemina, B. crassa, B. motasi, B. ovis, B. major, B. divergens, T. hirci, B. sp1 (Turchey), B. sp2 (Lintan)* (Schnittger et al., 2004).

Year	Step 1	Year	Step 2
2009	Search for carriers	2010	Search for carriers
2009	Splenectomization	2010	Splenectomization
2009	Infection of 8 Suffolk and 8 Comisana characterized by normal alpha globin gene arrangements and different beta genotypes	2010	Infection of 18 Altamurana characterized by different alpha globin gene arrangements

Table 7. Experimental design.

[1] Richard Phillips Feynman (May 11, 1918 – February 15, 1988) was an American physicist who received the Nobel Prize in Physics in 1965.

Thus, a project was set up to evaluate the response to anaplasmosis in susceptible and tolerant sheep breeds including the use of haemoglobin genetic systems as genetical markers of tolerance to the disease. Summarized actions are described in table 7.

5.1 Materials and methods

5.1.1 Search for carriers and parasites

Sixty ewes were sampled from a flock extensively reared in the countryside near Bari. The flock consisted of approximately 250 heterogeneous subjects belonging mainly to TBD tolerant breeds and crossbreds. The presence of TBPs was checked in the blood samples by a PCR-based molecular approach as described above. Most of the sampled animals were found to carry *A. ovis* mixed with other TBPs. Based on the results of the flock survey and the consent given by the breeder, three ewes carrying *A. ovis* and *T. ovis* were selected and purchased. Following the experimental design (table 7) Lina and Zoppina were splenectomized in 2009 while Gilda in 2010, as described in subsection 3.4.

5.1.2 Animals

Selected animals 7/8 months of age were involved in this study. Lambs less than six months of age were purchased and housed at the Medical Clinics of the Faculty of Veterinary Medicine of the University of Bary. Upon arrival at the Faculty of Veterinary Medicine, the animals were weighed and faecal samples were obtained to establish their worm burdens. Feet were checked for foot rot. The animals were dewormed with a broad spectrum anthelmintic. All of them were then housed in a tick proof isolation unit. In particular, in 2009 the lambs were selected based on different breed and equally divided between Suffolk and Comisana.

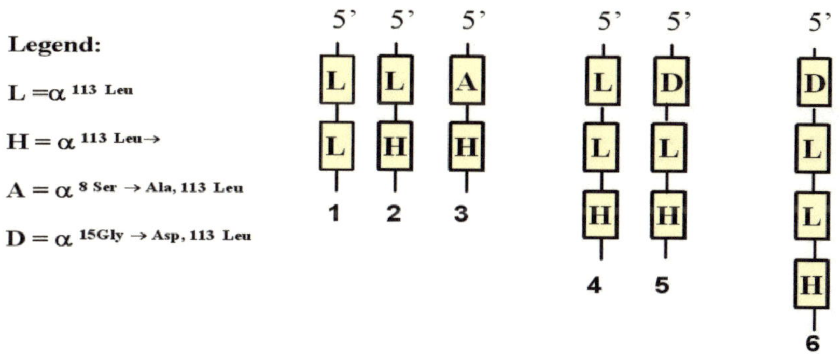

Fig. 5. Alpha-globin gene haplotypes detected so far in sheep, namely: haplotypes 1, 2 and 3 are normally duplicated (NH); haplotypes 4, 5 and 6 show extranumeral alpha gene arrangements (EH); particularly haplotypes 4 and 5 are triplicated while haplotype 6 is quadruplicated.

All the lambs were characterized by a normal duplicate alpha gene arrangement (Fig. 5) and most of them by homozigosity at the beta globin loci. Owing to high frequency of HBBA gene in the Suffolk breed, three out of the eight Suffolk lambs were HBBAB heterozygotes.
In 2010 eighteen Altamurana lambs less than six months of age, housed and treated as above described, were selected based on different alpha globin genetic arrangements. Nine lambs were homozygotes for the normal duplicate alpha gene haplotype (NH), the others carrying an extra-numeral alpha haplotype (EH) (Fig.5); most of the 18 lambs were homozygotes for the HBBB allele at the beta globin loci.

5.1.3 Experimental infection

A. ovis was isolated from one of the above splenectomized sheep. Lina was the donor for the 2009 lambs and Gilda for the 2010 lambs. Parasite density was estimated on thin blood film obtained by the buffy coat method and expressed as the percentage of parasitized red blood cells. At the peak of parasitaemia in the donor sheep (36% and 60% of red blood cells parasitized respectively), about 400 ml of blood were obtained and each lamb in the breed groups was inoculated intraperitoneally with 25 ml of infected blood.

5.1.4 Clinical observations

Clinical evaluation was done on a daily basis and rectal temperatures were recorded every morning for 8 weeks post infection. Blood and serum samples were collected twice a week during the observation period. Haematological variables were evaluated using a haematology analyzer. Parasite density was estimated on thin blood film as above described.

5.1.5 Haemoglobin phenotype

The reversible switch from haemoglobin A to C was observed in the above HBBAB Suffolk lambs. The expression of the silent gene encoding for Hb C was detected by isoelectric focusing and quantified by high performance liquid chromatography (Alloggio *et al.*, 2009).

5.1.6 Statistics

First, differences between breed groups for clinical and haematological data were assessed using analysis of variance (ANOVA) by GLM procedure (SAS, 1990). A second ANOVA was carried out only for the Altamurana group, considering the interaction between the alpha globin type (2 levels: NH and EH) and each clinical variable. The last ANOVA was carried out only for the Suffolk group considering the interaction with the beta globin type (2 levels: AB and BB) of the linear and quadratic regression of each haematological variable on the number of days from the infection, with three of the Suffolk that were AB compared to as many BB. This analysis was performed for the Suffolk, where, as cited above, both AB and BB genotypes were found, whereas only BB animals occurred in the Comisana.

5.2 Results and discussion

The following is an overall picture of the findings where they are reported and discussed relating to the different approaches.

5.2.1 Clinical findings

Host responses in the three experimentally infected sheep groups were first compared mainly according to typical high fever periods, microscopic observation and haematological values. *A. ovis* began to appear in the blood a week before the fever and the following records showed that the maximum of erythrocytes parasitized by *A. ovis* in any case did not exceed 2%.

All the animals developed the disease (Table 8) but symptoms varied in terms of severity and duration and none died. Fever syndrome (listlessness, anorexia, weakness, ruminal stasis, respiratory distress, increased heart and respiratory rates) and pallor of the mucous membranes were recorded in seven of the Suffolk group, in only one of the Comisana group and in none of the Altamurana.

Breed	Dose of infection	Symptoms	Need for therapeutic intervention	Morbidity	Expected Mortality
Suffolk	36%	very severe	7 out of 8 subjects	100%	87.5%
Comisana	36%	severe	1 out of 8 subjects	100%	12.5%
Altamurana	56%	mild	none	100%	0%

Table 8. Overview of responses to anaplasmosis in the three analyzed breeds.

The haematological patterns were then analyzed in detail comparing the intra breed variations between the different physiopathological moments - normal health status (time 0=T_0), acute phase (time 1=T_1) recovery phase (time 2=T_2) - and the between breed variations intra physiopathological moments (table 9). Finally, clinical parameters, such as incubation time (I.T) after infection, temperature peak (T.P.), percentage decrease in haematocrit (Δ HCT), percentage decrease in haemoglobin content (Δ Hb) expressed as gr Hb/dl blood, percentage decrease in red blood cells (Δ RBC) were evaluated for each breed (Table 10).

Breed	Parameter	T_0				T_1				T_2			
		Mean		SD		Mean		SD		Mean		SD	
	PCV (g/dl)	31.9	±	2.8	a	12.7	±	2.7	A	23.9	±	2.3	a
	Hb (g/dl)	11.5	±	1.0	a	4.7	±	0.7	A	7.7	±	0.7	a
	RBC ($10^6/\mu l$)	12.5	±	1.2	A	4.5	±	0.8	a	7.2	±	1.0	
Suffolk	MCV (fl)	25.0	±	1.0	A	32.3	±	1.6	A	33.3	±	3.0	A
	MCH (pg)	9.2	±	0.3	B	10.5	±	0.6	A	10.7	±	0.6	A
	MCHC (g/dl)	36.8	±	1.0	A	32.5	±	1.2		32.3	±	0.8	
	WBC ($10^3/\mu l$)	8.6	±	1.1		10.9	±	2.4		0.3	±	1.1	a
	PCV (g/dl)	35.0	±	2.4	b	11.3	±	2.7	A	26.2	±	1.7	b
	Hb (g/dl)	12.6	±	1.0	b	4.7	±	0.5	A	8.6	±	0.7	b
	RBC ($10^6/\mu l$)	11.9	±	1.3	A	5.1	±	0.8	a	6.9	±	0.7	
Comisana	MCV (fl)	29.7	±	2.3	B	29.1	±	3.2	B	38.4	±	3.2	B
	MCH (pg)	10.7	±	0.7	A	9.4	±	1.1	B	12.5	±	0.9	B
	MCHC (g/dl)	35.9	±	1.3	A	32.1	±	0.4		32.5	±	1.0	
	WBC ($10^3/\mu l$)	10.1	±	2.7		7.5	±	1.4		10.4	±	2.9	b
	PCV(g/dl)	31.2	±	3.2	a	21.6	±	3.1	B	25.8	±	2.4	b
	Hb (g/dl)	0.4	±	1.0	C	7.1	±	1.0	B	8.2	±	0.8	b
	RBC ($10^6/\mu l$)	9.4	±	1.0	B	6.2	±	1.0	b	7.1	±	0.8	
Altamurana	MCV (fl)	33.2	±	1.9	C	34.7	±	1.7	C	36.6	±	2.0	B
	MCH (pg)	10.6	±	0.5	A	11.4	±	0.5	C	11.6	±	0.5	B
	MCHC (g/dl)	31.7	±	0.7	B	32.8	±	0.9		31.9	±	1.0	b
	WBC ($10^3/\mu l$)	10.1	±	2.6		9.6	±	2.0		10.1	±	1.4	B

Table 9. Haematological parameters assessed for the three analyzed breeds, namely normal health status before infection (time 0=T_0), during the acute phase (time 1=T_1) and during the recovery phase (time 2=T_2). Means within columns with different letters significantly differ: capital letters: $P < 0.01$; small letters: $P < 0.05$.

As already reported, none of the animals had more than 2% erythrocytes parasitized by *A. ovis*. This confirms the role the spleen plays in the phagocytosis and clearance of parasitized erythrocytes; otherwise only splenectomized sheep showed significant percentages of parasitized erythrocytes (table 5).
Mean parasitaemia in the single group could theoretically be inferred from the Δ RBC and conclude that the higher the Δ RBC value, the higher the suceptibility of the erythrocytes to *Anaplasma* infection. According to the results shown in table 8 depicting the response of the three breeds to infection, broken down according to the dose of infection, symptoms, need for therapeutic intervention and expected mortality, seven out of the Suffolk group recovered after being treated every two days for a week with oxytetracycline and dexamethasone whereas seven subjects of the Comisana group recovered from clinical anaplasmosis with no drug treatment other than a single dose of dexamethasone. The highest degree of tolerance was observed in the Altamurana group where all the subjects showed only mild alteration of behaviour and basic life functions. Comparison of the haematological patterns of the three breeds at T_0 in table 10 revealed that, in normal health conditions, the differences which may be noticed are consistent with those of earlier studies described in section 2, indicating that both environmental and productive specialization seem to account for the different physiological results.
Hence the Altamurana breed is characterized by significantly lower RBC and Hb values and by significantly higher MCV, MCH and MCHC values than Suffolk, a northern meat breed, while Comisana, a Mediteranean dairy breed has intermediate values. At T_1 and T_2 the same variation pattern may be observed, that is:

- haematologically, *A. ovis* infection does not seem to seriously affect Altamurana whose response may be described as a moderate normochromic normocytic anemia followed by a normochromic macrocytic pattern representing an active regeneration phase.
- conversely, the Suffolk and Comisana animals exhibited a violent response to *A. ovis* with a severe anaemia. The hyperchromic and macrocytic anaemia in the Suffolk was followed by a slow regeneration and the hypochromic normocytic anaemia of the Comisana by an active regeneration phase, similar to the Altamurana pattern, as documented by the high MCV values.

The results shown in table 10 confirmed the differences among the three breeds both in terms of quantitative (Altamurana *vs* Suffolk) and temporal (Comisana *vs* Suffolk) variation in haematological parameters. While Suffolk animals displayed the most severe reduction in the number of erythrocytes and haemoglobin content, Altamurana was characterized by a more controlled response, with only a minor and more gradual decline in RBC and Hb values. Comisana experienced a more severe reduction in the number of erythrocytes than did Suffolk, though the decline in RBC values was not accompanied by a decrease in the total haemoglobin content as severe as that observed in Suffolk. This could be due to the significantly higher MCH values characterizing the Comisana haematological pattern as compared to the Suffolk.
Considering the overall responses shown in table 8 and detailed in table 9 and 10, there is no doubt that we are dealing with very different animal groups exhibiting different physiopathological phenotypes where a healthy haematological picture plays a relevant role.

Breed	I.T (days)	T.P. (°C)	ΔHCT (%)	ΔHb (%)	ΔRBC (%)
Suffolk	24.2^{A}	40.5^{A}	65.4^{A}	60.2^{A}	60.3^{A}
Comisana	38.8^{B}	39.9^{B}	57.7^{B}	56.9^{A}	55.9^{A}
Altamurana	25.3^{A}	39.9^{B}	19.2^{C}	19.8^{B}	33.7^{B}

Table 10. Clinical parameters assessed for the three breeds analyzed at the peak of the disease, namely incubation time (I.T) after infection, temperature peak (T.P.), percentage decrease in haematocrit (ΔHCT), percentage decrease in haemoglobin content (ΔHb), percentage decrease in red blood cells (ΔRBC).

5.2.2 Functional effect of beta globin genes on the recovery from anemia

As to the functional effect of beta globin genes on the recovery from anemia, Figure 6 shows the results of the analysis performed in the Suffolk, where both AB and BB genotypes were found.

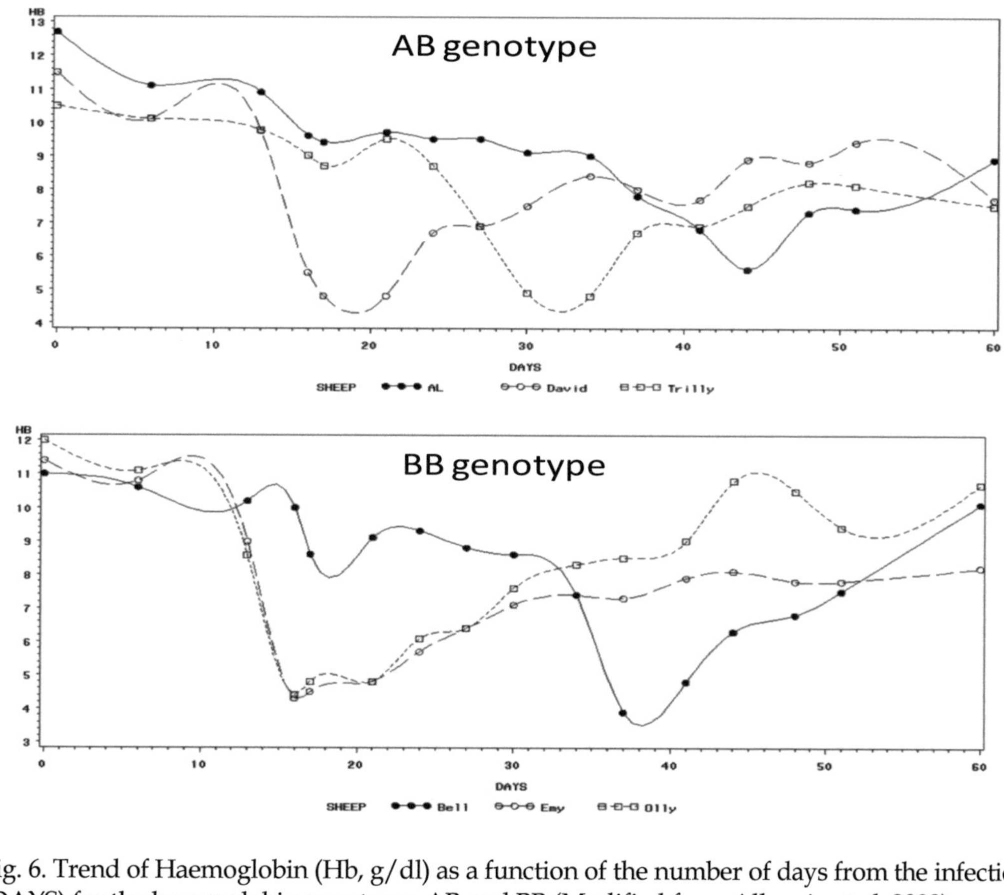

Fig. 6. Trend of Haemoglobin (Hb, g/dl) as a function of the number of days from the infection (DAYS) for the haemoglobin genotypes AB and BB (Modified from Alloggio et al. 2009).

Goats and some sheep under conditions of erythropoietic stress (anaemia) or hypoxia, synthesize a juvenile haemoglobin (Hb) type, Hb C, where β-globin is encoded by the silent gene *HBBC*. Anaemia causes a change in the type of circulating haemoglobin only in sheep carrying βA-globin haplotype, where Hb A is replaced by Hb C. Pioneered by the work of van Vliet and Huismam (1964), the Hb C in Caprini species has been thoroughly studied and particularly the mechanism of reversible switching has triggered focused research in the 70's (Nienhuis and Anderson, 1972; Nienhuis and Bunn, 1974). Little information is available on the effect of Hb A replacement by Hb C. Owing to the high oxygen affinity of Hb C (Huisman and Kitchens, 1968), the reversible switch from Hb A to Hb C may be considered a way to cope with the reduced amount of oxygen available at higher altitudes and thus suggest a positive effect on the fitness of mountain Caprini. Conversely, in the case of erythropoietic stress, it was suggested (Pieragostini et al., 1994; Pieragostini et al., 2006) that Hb C might negatively affect peripheral oxygen delivery and worsen the clinical picture of sheep breeds native of areas with endemic haemotropic pathogens. Hence, in the present case, the *conditio sine qua non* for checking the effect of beta globin genotype was the detection of Hb C switched on in AB individuals following a strong erythropoietic stress. As an example, figure 6 also shows the different trend after infection (days = 0) of the Hb content for the AB and BB ewes. Apart from individual differences observed in reaching the lowest Hb values, the recovery was always faster in BB sheep, as also indicated by the significantly higher quadratic regression coefficient of Hb for BB *vs* AB genotype (0.0045 *vs* 0.0027, $P < 0.03$). The different behaviour of one of the three heterozygous subject (Figure 6) may be justified by its less severe haematological picture due to a lower anoxaemic stress, also confirmed by the lack of the Hb A to Hb C switch in the same animal.

5.2.3 Functional effect of alpha globin system on the response to the anaplasmosis

As mentioned before, the extra numeral alpha globin haplotypes (EH) were suggested to be related to the host's response to TBDs. The unusual frequency of EH recorded in southern Italian sheep breeds and the peculiar haematologic pattern exhibited by the EH homozygous subjects may be taken as evidence of a selective advantage of the corresponding phenotypes in endemic TBD areas. Individuals carrying extra alpha-globin genes exhibit an overall blood picture mimicking a thalassaemia-like syndrome. In greater detail, when the erythrocytes of EH homozygotes were compared with those of NH individuals, the former had fewer erythrocytes that were bigger in size and had a higher Hb content and a greater erythrocyte osmotic fragility. These changes in EH homozygotes were assumed to produce an unfavorable environment for the parasites.

Thus, the trial checked this hypothesis as the different haematological patterns and the accelerated turnover of erythrocytes of EH individuals compared to the NH ones were expected to produce differences in the spread of the pathogen into the host blood.

Unfortunately a relevant element of prejudicial questions to obtain maximum results was the fact that only EH heterozygotes were present in the Altamurana group, since no homozygous lambs were found during the population survey. In normal health conditions, such as those recorded in the experience reported by Pieragostini et al. (2003), the EH heterozygotes showed an intermediate pattern, between that of EH homozygotes and that of NH homozygotes (Pieragostini, unpublished data).

The second relevant element was the level of response which undoubtedly is a limiting factor in checking the results.
Thirdly, owing to experimental constraints, the sample size was of nine subjects per each alpha haplotype group. Hence, based on these considerations, we could not expect striking results as to the functional effect of the alpha globin gene arrangements, except in the case of a strong interaction with the response to experimental infections. Despite our hopes, our concerns were well-founded because all the above elements of prejudicial questions affected the results.

α-globin gene arrangements	N	T.P. (°C)	PCV (g/dl)	Hb (g/dl)	RBC ($10^6/\mu l$)	MCV (fl)	MCH (pg)	MCHC (g/dl)	WBC ($10^3/\mu l$)
NH	9	40.1 A ± 0.18	25.9 ± 1.55	8.1 ± 0.89	7.8 ± 0.85	33.1 ± 1.03	10.4 ± 0.51	31.4 ± 0.51	10.3 ± 1.29
EH	9	39.8 B ± 0.12	26.3 ± 1.18	8.5 ± 0.39	8.0 ± 0.31	33.7 ± 0.73	10.6 ± 0.43	31.4 ± 0.47	10.5 ± 1.17

Table 11. Temperature peak and haematological parameters assessed during the acute phase of the disease, for the two Altamurana groups classified on the basis of the α-globin gene arrangement. Means within columns with different letters significantly differ; capital letters: P <0.01.

Altamurana subjects exhibited a very mild symptoms and no patent differences could be recorded in terms of haematological pattern between the EH and NH individuals within the Altamurana group. The EH group had a temperature peak that was significantly lower (P<0.001) than that of the NH group. This suggested that the level of response to infection in the EH group was lighter than in the NH group (Table 12). Morever, as shown in table 11, though no significance was attained by the ANOVA when the mean values of the haematological parameters of the two groups were compared, a univocal trend emerged whereby the RBC, PCV and Hb values in the EH group decreased less than in the NH group. These two phenomena seem to indicate a milder *Anaplasma* infection in EH subjects than in the NH individuals.

6. Conclusions

Several examples of breed-related tolerance to diseases have been reported worldwide but often the claims made for specific breeds have not been subject to scientific investigation. As to small ruminants, only tolerance to Heartwater (Cowdriosis) has been documented for Damara, a South African native sheep breed (Commission on Genetic Resources for Food and Agriculture, 2007). This report extends our knowledge about tolerance to tick borne diseases. The main findings can be summarized in the following points:

- Tolerance to piroplasmosis is documented for Apulian (Altamurana, Gentile di Puglia and Leccese) and Italian islander (Comisana and Sarda) sheep breeds.
- Non-tolerance to piroplasmosis is documented for Finnish, Friesian and Romanov breeds.
- Suffolk breed is shown to be not tolerant to anaplasmosis.
- Different physiological pattern and environment of origin may explain breed-specific haematological characteristics.
- Altamurana sheep breed is tolerant to anaemia *per se.*
- The response of Altamurana to simultaneous *B. ovis* and *A. ovis* infection results in a mild anaemia.
- There seems to be confirmatory evidence that haemoglobin genetic systems underlie the host response in the acute phase of disease and in recovery.

7. Aknowledgements

The earlier experiences reported in this work were supported by Bari University and/or the Italian Ministry for University and Research. The last section is part of a project sponsored by the Italian Ministry for Agriculture, Food and Forestry Policies (MIPAAF) for the improvement of animal breeding by means of molecular genetics (SELMOL). As far as the expert identification of TBP, the Authors are deeply endebted to Dr. Alessandra Torina head of the national reference laboratory for *tick-borne* diseases (C.R.A.BA.R.T.- Istituto Zooprofilattico Sperimentale della Sicilia "A. Mirri", Palermo, Italy). The authors are grateful to Dr. Rosanna Lacinio for the quality of her technical support at the haematology laboratory of the Veterinary Clinic of Bari University along years of collaboration. The authors are also grateful to Dr. Athina Papa for her accuracy in revising the English of the manuscript.

8. References

Aguilar-Delfin, I., Homer, M.J., Wettstein, P.J. & Persing, D.H. (2001). Innate resistance to Babesia infection is influenced by genetic background and gender. *Infection and Immunity*, Vol. 69, No. 12, December 2001, pp. 7955-8. ISSN 0019-9567

Agyemang, K., Dwinger, R.H., Touray, B.N., Jeannin, P., Fofana, D. & Grieve, A.S. (1990). Effects of nutrition on the degree of anaemia and liveweight changes in N'Dama cattle infected with trypanosomes. *Livestock Production Science,* Vol. 26 No. 1, September 1990, pp. 39-51, ISSN 0301-6226

Alderson, L. (2009). Breeds at risk: Definition and measurement of the factors which determine endangerment. *Livestock Science,* Vol. 123, No. 1, July 2009, pp. 23-27, ISSN 1871-1413

Alloggio, I., de Ruvo, G., Torina, A., Caroli, A., Petazzi, F. & Pieragostini E. (2009). Reversibile switch from haemoglobin A to C in sheep and recovery from anemia following experimental infection with *Anaplasma ovis*. *Italian Journal of Animal Science,* Vol. 8, No. S2, January 2010, pp. 27-29 ISBN/ISSN 1594-4077

Ariely, R., Heth, G., Nevo, E. & Hoch, D. (1986). Haematocrit and haemoglobin concentration in four chromosomal species and isolated population of actively speciating subterranean mole rats in Israel. *Experientia,* Vol. 42, No. 4, April 1986, pp. 440-443, ISSN 0014-4754

Bennison, J.J., Clemence, R.G., Archibald, R.F., Hendy, C.R.C. & Dempfle, L. (1998). The effect of work and two planes of nutrition on trypanotoleralt draught cattle infected with *Trypanosoma congolense. Animal Science,* Vol. 66, No. 3, June 1998, pp. 595-605, ISSN 1806-2636

Ceci, L & Carelli, G. (1999). Tick-borne diseases of livestock in Italy: general review and results of recent studies carried out in the Apulia region. Parassitologia. Sep; 41 Suppl 1:25-9.

Commission on Genetic Resources for Food and Agriculture, Food and Agriculture Organization of the United Nations (2007). *The State of the World's Animal Genetic Resources for Food and Agriculture.* Barbara Rischkowsky & Dafydd Pilling, eds. ISBN ISBN 9789251057629, Rome, Italy

Correia De Almeida Regitano, L. & Prayaga, K. (2010). Ticks and tick-borne diseases in cattle, In: *Breeding for Disease Resistance in Farm Animals,* Bishop, S.C., Axford, R.F.E., Nicholas, F.W. & Owen, J.B., pp. 295-314, CAB International, ISBN 978 1 84593 555 9, UK

Cresswell, E. & Hutchings, H. (1962). A comparison of production on blood values between the Romney Marsh and the Cheviot ewes in New Zealand. *Research in Veterinary Science,* Vol. 3, pp. 209–214, ISSN 00345288.

de la Fuente, J., Van Den Bussche, R.A., Prado, T.M. & Kocan, K.M. (2003). *Anaplasma marginale* msp1α genotypes evolved under positive selection pressure but are not markers for geographic isolates. *Journal of Clinical Microbiology,* Vol. 41, No. 4, April 2003, pp. 1609–1616, ISSN 0095-1137

de la Fuente J., Massung R. F., Wong S. J., Chu F. K., Lutz H., Meli M., von Loewenich F. D., Gzeszczuk A., Torina A., Caracappa S., Mangold A.J., Naranjo V., Stuen S., Kocan K.M. (2005). Sequence Analysis of the msp4 Gene of Anaplasma phagocytophilum Strains. J. Clin. Microbiol., 43, 1309–1317.

de la Fuente, J., Atkinson, M.W., Naranjo, V., Fernández de Mera, I.G., Mangold, A.J., Keating, K.A., Kocan, K.M. (2007). Sequence analysis of the msp4 gene of Anaplasma ovis strains. Vet. Microbiol. 119: 375-381.

Dumler, J.S., Barbet, A.F, Bekker, C.P., Dasch, G.A., Palmer, G.H., Ray, S.C., Rikihisa, Y. & Rurangirwa, F.R. (2001). Reorganization of genera in the families *Rickettsiaceae* and *Anaplasmataceae* in the order *Rickettsiales*: unification of some species of *Ehrlichia* with *Anaplasma, Cowdria* with *Ehrlichia* and *Ehrlichia* with *Neorickettsia,* descriptions of six new species combinations and designation of *Ehrlichia equi* and 'HGE agent' as subjective synonyms of *Ehrlichia phagocytophila. International Journal of Systematic and Evolutionary Microbiology,* Vol. 51, No. 6, November 2001, pp. 2145–2165, ISSN 1466-5026.

Evans, A. G. & Wellems, T. E. (2002). Coevolutionary genetics of *Plasmodium malaria* parasites and their human hosts. *Integrative and Comparative Biology,* Vol. 42, No. 2, April 2002, pp 401–407, ISSN 1557-7023.

Greenwood B. (1977). Haematology of the sheep and the goat, In: *Comparative Clinical Haematology,* Archer R.K., Jeffcott L.B., pp.305-308, Blackwell Scientific Publications, ISBN 0 632 00289 1, Oxford, UK .

Horin, P. (1998). Biological principles of heredity of and resistance to disease. *Revue scientifique et technique,* Vol. 17, No. 1, April 1998, pp. 302-314, ISSN 0253-1933.

Huisman, T.H. & Kitchens, J. (1968). Oxygen equilibria studies of the haemoglobins from normal and anemic sheep and goats. *American Journal of Physiology,* Vol. 215, No. 1, July 1968, pp. 140-146, ISSN 0002-9513

Jain, N.C. (1993). *Essential of Veterinary Haematology.* Lea & Febiger, ISBN 081211437X, Philadelphia, PA.

Jongejan, F. & Uilenberg, G. (2004). The global importance of ticks. *Parasitology,* Vol. 129, No. S1, October 2004, pp. S3–S14, ISSN 0031-1820

McCosker, P.J. (1979). Global aspects of the management and control of ticks of veterinary importance, In: *Recent Advances in Acarology,* Rodriguez, J.G., pp. 45–53, Academic Press, ISBN 0125922027, New York

Nienhuis, A. W. & Anderson, W. F. (1972). Haemoglobin switching in sheep and goats: change in functional globin messenger RNA in reticulocytes and bone marrow cells. *Proc. Natl. Acad. Sci.,* Vol. 69, No. 8, August 1972, pp. 2184-2188, ISSN 1091-6490

Nienhuis, A.W. & Bunn, H.F. (1974). Haemoglobin switching in sheep and goats: occurrence of haemoglobins A and C in the same red cell. *Science.* Vol. 185, No. 9, August 1974, pp. 946-948, ISSN 0036-8075

Oppliger, A., Clobert, J., Lecompte, J., Lorenzon, P., Boudjiemadi, K. & John-Alder, H.B. (1998). Environmental stress increases the prevalence and intensity of blood parasite infection in the common lizard *Lacerta vivipara. Ecology Letters,* Vol. 1, No. 2, September 1998, pp. 129-138, ISSN 1461-0248

Pieragostini, E., Dario, C. & Bufano, G. (1994). Haemoglobin phenotypes and hematological factors in Leccese sheep. *Small Ruminant Research,* Vol. 13, No. 2, March 1994, pp. 177-185, ISSN 0921-4488

Pieragostini, E., Dario, C., Petazzi, F. & Bufano, G. (1996). La piroplasmosi negli ovini pugliesi: una malattia da scarso reddito. Nota III. Profilassi e performance riproduttive. *Proceedings of the XIII International Congress of Mediterranean Federation for Ruminant Health and Production,* Murcia (Spain), 27-28 May 1996.

Pieragostini, E. & Petazzi, F. (1999). Genetics and tolerance to tick borne diseases in South Italy: experience in studying native Apulian and exotic sheep breeds. *Parassitologia,* Vol. 41, No. S1, September 1999, pp. 89-94, ISSN 0048-2951

Pieragostini, E., Petazzi, F. & Rubino, G. (1999). Haematological values in Apulian native sheep breeds. *Proceeding of the VII International Congress of Mediterranean Federation for Ruminant Health and Production,* ISBN/ISSN: 972-8126-05-0, Santarem, Portugal, 22–24 April 1999

Pieragostini, E., Petazzi, F., Rubino, G., Rullo, R. & Sasanelli, M. (2000). Switching emoglobinico, quadro ematologico e primo incontro con i parassiti endoeritrocitari enzootici in agnelli autoctoni pugliesi. *Obiettivi e Documenti Veterinari.* Vol. 7/8, pp. 31-40, ISSN 0392-1913.

Pieragostini E, Petazzi F, Di Luccia A. 2003 The relationship between the presence of extra alpha-globin genes and blood cell traits in Altamurana sheep. Genetic Selection Evolution, Vol. 35 No. 1, July 2003, pp. S121-133, ISSN 0999-193X.

Pieragostini, E., Rubino, G., Bramante, G., Rullo, R., Petazzi, F. & Caroli, A. (2006). Functional effect of haemoglobin polymorphism on the haematological pattern of Gentile di Puglia sheep. *Journal of Animal Breeding and Genetics,* Vol. 123 No. 2, April 2006, pp. 122-130, ISSN 0931-2668

Rubino, G., Cito, A.M., Lacinio, R., Bramante, G., Caroli, A., Pieragostini, E. & Petazzi, F. (2006). Hematology and some blood chemical parameters as a function of tick-borne disease (TBD) signs in horses. *Journal of Equine Veterinary Science,* Vol. 26, No. 10, October 2006, pp. 475-480, ISSN 0737-0806

Radostits, O. M., Arundel, J. H. & Gay, C.C. (2000). *Veterinary medicine: a textbook of the diseases of cattle, sheep, pigs, goats and horses* (9th ed.). W. B. Saunders & Co. ISBN 0702026042, Philadelphia, PA.

SAS, 1990: SA/Stat User's Guide, Version 6, 4th ed. SAS Institute Inc., Cary, NC.

Sayin, F., Dyncer, S., Karaer, Z., Cakmak, A., Yukary, B.A., Eren, H., Deger, S. & Nalbantoglu S. (1997). Status of the tick-borne diseases in sheep and goats in Turkey. *Parassitologia.* Vol. 39, No. 2, June 1997, pp. 153-156, ISSN 0048-2951

Schnittger, L., Yin, H., Qi, B., Gubbels, M.J., Beyer, D., Niemann, S., Jongejan, F., Ahmed, J.S. (2004). Simultaneous detection and differentiation of Theileria and Babesia parasites infecting small ruminants by reverse line blotting. Parasitol Res, 92:189-96.

Stuen, S., Nevland, S. & Moum T. (2003). Fatal cases of tick-borne fever (TBF) in sheep caused by several 16S rRNA gene variants of Anaplasma phagocytophilum. *Annals of the New York Academy of Sciences,* Vol. 990, June 2003, pp. 443-444 ISSN 1749-6632

Townsend, R.F. & Thirtle, C.G. (2001). Is livestock research unproductive? Separating health maintenance from improvement research. *Agricultural Economics,* Vol. 25, No. 2-3, October 2001, pp. 177-189, ISSN 0019-5014

van Vliet, G. & Huisman, T.H.J. (1964). Changes in the haemoglobin types of sheep as a response to anemia. *Biochem. J.* Vol. 93, No. 2, November 1964, pp. 401–409, ISSN 0264-6021

Whitelock, J.H. (1963). The influence of heredity and environment on maximum haematocrit values in sheep. *Cornell Veterinarian,* Vol. 53, October 1963, pp. 534–550, ISSN 0010-8901

Yeruham, I., Hadani, A. & Galker, F. (1998). Some epizootiological and clinical aspects of ovine babesiosis caused by *Babesia ovis.* A review. *Veterinary Parasitology,* Vol. 74, No. 2-4, January 1998, pp. 153-63, ISSN 0304-4017

Yin H & Luo J. (2007). Ticks of small ruminants in China. *Parasitol Res.,* Vol. 101, No. 2, September 2007, pp S187-189, ISSN 0932-011.

Youatt, W. (1867). *Sheep: their breeds, management, and diseases*. Orange Judd & Co., New York.

25

The Foragining Ecology of the Green Turtle in the Baja California Peninsula: Health Issues

Rafael Riosmena-Rodriguez[1], Ana Luisa Talavera-Saenz[1], Gustavo Hinojosa-Arango[2], Mónica Lara-Uc[3] and Susan Gardner[4]
[1]*Programa de Investigación en Botánica Marina, Departamento de Biología Marina, Universidad Autónoma de Baja California Sur, La Paz Baja California Sur,*
[2]*The School for Field Studies, Puerto de Acapulco s/n, Puerto San Carlos, Baja California Sur*
[3]*Depto. de Virología, Facultad de Medicina Veterinaria y Zootecnia, UADY, Mérida, Yucatán,*
[4]*Centro de Investigaciones Biológicas del Noroeste, La Paz Baja California Sur, México*

1. Introduction

Conservation of threatened species, such as the green turtle (*Chelonia mydas*), is closely related to habitat quality. In particular there are issues related to heavy metals, the presence of epibionts, parasites and fibropapiloms who might play a crucial role in the species survivorship. Heavy metals occur naturally in the environment (Sparling et al., 2000) as part of the biogeochemical cycles (Valiela, 2009), and it is often difficult to differentiate between natural and anthropogenic sources (Kieffer, 1991; Moreno, 2003). In marine systems, natural processes (e.g., upwelling, river runoff) can redistribute and concentrate heavy metals in the environment, occasionally reaching toxic levels (Sparling et al., 2000; Machado et al., 2002). The effects of these processes may vary over seasonal and spatial scales (Sawidis et al., 2001) and their understanding can aid in determining the sources as biomonitors (Szefer et al., 1998; Páez-Osuna et al.,2000), and ultimately their effects on wild life (Sparling et al., 2000; Talavera-Saenz et al., 2007). Also, they can be used for bioabsorption in contaminated waters (Kumar and Kaladharan, 2006). Caliceti et al. (2002) found a decrease in Zinc and Cadmium concentrations from the center of a lagoon, close to an industrial district, towards the Venice lagoon (Italy) openings to the sea, suggesting anthropogenic sources, while Villares et al. (2002) found that seasonal and spatial variation in metals was related to algal growth cycles and river runoff. Riosmena-Rodriguez et al. (2010) determined that heavy metals are related to the physiological features of each major analyzed taxon (green algae, red algae and seagrasses).

The processes controlling the concentration and distribution of metals in coastal environments and their consequences in the species health are poorly understood. It is generally assumed that diet is the main source of metals to sea turtles (Caurant et al., 1999; Anan et al., 2001), but little is known of the process of metal accumulation in these species because data on metal residues in most components of sea turtles' diet has been lacking. As adults, green turtles forage largely on marine algae and seagrasses with variation in the diet due to the relative availability of food types over geographic and temporal scales (Garnett et al., 1985; Brand-Gardner et al., 1999; Seminoff et al., 2002). In the process of metal bioaccumulation in marine food chains is poorly understood because very little data is available on metal concentration at different trophic levels (de la Lanza et al. 1989; Talavera-Saenz et al. 2007) or their temporal (Abdallah et al., 2006; Rodriguez-Castañeda et al., 2006) or spatial variation (Kalesh and Nair, 2006) and their effects on the photosynthetic process (Catriona et al. 2002). High concentrations of heavy metals have been found in sea turtles from many regions of the world (Storelli and Marcotrigiano, 2003). Although metal concentrations vary greatly by region and tissue type, green turtles (*Chelonia mydas*) have been found to have exceptionally high kidney cadmium concentrations. Elevated Cadmium levels have been measured in green turtles from around the world including Japan (Sakai et al., 2000; Anan et al., 2001), China (Lam et al., 2004), Europe (Caurant et al., 1999), Australia (Gordon et al., 1998) and the Arabian Sea (Bicho et al., 2006). Gordon et al. (1998) found that Cadmium concentrations in green turtles from Australia were up to three times higher than the levels reported in commercial seafood products. The presence of epibionts, parasites (internal and external) might occasionally cause the death of some marine turtles and being predecessors of fibropapiloms (Aguirre y Lutz, 2004; Work, 2000, Work *et al.*, 2005). The presence of fibropapiloms in Hawaiian waters was related with the presence of hirudineans (Díaz, *et al.*, 1992). This kind of infections are might be related with their foraging habitat and its conservation condition, their health condition to escape predators and, for the females, the fecundity reduction (Gámez et al., 2006; Alfaro, et al., 2006; Badillo, 2007).

The Baja California Peninsula serves an important role as foraging grounds for five of the world's seven sea turtle species (Gardner and Nichols, 2001). Although much of the peninsula is considered pristine, exploitation of mineral deposits has occurred since the 19th Century and concentrations of Cadmium, Zinc, Copper and Plumb in sediment and marine fauna have been observed above those in more industrialized regions (Gutiérrez-Galindo et al., 1999; Shumilin et al., 2000). In the mid 1970's, Martin and Broenkow (1975) reported that concentrations of Cadmium along the coast of the Baja California Peninsula were remarkably elevated as compared to other regions of the eastern Pacific. Sources of heavy metals in Baja California have been generally attributed to natural factors related to upwelling and the biogeochemistry of the region, however, the potential contribution from anthropogenic sources (e.g. mining and urbanization) cannot be entirely dismissed (Martin and Broenkow, 1975; Sañudo-Wihelmy and Flegal, 1996; Méndez-Rodríguez et al., 1998; Gutiérrez- Galindo et al., 1999; Shumilin et al., 2001). Rodríguez-Meza et al. (2008) developed an extensive evaluation of the heavy metals in sediments and seaweeds along ten sites in the bay. They suggested that the high levels of some heavy metals are related to terrigenous input from the arroyos and biogenic origin by the upwelling. In order to better understand the sources of heavy metals to marine species, more information is needed on metal concentrations in primary producers that make up the base of the food chain. However, few (Riosmena-Rodriguez et al., 2010) papers have approached the study of natural levels of heavy metals in seaweed communities and their temporal and spatial variation. Previous studies in Magdalena Bay, Mexico (Méndez et al., 2002; Gardner et al., 2006) have found high concentrations of metals in marine vertebrates, despite the lack of obvious anthropogenic sources. For example, Cadmium, Zinc, and Iron concentrations in the herbivorous green turtle, *Chelonia mydas*, were the highest ever reported in sea turtles globally (Gardner et al., 2006). In Magdalena Bay, like other regions of the Baja California

Peninsula (Seminoff et al., 2002), juvenile and adult green turtles preferentially consume soft red algae, especially species of Gracilaria (López-Mendilaharsu et al., 2005). Studies in Baja California have demonstrated that these same species of red algae tend to have higher enrichment factors of metals than other groups of seaweeds (Sánchez-Rodríguez et al., 2001), which could account for the high accumulation of metals in foraging green turtles in this region.

2. Materials and methods

2.1 Study area

Magdalena Bay is located on the Pacific coast of the Baja California Peninsula, Mexico between 24° 15′ N and 25° 20′ N, and 111° 30′ W and 112° 15′ W. It is a shallow lagoon protected from the Pacific by barrier islands, with high productivity resulting from seasonal marine upwelling along the coast. Diverse marine habitats within the bay include sandy bottoms and rocky margins, extensive beds of the seagrass *Zostera marina* and a diverse assemblage of macroalgae. A sea turtle refuge area known as Estero Banderitas is located within the mangrove channels in the northwest region of the Bay where green turtles reside year-round (Fig. 1). Because of the perceived importance of this area for green turtle foraging, its protection has been identified as a priority for conservation efforts (Arriaga et al., 1998; Nichols et al., 2000). Rodríguez-Meza et al. (2008) has found that the presence of heavy metals in the bay is heavily influenced by sediment type, organic material, and carbonates and concluded that there was no evidence of human impacts.

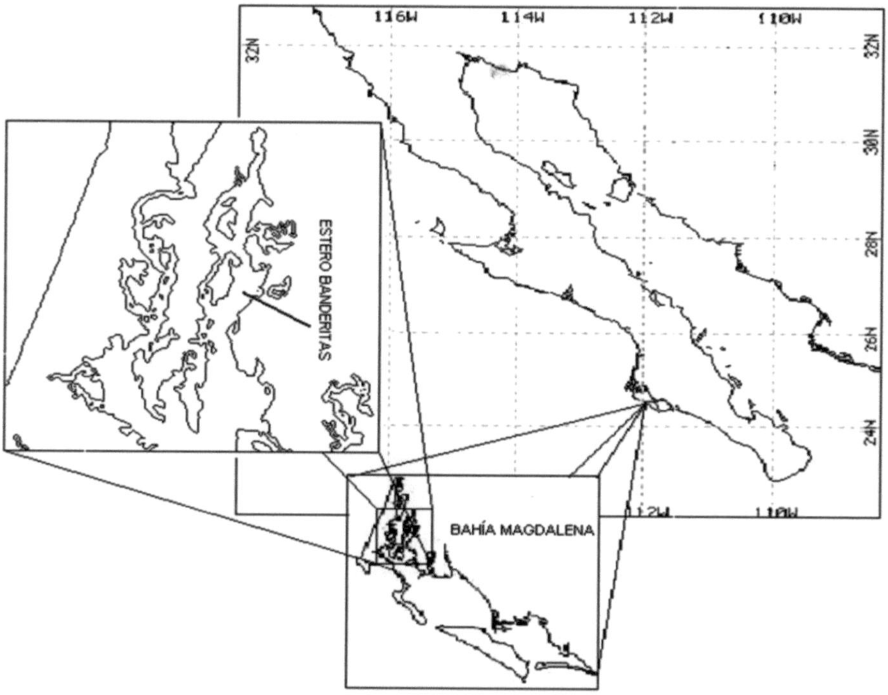

Fig. 1. Study area in Estero Banderitas (24° 50′ - 25° 00′ N and 112°08′ W) located in Bahía Magdalena, Baja California Sur, Mexico.

2.2 Marine plant collection

Three separate sampling trips were made in Estero Banderitas (November 2004, February, 2005 and April, 2005) in order to collect marine plants available during different seasons. Algae and seagrass samples were collected along the length of the mangrove channel using 16 transects of 30 m length. Every 6 m along the transects, plants were manually collected within a 25 cm2 to 1 m2 area, depending on the density of the flora at that location, for a total of 80 samples per trip. The samples were stored in labeled plastic bags and contents were separated by species using taxonomic keys (Riosmena Rodríguez, 1999). Samples were sun-dried in the field and then pressed to further remove moisture.

2.3 Sea turtle tissue collection

Liver and kidney tissues were collected from 8 dead green turtles that incidentally drowned in commercial fishing nets set in Magdalena Bay between February 2002 and April 2003. The straight carapace length of the turtles ranged from 47–77 cm, which is representative of the size range of green turtles in the region (Gardner and Nichols, 2001). The samples were collected within 24 h after the time of death from carcasses with minimal decomposition. Tissue samples were stored in plastic bags and placed on ice for transport to the laboratory where they were frozen at − 80°C until analyzed. From five turtles, intact stomachs were also collected.

2.4 Stomach content analyses

All stomach contents were collected and identified to the lowest possible taxonomic level based on published keys (Abbott and Hollenberg, 1976; Riosmena-Rodríguez, 1999). Entire sample volume and the relative sample volume of each plant species were calculated by the procedure of water displacement in a graduated cylinder. Voucher material was housed in Herbario Ficológico of the Universidad Autónoma de Baja California Sur (UABCS), La Paz, México.

2.5 Laboratory analyses

Tissue and plant samples (0.5 g) were dried in an oven at 70 °C until a dry weight was obtained. Dried samples were digested in acid-washed Teflon tubes with concentrated nitric acid in a microwave oven (CEM modelMars 5X, Matthews, NC). Samples were analyzed by atomic absorption (GBC Scientific equipment, model AVANTA, Dandenong, Australia) using an air-acetylene flame. The certified standard reference material, TORT-2 (National Research Council of Canada, Ottawa) was used to verify accuracy, and that the analytical values were within the range of certified values. All recoveries of metals analyzed were over 95%. Detection limits were: Zinc=0.0008, Cadmium = 0.0009, Mn= 0.002, Cu= 0.0025, Ni = 0.004, Fe=0.005, Pb=0.006 µg/g.

2.6 Quantitative analyses

We analyzed the data based on taxonomic group (red algae, green algae, and seagrass), season, spatial area, and dominant species. Reported statistics are medians (nN2) and ranges in µg/g on a dry weight basis. The Mann–Whitney test was used for conducting two-tailed sample comparisons of tissues for each metal separately and for comparing metals in marine plants collected in Magdalena Bay with those found in the stomach contents. The Kruskal–Wallis test was used to compare the median metal concentration across all plant species. The null hypothesis was rejected if $p \leq 0.05$. The influence of concentration differences among samples was removed by converting data to the percent contribution of each metal to the total metal signature of the individual sample. Fe was removed from these analyses because of its high Concentration and dominance of the metal signature profile. Principal Components Analysis (PCA) of the percent contribution of the metals in plants and turtle tissues. Additionally, factorial analysis was used to determine trends in the presence of heavy metals in the seaweed samples and the relative spatial and/or temporal variation. All analysis was conducted using the Statgraphics Plus software program (Version 5, Rockville, MD).

2.7 Prescence of fibropapiloms and epibionts

Monthly sampling has been develop in the Estero Banderitas and more recently in Estero San Buto as part of the monitoring efforts in was the prescence of fibropapiloms and epibionts by a physical inspection of each animal by region as head, neck, carapace, front or back fins, anus or tail. Comparative analysis was done of the proportion of animals with fibropapiloms and epibionts using the database and literature described in Lara-Uc (2011) in relation to the Bahía Madalena population information (Hinojosa-Arango unpublished data).

3. Results

3.1 Temporal and spatial variation of metal concentration in plant species

Based on our analysis, we found temporal and spatial variations in the concentration in several of heavy metals in seaweeds and seagrasses. In comparisons between the profiles of heavy metals in major plant groups, we found that Nickel differed significantly between the major groups (P=0.01), wherein seagrasses had lower concentrations (Tables 1 and 2). Analyzing all of the species (all sites combined), we found significant seasonal differences in the heavy metal concentrations with the exception of Zinc (P=0.53). Samples collected in April had a higher concentration of Cadmium (P<0.001) and Iron (P=0.002) and a lower concentration of Plumb (P<0.001) and Nickel (P=0.002) than the other months. Manganese was highest in November (P=0.049) and Copper was higher in November compared to February (P=0.01). In comparisons of the metal concentrations between plant species, the only significant differences were detected for Cadmium (p=0.009) in *Ruppia maritima* than all other species. In the case of the analysis of green algae alone, using all species combined, we found temporal significant differences of Cadmium in April (P=0.01).

In the case of other metals, we found significantly temporal differences in Plumb (Pb) concentration in *G. vermiculophylla* (P=0.02) in November but this species also had the highest concentration of Ni (P=0.03) in relation to the other species. Also, there were significant differences in the concentrations of Cadmium (P=0.001), Iron (P=0.01), and Nickel (P=0.002), while Plumb (P<0.001) and Copper (P=0.03) were significantly different than the same metals in November. In the same month, highest Nickel concentrations were recorded in *Codium amplivesiculatum*, while in April, *C. amplivesiculatum*, *Codium cuneatum*, and *Caulerpa sertularioides* from the middle region had the highest concentrations of Copper (7.3μg g−1 dw), Ni (11μg g−1 dw), and Mn (61.4μg g−1 dw), respectively. In February, like November, we had the highest Iron concentration and several species were responsible for this difference (in *H. johnstonii*; 567.5μg g−1 dw) and Zinc concentration (in *G. textorii*; 46.8μg g−1 dw). However, the lower zone had the highest concentrations of Cadmium (in *G. textorii*; 4.4μg g−1 dw) and Ni (*L. pacifica* and *Chondria nidifica*; 13.3 and 13.3μg g−1 dw). Copper (in *L. pacifica*; 2.9μg g−1 dw) and Plumb concentrations were highest in *G. andersonii* from the middle zone (3.8μg g−1 dw).

Season	Species	Cadmium	Plumb	Nickel	Manganese	Iron	Copper
November	*Codium amplivesiculatum*	0.2	1.8	8	52.9	362.2	0.9
		(nd - 0.5)	(1.3 - 2.3)	(6 - 9.9)	(42.2 - 63.5)	(349.8 - 374.7)	(0.7 - 1.2)
	Gracilaria textorii	1.5	1.4	4.8	48.5	325	1.6
		(nd - 3.9)	(nd - 1.9)	(3 - 5.1)	(45.3 - 51.1)	(100.9 - 1231.2)	(0.7 - 4.8)
	Gracilaria vermiculophylla	0.6	2.7	5.3	22.4	302.7	1.3
		(0.5 - 1.4)	(1 - 3.3)	(4.9 - 5.5)	(13 - 23.9)	(185.9 - 372.2)	(1 - 1.6)
	*Gracilariopsis andersonii**	0.5	2	5.7	28.5	195.2	2.5
		-	-	-	-	-	-
	Hypnea johnstonii	0.4	1.8	6.7	26.7	263.9	1.8
		(0.3 - 1.5)	(1.1 - 8.5)	(6 - 6.9)	(23.7 - 282.5)	(227.8 - 1424.1)	(0.9 - 4.4)
February	*Codium amplivesiculatum*	nd	0.8	6.6	12.6	190.2	0.8
			(0 - 2.3)	(6.2 - 7.3)	(12.1 - 20.4)	(189.5 - 522.7)	(nd - 1.3)
	*Codium cuneatum**	nd	1.6	5.9	17.2	241.7	0.4
		-	-	-	-	-	-
	Chondria nidifica	1	1.6	9.3	15.6	291.5	1.3
		(nd - 1.7)	(1.5 - 1.6)	(5.1 - 13.3)	(14.40- 21)	(88.8 - 557.8)	(0.2 - 1.4)
	Gracilaria textorii	3.4	1	6	49.1	139.9	0.5
		(2.7 - 4.4)	(0.7 - 2)	(4.5 - 6.2)	(43.5 - 54.8)	(81.8 - 476.3)	(0.4 - 1.2)
	Gracilaria vermiculophylla	1.1	0.8	4.3	19.3	206.2	0.6
		(1.1 - 1.6)	(0.7 - 0.9)	(3.6 - 5.1)	(14.4 - 19.5)	(139.4 - 269.9)	(0.3 - 1.6)
	*Gracilariopsis andersonii**	1.6	3.8	4.5	23.5	160.4	2.1
		-	-	-	-	-	-
	*Hypnea johnstonii**	nd	nd	11.3	20.6	567.5	nd
		-	-	-	-	-	-
	*Laurencia pacifica**	3	1.7	13.3	25.2	195.8	2.9
		-	-	-	-	-	-
	*Sarcodiotheca gaudichaudii**	0.9	1	5.4	17.2	121.8	0.1
		-	-	-	-	-	-
	*Zostera marina**	nd	2.5	3.1	78.6	51.1	0.4
		-	-	-	-	-	-
April	*Codium amplivesiculatum*	1.6	0.5	7.8	18.7	399.2	4.1
		(1.2 - 1.9)	(0.4 - 0.7)	(7.6 - 7.9)	(15.3 - 22.1)	(298.1 - 500.4)	(1 - 7.3)
	Codium cuneatum	2.1	0.3	7.1	16.7	284.3	1.2
		(1.9 - 2.2)	(0.1 - 0.5)	(3.2 - 11)	(10.5 - 23)	(141.5 - 427.1)	(0.5 - 1.8)
	Caulerpa sertularioides	2.1	0.2	2.6	34.3	374	1.8
		(1.8 - 2.3)	(nd - 0.4)	(1.8 - 3.4)	(7.3 - 61.4)	(223.9 - 524.1)	(1.1 - 2.6)
	*Gracilaria crispata**	4.6	nd	3.9	40.3	576.8	1.6
		-	-	-	-	-	-
	Gracilaria textorii	4.5	0.4	5.3	41.5	579.5	1.7
		(4.3 - 4.8)	(0.1 - 0.6)	(3 - 7.6)	(37.6 - 45.4)	(578.4 - 580.6)	(1.5 - 1.8)
	Gracilaria vermiculophylla	2.9	0.2	2.9	18.1	236.2	0.9
		(2.7 - 2.9)	(nd - 0.6)	(1.1 - 2.9)	(14.7 - 23.6)	(214.4 - 771.5)	(0.9 - 1.6)
	*Gracilariopsis andersonii**	3.8	0.1	2.3	25.5	322.3	1.5
		-	-	-	-	-	-
	*Hypnea johnstonii**	2.7	0.6	1.8	41.9	774.5	2.1
		-	-	-	-	-	-
	*Laurencia pacifica**	4.6	nd	1.9	22.9	497.6	1.8
		-	-	-	-	-	-
	Ruppia maritima	4.5	2.1	2.3	30.6	1230.2	0.5
		(2.1 - 7)	(0.5 - 3.8)	(1.7 - 2.9)	(28.6 - 32. 6)	(1017.4 - 1443)	(nd - 0.9)
	*Zostera marina**	2.2	nd	2.8	33.9	630.3	1.6
		-	-	-	-	-	-

* The values are referred to 1 specimen. nd signifies not detected.

Table 1. Temporal variation of heavy metal concentrations µg.g-1 dry weight in seaweeds and seagrasses collected at the Estero Banderitas. Values are expressed as medians and ranges given in parenthesis.

Site	Species	Cadmium	Plumb	Nickel	Manganese	Iron	Copper
Head	*Codium amplivesiculatum**	nd	2.3	6.6	20.4	522.7	0.8
		-	-	-	-	-	-
	*Chondria nidifica**	nd	1.5	5.1	14.4	88.8	0.2
		-	-	-	-	-	-
	Gracilaria textorii	1.3	1	4.5	50.1	853.7	3
		(nd - 2.7)	(nd - 2)	(3 - 6)	(45.3 - 54.8)	(476.3 - 1231.2)	(1.2 - 4.8)
	Gracilaria vermiculophylla	1.1	0.7	5	22.4	236.2	0.8
		(0.6 - 2.9)	(0.2 - 3.3)	(1.1 - 5.1)	(19.5 - 23.6)	(206.2 - 372.2)	(0.3 - 1.6)
	*Gracilariopsis andersonii**	0.5	2	5.7	28.5	195.2	2.5
		-	-	-	-	-	-
	Hypnea johnstonii	0.7	4.3	9.1	151.6	995.8	2.2
		(nd - 1.5)	(0 - 8.5)	(6.9 - 11.4)	(20.6 - 282.5)	(567.5 - 1424.1)	(nd - 4.4)
	*Ruppia maritima**	6.9	3.8	2.9	32.6	1017.4	nd
		-	-	-	-	-	-
Medium	*Coduim amplivesiculatum*	0.5	0.7	7.9	22.1	349.8	1.2
		(nd - 1.2)	(nd - 1.3)	(7.3 - 10)	(12.1 - 63.5)	(190.2 - 500.4)	(nd - 7.3)
	Codium cuneatum	0.9	1	8.4	20.1	334.4	1.1
		(nd - 2.3)	(0.5 - 1.6)	(5.9 - 11)	(17.2 - 22.9)	(241.7 - 427.1)	(0.4 - 1.8)
	*Caulerpa sertularioides**	2.3	0.4	3.4	61.4	524.1	2.5
		-	-	-	-	-	-
	*Chondria nidifica**	1	1.6	9.3	20.9	557.8	1.4
		-	-	-	-	-	-
	Gracilaria textorii	3.9	1	4.8	45.4	325	0.7
		(3.4 - 4.8)	(0.6 - 1.4)	(4.5 - 7.6)	(43.5 - 51.2)	(139.9 - 580.6)	(0.4 - 1.8)
	Gracilaria vermiculophylla	1.4	0.9	3.5	18.1	302.7	1.4
		(1.1 - 1.6)	(0.6 - 1)	(2.9 - 5.5)	(13 - 19.3)	(269.9 - 771.5)	(1 - 1.6)
	*Gracilariopsis andersonii**	1.6	3.8	4.5	23.5	160.4	2.1
		-	-	-	-	-	-
	*Hypnea johnstonii**	0.3	1.1	6.7	26.7	263.9	1
		-	-	-	-	-	-
	*Ruppia maritima**	2.1	0.5	1.7	28.6	1443	0.9
		-	-	-	-	-	-
	*Sarcodiotheca gaudichaudii**	0.9	1	5.4	17.2	121.8	0.1
		-	-	-	-	-	-
Mouth	*Codium amplivesiculatim*	nd	0.8	6.2	15.3	298.1	1
		(nd - 1.9)	(0.4 - 2.3)	(6 - 7.6)	(12.6 - 42.2)	(189.5 - 374.7)	(0.7 - 1.3)
	*Codium cuneatum**	2.2	0.1	3.2	10.5	141.5	0.5
		-	-	-	-	-	-
	*Caulerpa sertularoides**	1.8	nd	1.8	7.3	223.9	1.1
		-	-	-	-	-	-
	*Chondria nidifica**	1.7	1.6	13.3	15.6	291.5	1.3
		-	-	-	-	-	-
	*Gracilaria crispata**	4.6	nd	3.9	40.3	576.8	1.6
		-	-	-	-	-	-
	Gracilaria textorii	4.3	0.7	5.1	48.5	100.9	1.5
		(1.5 - 4.4)	(0.1 - 1.9)	(3 - 6.2)	(37.6 - 49.1)	(81.8 - 578.4)	(0.5 - 1.6)
	Gracilaria vermiculophylla	1.6	0.8	4.3	14.7	186	0.9
		(0.5 - 2.9)	(0 - 2.7)	(2.9 - 5.3)	(14.4 - 23.9)	(139.4 - 214.4)	(0.6 - 1.3)
	*Gracilariopsis andersonii**	3.8	0.1	2.3	25.5	322.3	1.5
		-	-	-	-	-	-
	Hypnea johnstonii	1.6	1.2	3.9	32.8	501.1	1.9
		(0.4 - 2.7)	(0.6 - 1.8)	(1.8 - 6)	(23.7 - 41.9)	(227.8 - 774.5)	(1.8 - 2.1)
	Laurencia pacifica	3.8	0.8	7.6	24	346.7	2.3
		(3 - 4.6)	(nd - 1.7)	(1.9 - 13.3)	(22.9 - 25.2)	(195.8 - 497.6)	(1.8 - 2.6)
	*Zostera marina**	2.2	nd	2.8	33.9	630.3	1.6
		-	-	-	-	-	-

* The values are refered to 1 specimen. nd signifies not detected.

Table 2. Heavy metal concentrations (µg.g-1 dry weight) in seaweeds and seagrasses collected in the three sites. Values are expressed as medians and ranges given in parenthesis.

Spatial differences in metal concentrations were dependent on the major taxa. In the case of seagrasses, we found a high concentration of Iron (Table 2) who was significant different from Manganese (in *Z. marina*; 78.6 μg g−1 dw) concentrations were highest in the upper zone (P=0.01) because their uneven distribution in the area. Consistent with the above analysis were the multifactorial analysis (Fig. 2) wherein the extreme values are represented by Iron and Manganese with no association among seasons or areas. In the green algae (Table 2), we were able to find many metals in the entire area, but the significant difference was found in Cadmium in April (P=0.01), when all species combined, because the low value in relation to other metals are highly concentrated. There is no consistent pattern in relation to the area of the highest concentration of any metal; they tend to present a group lower in relation to higher concentration in different areas or times (Tables 1 and 2).

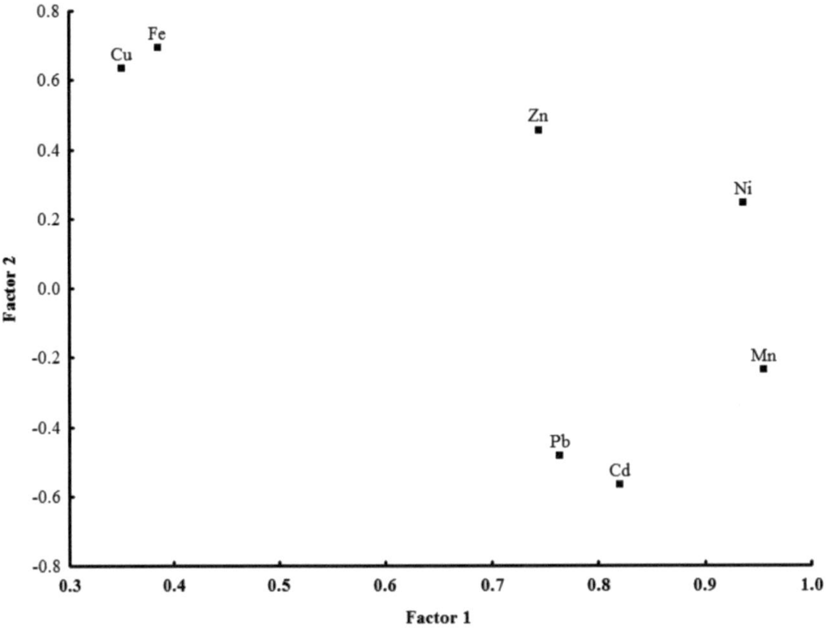

Fig. 2. Multivariate analysis of heavy metals contents in seagrasses.

This is well supported by the multivariate analysis (Fig.3) wherein most of the observed metals show a combination among them and the areas of sampling. We found an extremely high variability in the median content in the red algae (Table 2) but there were no significant differences between sites, with the exception of Zinc which was significantly higher in the upper zone (P=0.02). The highest concentration of any metal was Iron in *Hypnea johnstonii* from the upper zone (1,424.1μg g−1 dw). The highest concentration of Manganese (282.5μg g−1 dw) and Plumb (8.5) μg g−1 dw) were also detected in *H. johnstonii* from the upper zone. Similarly, Zinc (58.8μg g−1 dw) and Copper (4.8μg g−1 dw) concentrations were highest in *G. textorii* in the same zone. The highest Cadmium concentrations were measured in *G. textorii* (4.8μg g−1 dw).

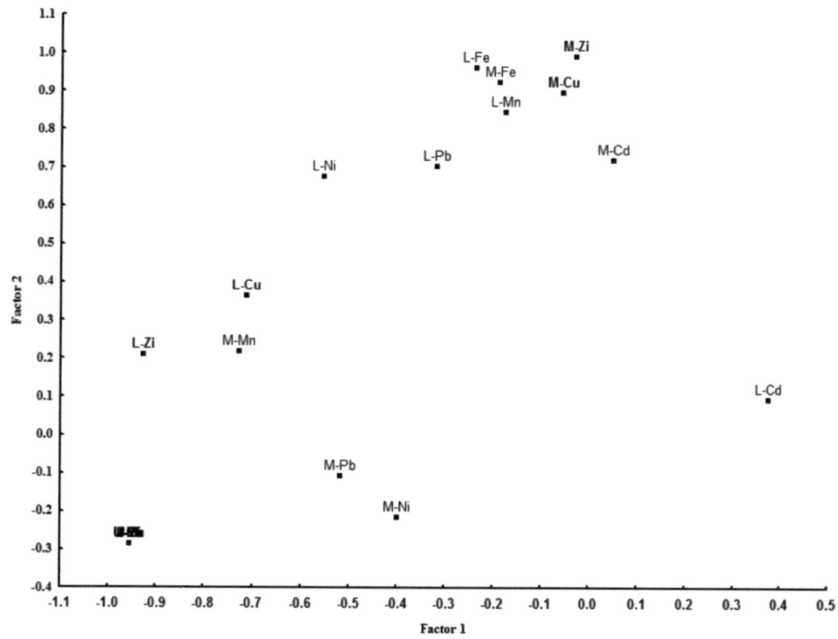

Fig. 3. Multivariate analysis of the spatial concentration of heavy metal in green algae.

Multivariate analyses show the same path in red algae (Figs. 4 and 5) with the clump of areas within metals and a group of metals with high concentration (Fig. 4) in relation to metals with low concentration (Fig. 5).

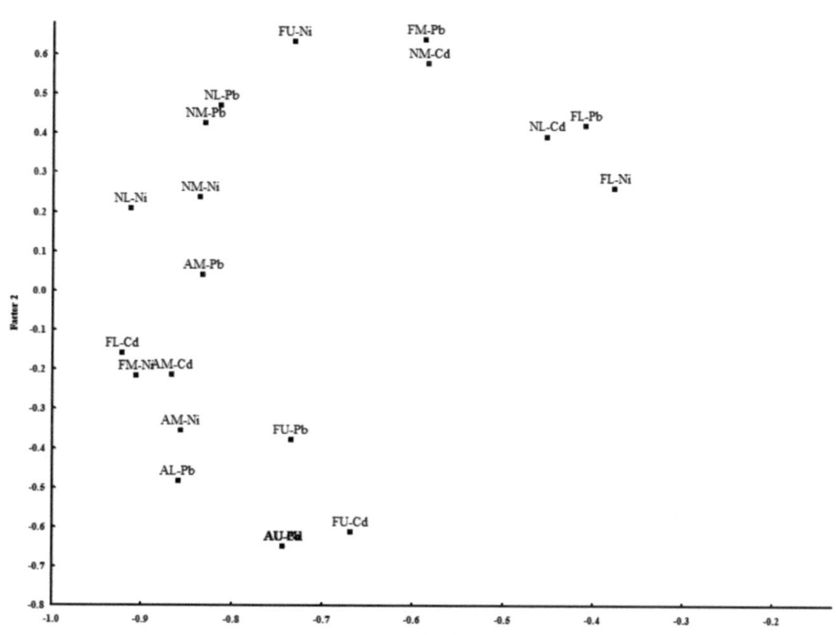

Fig. 4. Multivariate analysis of the spatial concentration of heavy metal in red algae.

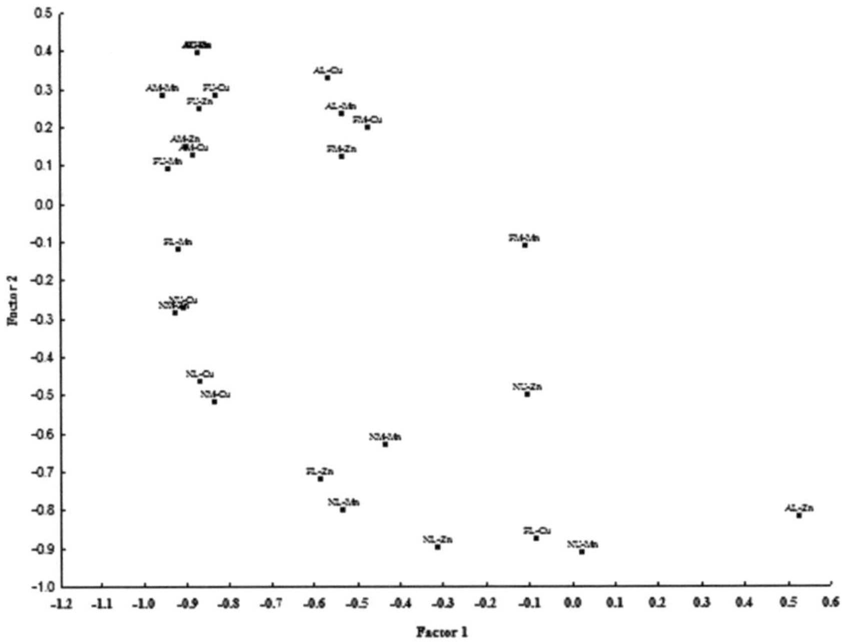

Fig. 5. Multivariate analysis of the spatial concentration of heavy metal in red algae.

3.2 Metals in sea turtle tissues, stomach contents, and plants from the bay

Concentrations of Cadmium and Zinc in flora from the sea turtle stomach contents were greater than the same species of marine plants collected in the bay ($p<0.001$ and $p=0.003$, respectively) (Figure 6). For both metals, the concentrations in sea turtle liver were not significantly different from the stomach contents. Sea turtle kidney Cadmium concentration was significantly higher than liver ($p=0.002$), while Zinc was the same in both tissues. Plumb, Manganese and Fe in flora from the stomach contents were significantly lower than in flora collected from the bay ($p<0.001$ for each) (Figure 6). The stomach contents had higher Plumb and Manganese concentrations than liver ($p=0.04$ and $p<0.001$, respectively) but were not significantly different in Fe. There were no differences in the concentrations of these metals in liver and kidney. Nickel and Copper concentrations did not differ in plants from the two sources. Nickel concentration in liver was similar to kidney concentrations, but significantly lower than the stomach contents ($p=0.005$). Copper was higher in liver than stomach contents ($p<0.001$) and higher than kidney ($p<0.001$). These same trends persisted when the data were transformed to the percent contribution of the metals in each plant species in the stomach contents as compared to the bay samples (Fig. 6). For each of the five plant species, the percent contribution of Manganese and Plumb was greater in the bay-collected plants, while Cadmium and Zinc consistently contributed more to the total metal profile in plants from the stomach contents. Fig. 7 shows the percent contribution of each metal in paired samples of liver, kidney and stomach contents (all flora combined) from the same turtles. Cadmium and Zinc contributed most to the overall metal profile in the kidney, while Copper contributed more in liver. The percent contribution of Manganese and Nickel were greatest in the plants from the stomach contents.

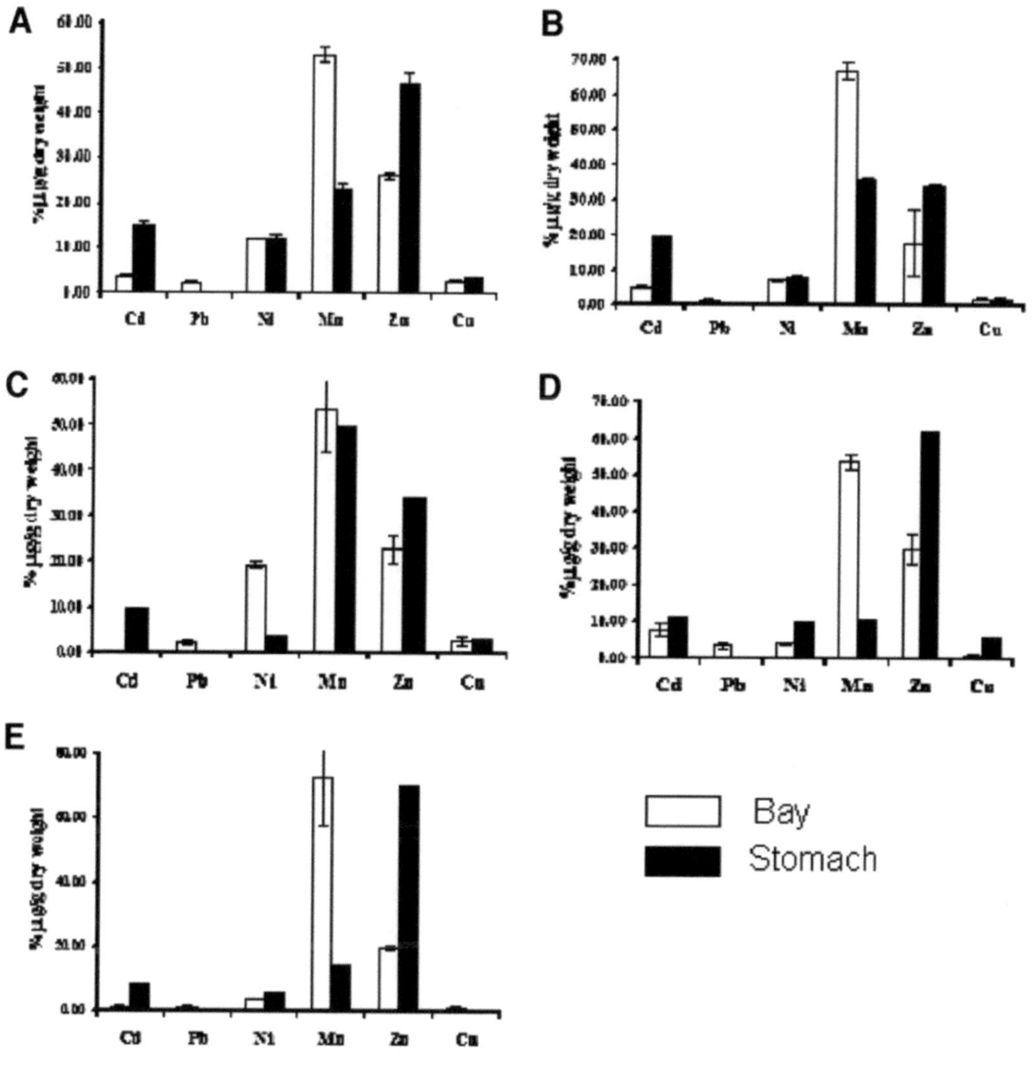

Fig. 6. Percent contribution of metals in species of marine flora collected in the Magdalena Bay and in green turtle (*Chelonia mydas*) stomach contents. A) *G. vermiculophylla*, B) *G. textorii*, C) *C. amplivesiculatum*, D) *R. maritima* and E) *Z. marina*.

Eight species of marine flora were identified within the green turtle stomach contents (Table 3). These same species were also collected from the mangrove channel of Estero Banderitas with the exception of *Neoagarddhiella baileyi*, *Pterocladiella capillacea* and *Ulva lactuca*. *Hypnea johnstonii*, which has been previously reported as a major food item in green turtle diet (López-Mendilaharsu et al., 2005), was available in the bay but not found in the stomachs of the turtles. *Gracilaria vermiculophylla* was present in 60%of the turtle stomachs analyzed and made up the greatest total percent volume (36%). Gracilaria textorii was present in the second greatest percent volume (16.5%).

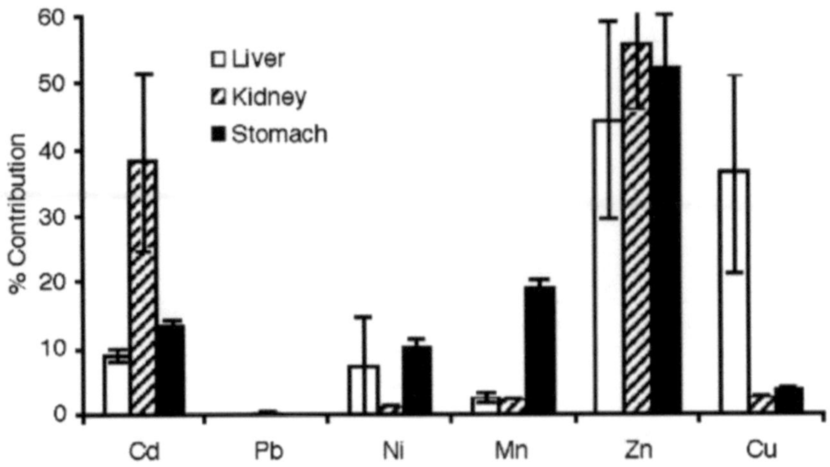

Fig. 7. Percent contribution of metals in tissues and the stomach contents of green turtles (*Chelonia mydas*) from Magdalena Bay, Mexico.

	Stomach Contents					
Species	1	2	3	4	5	TOTAL
Codium amplivesiculatum	69.1%					13.8%
Gracilaria textorii	30.9%	51.6%				16.5%
Gracilaria vermiculophylla		48.4%	33.6%		100%	36.4%
Neoagarddhiella baileyi				36.2%		7.2%
Pterocladiella capillacea				20.5%		4.1%
Rupia maritima				43.3%		8.7%
Ulva lactuca			31.8%			6.4%
Zostera marina			34.5%			6.9%

Table 3. Percent volume of macroalgae and sea grasses in the stomach contents of five green turtles (*Chelonia mydas*) collected in Estero Banderitas, Magdalena Bay, Mexico.

3.3 Principal components analysis

Principal components analysis (PCA) of the percent contribution of individual metals to the overall metal signature of each plant or tissue sample generated three principal components (PC) that explained 80.7% of the total variance in the data (50.1%, 17.6%, and 13.1%, respectively) (Fig. 8). Plots of the sample scores on the first and second principal components produced four groupings. Bay and stomach plant samples were separated by their scores on PC(1), while kidney and liver samples were separated by their scores on PC(2) (Fig. 8A). All but one of the bay plant samples obtained negative scores on PC(1), whereas plants from the stomach contents generally scored greater than 0. The loadings plot, which illustrates the influence of each metal on sample scores, indicated that the bay and stomach samples separated on PC(1) based on the dominance of the stomach samples' metal signatures by Zinc and Cadmium. The separation of liver and kidney samples appeared to be influenced by the greater contribution of Cadmium to the metal profile in kidney, and the dominance of Cu in liver samples which scored higher on PC(2) (Fig. 8B).

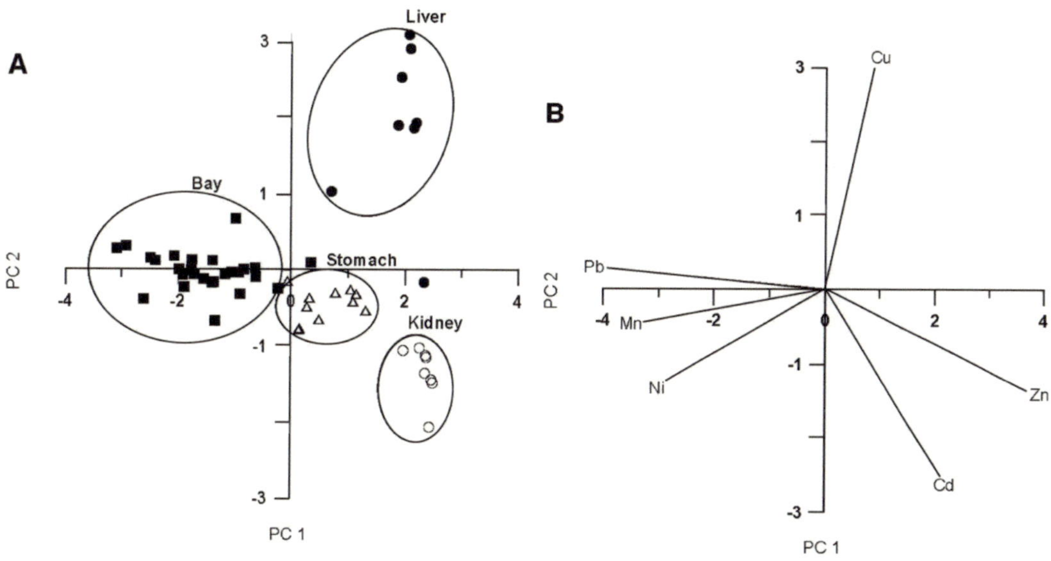

Fig. 8. A) Plot of sample scores of a Principle Component Analysis of the percent contribution of individual metals to the overall signature of marine flora from Magdalena Bay, kidney, liver and stomach contents samples from green turtles (*Chelonia mydas*). B) Loadings plot

3.4 Prescence of fibropapiloms and epibionts

In our study we found less of 1% of the animals with some fibropapiloms but at least 20% with epibionts. This is consistent with the data from Caribbean populations in where 2% had tumors present. The main observed difference was the degree of development between the populations in Bahía Magdalena (Fig. 9a) with very few in the carapace, frontal fins and head. In Caribbean populations bibber tumors (Fig. 9b) were observed and more concentrated in the head or in the frontal fins.

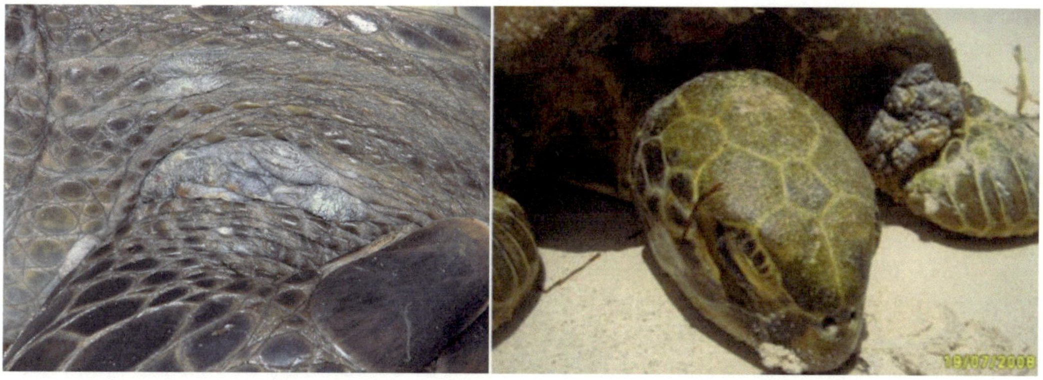

Fig. 9. A) Population in Bahía Magdalena (Fig. 9a) with very few in the carapace, frontal fins and head. B) Caribbean population's bibber tumors were observed and more concentrated in the head or in the frontal fins.

4. Discussion

Much of the literature on sea turtles has worked with absolute concentrations of metals, which is appropriate for comparisons of very similar sample types such as different sea turtle tissues or the same tissue in different sea turtle species. In the present paper we used absolute concentrations to compare metals in tissues (kidney vs. liver) and to compare metal concentrations in different plant species. However in order to better understand the source of metals to turtles in this region, the profile of all metals combined was used as an environmentally acquired marker. For this objective, we removed the influence of concentration differences among samples by converting the data to percent contribution of each metal to the total metal signature of the individual sample. This approach enabled the comparison of metal profiles across greatly different samples and was more appropriate than comparisons of absolute concentrations alone. For example, a single plant species located in two different areas will accumulate metals using the same physiological mechanisms. Therefore, a difference in metal profiles of the plant species from two different locations is an indication of differences in the availability of the metals from the environment. However, differences in the absolute concentrations of metals in plants would not necessarily indicate environmental difference because other factors might also be at play (e.g. age of the plant).

4.1 Comparison of metals in marine plant species

Metal concentrations in marine flora are controlled by both the bioavailability of metals in the surrounding water and the uptake capacity of the particular plant species. Marine algae have the capacity to accumulate trace metals several thousand times higher than the concentration in seawater (Bryan and Langston, 1992; Sánchez-Rodríguez et al., 2001). Red algae, such as Gracilaria sp tend to reflect the environmental availability of metals but have higher bioaccumulation of Cadmium, Copper and Zinc than other macroalgal groups (Sánchez-Rodríguez et al., 2001; Roncarati, 2003). These same species are a major component of the green turtle diet along the Baja California Peninsula (Seminoff et al., 2002; López-Mendilaharsu et al., 2005), and we proposed previously (Gardner et al., 2006) that their foraging habits could account for the high metal concentrations found in this population. However, comparisons across plant species in the present study suggest that species differences in metal concentrations are minimal. The only significant difference detected between plant species was that Cadmium was higher in *Ruppia maritima* than all other species, and higher in *Gracilaria textorii* than *Codium amplivesiculatum*. *R. maritima* was encountered in only one of the sea turtle stomachs analyzed, contributing a relatively small percentage of the overall diet (8.7%) in this study, and was absent from the diet of 24 green turtles analyzed in previous work (López-Mendilaharsu et al., 2005). *Gracilaria textorii* made up a larger proportion of the turtles' stomach contents (16.5%), but was similar in Cadmium concentration to most other plant species ingested by the green turtles. The results of the PCA also support this conclusion since the bay-collected plant samples grouped separately from the samples in the stomach contents despite that both groups consisted of the same five plant species.

We found significant spatial and temporal variations in heavy metal concentrations in marine plants as previous spatial studies has shown in the region (Páez-Osuna et al., 2000; Sánchez-Rodríguez et al., 2001; Rodriguez-Castañeda et al., 2006, Rodríguez-Meza et al., 2008). The high concentration of Zinc and Fe in the upper region might be related to the isolation of the site (Rodríguez-Meza et al., 2008). Heavy metal concentration was, in some

cases, in the levels of toxicity. Temporal variations in metal concentrations, such as high concentrations in Cadmium and other metals observed in April, may be related to local upwelling events. Surface water Cadmium concentrations have been strongly correlated with upwelling (Lares et al. 2002) which occurs during spring and early summer off the coast of Magdalena Bay (Zaytsev et al., 2003). These levels of Cadmium in seaweeds has not been observed in the Gulf of California studied populations but strong species and spatial variations where observed (Páez-Osuna et al., 2000; Sánchez-Rodríguez et al. 2001; Rodriguez-Castañeda et al., 2006). The differences in heavy metal concentrations that we found in the seaweeds did not generally correspond with patterns of those elements previously observed in the sediment from the same region or seaweed species (Rodríguez-Meza et al., 2008), contrary to the studied sites in the Gulf of California near a mine (Rodriguez-Castañeda et al., 2006) or near industrial ports (Páez-Osuna et al., 2000; Sánchez-Rodríguez et al., 2001; Rodriguez-Castañeda et al., 2006). This finding, together with the observed species differences, suggests that the metabolic condition and life cycle stage of the individual species might influence metal uptake and accumulation (Lobban and Wynne 1981). Similarly, Riget et al., (1995) found differences between seaweed species *Ascophyllum nodosum, Fucus vesiculosus,* and *Fucus distichus*. We found lower levels of Ni and Zinc in *H. johnstonii* than in the environment as reported by Rodríguez-Meza et al., (2008). Based on our data, there are similarities between the composition and concentration of heavy metals between the plant species reviewed and the sediment; except in the case of Cu, Fe, and Mn (Rodríguez-Meza et al., 2008). All those elements are considered critical in the photosynthetic metabolism (Lobban and Wynne, 1981). We might assume that those elements are more easily assimilated by the plants because of their use in photosynthesis.
The role of seaweeds and seagrasses in coastal lagoons (like Banderitas or any other along the Baja California Peninsula) are relevant because they are feeding grounds for black turtles (*C. mydas*), loggerhead turtles (*Caretta caretta*), olive Ridley turtles (*Lepidochelys olivacea*), and hawksbill turtles (*Eretmochelys imbricata*) and migratory birds like Brant geese (*Branta bernicla*; Seminoff, 2000; Herzog and Sedinger, 2004). All of the species are included in the Mexican endangered species list (NOM ECOL 059) and on the red list in the UICN endangered species (www. uicnredlist.org). They are high productivity areas for fishing all kind of products (CONABIO, 2000; Carta Nacional, 2005). The fact that we found more significant variation in the spatial than temporal heavy metal concentrations in most of the species show that they might be constantly incorporated in the diet of many herbivorous animals (Gardner et al., 2006) with severe consequences in their health. Management strategies for these species should consider monitoring the levels of metals.

4.2 Sea turtle tissue comparisons

Pb, Cu and Mn concentrations in tissue from this study were within the range of those reported for sea turtles in other parts of the world (Lam et al., 2004; Storelli and Marcotrigiano, 2003). However, the average concentrations of Cadmium, Zinc and Ni in kidney of green turtles from Magdalena Bay were high compared to previously reports for sea turtle tissues (Sakai et al., 1995, 2000; Storelli and Marcotrigiano, 2003). Studies of loggerhead turtles (Maffucci et al., 2005) suggest that sea turtles can regulate Copper and Zinc concentrations through homeostatic processes but that Cadmium uptake is not controlled by active process and thus tissue concentrations of this metal reflect exposure. In agreement with these findings, we observed that Cadmium concentrations in green turtle liver were similar to their food and that the Cu concentration in sea turtle liver was greater than in the stomach content. Similar relationships have been observed in green turtles from Japan (Anan et al., 2001). However, contrary to the findings of Maffucci et al., (2005), Zinc concentrations in the livers and kidneys of green turtles in our study were not significantly different from their stomach contents. The distribution of metals among organs is influenced by both duration and concentration of exposure. Liver is a major site of short-term Cadmium storage, whereas during long-term exposure, Cadmium is redistributed from the liver to the kidney where it is absorbed and concentrated (Thomas et al., 1994; Linder and Grillitsch, 2000; Rie et al., 2001). Therefore a significantly greater concentration of Cadmium in green turtle kidney than liver is often observed (Storelli and Marcotrigiano, 2003; Maffucci et al., 2005; Gardner et al., 2006) and likely results from years of accumulation in this long-lived species. While kidney Cadmium concentration may serve as a good indicator for assessments of sea turtle health, liver more closely reflects the concentration of this metal in the food and so analyses of liver may provide a better indication of recent environmental exposure. Accordingly, Cadmium concentrations in the livers analyzed in the present study were not different from the food in the sea turtles' stomachs. Concentrations of Fe and Zinc in liver were also similar to the stomach contents. Whereas, Plumb, Nickel and Manganese concentrations in liver were similar to kidney, but were lower than in the stomach contents, which may indicate metabolic processing of these metals. Alternatively, Copper concentration was higher in liver than in the turtles' food and appeared to be preferentially accumulated in liver over kidney.

4.3 Metals in sea turtle stomach contents and marine plants from the bay

Two principle components, PC(1) and PC(2), explained 68%of the total variance in the data.When plotted relative to PC(1) and PC(2), the plant samples collected in the bay formed a grouping at the left side of the plot while the green turtle tissue samples and the plants from the stomach contents plotted higher on PC(1) (Fig. 4A). Examination of the loadings plot for each of the metals confirmed that samples scoring high on PC1 had signatures dominated by Cadmium and Zinc (stomach contents and kidney) or Cu (liver) (Fig. 4B). This agrees with the observation that the plants in the stomach contents contained greater percent contributions of Cadmium and Zinc than the samples collected in the bay, while Pb and Mn contributed more to the metal profiles in the bay samples as shown in Fig. 2; a tendency that was consistent in all five plant species. The metal profiles in the sea turtle tissues more closely resembled the plants in the stomach contents than the same species of plants collected within Estero Banderitas. The fact that the concentrations of Cadmium, Fe and Zinc in green turtle liver were the same as the stomach contents but different from the plants collected in the bay suggests that sea turtles collected inside of Magdalena Bay use foraging resources outside of the Estero Banderitas region. Further support of this conclusion is provided by the fact that three algal species (*N. baileyi*, *P. capillacea* and *U. lactuca*) in the stomach contents were not found in Estero Banderitas. Franzellitti et al. (2004) proposed that tissue metal profiles can be used as "environmentally acquired markers" to determine sea turtle feeding areas. Similarly, principle component analyses have been applied previously to determine sources of metals in aquatic environments (Ruiz-Fernández et al., 2001). Comparison of the metal signature profiles in plants from the bay and the sea turtle stomach contents indicate that the plant species contained inside the sea turtle stomachs originated from a location outside of Estero Banderitas, in an area where Cadmium and Zinc concentrations dominate the metal profiles in the environment. Surface water metal concentrations have been strongly correlated with upwelling events and natural components of regional biogeochemistry (Daesslé et al., 2000; Lares et al., 2002). Similar to the distribution of nutrients in the water column, metals such as Cadmium and Zinc are depleted in the surface and enriched in deeper water. Upwelling processes are an important mechanism that brings elevated concentrations of both nutrients and metals to the surface and thus available for marine floral accumulation. Therefore it is highly probable that the sea turtles collected within Magdalena Bay are utilizing foraging areas in an upwelling-rich coastal region outside of the Bay. Coastal lagoons of the Baja California Peninsula such as Magdalena Bay have been identified as priority areas for sea turtle conservation programs (Nichols et al., 2000). Long-term sea turtle monitoring studies have demonstrated high site fidelity to Estero Banderitas over time, and low emigration of sea turtles from Magdalena Bay to other coastal lagoons along the Baja California Peninsula (Grupo Tortuguero, unpublished data). Efforts to protect areas within Magdalena Bay have focused on the creation of a refuge in the mangrove channels of Estero Banderitas, in part, because of the perceived importance of this habitat for sea turtle foraging (Nichols and Arcas, 2001). However, data generated by our work suggest that sea turtles residing in Estero Banderitas are feeding in areas outside of the bay, most likely in coastal regions with high upwelling. These findings support those of López-Mendilaharsu et al. (2005) and indicate that green turtles utilize spatially distinct feeding habitats within coastal areas. Therefore, we recommend that sea turtle protected areas be designed with an appreciation of regional rather than local scales in order to protect broader foraging areas.

4.4 Fibropapiloms and epibionts

The prescence of fibropapiloms are variable from 1.4% up to 90% of the population (Herbs *et al.*, 1999, Quackenbush et al., 2001, Chaloupka et al., 2009). The observed low proportion of the green turtles in Bahía Magdalena (less than 1%) agree with a well preserved environment and less stress situation for the animals. In the case of the epibionts we found a continuously prescence of cirripedia and balanus but not a diverse fauna like in the Atlantic that even polychaetes has been reported (Lara Uc, 2011).

5. Conclusions

Conservation of threatened species, such as the green turtle (*Chelonia mydas*), is closely related to habitat quality. In particular there are issues related to heavy metals, the presence of epibionts, parasites and fibropapiloms who might play a crucial role in the species survivorship. The process of metal bioaccumulation in marine food chains is poorly understood because very little data is available on metal concentration at different trophic levels and their temporal or spatial variation and its influence in turtle health. The Baja California Peninsula, Mexico serves an important role for feeding and developing sea turtles. High concentrations of metals detected in food items (seaweeds and seagrasses) and in green turtles (*Chelonia mydas*) from Magdalena Bay prompted an investigation into the sources of metals in the region in relation to the health issues of the animals. We compared metal concentrations in sea turtle tissues in relation to plant species found in their stomach contents, and with the same species of plants collected inside a sea turtle refuge area known as Estero Banderitas and determine the health state of turtles based on our long term monitoring efforts. Our results showed that Iron, Copper, and Manganese were the most significant metals found in seagrasses, red, and green algae. We found significant more variation in temporal heavy metal concentrations in relation to the maximum abundance in the samples and spatial variation in relation to the studied taxa suggesting that herbivores' have a differential intake of the metals. Also, our results suggest that heavy metals might be incorporated regularly in the diet of many herbivorous animals with severe consequences to their health. Differences in the metal concentrations between marine plant species in relation to animal tissue were minimal. Principal components analysis of the percent contribution of individual metals to the overall metal signature of each plant or tissue sample generated three principal components that explained 80.7% of the total variance in the data. The plant samples collected within Estero Banderitas formed a separate grouping from the green turtle tissue samples and the plants from the stomach contents. The plants in the stomach contents contained greater percent contributions of Cadmium and Zinc than the plants collected inside the bay, while Plumb and Manganese contributed more to the metal profiles in the bay samples. The metal profiles in the sea turtle tissues more closely resembled the stomach contents than the same species of plants collected within Estero Banderitas, and suggest that sea turtles collected inside Magdalena Bay use foraging resources outside of the Estero Banderitas region. Green turtle from Estero Banderitas seems to be healthy at this stage in comparison with nesting areas in the Pacific and Atlantic of Mexico our data on fibropapilomas and epibionts strongly support this idea. Our data supports the suggestion that metal profiles can be used as "environmentally acquired markers" to improve our understanding of the extent of sea turtle foraging areas. Management strategies for these species should consider monitoring the levels of metals.

6. Acknowledgements

Funding for this project was provided by a grant to SC Gardner from the Consejo Nacional de Ciencia y Tecnología (Conacyt, SEP-2004-CO1-45749) and the Centro de Investigaciones Biológicas del Noroeste, S.C. (CIBNOR). The authors express their appreciation to Dr. Wallace J. Nichols, Rodrigo Rangel and the Grupo Tortuguero for their assistance in this project. We also appreciate the expertise of Dr. Samuel Chávez Rosales and Griselda Peña Armenta for their help with the quantitative analyses. This research was conducted in accordance with Mexican laws and regulations, under permits provided by the Secretaria de Medio Ambiente y Recursos Naturales (SGPA/DGVS/002-2895).

7. References

Abbott IA, Hollenberg GJ. (1976)Marine algae of California. U.S.A.: Standford University Press; 1976. 827 pp.

Abdallah AMA, Abdallah MA, Beltagy A, Siam E (2006) Contents of heavy metals in marine algae from egyptian red sea coast. Tox Env Chem 88: 9-22.

Aguirre, A.A.; Lutz, P.L. (2004), Marine turtles as Sentinels of Ecosystem Health: Is Fibropapilomatosis an indicator EcoHealth 1:275-283.

Alfaro, A. Koie, M. Buchmann, Kurt. (2006). Synopsis of infections in sea turtles caused by virus, bacteria and parasites: an ecological review. University the Copenhagen. Report.30

Anan, Y, Kunito T, Watanabe I, Sakai H, Tanabe S. (2001)Trace element accumulation in hawksbill turtles (Eretomochelys imbricata) and green turtles (*Chelonia mydas*) from Yaeyama Islands, Japan. Environ Toxicol Chem 20:2802–14.

Arriaga, CL, Vázquez-Domínguez E, González-Cano J, Jiménez-Rosenberg R, Muñoz-López E, Aguilar-Sierra V. (1998). Regiones marinas prioritarias de México. México: Comisión Nacional para el Conocimiento y uso de la Biodiversidad;. 198 pp.

Badillo, A.F.J. (2007). Epizoítos y Parásitos de la tortuga Boba (*Caretta caretta*) en el mediterráneo occidental. Tesis de Doctorado, Universidad de Valencia. 264

Bicho, R, Joaquim N., MendoncaV., AlKiyumi A., Mahmoud .IY., AlKindi A. (2006). Levels of heavy metals and antioxidant enzymes in green turtle (Chelonia mydas) in the Arabian Sea, Sultanate of Oman. Twenty sixth annual symposium on sea turtle biology and conservation. Athens, Greece: International Sea Turtle Society.

Brand-Gardner, S.J., Lanyon J.M., Limpus C.J. (1999). Diet selection by immature green turtles, Chelonia mydas, in subtropical Moreton Bay, South-east Queensland. Aust J Zool;47:181–91.

Bryan , G.W., Langston W.J. (1992). Bioavailability, accumulation and effects of heavy metals in sediments with special reference to United Kingdom estuaries: a review. Environ Pollut 76:89-131.

Caliceti, M., Argese E., Sfriso A., Pavoni B. (2002). Heavy metal contamination in the seaweeds of the Venice lagoon. Chems 47:443-454.

Carta Nacional Pesquera (2005) Carta Nacional Pesquera, SEMARNAT México D.F. 120 pp.

Caurant F, Bustamante P, Bordes M, Miramand P. Bioaccumulation of cadmium, copper and zinc in some tissues of three species of marine turtles stranded along the French Altantic coasts. Mar Pollut Bull 1999;38:1085–91.

Catriona MO, Macinnis-Ng CMO, Peter JR (2002) Towards a more ecologically relevant assessment of the impact of heavy metals en the photosynthesis of the seagrass, *Zostera capricorni*. Mar Poll Bull 45: 100-106.

CONABIO 2000. Plan Nacional sobre Biodiversidad. CONABIO México D.F. 250 pp,

Daesslé, L.W., Carriquiry J.D., Navarro R., Villaescusa-Celaya J.A. (2000). Geochemistry of surficial sediments from Sebastian Vizcaino Bay, Baja California. J Coast Res 16:1133–45.

Díaz, M.M.; Gutiérrez, B.J.; Jasso, L.D.; López, S.C.; Sarti, M.L.; Vallejo, A.C. (1992). Epibiontes y estado físico de las tortugas *Lepidochelys olivacea* y *Dermochelys coriacea* en el playón de Mexiquillo, Michoacán, durante la temporada de anidación 1988-1989; Publ. Soc. Herpetol. Mex. 19-25.

Franzellitti, S., Locatelli C.,Gerosa G., Vallini C., Fabbri E. (2004). Heavymetals in tissues of loggerhead turtles (Caretta caretta) from the northwestern Adriatic Sea. Comp Biochem Physiol C 138:187–94.

Gámez, S.V., Osorio, D.S., Peñaflores, C.S.; García, A.H.; Ramírez, J.L. (2006). Identification of parasites and epibionts in the Olive Ridley Turtle (*Lepidochelys olivacea*) that arrived to the beaches of Michoacán and Oaxaca, Mexico. *Vet. Méx.* 37:431-440.

Gardner, S.C., Nichols W.J. (2001). Assessment of sea turtle mortality rates in the Bahía Magdalena region, Baja California Sur, México. Chelonian Conserv Biol 4:197–9.

G ardner, S.C., Fitzgerald S.L., Acosta-Vargas B., Méndez-Rodríguez L. (2006) Heavy metal Accumulation in four species of sea turtles from the Baja California Peninsula, Mexico. Biomet. 19(1): 91-99.

Garnett, ST, Pirce IR, Scott FJ. The diet of the green turtle, Chelonia mydas (L.), in Torres Strait. Aust Wildl Res 1985;12:103–12.

Gordon, A.N., Pople A.R., Ng. J. (1998). Trace metal concentrations in livers and kidneys of sea turtles from south-eastern Queensland, Australia. Mar Freshw Res 49:409–14.

Gutiérrez-Galindo , E.A., Villaescusa-Celaya J.A., Arrelola-Chimal A. (1999). Bioaccumulation of metals in mussels from tour sites of the coastal region of Baja California. Cienc Mar 25:557–77.

Herbst, L.H., Jacobson E.R., Klein P. A., Balazs G., Moretti R., Brown T. and Sndberg J.(1999).Comparative Pathology and Pathogenesis of Spontaneous Experimentally Induced Fibropapillomas of Green Turtle (*Chelonia mydas*). Vet Pathol 36:551-564

Herzog, M.P., Sedinger J.S. (2004) Dynamics of foraging behavior associated with variation in habitat and forage availability in captive black brant (*Branta bernicla nigricans*) Goslings in Alaska. Auk 121:210-23.

Kalesh, NS, Nair SM (2006) Spatial and temporal variability of copper, zinc, and cobalt in marine macroalgae from the southwest coast of India. Bull Environ Contam Toxicol 76:293-300.

Kieffer, F. (1991). Metals and their compounds in the environment. Weinheim: VCH: 481 pp.

Kumar, V.V., Kaladharan P. (2006) Biosorption of metals from contaminated water using seaweed. Curr Sci 90:1263-7.

Lam, J.C.W., Tanabe S., Chan S.K.F., Yuen E.K.W., Lam M.H.W., Lam P.K.S. (2004). Trace element residues in tissues of green turtles (Chelonia mydas) from South China waters. Mar Pollut Bull 48:164–92

Lanza, G, Ortega MM, Laparra JL, Carrillo RM, Godinez JL (1989) Chemical analysis of heavy metals (hg, pb, cd, as, cr and sr) in marine algae of Baja California. An Inst Biol Univ Nac Auton Mex (Bot) 59:89-102.

Lara-Uc, M. (2011). Establecimiento de valores hematológicos y bioquímicos de las tortugas carey (*Eretmochelys imbricata*) y blanca (*Chelonia mydas*), con y sin parásitos o fibropapiloma, que anidan en Yucatán. Upublised Ph.D. thesis Universidad Autónoma de Yucatán, Merida, 105 pp.

Lares, ML, Flores-Munoz G, Lara-Lara R (2002) Temporal variability of bioavailable cd, hg, zn, mn and al in an upwelling regime. Environ Pollut 120:595-608.

Linder, G., Grillitsch B. (2000) Ecotoxicology of Metals. In: Sparling DW, Linder G, Bishop CA, editors. Ecotoxicology of amphibians and reptiles. Society of Environmental Toxicology and Chemistry SETAC press; p. 325–459

Lobban, C.S., Wynne M.J. (1981) The Biology of Seaweeds. Botanical Monographs Vol. 17. Blackwell Scientific Publications, USA,786 p.

López-Mendilaharsu, M, Gardner SC, Riosmena-Rodríguez R, Seminoff J (2005) Identifying critical foraging habitats of the GreenTurtle (*Chelonia mydas*) along the Pacific Coast of the Baja California Peninsula, México. Aqu Conserv: Mar and Fresh Ecosys 15: 259-269.

Machado, W, Silva-Filho EV, Oliveira RR, Lacerda LD (2002) Trace retention in mangrove ecosystems in Guanabara Bay, SE Brazil. Mar Poll Bull 44: 1277-1280.

Maffucci, F, Caurant F, Bustamante P, Bentivegna F. Trace element (Cd, Cu, Hg, Se, Zn) accumulation and tissue distribution in loggerhead turtles (Caretta caretta) from the Western Mediterranean Sea (southern Italy). Chemosphere 2005;58:535–42.

Martin, J.H., Broenkow W.W. (1975). Cadmium in plankton: elevated concentrations off Baja California. Science 190:884–5.

Méndez-Rodríguez, L., Acosta-Vargas B., Alvarez-Castañeda S.T., Lechuga-Devéze C.H. (1998). Trace metal distribution along the southern coast of Bahia de La Paz (Gulf of California), Mexico. Bull Environ Contam Toxicol 61:616–22.

Méndez, L., Álvarez-Castañeda S.T., Acosta B., Sierra-Beltrán A. P. (2002) Trace metals in tissues of gray whale (*Eschrichtius robustus*) carcasses from the Northern Pacific Mexican Coast. Mar Poll Bull 44, 217-221.

Moreno, M (2003) Toxicología ambiental, evaluación de riesgo para la salud humana. Mc Graw- Hill. España. 370 pp.

Nichols ,WJ, Arcas F. Third Annual Meeting of the Sea Turtle Conservation Network of the Californias (Grupo Tortuguero de las Californias). Mar Turt Newsl 2001;93:30–1.

Nichols, W.J., Bird K.E., Garcia S.(2000). Community-based research and its application to sea turtle conservation in Bahia Magdalena, BCS, Mexico. Mar Turt Newsl 89:4–7.

Páez-Osuna, F., Ochoa-Izaguirre M.J., Bojórquez-Leyva H., Michel-Reynoso I.L. (2000). Macroalgae as Biomonitors of Heavy Metal Availability in Coastal Lagoons from the Subtropical Pacific of Mexico. Bull of Env Cont Tox 64:846-851.

Quackenbush, S. L., Casey R. N., Murcek R. J., Paul T. A., Work T. M., Limpus C. J., Chaves A., duToit L., Vasconcelos P. J., Aguirre A. A., Spraker T. R., Horrocks J. A., Vermeer L. A., Balazs G. H., Casey J. W. (2001). Quantitative análisis of Herpesvirus Sequences from normal tissue and Fibropapillomas of marine Turtles with Real-Time PCR. J. Virology. 287:105-111.

Rie, M.T., Lendas K.A., Callard I.P. (2001). Cadmium: tissue distribution and binding protein induction in the painted turtle, Chrysemys picta. Comp Biochem Physiol C 130:41–51.

Riget ,F., Johansen P., Asmund G. (1995) Natural seasonal variation of cadmium, copper, lead and zinc in brown seaweed (*Fucus vesiculosus*). Mar Poll Bull 30; 409-414.

Riosmena-Rodríguez, R. (1999) Vegetación subacuatica. In: Gaytán, J.,Informe Final de Actividades del Proyecto Bahía del Rincón . UABCS-S&R. 350 pp,

Riosmena-Rodríguez, R., Talavera-Saenz A.L., Gardner S.C., Acosta-Vargas B. (2010). Heavy metals dynamics from Seaweeds and Seagrasses in Bahía Magdalena, B.C.S., México. *J. App. Phyc.* 22; 283 -291.

Rodríguez-Meza, G. D. (2005) Caracterización geoquímica de componentes mayores y elementos traza de sedimentos de los ambientes marinos costeros adyacentes a la península de Baja California. Ph D. thesis, IPN-CICIMAR.

Rodriguez-Castaneda, A.P., Sanchez-Rodriguez I., Shumilin E.N., Sapozhnikov D. (2006) Element concentrations in some species of seaweeds from La Paz bay and La Paz lagoon, south-western Baja California, México. J App Phyc 18: 399-408.

Roncarati, F. (2003). Utilizzo di macrofite marine come indicatori di stress ambientali. Thesis in Environmental Sciences. University of Bologna, Campus Ravenna, Italy.

Ruiz-Fernández, A.C., Páez-Osuna F., Hillaire-Marcel C., Soto-Jiménez M., Gheleb B. (2001). Principle component analysis applied to the assessment of metal pollution from urban wastes in the Culiacán river estuary. Bull Environ Contam Toxicol 67:741–8.

Sakai, H., Ichihashi H., Suganuma H., Tatsukawa R. (1995). Heavy metal monitoring in sea turtles using eggs. Mar PollutBull 30:347–53.

Sakai, H., Saeki K., Ichihashi H., Suganuma H., Tanabe S, Tatsukawa R. (2000). Species-specific distribution of heavy metals in tissues and organs of loggerhead turtle (Caretta caretta) and green turtle (*Chelonia mydas*) from Japanese coastal waters. Mar Pollut Bull 40:701–9.

Sánchez-Rodríguez, I, Huerta- Díaz MA, Choumiline E, Holguín-Quiñones O, Zertuche-Gonzáles JA (2001) Elemental concentration in different species of seaweeds from

Loreto Bay, Baja California Sur, Mexico: implications for the geochemical control of metals in algal tissue. Env Poll 114: 145-160.

Sañudo-Wihelmy , S.A., Flegal A.R. (1996).Trace metal concentrations in the surf zone and in coastal waters off Baja California, Mexico. Environ Sci Technol 30:1575–80.

Sawidis ,T., Brown M.T., Zachariadis G., Sratis I. (2001). Trace metal concentrations in marine macroalgae from different biotopes in the Aegean Sea. Env Int 27: 43-47.

Seminoff J.A., Resendiz A., Nichols W.J. (2002). Diet of the East Pacific green turtle, Chelonia mydas, in the central Gulf of California, Mexico. J Herpetol 36:447–53.

Seminoff, J. A. (2000). Biology of the East Pacific green turtle, *Chelonia mydas agassizii*, at a warm temperate feeding area in the Gulf of California, Mexico. Dissertation, University of Arizona.

Shumilin, E.N., Rodriguez-Figueroa G., Bermea O.M., Baturina E.L., Hernandez E., Rodríguez-Meza G.D. (2000). Anomalous Trace Element Composition of Coastal Sediments near the Copper Mining District of Santa Rosalia, Peninsula of Baja California, Mexico. Bull Environ Contam Toxicol 65:261–8.

Shumilin, E., Paez-Osuna F., Green-Ruiz C., Sapozhnikov D., Rodriguez- Meza G.D., Godinez-Orta L. (2001). Arsenic, antimony, selenium and other trace elements in sediments of the La Paz lagoon, Peninsula of Baja California, Mexico. Mar Pollut Bull 42:174–8.

Storelli, M.M., Marcotrigiano G.O. (2003). Heavy metal residues in tissues of marine turtles. Mar Pollut Bull 46:367–400.

Sparling, D., Bishop C., Linder G. (2000) Ecotoxicology of amphibians and reptiles. Pensacola FL: Society of Environmental Toxicology and Chemistry.

Szefer, P., Geldon J., Anis-Ahmed A., Paéz-Osuna F., Ruiz-Fernandez A.C., Guerrero-Galvan S.R. (1998). Distribution and association of trace metals in soft tissue and byssus of *Mytela strigata* and other benthal organisms from Mazatlan Harbour, Mangrove Lagoon of the northwest coast of México. Env Inter 24: 359-374.

Valiela, I. (2009) Ecology of Coastal Ecosystems, in Fundamental of Aquatic Ecology, Second Edition (eds R. S. K. Barnes and K. H. Mann), Blackwell Publishing Ltd., Oxford, UK. doi: 10.1002/9781444314113.ch3

Villares , R., Puente X., Carballeira A. (2002). Seasonal variation and background levels of heavy metals in two green seaweeds. Env Poll 119: 79-90.

Talavera-Saenz ,A.L., Gardner S.C., Riosmena-Rodríguez R., Acosta-Vargas B. (2007). Metal Profiles Used as Environmental Markers of Green Turtle (*Chelonia mydas*) Foraging Resources. Sci Tot Env 373: 94-102.

Thomas, P., Baer K.N., White R.B. (1994). Isolation and partial characterization of metallothionein in the liver of the red-eared turtle (*Trachemys scripta*) following intraperitoneal administration of cadmium. Comp Biochem Physiol C 107:221–6.

Work, T. M. Balazs, G. H., Rameyer, R. A., Chang, S. P., Berestecky, J. 2000. Assessing humoral and cell-mediated immune response in Hawaiian green turtles, Chelonia mydas. Veterinary Immunology and Immunopathology 74:179–194.

Work, T.M.; Balazs, G.H.; Schumacher, J.L.; Marie, A. 2005. Epizootiology of spirorchiid infection in green turtles (*Chelonia mydas*) in Hawaii. *J. Parasitol.* 91:871-876.

Zaytsev, O., Cervantes-Duarte R., Montante O., Gallegos-Garcia A. (2003): Coastal upwelling activity on the Pacific shelf of the Baja California Peninsula. J of Ocean 59, 489-502